Prescribing Mental Health Medication

Prescribing Mental Health Medication is a comprehensive text for all practitioners who treat mental disorders with medication. This new (third) edition is fully updated and includes a variety of additional chapters.

Prescribing Mental Health Medication covers the latest digital methodologies including Internet-based mental health treatment, electronic medical records and prescriber use of social media. Including information on all psychotropic medications in use in the United States and the United Kingdom, the book incorporates clinical tips, sample dialogues for talking about mental health medications to patients, and information specifically relevant in primary care settings. It looks at:

- how to determine if medication is needed, proper dosing and how to start, stop and change medication
- specific mental health symptoms and appropriate medication
- special populations including non-adherent patients, medication abusers, those mixing alcohol and psychotropics, confused patients, children, adolescents, pregnant women and seniors
- management of medication side effects and avoidance of medication risk
- prescription of generic preparations
- organizing a prescriptive office and record keeping.

The additional chapters in this new edition of *Prescribing Mental Health Medication* cover topics such as combining specific medications, combining medications and psychological therapies, use of 'natural' substances in mental health treatment, successfully managing patient relapse, and appropriate prescriptions of potentially controversial medications such as stimulants and benzodiazepines.

This practical text explains the entire process of medication assessment, management and follow up for general medical practitioners, mental health practitioners, students, residents, prescribing nurses and others perfecting this skill.

Christopher M. Doran MD is a Psychiatrist and Distinguished Fellow of the American Psychiatric Association. He has been a Clinical Associate Professor at the University of Colorado School of Medicine and Nursing, USA.

Prescribing Mental Health Medication

The Practitioner's Guide

Third edition

Christopher M. Doran MD

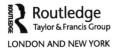

Routledge
Taylor & Francis Group

LONDON AND NEW YORK

Third edition published 2022
by Routledge
2 Park Square, Milton Park, Abingdon, Oxon OX14 4RN

and by Routledge
605 Third Avenue, New York, NY 10017

Routledge is an imprint of the Taylor & Francis Group, an informa business

First edition published by Routledge 2003
Second edition published by Routledge 2013

British Library Cataloguing-in-Publication Data
A catalogue record for this book is available from the British Library

Library of Congress Cataloging-in-Publication Data
A catalog record has been requested for this book

ISBN 13: 978-0-367-46692-3 (hbk)
ISBN 13: 978-0-367-46691-6 (pbk)

Typeset in Times New Roman
by Newgen Publishing UK

To my patients whose patience, strength and perseverance have taught me much of what is written here.

Contents

List of figures   xvii
List of tables   xviii
List of clinical tips (boxed material)   xxii
Preface   xxv
A note on the icons used in this book   xxvii
Acknowledgments   xxviii

PART I
The need for this book   1

1   General principles of medication management   3
Mental health medication is not like other medication 3
The scope of the problem 6
Mental health in the spotlight 7
References 7

2   Medication myths, truths and likely patient questions   9
Is mental health medication a placebo? 10
Is mental health treatment expensive? 11
These medications may change my personality 15
Stopping mental health medicine as soon as possible is competent practice 16
Taking medication for depression means personal weakness 17
If I am abusing alcohol, will starting mental health medication treat my
  alcoholism? 17
How do I know if my child needs treatment or medication? 18
References 19

PART II
Medication management start to finish   21

3   The initial prescriptive interview   23
What to say after "Hello" 26
General issues of history taking 28

Essentials that must be obtained for medication prescription 30
Mental status exam 31
Suicide and homicide assessment 32
Useful but optional information 32
Target symptoms 33
Historical information from others 33
The medical work-up 34
The next decision 35
Assessment and formulation 36
Length of an initial prescriptive interview 38
Sample clinician guidelines 40
Diagnostic and medication bias 40
References 44

4   Helping a patient decide to try medication   45
Shared goals 45
Common patient concerns about psychotropic medication 46
Other resistances to psychotropic medication 48
The use of levers 49
Reasons that patients take psychotropic medication 50
The use of metaphor 51
Reference 52

5   Starting medication   53
Monotherapy 54
Overlap and "indications" 54
What is the target of the medication? 56
Choosing a starting dose 56
Loading doses 57
The art of choosing a medication 58
Selecting medication in the previously treated patient 61
The liver-impaired patient 62
The kidney-impaired patient 63
How many pills to prescribe? 64
Polypharmacy – from the doghouse to the penthouse 64
Typically helpful combinations 66
The five points of education about psychotropics 67
Other issues to be discussed 69
Special consideration when prescribing an antipsychotic 70
Informed consent 70
Involuntary medication 71
Education as treatment 72
The use of placebo 72
References 73

6   Follow-up appointments and strategies   75

When do I schedule follow up? 75
How long does it take? 76
Inpatient medication follow up 77
Preparing for a follow up 77
Goals of a follow up 78
Two simple, powerful questions 79
Mental health prescriber and/or primary care provider 83
The power of positive comments 85
What is an adequate trial? 86
Switching medication and side effects 87
Feedback from others 89
Helping a patient stay on medication – the adherence dilemma 91
Antipsychotics and movement disorders at follow up 95
For primary care providers – how and when to refer to a mental health
  specialist 95
Missed doses 97
Parenteral medications 99
Information and tips for prescribing practice 99
References 101

7   Medication, psychotherapy and "What else helps?"   102

The first session dilemma 103
Patient's preference 104
What can medication do? 105
Who prescribes psychotropic medication? 105
Other adjunctive therapies 107
Beyond medication and helping the patient stay well 107
Work–life balance 109
References 111

8   Stopping medication   113

When to stop a psychotropic 114
Tapering medications 116
"When I stopped, I got worse" 116
Benzodiazepine withdrawal 118
Management of discontinuation syndromes 122
Relapse versus discontinuation syndrome 122
When to stop medication more quickly 123
New episode or relapse? 124
Side effects pass quickly 124
Unplanned stoppages of medication 124
Complex discontinuation 126
Reference 126

9 The long-term patient 127

Who should receive long-term treatment? 128
A symptomatic crisis in a stable patient – general principles 129
"The medicine stopped working" – getting back on TRAACCC 130
Inappropriate requests 134
Is newer medication better? 135
Periodic reassessment 137
Concurrence for a change of medication 137
Conflicting advice from others 138
References 139

10 Benzodiazepines and stimulants – useful, but controversial 140

History of benzodiazepines 140
Uses and side effects of benzodiazepines 141
Stimulant medication and its appropriate uses 144
Other uses of stimulant medication 145
Why so many? The "me too" concept of medication development 145
Dosing of stimulants 146
Side effects of stimulants 147
Abuse of stimulants 147
Notes and references 150

11 "Natural" substances – do they help? 151

Are natural substances superior to prescription medicines? 152
The shopping bag presentation 152
Potentially helpful natural substances 154
Potentially harmful natural substances 159
Notes and references 160

PART III
Medicating special populations 163

12 Using medication with children and adolescents 165

Outdated views of pediatric mental health prescription 166
The scope of pediatric psychopharmacology 167
Principles of psychotropic prescription with children and adolescents 167
Diagnostic and conceptual issues in the pediatric prescriptive process 169
A child's goals differ from those of adults 173
Parental power struggles over medication 173
The medical work-up prior to psychotropics 174
Practical issues in child/adolescent prescription 174
Notes and references 177

13 Pregnancy and psychotropics – rewards and risks   180
Clinician principles for prescribing to the pregnant woman 181
The A, B, C, D, X classification of medication in pregnancy and lactation 183
Working with the fertile woman, pre-pregnancy 185
When the patient wishes to become pregnant 186
While the patient is actively trying to become pregnant 187
When pregnancy occurs 188
During pregnancy 188
Medication prescription for symptoms occurring during pregnancy 189
Specific conditions and medication groups 190
Postpartum 196
Lactation and psychotropics 196
Specific medicines and medication groups in breastfeeding 198
Data will change; the decision process will not 201
Notes and references 202

14 Prescribing psychotropics for older patients   208
Seniors at risk 209
Non-adherence – a major problem 210
Principles of psychotropic medication prescription with the elderly 211
Regular re-evaluation 212
Senior medication problems – general strategies 212
Specific psychotropic medication considerations in the elderly 215
References 217

15 Medication of sleep problems   219
Facts and definitions 220
Stages of sleep 220
Evaluating a sleep problem 221
Principles of treating sleep disorders 224
Treatment of sleep problems 225
Necessity of follow up 229
Sleep problems in special populations 229
Notes and references 231

16 Alcohol, tobacco, recreational drugs and psychotropic medication   233
Ingesting chemicals – a human activity 233
Alcohol use 234
*Routine warnings regarding alcohol use and psychotropics in the non-substance
   abusing patient 238*
Early detection of substance abuse 239
The CAGE assessment tool 241
Polysubstance abuse 241

Evaluation of the intoxicated and withdrawing patient 242
Psychotropic medications and dual diagnosis patients 242
Psychotropics used in the treatment of substance use disorders 245
Psychotropics in the treatment of alcohol withdrawal 249
Other interventions for the prescriber with a substance abusing patient 249
Smoking, tobacco and nicotine 250
Routine warnings for other recreational drugs 252
References 255

17 The confused and cognitively impaired patient – medication pitfalls   257
General principles of dealing with the confused patient 258
Cognitive disorders – delirium and dementia 259
Management of delirium and dementia 262
Medication use in delirium and dementia 263
Dementia of the Alzheimer's type 265
Current medications for Alzheimer's dementia 267
Mild cognitive impairment 268
Psychiatric diseases that may present with confusion 270
References 270

18 Inattention and hyperactivity – ADHD and stimulants   272
ADHD – a diagnosis which is increasing rapidly 272
What are the syndromes of ADHD and why is it confusing? 274
What are the causes of ADHD? 274
How is ADHD diagnosed in children? 276
ADHD in adults 277
Stimulant medication and its appropriate uses 279
Other medications used in ADHD 280
Additional treatments for ADHD beyond medication 281
Other alternative/home remedies for ADHD 282
Abuse of stimulants 284
Notes and references 284

PART IV
Medication dilemmas and their clinical management   287

19 Side effects of psychotropic medications and their treatment   289
During the initial evaluation 290
Useful advice to patients 292
Side-effect assessment in follow-up visits 293
How much of a problem is it? 293
Other issues to consider in evaluating side effects 294
Changing medication due to side effects 295

Severity of side effects 295
Side effects and clinical response 296
The novice clinician and side effects 296
Side effects seen most frequently 297
Sedation 298
Overactivation/anxiety 299
Nausea and gastrointestinal problems 304
Sexual interference 306
Weight gain 311
Headaches 318
Asthenia/weakness 318
Dry mouth 319
Hair loss 319
Skin reactions 321
Prolactin elevation 322
Hypotension 324
Falls 324
Elevation of blood sugar and lipids 325
Hyponatremia 326
Suicidality 328
Side effects and medication combinations 329
References 329

20   Danger zones – areas of risk with psychotropics   333
P-450 issues made easy 333
Serotonin syndrome 340
Anticholinergic intoxication 343
Lithium toxicity 346
QTc interval issues 349
Sudden death and antipsychotics 354
*Extrapyramidal symptoms, neuroleptic malignant syndrome and tardive
    dyskinesia 355*
Extrapyramidal symptoms 356
Neuroleptic malignant syndrome 359
Tardive dyskinesia 361
Monoamine oxidase inhibitor reactions 364
Other potentially dangerous side effects 368
Notes and references 373

21   Medication allergies   378
Identification of allergic responses 378
Management of allergy symptoms 380
Other issues of evaluation when allergy is suspected 380

Stopping the offending medication 381
What else to do 381
Pills contain more than just the active ingredient 382
Reference 382

PART V
Competent clinical practice   383

22 Misuse of medication – taking too much and taking too little   385
How medication misuse presents 387
Accidental and careless overutilization 388
Intentional overdose 389
Serious overdose 390
Minor overdose 391
Using too little medication 392
Fraud and abuse with psychotropic medications 392
Practitioner protections against abuse of prescription medications 393
The development of abuse 396
If abuse is suspected 396
The pharmacist as ally 397
What to do when abuse occurs 397
References 399

23 "Difficult" medication patients and how to treat them   400
Overriding principles of managing difficult patients 400
The patient who abuses the telephone 403
The overly anxious patient 404
The patient preoccupied with side effects and negative reactions 405
The minimal contact patient 407
The non-adherent patient 408
The patient who needs to be in charge 410
The information overload patient 412
The "naturalist" 413
The borderline patient 414
Consultation and disengagement 419
The patient is not always the problem 420
Notes and references 420

24 Prescription writing and record keeping   422
The written prescription 422
Stylistic elements and recommendations 422
Record keeping 424
Elements of a clinician's prescriptive note 424
Systems for note taking 426

Style items in a medication note 426
Separate medication lists 427
Ongoing laboratory monitoring 427
Confidentiality and security of records 429
Discussing clinical matters 430
Record every encounter, not every fact 430
Documenting unusual treatment 431

25 Blood levels of psychotropics   433
When blood levels help 433
Instructions to patients 435
Frequency of blood levels 436
Using clinical judgment 437
When blood levels do not help 437
Necessary documentation 438
References 438

26 Generic medications   439
Generic substitution problems 441
Generic change without the clinician's knowledge 442
Tips for generic use 442
Serum blood levels and generic substitution 443
Mandated generics 443
References 444

27 The digital prescriber   445
The Internet and the digital revolution 445
E-mail and the medication prescriber 446
Texting 449
A Communications Information Sheet for patients 449
Electronic medical records (EMRs) 450
Electronic prescribing and prescriptions 452
Telepsychiatry – medication management via the computer 453
Internet-based mental health treatment modalities 454
Internet-based medication reference and educational information for
   practitioners 455
Internet medication information for patients 457
Websites maintained by practitioners for patient information 457
Data collection, protocols and oversight 459
Online patient access to medical records 460
Computer and Internet security 460
Social media and the prescriber – gold mine or mine field? 461
The nasty underside of the Internet 463
Notes and references 464

28 The prescriber and the telephone – mainstay and millstone 466
Being available by telephone 466
Appropriate use of the telephone by clinicians 467
Telephone appointments 467
Inappropriate use of the telephone 468
When a patient calls too much 471
Clinicians' over usage of the phone 472

29 The pharmacist, the pharmaceutical industry and the clinician 473
Interacting with the pharmacist 473
Preauthorization – a fact of American practice 474
The pharmaceutical industry 474
Indigent care medication programs 476
Media advertising and mental health medications 476
Reference 477

30 Preparing an office for mental health prescribing 478
Mandatory issues 478
Optional measures 481
Personal presentation 482
Periodic re-evaluation of image 483
References 483

31 The way forward 484
Practice guidelines 484
Genetics – the next big frontier 485
Lifestyle prescribing 486
Summary 487
References 487

Appendices 489
Index 537

Figures

6.1 Oral-to-LAI dose equivalency recommendation 94
8.1 Survival analysis for maintenance therapies in the recurrent depression extended study 115
13.1 Prescription Drug Labeling Sections – use in specific populations 184
15.1 Sample sleep graphs of children, young adults and seniors 222
20.1 QT interval 350
24.1 Sample prescription 423

Tables

1.1	Factors that make mental health medications unique	4
3.1	Framework of a prescriptive interview	26
3.2	Important elements of history taking	28
3.3	Essentials to be obtained for medication prescription	30
3.4	Other factual information that may be useful	32
3.5	Depression issues checklist	41
3.6	Mania/bipolar issues symptoms checklist	42
3.7	Anxiety issues checklist for panic disorder/generalized anxiety disorder (GAD)/obsessive–compulsive disorder (OCD)/social anxiety disorder	43
5.1	Other common mental health uses of FDA-approved drugs	55
5.2	The art of choosing a medication	59
5.3	Preferred choices of psychotropics for the hepatically impaired patient	63
5.4	Recommended medications for the renally impaired patient	64
6.1	Recommended laboratory monitoring for psychotropic medication for antipsychotics	82
6.2	When to change antidepressants	88
6.3	Medication changeover sheet	89
6.4	Completed medication changeover sheet (dosage)	90
6.5	Completed medication changeover sheet (number of pills)	90
6.6	Factors that can increase adherence with psychotropic medication	91
6.7	Using long-acting depot preparations of traditional neuroleptics	93
6.8	Second-generation long-acting injectable antipsychotics: a practical guide	94
7.1	One-stop shopping – psychiatrist or advanced practice mental health nurse only	106
7.2	Non-medical psychotherapist with mental health specialist prescribing (psychiatrist or advanced practitioner nurse)	106
7.3	Non-medical psychotherapist with primary care provider prescribing psychotropics	106
7.4	Mental health treatments and modalities that might be combined with medication	107
7.5	Mediterranean Diet	108
7.6	General Dietary Recommendations	108
8.1	Issues related to stopping medication	115
8.2	Discontinuing medications	116
8.3	Psychotropics that may cause discontinuation syndromes	116

8.4	Psychotropics that do **not** cause discontinuation syndromes	117
8.5	Tip-offs that a discontinuation syndrome may be occurring	117
8.6	Symptoms of an SSRI discontinuation syndrome	117
8.7	Symptoms of a TCA discontinuation syndrome	118
8.8	Symptoms of stimulant withdrawal	118
8.9	Benzodiazepine comparison chart	119
8.10	Symptoms of benzodiazepine withdrawal	120
8.11	Slow benzodiazepine taper from high dose	121
8.12	Management strategies for discontinuation syndromes	123
8.13	Possible causes of unplanned stoppages	125
9.1	Getting back on TRAACCC (RAATCCC)	131
10.1	Benzodiazepines available in the United States and their half-lives	141
10.2	Common uses for benzodiazepines	142
10.3	Common side effects of benzodiazepines	142
10.4	List of available stimulants grouped by underlying active ingredient	145
10.5	Warning signs of possible stimulant misuse	148
12.1	Children and adolescents aged 9–17 with mental or addictive disorders, combined MECA sample, 6-month (current) prevalence from 2005 to 2011–2012	166
12.2	Some psychiatric disorders in children and adolescents for which pharmacotherapy has been used	168
12.3	Child and adolescent prescriptive issues	168
14.1	Psychotropic medications to be used with caution in elderly patients	215
14.2	Possible adverse effects of mood stabilizing medications	216
15.1	Factors in a sleep evaluation	223
15.2	Non-benzodiazepine sedative hypnotics	228
16.1	Common drugs of abuse	235
16.2	The CAGE questionnaire to detect alcohol use disorders	241
16.3	Examples of diazepam and lorazepam protocols	250
16.4	The 5 As of brief interventions for alcohol use	251
17.1	Signs and symptoms that can alert the clinician to patient confusion	258
17.2	Causes of confusion	258
17.3	Symptoms of delirium	260
17.4	Causes of delirium	261
17.5	Symptoms of dementia	262
17.6	Causes of dementia	263
17.7	Medical work-up for delirium and dementia	264
17.8	Dosing schedules of medication in medications used to treat dementia of the Alzheimer's type	268
18.1	Signs of inattention	273
18.2	Signs of hyperactivity and impulsivity	273
18.3	ICD-10 wording of criteria for hyperkinetic disorders	278
18.4	Rating evaluation forms for ADHD in adults	279
18.5	Non-medication interventions for ADHD patients	281
18.6	ADHD therapy references	282
18.7	ADHD therapies that have some evidence-based support	283
18.8	Purported ADHD therapies that in general are *not* adequately evidence based	283

18.9   Warning signs of possible stimulant misuse   284
19.1   Facts regarding psychotropics and side effects   290
19.2   Common side effects of psychotropic medications   298
19.3   Potential causes of overactivation as a side effect   300
19.4   Medications used in mental health that can cause tremor   303
19.5   Medical and surgical causes of sexual dysfunction   307
19.6   Classes of medication that may affect sexual response   308
19.7   Phase I: first responses to medication-induced sexual interference   309
19.8   Phase II: remedies for medication-induced sexual interference   310
19.9   Drugs used to treat antidepressant-induced sexual dysfunction   311
19.10   Psychotropics and weight gain   312
19.11   Psychotropic medications causing hair loss with significant frequency   320
19.12   Psychotropic medications with at least one case of possible
        medication-related hair loss   320
19.13   Psychotropic medications with an incidence of skin rash greater
        than 3 percent   321
19.14   Clinical effects of elevated prolactin   323
19.15   Metabolic effects of atypical antipsychotics   326
19.16   Monitoring protocol for patients on second-generation antipsychotics   326
20.1   Drugs with known P-450 enzyme metabolism   337
20.2   Symptoms associated with serotonin syndrome   341
20.3   Drugs that affect serotonin levels and have been implicated in
        serotonin syndrome   342
20.4   Medications that have strong anticholinergic properties   344
20.5   Anticholinergic effect of commonly prescribed psychotropic drugs
        compared with trihexyphenidyl   345
20.6   Drugs that prolong the QTc interval and/or induce *torsades de
        pointes* (TdP)   351
20.7   Strongly serotonergic psychotropics prohibited in conjunction
        with MAOIs   365
20.8   Dietary restrictions for patients taking irreversible MAOIs   365
20.9   Drugs contraindicated for patients receiving irreversible MAOIs   366
20.10   Medications with known risk of agranulocytosis   369
20.11   Psychotropics associated with liver toxicity   370
20.12   Clinical symptoms of liver toxicity   371
20.13   Psychotropics with a low risk of seizure   371
20.14   Psychotropic medications associated with a higher-than-average
        seizure risk   372
21.1   Common allergy symptoms   379
21.2   Drug allergy assessment and treatment   380
22.1   Misuse of medication   386
22.2   Methods of obtaining medication fraudulently   393
22.3   Reporting drug misuse in the UK   399
23.1   Some "difficult" medication patients   401
23.2   Principles of treating "difficult" medication patients   401
24.1   The essential elements of a prescription   423
24.2   Optional elements on a prescription   423
24.3   Elements of a prescriptive note   425

24.4	Sample medication list	428
24.5	Sample laboratory test results form	428
24.6	Sample laboratory test results form (filled in)	429
25.1	Psychotropic medications for which serum blood levels are helpful	434
25.2	Therapeutic serum blood levels of commonly used psychotropic medications	434
25.3	Instructions for blood level testing	435
25.4	Reasons to obtain more frequent serum psychotropic levels	436
25.5	Psychotropic medications for which <u>serum blood levels are of no value</u>	438
26.1	Generic medications	440
26.2	Commonly used mental health medications that have a generic preparation	441
26.3	Potential generic problems	441
26.4	Common situations when different generics may have been substituted	442
27.1	Technological functions used by mental health prescribers and their patients	446
27.2	Expected advantages of linked, computerized electronic medical records	451
29.1	Services provided by pharmaceutical representatives	475

Clinical tips (boxed material)

2.1	Clinical tip	11
2.2	Talking to patients	17
3.1	Talking to patients	27
3.2	Talking to patients	27
3.3	Talking to patients	28
3.4	Talking to patients	36
3.5	Talking to patients	37
3.6	Primary care	39
4.1	Talking to patients	46
4.2	Talking to patients	47
4.3	Talking to patients	49
4.4	Talking to patients	51
5.1	Clinical tip	62
5.2	Talking to patients	68
5.3	Talking to patients	68
5.4	Clinical tip	70
6.1	Primary care	76
6.2	Talking to patients	79
6.3	Clinical tip	87
6.4	Clinical tip	88
6.5	Talking to patients	92
6.6	Talking to patients	96
6.7	Talking to patients	97
6.8	Clinical tip	99
7.1	Talking to patients	103
8.1	Talking to patients	114
9.1	Clinical tip	132
11.1	Talking to patients	153
12.1	Primary care	169
12.2	Talking to patients	171
12.3	Talking to patients	171
12.4	Clinical tip	175
12.5	Primary care	176
12.6	Primary care	176
13.1	Talking to patients	182
15.1	Clinical tip	224

16.1	Talking to patients	238
17.1	Primary care	259
18.1	Primary care	276
19.1	Talking to patients	290
19.2	Talking to patients	291
19.3	Talking to patients	291
19.4	Talking to patients	292
19.5	Clinical tip	293
19.6	Talking to patients	294
19.7	Primary care	297
19.8	Clinical tip	298
19.9	Talking to patients	313
19.10	Talking to patients	313
21.1	Danger	380
21.2	Danger	382
23.1	Talking to patients	403
23.2	Primary care	403
23.3	Talking to patients	405
23.4	Talking to patients	406
23.5	Talking to patients	408
23.6	Talking to patients	411
23.7	Talking to patients	411
23.8	Talking to patients	413
23.9	Talking to patients	413
23.10	Clinical tip	414
23.11	Talking to patients	419
24.1	Clinical tip	426
27.1	Talking to patients	458
28.1	Talking to patients	471
28.2	Talking to patients	471

Preface

The diagnosis and treatment of mental disorders have always been a part of healthcare treatment. Initially, diagnostic skills were minimal and "treatment" primarily consisted of incarceration in mental "hospitals" which did little besides housing patients. Over the first half of the twentieth century mental health treatment gradually took shape. Most of this consisted of procedures aimed at benefiting chronic and serious mental illnesses such as schizophrenia, dementia and other psychotic illnesses. With hindsight these treatments were at best cruel and at times almost barbaric. They would include trephination (removing a small part of the skull with a drill or saw), bloodletting and purging, insulin coma therapy, hot and cold hydrotherapy and the induction of an artificial fever. The treatment of mild to moderate mental health conditions such as depression and anxiety, particularly on an outpatient basis, only became a focus in the latter half of the twentieth century. Starting with only a few medications such as lithium carbonate, chlorpromazine and imipramine, medication treatment gradually became a juggernaut with a wide variety of psychotropic medications. There are many texts that describe dosages, side effects and indications for various medications, but there are virtually no other texts which attempt to teach the process of a practitioner evaluating and treating a patient with medication.

Therefore, this is a unique book about psychopharmacology. It is written with the intent of teaching principles and guidelines to clinicians which will result in successful, rational and evidence-based prescribing. Step by step, it will take the reader from the initial prescriptive evaluation for mental health medication through follow-up sessions, to the ending of a course of medication. Special populations such as children and adolescents, pregnant women and older patients are discussed, noting the adaptations in practice necessary for these populations. Common clinical situations in which psychotropics may be considered, such as patients with sleep problems, the cognitively impaired patient and the treatment of alcohol abuse, are also addressed. Other essentials of prescribing such as measuring serum blood levels, use of generic medications, record keeping, use of digital technologies, the telephone and the Internet are discussed as they apply to the prescription of psychotropics.

Throughout the book there are numerous examples of suggested ways to approach patients verbally, giving the clinician possible scripts and analogies for clinical psychotropic prescription. These suggestions are highlighted under the "Talking to Patients" icon. Specific remedies are detailed for potential problem situations such as intrusive side effects and patients who are unusually difficult to treat.

This work is not intended to be a textbook of psychiatry, or to cover in depth the issues of comprehensive psychiatric diagnosis, both of which are available in many other texts.[1-6] Although many medication specifics are documented in the text and appendices, this is much more than a compendium of drug facts, dosages or medication side effects, which can be found in other volumes.[6-8]

This book is a necessary precursor and companion to using drug information and mental health textbooks, since it helps the prescriber make sense of the facts. It is a manual for students to learn the essentials of competent clinical practice. The text also serves as an educational tool for current prescribers in helping to refine their clinical practice and to organize the process of prescribing psychotropic medications.

References

1   Geddes JR *et al.* (2020) *New Oxford Textbook of Psychiatry*, 3rd edn., Oxford University Press.
2   Sadock BJ and Sadock VA (2017) *Kaplan and Sadock's Comprehensive Textbook of Psychiatry*, Vol. 9, Lippincott, Williams & Wilkins.
3   Andreason NC and Black DW (2020) *Introductory Textbook of Psychiatry*, 5th edn., American Psychiatric Press.
4   Taylor D *et al.* (2018) *The Maudsley Prescribing Guidelines*, 10th edn., Informa Healthcare.
5   *The Physician's Desk Reference* (2020) Medical Economics Company Inc.
6   *U.S. Pharmacopeia* (2020) USP–NF.
7   *Drug Facts and Comparisons* (2020) Lippincott, Williams & Wilkins.
8   *British National Formulary*, 79th edn. (2020) British Medical Association and Royal Pharmaceutical Society.

A note on the icons used in this book

There are four icons used in this text to highlight special areas of interest to the reader. These are:

 This icon denotes a sample phrasing or dialogue that can be used by the practitioner in discussing a mental health prescribing issue with a patient or family member. Although not intended to be an exclusive way to introduce or discuss an issue, these sections provide the practitioner with simple, easily remembered concepts and phrases without excessive medical jargon. Novice clinicians will find these suggestions helpful as presented; others may modify them to meet their own style or the clinical situation.

 This icon points out particularly helpful clinical tips, ideas and approaches useful to prescribers.

 When this icon appears, it denotes a clinical consideration particularly helpful to those prescribing in a general medical/surgical or primary care setting. Mental health providers may find these suggestions useful as well.

 This icon alerts the reader to areas of special risk in the prescription of psychotropics. Most instances of its use are in Chapter 20 on Danger Zones, but others may be found elsewhere in the book.

Acknowledgments

To my wife, Maureen O'Keefe Doran RN APRN, who is an outstanding mental health clinician in her own right and one of the first mental health nurse prescribers in Colorado. I cannot thank you enough for your tireless first-line editing, and your emotional support when I have needed it most.

To my daughters, Alison O'Keefe Doran and Meghan Miller Macaluso. Your generation will see mental health and mental illness treatment with a clarity of vision and freshness of spirit.

To my parents, Kenneth and Kathleen Doran. Your reviews of this work brought the wisdom of lifetimes devoted to education and the practical perspective of healthcare consumers.

Part I

The need for this book

Part

Protect the Net Locol

1 General principles of medication management

- Mental health medication is not like other medication   3
- The scope of the problem   6
- Mental health in the spotlight   7
- References   7

Mental health medication is not like other medication

Mental health medication is neither fundamentally chemically different nor necessarily more complicated than other prescription medication. Nevertheless, prescribing medication for the psyche is a very different process from prescribing antibiotics, pain medications, anti-hypertensives, cardiac medication, pulmonary medication or any other group of medications – for the patient and often for the practitioner.

Consider the practice of writing a prescription for penicillin. Once an assessment has been made and a medication selected, there is very little that need be considered beyond writing an accurate prescription and giving appropriate instructions. The patient has an illness, wishes to get better and comes to the prescriber for a treatment that will remedy the problem. Although patients may wish that they did not need medication, prescribing is a relatively simple and straightforward process.

When a patient comes for mental health medication, however, there are many additional issues intrinsic to the process that may complicate the prescription. Before patients even set foot in the clinician's office, they may obsessively worry for weeks, months or even years as to whether this is a reasonable, healthy or necessary decision. They may be embarrassed to present to a practitioner and feel that it reflects negatively on them to ask for help. Patients may have strong feelings about whether they wish to have a mental health diagnosis made and recorded in their chart. Even if a correct assessment is made, they may have mixed feelings about whether or not they will allow medication to be part of their treatment.

Once the prescription is written, patients may have fears that the medication will irrevocably change their mind, their behavior or personality. They can be concerned about whether it will be necessary to take the medication for life, and whether or not their lifestyle will be significantly altered or restricted. They often worry that the medication may be habit forming, and that they may become addicted to the simple pill they are being offered. They can be concerned about what their family, spouse or friends will think of them for taking a psychiatric medication. They begin to doubt their own abilities and wonder if they are weak for having started the treatment.

Thus, these medications – whether we call them mental health medications, psychotropics or psychiatric medications – are unique in the prescribing spectrum. Whether an antidepressant is prescribed for a diagnosis of depression or in the treatment of irritable bowel syndrome, chronic pain or fibromyalgia (to name a few other common indications), the use of an "antidepressant" has extra meaning to the patient. An anti-anxiety medication often carries a similar excess "charge," whether it is specifically for an anxiety disorder or is used as part of an anti-hypertensive regimen.

Because of their special character and meaning within our culture and practice (see Table 1.1), these medicines require the practitioner to have special knowledge, techniques and sensitivity in order to prescribe effectively. That is what this book addresses – describing and teaching the body of knowledge that, when incorporated into everyday practice, will transform a practitioner from someone who merely writes a prescription to a person skilled in mental health medication management.

The special nature of mental health prescription often begins with the practitioner. Many of us, in our personal or family lives, have been exposed to mental illness and/or the varying prejudices about it. On the basis of a family member's experience with medications, shared family beliefs, professional hearsay or media presentation about psychotropics, many practitioners have mistaken notions of the purpose, therapeutic potential and safety of psychotropic medication. Unfortunately, medical and nursing training is often inadequate in counteracting these misconceptions. Even when appropriately educated, some practitioners may dismiss the evidence concerning the effectiveness of psychotropic medication and continue to rely on data based on their family or personal experience. More unfortunately, in some areas of the world, "mental illness" is still regarded as a function of societal ills without any biological cause. Solutions to emotional problems are thought to lie solely in manipulation of the person's environment, with medications having no part to play in treatment. In parts of the UK, as recently as the early 1990s, nursing training had an explicit anti-psychiatry content, often leaving nurses highly critical of what they believed to be a malevolent medical model.[1]

Beyond the healthcare community, society at large continues to foster special ideas about mental health medication. Psychotropic medications such as diazepam (Valium), alprazolam (Xanax) and fluoxetine (Prozac) have, at various times, become the most frequently prescribed medications in the world. They also have become cultural icons – the butt of jokes, the material of night-time comedians and the front-page stories of news magazines. While recent media coverage has tended to be more accurate with regard to psychotropics, in a world of sensationalism and hype where a premium is placed on sales of magazines, increasing traffic to websites and social media sites as well as increasing viewership ratings for radio and TV programs, articles designed to grab

Table 1.1 Factors that make mental health medications unique

- Practitioner beliefs
- Media distortion
- Courtroom tactics
- Beliefs about the causes of mental illness
- Artificial separation of the "mind" and the "body"
- Conflicting beliefs about what constitutes treatment for mental health symptoms

the public's attention often ignore or distort the true facts. Such presentations reinforce erroneous beliefs and continue to make these medications uniquely mistrusted.

Courtroom cases that involve psychotropic medications, and the headlines which these cases create, further make these medications "special." An attorney with a defendant who has no other viable defense for a crime can make the taking of a psychotropic medication the focus of the defendant's case. While few cases have been won on this basis, the fact that psychotropic medications regularly receive headline attention as possibly being the cause of violent, suicidal, abnormal or criminal behavior does little to normalize their prescription and use. Such publicity heightens sensitivity and these medications remain potentially controversial in our medical repertoire.

We cannot discuss the prescription of psychotropics without briefly discussing the evolving (and often confused) beliefs about the causes of mental illness. Within the last century, Western civilization has struggled at different times with beliefs that mental illness is caused by demonic possession, willful sloth, religious error, poor social conditions, intemperance, poor parenting or brain dysfunction. It can be expected, then, that when we talk about medication treatment of mental illness, people's notions of what these medicines are, what their value is and how to prescribe them are also confused and evolving. Although many mental health conditions have an etiology which contains both chemical and genetic background as well as family nurturing and environmental toxins, we are learning more about potential biological underpinnings. Psychiatry has generally become seen as a medical science based on objective data. In this paradigm the use of psychotropic medications will become further demystified. This is, however, a long and slow process. Prejudice dies hard. For the majority of current practitioners' lifetimes, the prescription of these medications will continue to require special skills and sensitivities.

Even medical and nursing practitioners exposed to balanced teaching about mental health conditions are not strangers to misguided notions surrounding mental illness and mental health medication. They may have discussed, learned and believed "facts" that supported the now outdated notion of a split between mind and body. It has often been a standing joke in healthcare training that some practitioners treat the patient from the "neck down," while others treat from the "neck up." For many trainees, it has been an acceptable and routine part of medical treatment to provide medications for illnesses of the heart, kidney, liver, musculature, etc. Neurological and neurosurgical treatment can be comfortably included in this group as "normal," because defined physical symptoms of a neurobiological disorder can be observed outwardly or by laboratory testing. Brain tumors, degenerative disorders and seizures are also easily described and documented, and are all considered to be part of the "body." The mind, spirit and emotions, however, have been much more elusive and difficult to define, and this has been reflected in the history of our treatment of mental dysfunction.

Psychiatry's long-standing inability to objectify and make scientific its body of knowledge was particularly complicated in the 1930s, 1940s and 1950s, with the advent and ascendancy of psychoanalysis. Psychoanalytic teaching suggested that, given enough time and intensity of treatment, talking about one's problems in sufficient depth could remedy most, if not all, symptoms. Even major mental illnesses, which we now know to have strong fundamental biological underpinnings, were seen as expressing unresolved conflicts from childhood, neuroses or conflicts of the ego, id and superego. While useful in the treatment of certain neurotic conditions, psychoanalytic concepts only furthered the gulf between treatments for the "mind" and treatments for the "body."

We now understand much more about brain physiology, genetics and cellular signaling mechanisms. It is clear that abnormal brain functioning may have substantial effects on major physiological systems including sleep and wakefulness, appetite, energy, concentration, memory, orderly thinking, anxiety regulation, attention, affect regulation and social relatedness. In many ways, though, we have only scratched the surface of understanding the various aspects of brain function, and how our treatments can improve mental symptoms.

The scope of the problem

Mental health problems are a worldwide epidemic. The statistics are staggering and numbers are increasing rapidly.[2]

- 47.6 million American adults (representing 1 in every 5) and 450 million persons worldwide experience mental health problems.
- 4.6 percent of U.S. adults experienced serious mental illness in 2018 (11.4 million people). This represents 1 in 25 adults.
- At least 1 in 5 youths aged 9–17 years currently has a diagnosable mental health disorder that causes some degree of impairment; 1 in 10 has a disorder that causes significant impairment.
- 16.5 percent of U.S. youth aged 6–17 experienced a mental health disorder in 2016 (7.7 million people).
- 10–40 percent of primary care patients have a diagnosable mental disorder.[3]
- Depression is the single largest cause of disability worldwide – 12 percent of the total.[4]
- Mental health and substance abuse is estimated to cost the global economy $8.5 trillion and this is expected to double by 2030.[5]
- Five of the 10 top causes of disability in the 15–44-year-old age group are mental health disorders.[6]
- 37 percent of prisoners and 44 percent of jail inmates have a history of a mental health problem.[7]
- In the UK, 1 in 6 persons experienced mental health symptoms in the previous week.[8]
- Total spending on mental health in the UK was planned to be £11.9 billion in 2017/18.[9]
- In Europe, 27.1 percent of the population has some form of mental disorder. The percentage goes up to 38 percent if Attention Deficit Hyperactivity Disorder (ADHD), dementia and sleep disorders are included in the figure.[10]
- Antidepressant use in the United States has increased 400 percent over the last two decades and 12.7 percent of all Americans over the age of 12 take an antidepressant.[11]
- The number of prescriptions for antidepressants in England has almost doubled in the past decade. In 2018, 70.9 million prescriptions for antidepressants were given out, compared with 36 million in 2008.[12]
- Antidepressant use in the UK has risen from 34 million in 2007/08 to 43.4 million in 2010/11 – up 28 percent.
- One in 6 Americans take mental health medication and the number is growing.[13]

Mental health in the spotlight

Mental health medications and treatments have been "discovered." The spotlight of attention has now been firmly fixed on mental health medication by medical research, public opinion, pharmaceutical companies, the mental conditions caused by or associated with the COVID-19 pandemic, and, gradually, by society at large. Millions of dollars annually are now being poured into mental health research as the major mental illnesses are seen for what they are: public health crises whose incidence is rapidly increasing throughout the world.

There is now a sharply rising exponential curve of knowledge about mental illness, its connection to various areas of brain function and psychotropic medications that can affect the brain. In the last quarter of the twentieth century, and into the twenty-first, the amount of information available to the practitioner about mental illness and its treatments has grown from a trickle, to a river, to the beginnings of a flood. Mental health medications and mental health conditions are now not just confined to books, journals and Internet sites; such topics are regularly discussed in the evening news, newspapers, radio and magazines. A day does not go by when the informed reader or listener does not hear information about mental health medications or the illnesses that they treat. The COVID-19 pandemic with its associated lengthy quarantine has further increased the frequency of mental health problems, but has also increased the media coverage of these issues. As medical and nursing professionals, we can expect ever-increasing amounts of information from public health organizations, pharmaceutical companies and professional societies about mental health medications and psychiatric conditions.

As the use of mental health medication grows and the number of prescribers increases, it is more necessary than ever to learn the prescriptive process well. To do so means being sensitive to the special needs and beliefs of patients, objectively sorting through our own prejudices and incorporating the growing body of objective, evidence-based data into our work. This book is intended to serve as a manual for professionals to guide their understanding of the prescriptive process. There is little doubt that a gradual movement toward "normalization" of psychiatric conditions is slowly occurring. This will permit and encourage the general medical practitioner to treat a large segment of the growing number of individuals with various mental health conditions. Since the education of most general and family medical practitioners at present remains seriously limited with regard to aspects of mental health, it is hoped that this book will be particularly valuable to this group of professionals.

From the occupational standpoint of the prescriber, the prescription of psychotropic medications can be extremely rewarding. Gaining the ability to use medication to remedy mental health symptoms effectively and promptly reinforces the wish to heal that first attracted many of us to the healthcare field. The accurate targeting of psychotropics can, in some cases, elicit the response that health professionals desire, when a patient will return and say, "Your treatment has transformed my life." The knowledge that can be obtained in this text can increase a patient's ability to work, love, maintain nurturing interpersonal relationships and enjoy life.

References

1   Gournay K (2000) Role of the community psychiatric nurses in the management of schizophrenia. *Advances in Psychiatric Treatment* 6: 243–251.

2   Global Burden of Disease Study 2013 Collaborators (2015) Global, regional, and national incidence, prevalence, and years lived with disability for 301 acute and chronic diseases and injuries in 188 countries, 1990–2013: a systematic analysis for the Global Burden of Disease Study 2013. *Lancet* 386: 743–800.

3   Mental health care in the primary care setting, available at: www.ncbi.nlm.nih.gov/books/NBK232639/

4   Depression: key facts, available at: www.who.int/news-room/fact-sheets/detail/depression

5   Patel V *et al.* (2016) Global priorities for addressing the burden of mental, neurological, and substance use disorders. In V Patel *et al.* (eds.), *Mental, Neurological, and Substance Use Disorders* (pp. 1–27), The World Bank.

6   World Health Organization and OCD, available at: www.ocduk.org/ocd/world-health-organisation/

7   Mentally ill people in United States jails and prisons, available at: https://en.m.wikipedia.org/wiki/Mentally_ill_people_in_United_States_jails_and_prisons

8   Mental health statistics: prevalence, services and funding in England, available at: https://researchbriefings.parliament.uk/ResearchBriefing/Summary/SN06988

9   Ibid.

10 Nearly 40 percent of Europeans suffer mental illness, available at: www.reuters.com/article/us-europe-mental-illness/nearly-40-percent-of-europeans-suffer-mental-illness-idUSTRE7832JJ20110904

11 Antidepressant use in persons aged 12 and over: United States, 2005–2008, Centers for Disease Control and Prevention, available at: www.cdc.gov/nchs/products/databriefs/db76.htm

12 NHS prescribed record number of antidepressants last year, available at: www.bmj.com/content/364/bmj.l1508.full

13 Study reveals how many U.S. adults are taking psychiatric drugs, available at: www.cbsnews.com/news/psychiatric-drugs-study-reveals-widespread-use-women-men/

2 Medication myths, truths and likely patient questions

- Is mental health medication a placebo? 10
- Is mental health treatment expensive? 11
- These medications may change my personality 15
- Stopping mental health medicine as soon as possible is competent practice 16
- Taking medication for depression means personal weakness 17
- If I am abusing alcohol, will starting mental health medication treat my alcoholism? 17
- How do I know if my child needs treatment or medication? 18
- References 19

There are certain questions about mental health medication that are frequent or almost universal in potential patients. These questions are based on beliefs that are unfortunately commonplace in society. They can reflect partial or total misconceptions about psychotropic medications or at times reflect partial truths which need to be addressed early in the assessment process. These beliefs are so pervasive and can so strongly affect a patient's willingness to come to the office for an evaluation or accept a prescription for psychotropics that it is necessary to devote an early chapter in this text to understanding the facts. This chapter will contain accurate, brief answers to common questions of this sort. Some questions require a more in-depth explanation of the origins of the misconceptions to clarify why these myths came into being and remain very prevalent. Although any type of healthcare worker may be asked these questions, in this text, they will be proposed and answered as if they are being asked of a family medicine practitioner.

If I feel I have a mental health problem, where do I start?
Usually, the best place to start is with a family medicine practitioner who can perform a physical exam and when necessary refer you to a mental health specialist. Often in the twenty-first century, family practitioners prescribe medication with counseling provided by a separate mental health therapist.

How can I decide if I need medication, counseling or both?
I may be able to give you some input on that decision, but generally the best recommendation comes from the mental health professional to whom I will refer

you. Some people need one or the other, but mental health research shows that the fastest and most effective treatment for mental health conditions involves at least starting with both modalities. A mental health professional who has the specialized knowledge is best able to give you the most authoritative answer.

How can I find the best therapist for me?
Start with the person to whom I will refer you. I have worked with them in the past and the quality of their work is excellent. If you feel that for any reason you have difficulty relating to this person, it is perfectly appropriate to schedule an initial session with several therapists to see with whom you feel most comfortable.

How can I find a good practitioner whose office is close to where I live?
Although having a therapist in your neighborhood may be convenient, it is absolutely *not* an important criterion. Finding a therapist who is known to be a quality practitioner and with whom you feel comfortable is much more important. Generally, looking on the Internet for a practitioner whose office is close to you is not a good procedure to use

I need to find a practitioner who will take my insurance, can you help me?
Every insurance company keeps a list of practitioners and therapists who are covered by their insurance. Call the insurance company and ask for a list of "preferred or participating" providers. I would hope there will be a match with the name that I will give you. If not, tell me and I will try to find a suitable match.

Do I need to tell my boss or employment that I am getting mental health treatment?
No. If you prefer, it is perfectly appropriate to ask for sick leave for a "medical issue." It does not need to be specified that it is a mental health issue. It is also important to know that your workplace cannot terminate your employment just because you are getting mental health treatment as long as you continue to be able to perform your work adequately.

What is the best type of practitioner to prescribe mental health medication?
The therapist or counselor can generally give you the name of a provider who can prescribe medications. Sometimes it typically is a psychiatrist or mental health nurse practitioner. In some communities where specialists are in short supply, you will be able to come back to me for the initial prescription.

Is mental health medication a placebo?

While far from perfect, mental health medication has defined biological effects and can make a significant difference in patients' lives. While this placebo myth persists on the Internet or can be heard from other people (even some medical practitioners), it is totally untrue. Although there is a small subgroup of practitioners who believe that mental health medications are essentially expensive placebos and have no active value, often these individuals also believe that mental illness itself is not real, which is also untrue. They often espouse the belief that mental "illness" is just a construct of the person's imagination, or is a result of social circumstance. They further believe that there is no underlying chemical abnormality, and that the use of medications to treat this "imaginary" condition must itself be magical, suggestive, hocus-pocus and/or not scientific.

As modern science is better able to demonstrate the physiological changes associated with mental conditions through the use of biological and genetic assays, PET (positron emission tomography) scans, SPECT (single-photon emission computed tomography) scans and other imaging techniques, this myth will gradually fade away.

Box 2.1 Clinical tip

It is often useful to have SPECT scan images of individuals with biological mental health conditions – taken before and after treatment – available to show patients in the office, particularly if they are hesitant about trying medications. Such pictures "medicalize" the condition and will often reassure patients sufficiently that they can begin taking medication. Many mental health journals and/or pharmaceutical representatives are sources of such images.

Is mental health treatment expensive?

Costs for psychotherapy sessions and medication treatment can vary considerably with location. In general, costs for such treatment are higher in larger cities than in smaller towns or rural areas. Although the costs per session may seem high, virtually all medical costs have escalated over the past decades. Physical examinations, emergency room visits, x-ray procedures and other expenses now cost multiple hundreds or even thousands of dollars. If possible, do not allow finances to interfere with getting the help that you or your child need. In virtually all areas of the United States, there are federal- and state-supported mental health centers that offer treatment on a sliding scale depending on your income.

In addition to those questions above, there may be multiple questions about the medications themselves and any possible untoward effects. In general, these questions are best answered by the prescriber when a particular medicine is selected so that the most precise information can be provided. Nonetheless, some patients require at least general answers before they can continue with an evaluation. Appropriate answers are therefore provided here:

Will psychotropics interact with medications that I am already taking?
The prescriber as well as myself can look at specifics regarding any mental health medicine prescribed and what you are now taking. That being said, the vast majority of mental health medications *do not* interact with common medications in a problematic way. You will be able to safely take typical pain medications such as ibuprofen and acetaminophen (paracetamol in the UK) as well as over-the-counter preparations without problem.

Will I be able to perform my usual tasks of daily living? Will my sex life change?
Although most patients are advised to avoid operating machinery or climbing heights for the first few days to assess your response to the medication, after that you will be able to drive, operate machinery, and perform other tasks of daily living.

On occasion, certain mental health medications may cause you to be sleepy. If this occurs, you and your prescriber will decide what, if any, behavior should be avoided temporarily. If sleepiness is severe and/or does not pass, you will likely have your medication changed.

Some antidepressants can cause a decrease in sexual desire or responsiveness. Many people do not get this problem. If it does occur, it is *always reversible* by stopping the medication. We will decide what is the best course of action when and if it occurs.

Will I have to change my diet? What about using alcohol?

The vast majority of psychotropic medications do not require any dietary change and you will be able to eat and drink whatever you prefer. There is one type of antidepressant (an MAOI or monoamine oxidase inhibitor) which does require dietary restrictions, but this is not commonly used. I will tell you if this is necessary.

As to alcohol, most people can drink alcohol in moderation (no more than one drink in a day and no more than four in a week) without significant interference. Do be aware that some patients get increased intoxication effects from alcohol when they are taking psychotropic medications. Excessive use of alcohol or any type of street drug is not recommended.

Is mental health medication addictive?

There has been much misinformation about this topic. Virtually all medicines for depression, bipolar disorder or psychosis are not addictive. Two classes of medications – benzodiazepines for anxiety and stimulants for attention deficit disorder – can cause physical dependence if used in a higher dose or for longer periods of time. We would discuss these issues in more depth if it emerges that a medicine from one of these two groups is recommended. Even so, a carefully monitored prescription will minimize any risk or danger (see Chapter 10).

This myth has multiple roots. In the 1950s and 1960s, a large portion of psychotropic medications were, in fact, habit forming. The widespread use of barbiturates, certain addictive sedative/hypnotics and, eventually, benzodiazepines, led many practitioners to extrapolate from these classifications of drugs and to assume that all medicines for the mind were habit forming. The fact is that *benzodiazepines, stimulants and certain hypnotics are the only psychotropic medications on which a patient may become physically dependent*.

While there are individual patients who will overutilize habit-forming medications, practitioners are particularly sensitive to this possibility and often feel that such patients will take advantage of them. These instances often embarrass and anger the practitioner, and can have an excessive impact on the practitioner's willingness to prescribe psychotropics in the future. These experiences are often generalized in the practitioner's mind such that all psychotropics are seen as habit forming, even though this is not accurate. As the science of mental health medication has evolved over the past 50 years, a larger and larger percentage of psychotropic medications are not habit forming at all. There is, however, a residual belief that practitioners need to be "on guard" for patients who may try to overuse medication or try to "con" practitioners out of prescriptions for the mind.

Another important root of this myth is the chronic relapsing nature of mental health conditions. Many patients who stop medication will experience a return of symptoms. They request, sometimes strongly, to be placed back on the medication. Practitioners can erroneously interpret this request as indicating that the patient is becoming "addicted" to the medication, when in fact the mental disease re-emerged when the treatment was withdrawn. This is essentially no different from an insulin-dependent diabetic having insulin withdrawn and seeing the symptoms of blood sugar dysregulation recur. The patient is not "addicted" to insulin, but requires it in order to treat the underlying medical condition.

Benzodiazepines, stimulants and some sedatives/hypnotics *are* potentially habit forming, and may be abused by certain individuals. Vigilance on the part of the practitioner is reasonable in the appropriate use of these medications. However, the *vast majority of currently used antidepressants, mood stabilizers, antipsychotic and other medications used in a medical practice are not habit forming, are not abused and have no street value.*

What are the most common side effects of mental health medications?
Many medications have virtually no side effects at all. If there are side effects, the most common ones are sleepiness, upset stomach, nausea, headaches, changes in sleep, changes in appetite or weight, dizziness, tiredness, fatigue and sexual inter-ference. Any of the side effects may pass after you have been on the medication for a few days or weeks. If they do not pass, specific remedies will be offered or the medication will be changed. Almost all side effects are reversible and do not remain present when the medication is stopped.

How long will I have to stay on medication?
Although this answer depends on your response to the medication and the severity of your illness, almost all patients will be tried off medication after 6 to 12 months. The procedure thereafter is dependent on how you feel and function without medication. Some patients do have to stay on medicine long term, but this is only determined after several trials of stopping it and seeing that a significant recurrence of symptoms occurs.

Will medication make me suicidal, a danger to others or change my personality?
As an adult, it is very *unlikely* that you would experience suicidal ideation or become a danger to other people. It is hoped that some of your target symptoms will improve, but your underlying personality characteristics will remain the same.

Any effect from the medication causing or worsening suicidal ideation for adults is at most very small. There have been large cohorts of patients which have been carefully examined, and the results show that any increase in suicidal action or thoughts, if at all, remains controversial. In large numbers of patients, children and adolescents may be at slightly greater risk than adults of an increase in suicidal thoughts. Homicide is *not* a result of taking antidepressants.

Since most clinicians have successfully prescribed antidepressants for over 50 years with overwhelmingly positive results, they would be surprised at the idea that antidepressants could cause or worsen suicidal ideation or behavior. This was challenged in 2004 when the American Food and Drug Administration (FDA) issued an across-the-board "black box warning" for the use of antidepressants in children and adolescents. Two studies in 2003 and 2006 by Hammad et al.,[1-2] raised concerns from re-analyzing clinical trial data about this relationship. The publications stated that children and adolescents starting treatment with antidepressants had a 4 percent risk of developing suicidal ideation or behavior compared with a 2 percent risk in those receiving a placebo. These studies received much publicity in the media and resulted in a significant decrease in the prescription of antidepressants to this age group.

This concern continued to be active with a number of clinicians and the "black box warning" has remained in effect despite the fact that a series of subsequent studies[3–8] has shown that the use of antidepressants more likely *reduces* the risk of attempted suicide or death from suicide rather than the opposite. Evidence is particularly strong that antidepressants are helpful in adults and geriatric patients.[9–10] A follow-up review by Gibbons *et al.* in 2010 concludes that "Overall, the data do not support a risk of suicidality (ideation, attempts, or completion) in adults, and if anything, the data suggest protective effect."[11–12]

There are several other factors leading to this particular myth and ongoing controversy. A certain number of depressed individuals do attempt or complete suicide. Families and friends of these individuals find it difficult to see their relative "at fault" for this behavior and, in the search for other causes, medication becomes an easy scapegoat. Coroner reports of successful suicides may show antidepressants in the blood of the deceased. This does not necessarily mean that the medication "caused" the suicide; it merely shows that the patient was being treated with medication at the time the suicide occurred. *Many patients have suicidal ideation, which is part of the underlying illness, before they begin medication therapy.* When a depressed person does attempt or succeed with suicide while being medicated, it is often the case that the diagnosis was incorrect, the choice of medication failed, it was given in inadequate doses or it was taken only sporadically by the patient. While it is prudent for the clinician to carefully monitor every patient beginning antidepressant therapy, most knowledgeable clinicians believe that if, in fact, there is an increased risk of suicidality with the use of antidepressants, it is very small. Treatment with antidepressants is both appropriate and necessary in many depressed patients.

Regarding violent behavior and antidepressants, an attorney's legal defense may play a role in promoting or perpetuating this myth. Defense attorneys for persons who have committed violent crimes may have only a meager justification for the patient's actions. If the patient was taking a psychotropic medication, it may be very convenient for such an attorney to argue that the medication was to blame for the patient's behavior. Several studies and professional bodies have dismissed the possible link between antidepressants and homicide.[13–14] In many situations, when one investigates the past history of persons who have committed violent crimes, they have been found to be aggressive, violent or homicidal prior to the current act, and well before they were on medication.

Several other truths may also contribute to this myth:

1   Some, but not most, antidepressants may cause akathisia, a very disturbing but relatively rare sense of physical inner restlessness. Patients with akathisia have been noted to have a suicide rate above that of the general population. It is at least theoretically possible that the small percentage of patients who do develop akathisia while on medication could be at some increased risk for self-injury or violence. However, the jump from observing restlessness in an individual to suggesting that it causes the individual to commit homicide is a large one. No study has demonstrated a link between an activated state such as akathisia and homicide.[15]

2   In general, appropriately treated persons with depression become significantly less suicidal and the likelihood of a suicide attempt decreases dramatically. We have, however, long known that *the profoundly depressed, suicidal persons who have marked psychomotor slowing may be at some measure of increased risk for suicide in the first several days or weeks of treatment.* As the patient first begins to improve, he/she may become energized. If not carefully monitored and supported during this period, the increase in energy may precede the lessening of the other depressed symptoms, including suicidal thoughts. At this point, there may be an increased risk for a self-injury action that the patient was previously too anergic to attempt.

3   Finally, mental health medications are more frequently being prescribed in efforts to address a wide variety of problematic human behaviors, including aggression, violence and suicide. When other treatments have failed, psychotropics may be prescribed as a last resort in seriously violent and suicidal individuals. With the significant gaps in our ability to predict and remedy suicide and violence in general, medications too may fail to adequately correct the underlying factors that precipitate these problematic behaviors. With the increased use of psychotropics, it is to be expected that a percentage of people who do act violently or kill themselves may have medication in their bodies at the time of their destructive acts. It should not be assumed, however, that the medication is the underlying cause.

These medications may change my personality

One frequent question from patients about psychotropics is "Will this medication change me?" The answer to this question is not always simple; it depends on what the person means by the question.

To the extent that we see specific biological symptoms as part of the diagnosed condition (e.g., sleep disorder, appetite disturbance, poor concentration, fluctuations in energy and disordered thinking), it is hoped that these target symptoms will be improved or eliminated with medication. So, yes, the patient will be "changed." That is the therapeutic hope and intent.

It would be misleading, however, to assume that other underlying personality traits – personal likes and dislikes, hobbies, work interests or many of the elements that comprise personality – are likely to be changed in any direct way. Some patients with long-standing untreated illness may develop new interests, find new employment or change relationships as a consequence of feeling better, but this is not a direct chemical effect of the medication. Some patients with certain behaviors associated with their illness (e.g., excessive anger, unreasonable fears, lack of energy to work or be social) can also have these behaviors modified by therapeutic intent. Psychotropic medication does not, however, change fundamental personality structure by taking a pill. Introverts do not become extroverts, individuals with lack of motivation do not become workaholics, rude individuals do not become automatically polite, sportsmen and -women do not become bookworms and city dwellers do not become farmers.

Many people hope that by taking a pill they can eliminate all unpleasant emotions from their lives – not only diagnostically targeted symptoms such as depressed mood or anxiety, but also elements of life's unpleasantness. They hope that medication will make them "emotionally bulletproof," or compensate for other deficits in their life. There may be a wish on the part of anxious or depressed individuals that, once they are on medication, they will automatically overcome procrastination, inattention to detail, abrasive personal traits, social isolation, poor financial budgeting, self-centeredness, psychological resistance to change or unwillingness to approach difficult personal issues. These traits and behaviors, which fall under the rubric of "personality" and "personal style," are often not affected by psychotropic medications.

Other patients hope that by taking medication their relationship with their parents, their spouse, children or their boss will magically improve. In fact, some patients who take psychotropic medication *may significantly* improve their interpersonal relationships, although it often takes a considerable amount of psychological work. Individual, marital, family or group psychotherapy may help to achieve this goal. Part of our role as clinicians is to help the patient sort out realistic expectations of medication from wishful fantasies.

Stopping mental health medicine as soon as possible is competent practice

One underpinning of this notion is the universally held tenet of good medical prescriptive practice which states that we should prescribe the least amount of medication for the shortest period of time to achieve our medical aim. This is indeed good practice, but the decision to stop psychotropic medication can be more complex.

While, in general, no one should take any medication longer than needed, the practitioner's good intentions to accomplish this with psychotropics may be clouded by misconceptions. Some roots of these misconceptions have been identified in the previously identified myths that most psychotropic medications are addictive or placebos. Prescribers with this mindset will also subscribe to the corollary that if medication is used it should be used for a very brief period, and that it is inappropriate for a patient to take long-term medication. Clinicians who read statements such as those in the *Physician's Desk Reference* or other sources that "efficacy has not been proven beyond eight weeks" may use this information to support the misconception. Pharmaceutical companies must often make these statements because the initial clinical trials necessary to bring a medication to market were undertaken on a short-term basis and, at the time of initial medication release, longer-term maintenance medication trials had not yet been performed. It is only several years after the introduction of a medication that maintenance trials may be undertaken, and the results may take several more years to be completed and published.

What also reinforces this myth is the notion that many mental health problems are primarily or solely related to life stressors. The assumption is that once these stressors are resolved, the patient should no longer need to be medicated. If symptoms persist significantly after the resolution of a divorce, a job loss, a personal tragedy or some other stressor, the practitioner may assume that any symptoms should disappear, or at least not require medication. Within this belief, the practitioner acts as if the patient should automatically be treated with medication for a short period of time following the stressor. The clinician feels that he/she is practicing good medicine by recommending or insisting that the patient stop medication as soon as possible.

While no ethical practitioner would recommend that anyone be treated longer than needed, we cannot fail to appreciate the chronic nature of many mental conditions. Depression, bipolar disorder, schizophrenia, panic disorder, generalized anxiety disorder and many other mental health conditions are often chronic or relapsing illnesses. It is quite common to have flare-ups of these chronic illnesses triggered by environmental stressors. At times, even when the stressors resolve, symptoms requiring treatment may remain. The treatment of these conditions with medication may be episodic or, in some cases, continuous. *For many patients, it is safe, life-enhancing or even lifesaving, to remain indefinitely on medication.*

Taking medication for depression means personal weakness

This is one of the most common misconceptions about mental illness. For illustration we will use depression, but the principle applies to most emotional illnesses. Because many people with severe emotional illnesses do, in fact, have some difficulty with day-to-day functioning, job performance and interpersonal relationships, they arrive at the clinician's office already feeling inferior. They may have struggled for months, years or decades, feeling they were unable to "keep up" and perform in the way that they them-selves expected. This feeling may be reinforced by critical comments and attitudes from family or friends, or work sanctions from employers. Patients often may have tried a variety of home remedies, self-improvement techniques or just "trying harder." Now, with trepidation, they are seeking help. We, as clinicians, must understand their struggle and support the efforts they have already made. It is a fact that depression is an illness and that depressed individuals often have to try harder than most.

When a diagnosis is made and appropriate medication prescribed, most patients are quite capable of increased functioning in their lives. While very ill patients may remain handicapped by their emotional illness, the majority of outpatients can be helped sig-nificantly by targeted psychotropic medications. Quality of life can be enriched and the person's level of function improved. Adequate treatment can also help patients to redis-cover their strengths and abilities to further grow and prosper.

Box 2.2 Talking to patients

A very powerful and alliance-building message can be conveyed by clinicians in the statement: *"I think I know how difficult it may have been to make the decision to see me about medication today. You may have heard from others (or believed yourself) that all you needed to do was try harder and 'get over it.' After trying many methods that didn't work, you may have even begun to believe that you were just lazy or unmotivated. I believe you have an illness – depression – that has, as some of its symptoms, low motiv-ation, decreased energy and an inability to concentrate. You have been using a lot of energy just to get through the day and accomplish tasks that should be routine. One effect I expect from this medication is that it may not be as hard to lead your day-to-day life."*

If I am abusing alcohol, will starting mental health medication treat my alcoholism?

There is a significant overlap between many emotional illnesses and substance abuse, and many mental health patients "self-medicate" with alcohol or recreational drugs. Once they begin feeling better as a result of treatment, which may include psychotropic medication, some of these patients no longer need substances for self-medication. *It is not reasonable, however, to assume that all persons with substance abuse problems will necessarily decrease their use of substances when they are medicated.* Some may continue to abuse alcohol and/or recreational drugs despite their mental health improvement, and will need separate, independent substance abuse treatment.

Do I have to be substance-free to be assessed and treated accurately for mental illness?

The willingness of practitioners to medicate with psychotropics in those patients abusing alcohol or drugs will vary. There is a group of practitioners who will insist on patients being substance-free before they will medicate. Other practitioners are willing to prescribe for clearly diagnosed mental health conditions despite the presence of mild to moderate drug or alcohol usage. The hope in the latter situation is that when patients are appropriately medicated, they will be better able to give up or cut down their alcohol/drug usage. Some practitioners will refuse to write any prescriptions until a patient is totally substance-free.

Such a premise of reduced substance usage with medication requires constant re-evaluation, and certainly is not universally true. For those patients who, despite adequate medication, continue to abuse alcohol or drugs, continuing medication prescription may not be in their best interest, and may indeed present a medical hazard.

To expect that patients who have been using substances for a long time, particularly for self-medication, will totally cease their habit prior to being medicated is, in most cases, unlikely and unreasonable. Often such a prerequisite, if strictly and uniformly enforced, will drive such patients from treatment before medication can offer improvement. If, however, as a practitioner, you have a history that a patient is a heavy substance abuser or has abused the combination of medications and alcohol before, it may well be reasonable to insist that the patient be detoxified before medication is prescribed.

How do I know if my child needs treatment or medication?

Just because a child is very active, is not doing well academically, does not have a lot of friends or stays in his/her room a lot does not automatically indicate that a child needs mental health treatment. It sometimes can be difficult to distinguish "normal" rebellious, anxious or sad behaviors from symptoms of mental illness. This distinction will often require input from several sources and professionals. Appropriate actions to undertake to help in making this distinction include:

- taking the child to his/her pediatrician for an evaluation
- talking to the child's teacher to see if any concerning behaviors are occurring in the classroom.

Some symptoms that are of significant concern and should prompt an evaluation as soon as it can be scheduled include:

- suicidal thoughts, verbalizations, talk or actions threatening to harm another child or any other person
- repeated runaways from home
- cruelty to animals

- repeated behavioral outbursts in multiple locations including home, school, the playground or on athletic teams
- severe difficulty with sleep lasting longer than a week
- unexplained weight loss, vomiting or refusal to eat
- repeated impulsive behaviors leading to dangerous actions
- excessive fear, worry or anxiety for no obvious reason
- nightmares, recurrent memories or excessive anxiety following episodes in the child's life that involve violence, abuse, injury or trauma
- frequent headaches or stomach aches without medical cause
- avoiding or missing school on a regular basis
- repeated tantrums in multiple situations, not just at home
- using tobacco, drinking alcohol or using drugs
- verbalizations from the child that other people are trying to control his/her mind
- verbalizations of hearing voices or sounds that no one else hears
- long-lasting sadness, particularly with social withdrawal
- frequent severe changes in mood going from psychomotor slowing to excessive elevation of mood, grandiose thought, rapid speech and lack of need for sleep.

Whether the child is referred by a pediatrician or if multiple concerning symptoms are seen, ensure that he/she is seen by a behavioral health specialist in child psychology. Unfortunately, some communities have a very limited number of qualified child therapists. You may have only your pediatrician's evaluation on which to proceed or you may need to travel some distance to a nearby larger town that has a practitioner specializing in children's mental health. Expect that parents or guardians will be evaluated by the practitioner

It cannot be assumed that your child will or will not automatically be placed on medication by a general health practitioner. Some children respond well to psychotherapy or "play therapy" alone, while others are best treated by both therapy and appropriate mental health medication. You will be consulted by any prescriber to understand the side effects and expected outcome of using a medication. In contrast to some information on the Internet, when appropriately prescribed and dosed, psychiatric medication in children is safe and can be very helpful.

References

1 Hammad TA *et al.* (2003) Incidence of suicides in randomized controlled trials of patients with major depressive disorder. *Pharmacoepidemiological Drug Safety* 12 (Suppl. 1): S156.
2 Hammad TA *et al.* (2006) Suicidality in pediatric patients treated with antidepressant drugs. *Archives of General Psychiatry* 63: 332–339.
3 Simon GE *et al.* (2006) Suicide risk during antidepressant treatment. *American Journal of Psychiatry* 163: 41–47.
4 Rothschild A (2011) Do antidepressants cause suicide? *Psychiatric News* 1(14): 1–2.
5 Gibbons RD and Mann JJ (2011) Strategies for quantifying the relationship between medications and suicidal behavior: what has been learned. *Drug Safety* 34(5): 375–395.
6 Mulder R *et al.* (2008) Antidepressant treatment is associated with a reduction in suicide ideation and suicidal attempts. *Acta Psychiatrica Scandinavica* 118: 116–122.
7 Tondo L *et al.* (2008) Suicidal status during antidepressant treatment in 789 Sardinian patients with major affective disorder. *Acta Psychiatrica Scandinavica* 118: 106–115.

8   Gibbons RD *et al.* (2007) Early evidence on the effects of regulators' suicidality warnings on SSRI prescriptions and suicide in children and adolescents. *American Journal of Psychiatry* 164(9), available at: https://doi.org/10.1176/appi.ajp.2007.07030454

9   Fava M and Rosenbaum JF (1991) Suicidality and fluoxetine: is there a relationship? *Journal of Clinical Psychiatry* 152(3): 108–111.

10 Beasley CM Jr *et al.* (1991) Fluoxetine and suicide: a meta-analysis of controlled trials of treatment for depression. *British Medical Journal* 303: 685–692.

11 Gibbons RD *et al.* (2007) Relationship between antidepressants and suicide attempts: an analysis of the Veterans Health Administration data sets. *American Journal of Psychiatry* 164: 1044–1049.

12 Gibbons RD *et al.* (2010) Post-approval drug safety surveillance. *Annual Review of Public Health* 31: 419–437.

13 Bouvy PF and Liem M (2012) Antidepressants and lethal violence in the Netherlands 1994–2008. *Psychopharmacology* 222(3): 499–506. doi: 10.1007/s00213-012-2668-2

14 Tardiff K *et al.* (2002) Role of antidepressants in murder and suicide. *American Journal of Psychiatry* 159: 1248–1249.

15 The Irish College of Psychiatry (2010) Antidepressant medication: clarification, available at: www.irishpsychiatry.ie/wp-content/uploads/2016/12/10-CPsychI-Press-statement-antidressant-medicaiton-clarification-13-05-10-NO-Mobiles-.pdf

Part II

Medication management start to finish

3   The initial prescriptive interview

- What to say after "Hello"   26
- General issues of history taking   28
- Essentials that must be obtained for medication prescription   30
- Mental status exam   31
- Suicide and homicide assessment   32
- Useful but optional information   32
- Target symptoms   33
- Historical information from others   33
- The medical work-up   34
- The next decision   35
- Assessment and formulation   36
- Length of an initial prescriptive interview   38
- Sample clinician guidelines   40
- Diagnostic and medication bias   40
- References   44

Practitioners who are in the process of learning or improving their mental health prescribing expertise often feel that their primary goal in the initial and follow-up appointments is to select the "best" and most effective medication for the patient's problems. A provider with mental health expertise will often be collared by a colleague in the hallway or the parking lot for "Curbstone Consult." The nature of these inquiries often revolves around questions like: "What is the best medicine for X condition?" or "I have a patient with these symptoms. What should I prescribe?" In these circumstances, sharing the names of several possible medication choices is totally appropriate. However, as part of learning the medication prescription process, there is a totally different skill that this text will recommend and provide. It is not a "secret," but it is something that the vast majority of practitioners do not consider as perhaps *the* most important foundation to the success of their patient interactions and medication adherence.

Effective physician–patient communication is an integral part of clinical practice and serves as the keystone of physician–patient relationships and trust. Trust extends to many different aspects of the physician–patient relationship including, but not limited to: physicians' willingness to listen to patients; patients believing that physicians value patient autonomy and ability to make informed decisions; and patients feeling comfortable enough to express and engage in dialogue related to their health concerns.[1] Numerous studies[2-3] have shown that the approach taken by physicians to communicate information is equally important as the actual information that is being communicated. Enhancing communication can be accomplished by three skills – *improving one's listening skills; learning gentle but clear ways of communicating information to patients; and, lastly, including in the dialogue at least one or several complimentary phrases to the patient*. The quotations "They may forget what you said – but they will never forget how you made them feel" and "I can live for several months on one good compliment" contain valuable lessons for the clinician.

It cannot be stressed enough that these traits are crucial to successful communication and outcome. Learning and practicing these skills will provide exponential improvement to clinical appointments and far outweighs any reading or studying about specific medications

and diseases. The presence of this symbol will highlight suggested dialogues for

possible ways of speaking to patients. Sample positive complimentary phrases that can be used in the course of a dialogue are listed in Chapter 6.

Some people assume that the ability to be a good listener is an inborn trait which some people have and others do not. Nothing could be further from the truth! Good listening is a skill which absolutely can be learned and perfected. There are a few important elements to quickly improving one's listening ability. Below is a list of the most important considerations to becoming a good listener:

1   In any patient interaction, *the amount of time that the practitioner* **listens** *should be at least* **three times** *as long as the amount of time he/she spends* **talking**.

2   Set the scene to maximize the likelihood of good listening by minimizing distractions. This needs to be done well in advance by arranging your office furniture in a way that permits you to deal directly with the patient with minimal impediments, including your desk, table or other blocks. Setting up your office will be dealt with in more detail in Chapter 30, but a simple exercise is to sit in your patient's chair. Observe whether you feel he/she has direct line of sight and a reasonable amount of closeness to the practitioner.

     Think about minimizing distractions. This is both an internal mental process for you to avoid thinking about other issues than the patient's dialogue, as well as an external process to minimize noise and distraction. If necessary, consider a low-volume "white noise" machine to blur and diminish external sounds. Evaluate your posture – turn and face the patient, look at the patient even if he/she is not looking at you, look pleasant and smile. Avoid a rigid fixed stare whether seeing the patient face-to-face or through a computer monitor during telepsychiatry. Maintain an open and receptive posture such as sitting upright in a chair, feet on the floor and bending slightly toward the patient. Avoid closed postures, such as crossing your arms in front of your chest, tightly crossing your legs or raising your arms with your hands behind your head. A silent clue that you may observe when the patient is bonding well with you is that she/he starts replicating the posture that you are showing.

3   In addition to the patient's speech, observe his/her facial movements, eye movements, signs of tension and other body language

4   Make sure that your attention is totally focused on what the patient is saying and not wandering to other issues such as the last patient seen, the difficult patient upcoming or some other personal or professional issue. If a practitioner is preoccupied with a difficult clinical issue, it is better for her/him to spend a few moments in private thinking about the issue, even if it means coming to the exam room a few minutes late, but with a clear mind. Patients can easily detect practitioners who are distracted and not really listening to their complaints/speech. When this happens, the patient will consciously or sometimes unconsciously find themselves irritated with the practitioner.

5   It is not possible to do two things at once. You simply cannot effectively listen to the patient when talking, or listen well while mentally planning your response. Virtually all practitioners are intelligent and have ideas, potential treatment plans or therapies at their fingertips. You will be able to formulate them and discuss them better when the patient has finished talking.

6   If you find yourself feeling that the patient is talking too slowly, try to avoid being a "sentence grabber" by interrupting and finishing a sentence for the patient.

7   Wait for a pause in the patient's speech to ask clarifying questions.

8   Even though the patient is coming to you for your expertise, the old adage is still true – "what the patient wants to hear is more important than what you want to say." That is not to say that you need to alter the facts of your assessment and prescription, but it is important for you to make sure you have dealt with the patient's questions and uncertainties, as well as expressing your assessment in ways that the patient can understand and internalize.

9   Whenever possible, ask open-ended questions that encourage explanation, not a simple yes or no answer. Utilize "What do you mean when you say…?"

10 Try to feel what the patient is feeling. It is often helpful to form a mental picture in your mind.

11 If you regularly keep notes as the patient is talking, write down only key words or phrases to utilize when you later compose your record of the interview. Avoid turning to face the computer screen and keyboard.

12 Many practitioners worry that encouraging a patient to talk will result in excessively long consultations or talking about non-useful information. Clarification and encouragement can be useful, though, by periodically nodding or utilizing a phrase like "Tell me more about…" (your pain, your mood, your behavior, etc.)

13 Periodically summarize what the patient has said with phrases like "What I am hearing is…," "Let me see if I am following you…," "It sounds like you are saying…."

14 Look for signs of emotion. They are the portals to the essence of what the patient is saying and feeling. Tears (sadness), getting choked up, sweating, or trembling (anxiety), looking away (shame or guilt), smiling, or a twinkle in the eye (pleasure or pride), clenched fists, raised voice, clenched shoulders or jaw (anger) can be useful emotional identifiers.

15 Reflect the patient's feelings – "You look like you are feeling…," *not* "You must be feeling…." You may be wrong!

16 A dialogue between patient and practitioner has four parts – *Receive, Understand, Evaluate and Respond*. Note that three out of the four do not involve your talking.

It is suggested that the above sections be re-read now and periodically toward refreshing *the most important part of the prescriptive process.*

The rest of this chapter focuses on the elements of the initial patient contact for the purposes of determining if medication is indicated, and, if so, what kind of medication might be prescribed.

Performing an organized, thorough evaluation is crucial to success with psychotropic prescription. Whether conducted in an outpatient office or clinic, an inpatient or institutional setting, the process of this initial evaluation seldom changes. Although each individual is different and each of these initial evaluation sessions may take a slightly different course, it is important to have a general procedural process.

If a clinician is coming to the practice of prescribing psychotropics from a psychotherapy background, the directed, focused interview described in this chapter may seem somewhat foreign and overly structured. Those practitioners who come from a strong medical/surgical background will find this outline very similar to the initial evaluations done for medical problems in a primary care office.

A useful way to conceptualize the elements necessary in the initial prescriptive interview is *to start with the end in mind,* and think of *those items that would be included in a written report* following this initial interview. In many cases, a written report may, in fact, be necessary, not only as the record of contact but also for the purposes of discussion with a collaborating professional or for distribution to other medical personnel who may be caring for the patient. The overall framework of the elements of such a report is shown in Table 3.1 and is discussed in more detail below.

What to say after "Hello"

The first several minutes of a medication interview are often the most crucial time for an emotionally anxious patient. What is said and done in this initial period can set the stage for a comfortable, helpful experience for the patient, or negatively color the process from the start. After greeting the patient, there are several things a clinician can do in a brief period of time that will facilitate the task and relax the patient.

As simple as it may sound, making sure that the patient knows *who you are* and *why he or she is being seen* is crucially important, and surprisingly is often misunderstood by the patient. Clinicians, therefore, should state not only their name, but also their professional identifier, and why the patient is being seen today.

Table 3.1 Framework of a prescriptive interview

- Demographic data
- Chief complaint
- History of present illness
- Past history
- Previous mental health episodes
- Previous mental health treatment
- Medical/substance abuse history
- Mental status exam
- Assessment/diagnosis
- Treatment plan

Box 3.1 Talking to patients

"I am Mary Smith, psychiatric nurse practitioner. Your therapist, Frank Jones, has asked me to see you to determine if medication would be helpful for you as part of your treatment. How do you feel about coming to see me today?"

This latter simple question is exceptionally important. Patients coming to see a mental health professional or a primary care doctor about a mental health problem are often very anxious. Their emotions can run the gamut from marked positivity to profound negativity. They may feel relief and eager anticipation ("I am finally doing something about this"; "I should have done this a long time ago"). They may, however, be openly anxious and fearful about the process of seeing a mental health prescriber, and the possibility of being diagnosed and/or being prescribed medications, for all the reasons that are listed in Chapters 1 and 2. Patients may have significant uncertainty or misgivings, or blame themselves unnecessarily ("I never thought it would come to this"; "Just being here means that I couldn't handle things"). Other patients are considerably reluctant and show great resistance. Perhaps they are being seen under duress, complying with the wishes of others who insist they be evaluated ("I wouldn't be here except my wife said she would leave me if I did not come"; "My boss said that I needed to do something or I would lose my job").

The discussion regarding how a patient feels about being seen can be relatively simple and brief, or it may take some measure of time. The very fact that the clinician is interested in the patient's feelings is a good start. When patients are apprehensive, having an opportunity to say how anxious, reluctant or fearful they are, often sets them at ease. Sometimes they will say (and genuinely believe) that they do not have a lot of feelings about the evaluation. If so, this should be accepted at face value. Patients who have seen mental health professionals before may be accustomed to such consultations. For some patients, medication and mental health assessments have been conducted on many previous occasions.

If significant affect is revealed regarding the evaluation session, it is worthwhile spending several minutes allowing the patient to vent. The practitioner may also correct any possible misunderstandings or misconceptions. Generally, this will not take more than a few minutes.

Box 3.2 Talking to patients

In the rare circumstance where a patient seems to wish to talk for a long period of time about the lead-up to this evaluation, the discussion should be gently curtailed. The practitioner can suggest that: *"We need to move on to specific questions that will help us decide if medicine is for you."*

Following this discussion, another brief but very helpful intervention is to describe the process of the interview.

Box 3.3 Talking to patients

If you know beforehand that the visit is specifically for medication evaluation (and not for other mental health services), you can say: *"I will be seeing you today for approximately [number of minutes]. We will focus on the specific symptoms that are bothering you. We will not be spending as much time talking about the issues in your life even though these are important. For purposes of determining if medication is useful, it is essential that we understand what symptoms you have, and how long you have had them. Our overall plan is to define what the problem is, determine if medication can help and, if so, what medication would be best for you. How does that sound to you?"*

In the majority of circumstances this brief introduction, which will take as little as one or two minutes, will prepare the clinician to begin specific symptomatic inquiry.

General issues of history taking

Table 3.2 lists important elements of history taking. It is important in an initial prescriptive interview that this activity is *clinician directed*. The clinician must have an understanding of the information to be covered, and direct the conversation so that the appropriate information is gathered in the time allotted.

This notion opposes tenets taught in schools of psychotherapy about the initial *psychotherapeutic* interview. For therapy evaluations, clinicians are instructed to "let the patient tell his own story in whatever way he needs to." Patients are encouraged to associate freely, telling what is important to them. While this method may be helpful as a basis for psychotherapeutic "talking" therapy, it is an inefficient methodology for gathering necessary data for prescriptive purposes. If patients are allowed to direct the interview, the clinician is often left at the completion of the session trying to make decisions with inadequate information.

Most patients are quite familiar with a structured interview. They expect it from the clinician, and fall easily into a question-and-answer format. Other patients expect to tell their life story, or to spend a considerable amount of time talking about a personal crisis. For medication purposes, these latter patients need to be redirected by the clinician to specific historical elements or by specific symptom questions that will lead to the necessary assessment.

Table 3.2 Important elements of history taking

- Directed interview
- Ask open-ended questions
- Elicit facts and clarify the patient's words
- Framework and wording
- End product is a chronological symptom history, hopefully leading to a diagnosis

Questions should be asked *in a consistent manner* and *framed in an open-ended way*, omitting phrasing that suggests the answer. For example, asking "Have you had any problems with your sleep?" will elicit a more valid answer than "You haven't had any sleep problems, have you?" Similarly, asking "Have you had any difficulty with your concentration and mental focus?" is more helpful than "Given how depressed you've been, I'm sure you've been having trouble concentrating, haven't you?" Particular questions about a patient's symptoms should be phrased in ways that are familiar to the clinician and can be asked consistently.

An important item in evaluating a patient for medication is the *meaning of the patient's terms or jargon.* A patient may think he or she is "depressed" or "anxious," has "panic attacks," is "confused" or "doesn't sleep well"; this does not necessarily mean that the clinician's assessment of these problems will be similar.

Essential to performing a good medication evaluation is asking patients questions to elucidate what they mean by the terminology that they use. *The clinician needs to elicit and record behavioral facts, not the patient's assessment of the facts.*

For example, when someone comes in saying "I'm depressed," elucidate specifics with questions such as:

- What do you mean when you say you are depressed?
- How do you recognize when you are depressed compared to when you are not?
- What changes indicate to you that you are depressed?

If a person complains of "problems sleeping," ask:

- When do you go to bed?
- When do you fall asleep?
- How many times do you awaken?
- How long do you stay awake?
- When do you arise for the day?
- Do you nap? How often? For how long?
- Do you work different shifts or have a markedly variable sleep/wake cycle?

Similarly, with eating and appetite, if a patient complains of a poor appetite or of "not eating well," clarify using the following:

- How many meals do you eat in a day?
- What does a typical meal consist of?
- Does food taste normal? Has it lost its taste?
- Is your weight changing? By how much?
- If you do not measure your weight, do your clothes fit differently?
- Over what period of time has this change occurred?
- Are there periods of increased appetite?
- Have there been any food binges?
- Have you intentionally vomited food? How often?

The medication interview should be routinized. There should be a framework that the clinician is familiar with and has practiced over time, and that can be repeated with limited variations as necessitated by the patient. It is often helpful for clinicians to use a written outline of those elements to be included in the evaluation.

A checklist can be helpful, particularly for less experienced clinicians. Many clinicians with limited experience assume that using a written checklist indicates their inexperience to the patient, or that they will be seen as novices. They assume that experienced clinicians have all the needed information "in their head." This, in fact, is not true, and many patients see the use of a written format as thoroughness on the part of the clinician, not inexperience. Several examples of such checklists to guide clinicians in an initial interview are provided in Tables 3.5–3.7 at the end of this chapter.

Essentials that must be obtained for medication prescription

Demographic data include age, sex, ethnicity, marital status and occupation. The *chief complaint* (CC) is the patient's statement of the reason for seeking assessment. It is very useful, if possible, actually to quote the patient's words. The *history of present illness* (HPI) is a specific history of those complaints or symptoms that occurred with or led up to the CC. The time period covered by this HPI may be weeks, months, years or much of the patient's life, depending on how long the symptoms have been present. *Past history* (PH) for a psychotropic medication evaluation specifically focuses on previous episodes of symptoms, previous mental health treatment episodes including hospitalization, psychotropic medications previously used and response or non-response to medication (see Table 3.3). Elements of childhood developmental history, education, military service, marital history and chronological occupational history, while interesting and useful in other contexts, may not be initially crucial to assessing the adult patient for mental health medication.

The elements of the *medical history* portion should include:

- current medical problems for which the patient is being treated
- current medications taken, dosage and frequency (both prescription and over-the-counter [OTC] medications should be included)
- any history of medication/food/substance allergies
- use of caffeine/nicotine.

If the patient is female, a specific assessment of pregnancy status is essential.

- Are you sexually active?
- Is there a possibility you could be pregnant now?

Table 3.3 Essentials to be obtained for medication prescription[3]

- Symptom-focused psychiatric present illness
- History of past symptoms and episodes
- Previous treatment response to psychotropics
- Medical history
- Current medications used (prescription and OTC)
- Assessment of suicidal and homicidal risk
- Substance use – current and past
- Pregnancy status

- If not, how do you know?
- Is any form of birth control being used?
- When was the date of your last menstrual period?

The patient's substance use should be evaluated, not only currently, but also in regard to any previous history of overuse of alcohol or drugs.

- Do you drink alcohol? How much? How often?
- Do you use recreational drugs? Which ones? How much? How often? Orally, intra-venously or by other means?

If the patient does drink or use drugs, two useful screening questions can often detect a possible substance abuse problem:[1]

1   In the last year, have you ever drunk alcohol or used drugs more than you meant to?
2   Have you felt you wanted to or needed to cut down on your drinking or drug use in the past year?

If either of these questions is answered positively, follow up with:

- Have you ever drunk alcohol or used drugs to deal with your feelings, stress or frustration?
- As a result of your drinking or drug use, did anything happen to you that you wish hadn't happened?
- Does anyone else think you have a problem with substances?

Mental status exam

Most outpatients undergoing a medication evaluation for mild to moderate anxiety or mood disorders do not require formal mental status testing unless:

1   there are *signs of memory loss, poor concentration, confusion or disorientation*
2   *psychotic signs* or symptoms are present
3   it is *required by the clinic or institution* in which the evaluation occurs or, in the United States, it is requested by a third-party payer.

Patients with severe psychiatric symptoms and any patient admitted to an inpatient or custodial setting should have a full mental status exam on admission. Even if a full mental status exam is not or cannot be performed, a behavioral descriptive summary of the patient during the evaluation, including any outstanding elements of appearance, behavior, speech or thought pattern, is useful.

Depending on the time available and the clinician's index of suspicion for mental status abnormalities, practitioners may choose to perform a *Mini-Mental Status Exam* (MMSE), a full *Mental Status Exam* or the three-minute *Mini-Cog*. The formats for each of these evaluations of mental status are detailed in Appendix 1.

Suicide and homicide assessment

As part of the mental status assessment, evaluation of the patient's suicidal and homicidal risk must be included. If the patient has had suicidal ideation, estimation must be made of the frequency, intensity and lethality of these thoughts:

- Have you ever had thoughts of hurting or killing yourself?
- If suicidal thoughts have been present, how often?
- How easy/difficult has it been for you to deal with these thoughts?
- If there have been thoughts, do you have a plan for killing yourself?
- How would you commit suicide, if you were to attempt it?
- What is your plan?
- Do you have access to the materials/equipment/weapon needed to carry out the plan?
- Have you tried to kill yourself in the past? When? How was the attempt discovered?
- Was any medical or psychiatric intervention required?
- Were there any medical sequelae to the attempt?
- Is there anything that would prevent you from following through with such an attempt now?

If homicidal ideation or thoughts of direct harm to others are present:

- How often have they occurred?
- Toward whom are the thoughts directed?
- Have you made any specific plans to do this?
- Is there any direct plan to harm someone now?
- Is there anything that would prevent this from happening, now or in the future?

Prescribers will find the above screening questions brief and useful for the majority of medication evaluations. Some prescribers prefer a more detailed set of suicide screening questions. If so, a widely used and validated screening tool is the Columbia Suicide Severity Rating Scale, available at: https://cssrs.columbia.edu/

Useful but optional information

There is information that may be helpful, but is not essential for evaluation (see Table 3.4). If possible, it is reasonable for the clinician to ask about these items, knowing that in some cases there will be insufficient time to do so.

A *history of psychiatric illness in the patient's blood relatives*, particularly first-degree relatives, can be diagnostically helpful. For example, a child brought for evaluation of

Table 3.4 Other factual information that may be useful

- Family psychiatric history
- Use of psychotropics by family members and results
- Patient's thoughts about using medication
- Knowledge of, or concerns about, medication
- Sexual history

attention and behavior problems who has several relatives with a history of bipolar disorder raises the clinician's suspicion that this patient may have a bipolar diagnosis, rather than attention deficit disorder. In this case, more detailed questions about hypomanic behavior would be warranted. Whenever a family history is positive for psychiatric illness in blood relatives, it is useful to learn if any medications have been prescribed for these individuals and the effect of such medication. If the patient thinks that medications have been prescribed for close relatives, but does not know the details, the clinician can suggest that the patient try, if possible, to get this information to bring in at the second appointment.

Additionally, it is helpful to ask what the patient thinks about the use of psychotropic medications.

- What have you read?
- What have you heard from friends or relatives?
- Do you have any particular overriding concerns about how medication may affect you?
- Do you have any particular side effects or risks about which you are concerned?

These questions, when asked before recommending a particular medication, can be very helpful in assisting the clinician in choosing a medication. If the patient, for example, is very concerned about weight gain, then perhaps a medication can be chosen in which weight gain is a minimal side effect. If a blood relative has done well on a particular medication, the patient may be positively predisposed to that medication.

Target symptoms

As the chronological symptom history is being obtained, the clinician can begin to identify target symptoms to be treated with medication. Items such as sleep disturbance, appetite dysregulation, concentration difficulties, diminished energy, thought disorganization, hallucinations, delusions, anxiety, panic attacks, excessive ruminations, social avoidance, confusion, suicidal ideation/behavior, homicidal ideation/behavior, irritability and rage attacks are examples of possible target symptoms. When the information gathered leads the clinician to make a diagnosis, this should be made and recorded. When a positive diagnosis cannot be determined, a list of possible diagnoses or "rule outs" should be created.

Historical information from others

Input from other sources can be very helpful to the clinician in making decisions about medication, particularly when patients are:

- poor observers of their own behavior
- having trouble with memory or concentration
- having trouble verbalizing their symptoms
- frankly confused or psychotic
- intoxicated.

It can be assumed that anyone who accompanies a patient to an initial prescriptive interview is there for a reason, and should be at least offered the opportunity to provide input. This person may be a family member or spouse, a therapist, social worker, home health visitor, probation officer, friend or neighbor. If the patient has not asked to have the visitor come into the consultation room, the clinician should ask the patient's permission to speak with the accompanying party before completing the assessment. If, in the initial portion of the interview, it becomes clear that the patient is having significant concentration or memory problems, it is generally most efficient to bring in any accompanying visitor early in the interview.

Identify other important sources of information that need to be collected, including:

- psychotherapists
- medical colleagues
- psychological testing
- family input
- laboratory tests
- physical exam or assessments.

When another clinician is to be contacted, obtain a signed release of information from the patient.

The medical work-up

Prior to prescribing a psychotropic, a recent full physical examination is not mandatory for a healthy patient without medical problems. If, however, there are uncompensated medical issues or the patient has significant somatic complaints, a physical exam should be performed as part of the initial evaluation or soon thereafter. Attention should be paid to the organ systems about which the patient complains (e.g., back, headache, bowels, fatigue), with follow up of any abnormal findings. If the screening physical exam is negative, emotional causes are often hypothesized, at least initially, to be the cause of the somatic symptoms. In such situations, a further physical diagnostic work-up is not warranted unless new symptoms emerge or mental health treatment does not improve the symptoms.

- If there are signs, symptoms or a history suggestive of liver disease, a liver function panel should be obtained because almost all psychotropic medications are hepatically metabolized.
- Pregnancy testing should be performed on any menstruating female who cannot give a reliable history of consistent use of birth control measures or sexual abstinence for the previous menstrual cycle.
- In any depressed patient, the work-up should include a TSH (thyroid stimulating hormone) level, since up to 15 percent of depressed patients will have abnormal thyroid tests without any other symptoms of thyroid dysfunction.
- Prior to the anticipated use of a mood stabilizer such as lithium, valproic acid or carbamazepine, a full chemical panel, including liver functions, electrolytes, kidney functions, blood sugar, a CBC (complete blood count) and TSH level, is recommended.

- If there is a history of kidney disease, a urinalysis should also be obtained.
- If the patient is likely to be started on an atypical antipsychotic, a fasting blood sugar and a baseline lipid profile should be obtained.
- When the patient is deemed to be at high risk for HIV and/or hepatitis, testing for these two conditions is wise.
- If the patient is currently taking a mood stabilizer that the clinician is not going to discontinue, a serum blood level of that medication should also be drawn. (See Chapter 25 for details of blood level protocol.)
- If there is consideration of prescribing an antipsychotic medication, a baseline AIMS test should be performed and documented. (See Chapter 19 on Movement Disorders, and Appendix 6 for details of the AIMS examination.)

Thyroid evaluation

As to the issue of thyroid evaluation for mental health patients, recent opinion questions the relevance of thyroid abnormalities discovered during a mental health work-up to the hypothalamic–pituitary–thyroid axis and true thyroid disease.[1] The authors suggest that these laboratory abnormalities are part of what has been referred to as "non-thyroidal illness," are more referable to the underlying psychiatric illness and will resolve spontaneously with mental health treatment. This report concludes on page 130 that "current data are inadequate to definitively address the question of whether evidence of active non-thyroidal illness improves or worsens morbidity, mortality and psychiatric symptoms."[4]

True thyroid illness does co-exist in psychiatric patients with some frequency. Resolution of mental health symptoms also seldom occurs quickly and thoroughly in the presence of unresolved thyroid abnormalities. From an interpersonal standpoint, patients who become aware of having abnormal thyroid laboratory results will often be quite strong in their request to have their thyroid status treated, even to the point of going to another practitioner if it is not attended to. This author therefore disagrees with this report's authors and continues to recommend obtaining a TSH as part of an initial evaluation with further evaluation and/or thyroid supplementation when non-trivial TSH elevations are discovered, especially if T4 levels are equivocal or low.

Unlike most thyroid disease not associated with mental illness which does not spontaneously resolve, it may ultimately turn out that thyroid supplementation which has been part of a treatment that results in a good therapeutic outcome, is not permanently necessary. After a sustained remission therefore, competent practice would be to discontinue any thyroid supplementation and recheck a TSH level 3–4 months later. Unless the TSH is again elevated, further thyroid supplementation could be omitted.

Genetic testing

Although one of the holy grails of mental health medication prescription would be a genetic screen which would, in advance, determine which medication a patient might respond to, *this is not yet a reality* (see Chapter 5).

The next decision

Following information gathering, the next decision for the clinician is whether or not medications are indicated. Obviously, if the clinician decides that medications would not help the target symptoms or chief complaint, this should be stated and any other treatments that might be helpful discussed with the patient. Referral can be made to another clinician who might be consulted for the patient's particular complaint.

If medication is deemed appropriate, the first question is: what *category* of medication is useful for this patient – antidepressants, anti-anxiety medicine, antipsychotics, a mood stabilizer, another category or a combination? Once decided, a single category may have *several classes* from which to choose. For example, within the antidepressants, the clinician may choose an SSRI (selective serotonin reuptake inhibitor), a non-SSRI antidepressant, a tricyclic antidepressant or a monoamine oxidase inhibitor (MOAI). Within the antipsychotic category, the clinician may prescribe a traditional or atypical antipsychotic. Once the class is identified, the clinician must choose a *specific medication* within that class.

Although it is clearly desirable to use monotherapy whenever possible, in some cases it may be necessary to use more than one medication simultaneously or to prescribe one medication on a regular basis while providing another medication on a PRN (as needed) basis. Further information on selecting an initial medication is specified in Chapter 5.

Assessment and formulation

Having responded to the clinician's questions and having revealed significant personal information, the patient will eagerly, and often anxiously, await the practitioner's reaction. Many patients remain uncertain about presenting for medication evaluation, and are concerned as to how the clinician will react. A brief preface to your assessment and formulation can often set the patient further at ease.

 Box 3.4 Talking to patients

"Making an appointment for mental health medication is not always easy. Having heard what you have been experiencing, I think you have made a good decision to come today. Here is my assessment and what I think will help."

Summarizing the information, the clinician should then provide the patient with an assessment in layman's terms. For clarity, it is important that long diagnostic or medically complicated terms be avoided. When such language must be used, simple definitions are helpful.

The clinician can then make pharmacological and non-pharmacological recommendations to the patient. Non-pharmacological interventions may include psychotherapy, cognitive/behavioral therapy, relaxation training, biofeedback, light therapy, eye movement, social skills training (more information is documented in Chapter 7). Pharmacological recommendations from the clinician should include the name of the medication, its classification, which target symptoms the medication is likely to improve and the probable timetable for results.

A discussion of side effects is appropriate at this time. There is a delicate balance involved in any discussion of side effects. On the one hand, the patient must have enough information to be truly informed. However, overloading the patient with data will likely produce increased fear, anxiety and non-adherence. In general, mentioning the three or four most commonly experienced side effects of the medication chosen will suffice. A detailed explanation of all possible side effects will only confuse the patient, and will not be helpful to the prescriptive process. If there are any serious risks (for example, hypertensive crisis with MAO inhibitors, and/or alcohol/antabuse reaction with disulfiram), specific risks should be discussed in more detail. If there are particular medications to avoid because of possible medication interactions, they should be mentioned and included in written information given to the patient. (See Chapter 19 for a more in-depth discussion of side effects.)

A crucial point, often overlooked, particularly if the clinician is busy or new to the prescriptive process, is patient feedback and consent. It is critical to be sure that patients understand what the assessment is and what role medication may play; and most importantly, whether the patient concurs with the medication recommendations. A thorough examination, culminating in an accurate diagnosis followed by appropriate treatment recommendations will be futile if the patient deposits the carefully written prescription into the trash upon leaving!

Non-adherence with a prescription medication often results from:

- ignorance (the patient did not hear or understand what was said)
- disagreement (the patient disagreed with the use of medication at all or with the medication choice)
- fear (the patient has not been adequately reassured about the safety of medication)
- denial (the patient does not want to believe, or disagrees with, the diagnosis).

Completing the patient feedback loop is essential. Does the patient understand what has been said? Are there any fears that might interfere with adherence? Is the patient willing, with your support, to try medication?

Box 3.5 Talking to patients

Following your statement of diagnosis and treatment: *"That is my assessment of the problem and what I think will help. Does that sound reasonable? Do you have any concerns about what I said? Can you follow through with these recommendations?"*

Purely verbal instructions to patients are often misheard, misunderstood or totally forgotten in the midst of the probable anxiety present in the prescriptive interview. If the clinician verbally gives a quick set of instructions and asks "Do you understand?" or "Any questions?" patients will often nod "Yes," even when they are quite unsure. Therefore, _written instructions are extremely helpful_.

If there is agreement, the prescription is written, dosages and directions for use are reviewed and the patient should be given the opportunity to ask questions. If the clinician has done a competent, thorough job in the previous steps, questions are usually minimal. In some cases, though, the patient may have several questions held in abeyance for just this opportunity. Once the questions are answered, an appointment for a *follow-up evaluation* is made. A written appointment card given to the patient is beneficial. It is seldom appropriate to have the patient leave the office without a definite time agreed upon for follow up.

Immediately after the interview, the patient's written or electronic record should be completed. This will document the above-mentioned steps, including the chief complaint, present illness and target symptoms; negative responses to important questions within the assessment; mental status examination; medical history; medication history; alcohol and drug history; clinician assessment and recommendations; and a record of the specific medication and prescription data.

Although there are time pressures on all clinicians, it is crucial that the record be completed as soon as possible. Even an hour or two later, if the clinician has seen more patients, it will be difficult to remember details from an earlier evaluation. Whether the clinician handwrites, dictates or types the record is immaterial, as long as the information is documented quickly and substantively. (See Chapter 24 for further details about record keeping.)

Within 24–72 hours, with a signed release of information completed, the clinician should *telephone the patient's referral source* and also *contact any other treaters* who will be involved in the patient's medical care. Some clinicians prefer to dictate an evaluation and send a fax/e-mail copy to the referring clinician. In the United States, some third-party payers require the mental health prescriber to have contact with the primary care provider.

Length of an initial prescriptive interview

In reality, the initial prescriptive interview is of varying length depending on the complexity of the patient and the time that the clinician has to spend with the patient. Ideally, an experienced clinician can conduct a full, thorough evaluative interview, provide patient education, prescribe medication and devise an initial treatment plan in a 60-minute time period. There are some patients for whom this can be realistically compressed into a 45-minute time slot. In general, those clinicians who have less than 45 minutes to spend in an initial evaluation will almost certainly have to eliminate certain elements from the evaluation or have the information collected by other means. For example, some busy offices are organized such that another clinician gathers and records some information prior to seeing the prescriber who then reviews, clarifies and elaborates on this data. Under no circumstances should this information be collected by a non-clinically trained person. The primary care practitioner may also choose to retain in-house specialists, such as specially trained psychiatric nurses, physician's assistants, psychologists or social workers, to do all or part of an initial patient screening. In a situation where there is a prescriber such as a psychiatric nurse with prescriptive authority in the office, the nurse may be able to conduct the initial evaluation and write the prescription either independently or with the collaboration/supervision of the primary care physician. Alternatively, some offices will have the patient fill out a written questionnaire or symptom screen or enter responses on a computer. Both of these methodologies, while not ideal, do maximize the prescriber's valuable time.

When time is short

> ## Box 3.6 Primary care
>
> The timeframes described above are realistically necessary and appropriate for thorough mental health prescription. While primary care practitioners should strive to allow for sufficient time to perform a complete exam, busy primary care clinics may need to streamline the amount of clinician–patient contact. There is an ongoing concern about the length of time that primary care clinicians may make available for an initial psychotropic evaluation. *If the time is pared too greatly, important elements of effective prescription will be omitted or overlooked.* A reasonable assessment for mental health medications simply cannot be performed in 5 or 10 minutes.

Screening tools that have been developed and tested for reliability include:

- Prime-MD, developed in 1994 by Robert Spitzer *et al.*, is a very complete clinician tool for evaluation of mental conditions in a primary care office, but the original format was time-consuming to fill out. A shorter version, the Patient Health Questionnaire 2, is an abbreviated three-page version that is self-completed, and can be reviewed by the clinician in 3 minutes.[5–7]
- The Mini International Neuropsychiatric Interview, by David Sheehan *et al.*,[8–9] is a useful clinician-administered set of questions that lead the clinician to a specific mental health diagnosis. It has been tested and validated around the world and translated into a number of languages.
- The Beck Depression Inventory (BDI) is one of the most widely used and simple screens for depression. It consists of 21 multiple-choice questions that can be completed by the patient quickly. Repeated administration of the test can also reflect the extent of progress and symptom improvement. The original version was published in 1961,[2] and has been validated on multiple occasions. It was revised and copyrighted in 1978.[10] The copyrighted version and many other office screening tests are available for purchase at www.psychcorp.com

The most commonly used screens are copyrighted proprietary tests, and further sources are listed at the end of the chapter. Many pharmaceutical firms also have access to office screening questionnaires and evaluation tools.

A primary care provider may also choose to schedule patients with mental health concerns into a longer initial time slot. Sometimes an interview before the lunch hour or just before the workday's end will allow extra time for a more thorough interview. The extra time spent in this initial interview will often pay off in better patient communication, better treatment of the mental health problem and, ultimately, a diminished use of medical/surgical services and fewer demands on the professional's time in later months.

While most professionals like to complete an initial evaluation in a single session, it can sometimes be useful to complete the evaluation in two separate closely spaced appointments. A busy primary care physician can see a patient, gather initial information, order appropriate laboratory tests and see the patient again in several days to complete the diagnostic work-up. If the patient is particularly symptomatic, the prescription of a sleeping medication or an anti-anxiety medication can sustain the patient until he/she is seen for the second evaluation interview.

Written or multimedia education materials are abundantly available and can assist in the patient education portion of the interview, which is critical to adherence. Educational organizations and pharmaceutical companies have produced many pamphlets, videotapes, audiotapes, DVDs and CD-ROMs that can help the busy clinician avoid having to repeat baseline instructions, descriptions and warnings. Some clinicians may choose to devise their own instruction sheets that include educational information about common medications they prescribe. Preferably, the clinician will review such education sheets in the office personally with the patient; however, when this is not possible, the patient can read the information at a later time. At times in a busy primary care office, the physician or the prescribing nurse will write the prescription and then have the patient seen by another professional (another nurse, a physician's assistant or mental health technician), who will answer questions, review educational materials or perform other patient education tasks.

Sample clinician guidelines

The following are examples of formats for checklist reminder outlines that could be used by a clinician during an initial evaluation interview. Some prefer to use brief phrases on a single sheet to serve as an outline and prompt for thoroughness (e.g., the depression issues checklist in Table 3.5). Other prescribers prefer to devise multi-page sheets with spaces after each question to write in the patient's responses. This document is then included as part of the patient's record (e.g., the mania/bipolar issues shown in Table 3.6). Others may prefer to write out exact phrasing for questions so they can be asked in a routine way (e.g., the anxiety issues checklist in Table 3.7). Each format is useful, and clinicians will benefit from customizing a personal list of questions in a format and sequence that they prefer.

- The General Health Questionnaire-12 (GHQ-12)[11] and the Symptom Checklist-10 (SCL-10)[12] are other screens that have been validated and are widely used in Europe.
- Descriptions of a number of screening tests used by primary care practitioners for mood, anxiety, sleep, psychosis and substance abuse are available on the Internet at www.fpnotebook.com

Diagnostic and medication bias

Since competent medication prescription is based ideally on accurate, targeted diagnoses, mention must be made here regarding diagnostic bias. In the best of all worlds, every practitioner would see mental health syndromes with equal clarity and without preconceived notions. Of course, this can never be the case and all practitioners bring at least some measure of bias to their patient assessments. There are, however, some practitioners who carry this to the extreme and have an excessive sensitivity either toward or against making certain diagnostic conclusions, which then biases their medication choice.

Table 3.5 Depression issues checklist

- When were you last well?
- Describe your current symptoms:
  Depressed mood – crying spells, feelings of worthlessness
  Sleep
  Appetite, weight change, food not tasting good, binges, excessive concerns with eating
    or weight
  Concentration – school, work, reading, TV
  Any change in the way your mind works?
  Change in speed of thoughts
  Mental confusion, indecisiveness
  Inappropriate anger, irritability, violent feelings
  Excessive anxiety, agitation
  Change in activity level or energy
  Headache, head pains
  Mood reactivity – do positive events cheer you up?
  Sensitivity to rejection – "leaden paralysis"
  Loss of pleasure in activities
  Suicidal ideation – plan – attempts
  Social isolation
  Change in sexual interest, drive or performance
- Known life events/precipitants
- Rating of mood on scale of 1 to 10 – now, 1 month ago, 6 months ago, 1 year ago
- Patient's age at time of first episode – What were the symptoms? Similar or different from
  current episode?
- Subsequent episodes – length and timing
- Return to normal between episodes?
- Psychiatric hospitalizations?
- Previous treatments
  Medications – duration, response, side effects, dose, ECT?
  Psychotherapy – issues, results, who was therapist?
  Technique used?
- Current medications
- Ongoing medical problems
- Medical hospitalizations/surgeries
- Allergies
- Possibility of pregnancy
- Using any form of pregnancy prevention?
- When was last physical exam?
- Drug/alcohol usage
- Family history of substance abuse
- History of thyroid problems in self or family
- Family history of depression or psychiatric problems
- Is there a pattern to the onset or remission of depression (seasonal, with the menstrual cycle,
  postpartum)?
- Psychiatric medications used by family members – response?
- Hallucinations?
- Paranoia?
- Manic episodes? Describe length, frequency and intensity
- What have you read about treatments for depression?
- Preferences for treatment?
- Concerns about treatment?

Table 3.6 Mania/bipolar issues symptoms checklist

* Lack of need for sleep without loss of energy
* Unusual activity in the middle of the night (cleaning, writing, shopping)
* Speeded/racing thoughts, rapid speech
* Too many thoughts at once
* Impulsive decisions
* Increased spending/buying/generosity
* Start many projects, but finish few
* Rapid mood shifts, with or without precipitant
* Marked fluctuations in emotions/behavior
* Excess irritability, rages
* Unusual endurance when fatigue would be expected
* Inability to slow thoughts or behavior
* Family history of bipolar disorder
* Previous excessive/agitated/unusually rapid response to antidepressants
* Any pattern to these symptoms?

Some clinicians are extraordinarily reluctant to make certain diagnoses, feeling that they will label the patient, or that some diagnoses are not validly based on current research. Some providers, for personal reasons, tend to ignore signs, symptoms or criteria which would lead them to make a particular diagnosis. Equally problematic are practitioners who, for various reasons, "see" and diagnose the same condition in almost every patient and tend to use the same diagnosis for a large percentage of patients that they work with. Reasons for professional bias can vary but include:

* training bias which was passed on from previous educators or trainers
* the practitioner's personal or family history
* internal or external pressure to make certain diagnoses because of reimbursement or clinic policy
* an inflated sense of professional competence with the feeling that a practitioner is exceptionally trained or astute in recognizing conditions that others do not.

In settings which serve a general mental health population, one would expect to make a variety of diagnoses and to use a wide variety of medications based on patient need. There are, of course, clinical situations in which the mix of patients is atypical. In these situations, there may be a larger percentage of patients with a particular problem because they have been self-selected to attend a "Mood Disorder Clinic," a "Trauma Recovery Center," a clinic for substance abuse, a mental health clinic catering to military veterans or a mental health practice which "specializes in ADHD." Even in these circumstances, it would be unusual for all patients to have the same diagnosis and consequently be treated with similar and/or the same medications. Unfortunately, though, in specialty clinics, practitioners can often utilize "confirmation bias," attending to symptoms or behaviors which support the specialty diagnosis for which the clinic is known, but tend not to do a diligent job at looking for other potential signs or symptoms.

Another element of bias does not relate to diagnosis but to the prescription of certain medications or medication groups. Some practitioners are unnecessarily and extraordinarily concerned about the possibility of certain side effects, the possibility of habituation and addiction, or the feeling that they will be "taken advantage of"

Table 3.7 Anxiety issues checklist for panic disorder/generalized anxiety disorder (GAD)/
obsessive–compulsive disorder (OCD)/social anxiety disorder

- Have you had problems with anxiety or nervousness?
- Is the anxiety present almost all the time, or does it come in sudden bursts or attacks?
- What are these attacks like? Do you have any physical signs that go along with the anxiety (e.g., rapid heartbeat, shortness of breath, sweating) (panic disorder)
- Are there any places or activities that you avoid because of these attacks? (phobias)
- Have you had to alter your daily routine because of them? (panic disorder)
- Does the anxiety affect your eating or sleeping? (all)
- Do you have recurrent, repetitive worries, such that you are worrying about something almost all the time? (GAD)
- Do you have repetitive thoughts that you can't get out of your head (similar to getting a song "stuck in your head")? (OCD)
- What are these thoughts about? (OCD)
    Dirt/contamination
    Diseases
    Fear of harming self/others/pets
    Violent scenes/images
- Do you have repetitive behaviors that you do over and over, even if they are unnecessary or seem silly? (OCD)
    What kind of behaviors?
    Washing/showering/cleaning
    Collecting/hoarding
    Checking locks/appliances/for mistakes in writing or papers
    Excessive doubt or indecision
- How much time per day do you spend thinking these thoughts or performing these behaviors? (OCD)
- Do you have mental rituals or sequences that must be repeated in an exact way? (OCD)
- Do you regularly count items? (OCD)
- Do numbers have special meanings? (OCD)
- Do you pull or remove any hair on your head or body unnecessarily? (trichotillomania)
- Has anyone told you about or have you noticed recurrent facial movements that are hard to control? (tics – OCD)
- Are you fearful of speaking in large or small groups? (social anxiety disorder)
- Do you avoid social gatherings? (social anxiety disorder)
- Do you fear being watched closely by others when doing an activity? (social anxiety disorder)

- Which activity?
    Talking
    Eating
    Writing
    Voiding or bathroom issues
- Do you blush or sweat easily? Does this bother you? (social anxiety disorder)
- Do you use alcohol to "loosen up" before a social gathering? (social anxiety disorder)
- What treatment, if any, have you had for these problems? (all)
- Have you ever taken medication for this?
    What medication?
    For how long?
    Did it help?
    How did it help?
    What were the side effects, if any?
- Have you ever used alcohol or recreational drugs to deal with these problems?

by patients if they prescribe certain medications. Most commonly this bias applies to potentially habit-forming medication including benzodiazepines, sleep medications or stimulants.

Prescribing clinicians should be aware that biases can and do exist even in the most competent of practitioners. It is wise to periodically sit back with perspective and assess one's own behavior for the possibility of diagnostic and/or medication bias. If the clinician suspects that bias may be present, notes that a large percentage of patients carry the same diagnoses, and/or are prescribed the exact same medications, it would be prudent to utilize the consultation of an experienced colleague to help assess the situation.

References

1   The importance of physician–patient relationships[,] communication and trust in health care, available at: https://dukepersonalizedhealth.org/2019/03/the-importance-of-physician-patient-relationships-communication-and-trust-in-health-care/

2   Lee SJ *et al.* (2002, January 1) Enhancing physician–patient communication, available at: www.ncbi.nlm.nih.gov/pubmed/12446437

3   Stewart MA (1995, May 1) Effective physician–patient communication and health outcomes: a review, available at: www.ncbi.nlm.nih.gov/pubmed/7728691

4   Dickerman AL and Barnhill JW (2012) Abnormal thyroid function tests in psychiatric patients: a red herring? *American Journal of Psychiatry* 169: 127–133.

5   Staab JP *et al.* (2001) Detection and diagnosis of psychiatric disorders in primary medical care. *Medical Clinics of North America* 85(3): 579–596.

6   Kroenke K *et al.* (2003) The Patient Health Questionnaire-2: validity of a two-item depression screener. *Medical Care* 41(11): 1284–1292.

7   Goldberg D (1978) General Health Questionnaire (GHQ 20), available at: www.mapi-trust.org/services/questionnairelicensing/cataloguequestionnaires/52-GHQ

8   Lecrubier Y *et al.* (1997) The MINI International Neuropsychiatric Interview (M.I.N.I.). A short diagnostic structured interview: reliability and validity according to the CIDI. *European Psychiatry* 12: 224–231.

9   Sheehan DV *et al.* (1998) The Mini International Neuropsychiatric Interview (M.I.N.I.): the development and validation of a structured diagnostic psychiatric interview. *Journal of Clinical Psychiatry* 59 (Suppl. 20): 22–33.

10 Beck AT *et al.* (1961) An inventory for measuring depression. *Archives of General Psychiatry* 4: 561–571.

11 Gureje O and Obikoya B (1990) The GHQ-12 as a screening tool in a primary care setting. *Social Psychiatry and Psychiatric Epidemiology* 5: 276–280.

12 Rosen CS (2000) Six- and ten-item indexes of psychological distress based on the Symptom Checklist-90. *Assessment* 7(2): 103–111.

4 Helping a patient decide to try medication

- Shared goals   45
- Common patient concerns about psychotropic medication   46
- Other resistances to psychotropic medication   48
- The use of levers   49
- Reasons that patients take psychotropic medication   50
- The use of metaphor   51
- Reference   52

Shared goals

It is most desirable for a patient and a prescriber of psychotropic medication to mutually share a contract to begin medication with commonly accepted goals. It is decidedly advantageous for the clinician to attempt to reach this consensus during the initial evaluation interview as the clinician begins to make therapeutic recommendations. In addition to the clinician's assessment and diagnosis, he/she can begin the medication discussion with a simple statement: *"I believe that some medication could be helpful to you in feeling better. How do you feel about that?"*

Although many patients will want specifics about what medication is being recommended before they consent, obtaining the patient's agreement to consider the possibility of medication is the first step. If the patient is agreeable to considering medication as part of his/her treatment, the best follow-up question is: *"What are the top two problems that you would like medication to help?"*

Usually at this point the patient will mention several issues associated with their target symptoms. It is then easy for the clinician to be in agreement, and suggest that the recommended medication will likely help in those areas which are of the greatest concern to the patient. This creates a strong foundation for further medication treatment.

In some situations, as soon as the concept of psychotropic medication is raised, the patient will be reluctant or resistant. It is crucial at this point for the clinician to deal with these resistances before proceeding. Some of the common hesitations are detailed in the section below, with recommendations on how to approach these potential stumbling blocks.

Box 4.1 Talking to patients

In some cases, the patient may be looking for medication assistance with a problem that the clinician feels is unlikely to be affected by medication. It is useful to suggest gently, but clearly, that medication may not result in that benefit. At the same time, the clinician can reinforce the realistic potential benefits of a medication prescription. For example, if the patient hopes that medication will make them "smarter," the prescriber can say: *"I don't think this medication will raise your IQ but I do think it may help you be less depressed and be able to concentrate better. If you can concentrate better, I do think that you will find that you will feel mentally sharper."*

The patient may wish that medication will help them have more friends. The prescriber can say: *"I don't think that the medication will change your personality. I do, however, expect that as you take the medication, you will have more energy and will be better able to put yourself in social situations where you can make friends. If we find that you are still having difficulty connecting with people as you feel better, we can look into specific behaviors and interventions which may help."*

If the patient wants the medication to fix his relationship with his boss, the prescriber can say: *"I don't expect that will be a direct effect of the medication, but I do think if you are less anxious, your work performance will improve and you may need to take fewer sick days. If you are more confident and performing better at work, it is likely that your boss will notice. You will also be in a better mental state to deal with him about any concerns you have on the job."*

In rare circumstances, the patient may be positively predisposed to taking medication, but is doing so for an unusual or even psychotic reason. This circumstance is discussed later in the chapter and requires a slightly different approach by the clinician.

Common patient concerns about psychotropic medication

There are multiple resistances and obstacles to a patient beginning psychotropic medication. Specific concerns regarding this class of medication typically exceed concerns regarding medical/surgical medications. Some of these worries are enmeshed in the myths described in Chapter 2; others are based on other beliefs about how medication might affect personality.

When the clinician raises the concept of beginning psychotropic medication and there is resistance from the patient, there are several common issues that are likely to be present, alone or in combination. A brief discussion can often allay concerns or fears.

The following issues should be addressed, even if the patient does not raise them directly:

1   Is this medicine for life?
2   Is this medication addictive?
3   Will I be different?

4   Will I get side effects?
5   Can I drink alcohol while taking this medicine?

Is this medicine for life?

Many patients know of relatives or friends who have been on medication indefinitely. Their fear is that if a medication is started, it means a life-long commitment. In fact, while some patients may need long-term medication, many patients will take medication intermittently or for an isolated period. Explaining that virtually all patients will be given a trial period without medication at some point in their care is reassuring to the patient. The approximate timeframe for when this trial will occur should be defined, and should be part of the treatment plan that the clinician describes. More detail on this issue is described in Chapter 8.

Is this addictive?

Many patients (and some clinicians) consider all mental health medications to be addictive or habit forming. There may be an assumption that patients will need (or want) to take more of the medication than prescribed. While this is true for some addictive personalities, as well as some people with substance abuse problems, the vast majority of patients will not only *not* abuse medication, they will also not feel the need to. They will also not develop any physical dependence on the medication. It is often very useful to state specifically that antidepressants, mood stabilizers, antipsychotic medications and many other psychotropics have no potential whatever for physical tolerance or addiction. Benzodiazepines and stimulants are the primary medications that can have habit-forming potential, and should be differentiated from other types of medication for the patient.

Will I be different?

This is often a difficult question to answer, since both clinician and patient obviously want the patient to be different, at least in terms of symptom relief. Usually, this question actually overlies the concern, "Will my personality be altered? Will I be a different person?" This, too, is not easily answered, since many mood, psychotic and anxiety disorders, when properly treated, can lead to significant differences in behavior, attitude and interrelatedness. No evidence exists, however, to suggest that antidepressants, antipsychotics or anti-anxiety medication will alter a person's fundamental personality.

Box 4.2 Talking to patients

When a patient asks "Will I be different?" a possible response is: *"You will be the same person, but I am hopeful that you will not be experiencing these troublesome symptoms that you are now having."* Then list the target symptoms that have been identified earlier in the interview.

Will I get side effects?

The details of discussing side effects with patients are covered in Chapter 19. As indicated there, the clinician needs to address several common side effects that occur with the medication selected. Examples might be drowsiness, dizziness, nausea or interference with sexual arousal. Fortunately, although the vast majority of these side effects can be annoying, they are physiologically not life-threatening. In the initial interview, clinicians can ask patients what they have read or heard about side effects, both to the class medication prescribed and/or the specific medication. If so, are these side effects of concern to the patient? When specific side-effect concerns are raised, the clinician should address them directly.

Can I drink alcohol while taking this medication?

As discussed in more depth in Chapter 16, the answer to this question is that usually it is not desirable to drink alcohol during the first several weeks of medication so that the patient can adjust to the medication's effects and any side effects without alcohol's confounding effects. Thereafter, most patients *without* a history of substance abuse can drink in moderation. "Moderation" must be specifically defined by the clinician, since people have distinctly different ideas of what it means to be "moderate" in their drinking. For a majority of patients, this is no more than one drink in an evening and no more than four drinks in a week. Patients should be cautioned about the possibility of increased reaction/intoxication when drinking while taking medication, and the risks of exceeding recommended limits. Chapter 16 contains a specific *Talking to Patients* dialogue for discussing this issue.

Other resistances to psychotropic medication

Some other common resistances are:

1   You should not tinker with "Mother Nature."
2   "Natural" remedies are always best.
3   The cure (with its side effects) will be worse than the illness.
4   I mistrust doctors, nurses and hospitals in general.
5   On medication, my life will not be the same.
6   Medication will control me.
7   Medication is only for "crazy" people.

Other more "psychological" reasons for resisting psychotropic medication are not always conscious, or verbalized by the patient, but are nonetheless powerful roadblocks to beginning a course of medication treatment. Some examples of intrapsychic reasons include:

1   Because of my past behavior or my lack of self-confidence, I do not deserve to feel better.
2   If I take medication and get better, I will have to confront … [some element of my life], such as:
   • I will have to deal with the lack of intimacy in my marriage.

- I will have to confront the fact that my job is repetitive, boring, stressful or inappropriate to my skills.
- To solidify my recovery, I may have to make substantial lifestyle changes.
- I will have to confront the fact that my social acquaintances and social behaviors may be contributing to my problem.
- If I feel better, I may have to reassess the nature of, and with whom I have, interpersonal relationships.

While these issues are not often overtly brought up, it is important that the clinician be aware of some of these common resistances and be alert to cues that resistance may be occurring in a particular patient. When patients resist trying or continuing with medication, it is worth asking whether any of these reasons may be present.

The use of levers

Even when the above issues have been addressed and discussed, and some of the more psychological reasons considered, some patients may remain resistant to the concept of using medication for emotional illness. In these situations, the clinician who has obtained a history of symptoms – and (more importantly) the activities, behaviors or lifestyle alterations that have occurred because of the symptoms – can utilize this information to help convince the patient to try medication. Simply put, *what has the patient given up because of the symptoms of this illness? What does he or she avoid or no longer enjoy because of the symptoms?* When clinicians know which significant parts of the patient's life are being affected, they can use these "levers" as reasons to try medication.

Box 4.3 Talking to patients

A 60-year-old grandmother may resist the concept of taking a medication for her anxiety disorder; however, she may be quite upset that her anxiety is keeping her from being able to cook the holiday meal that she has traditionally been proud to prepare for her family. Therefore, proposing medication to such a person could include: *"I want you to feel less anxious so you can do the good job of cooking your usual Christmas dinner."* This can be much more powerful than: *"I think we need to treat your anxiety disorder."*

Similarly, a 35-year-old man who has no belief that he has bipolar disorder, but is on probation at work and on the verge of losing his job, may be willing to try medication solely for the purpose of maintaining his employment and livelihood despite the fact that, if pressed, he would say he doesn't have a psychiatric condition. The clinician may say: *"I know how important it is for you to be a good provider for your wife and children. I would like to help you do that. I know that medication for this problem is probably not your first choice, but I strongly suspect that, if we start medication now, it may help you feel well enough to stay on the job."*

A third example is a 27-year-old single mother with depression who presents only at the insistence of her boyfriend, Mark, who is considering breaking up with her because she is so lethargic, has repeated crying spells and "is no fun anymore." Although she does not recognize her depression, she does worry that, at times, she is so tired she cannot manage to play with her 3-year-old son, Bobby. The clinician may say: *"I know you want to be the best Mom for your son that you can be. Right now, this fatigue and crying is keeping you from being the kind of parent you always imagined yourself to be. I am suggesting this medication to help reduce these crying spells and increase your energy so you can be a bigger part of Bobby's life. If you can feel more like your old self, and I think the medicine will help, perhaps you and Mark can get out more and you will enjoy it."*

This process involves determining what behaviors are important to *this* patient. These factors may be very different from patient to patient. It may be far less important to patients that a diagnosis is made, than how the illness specifically impacts their life. At other times, the patient's symptoms may be of far greater concern to someone other than the patient. Understanding how the condition impacts the relationships within the person's family may also provide powerful tools for encouraging appropriate treatment.

Reasons that patients take psychotropic medication

Clinicians usually assume that patients take medications to resolve their symptoms. While this may be true for many patients taking psychotropics, there may be many other reasons as well. Some of these include:

- to please their spouse
- to save their marriage
- to keep their children happy
- to allow them to interact with their children in a way that they find appropriate
- to save their job
- to please the clinician
- to prove someone else wrong (e.g., I'll try this medication to show my girlfriend that it is not going to work)
- to have a longer life
- for "general improvement"
- to satisfy the courts or the law
- to help in a lawsuit, claim for disability or child custody
- because someone else they respect has already tried medication and found it helpful (a friend, relative or celebrity)
- because they are totally desperate and must do something.

Although it is desirable that the clinician and patient agree on the reason for the patient taking the medication, it is not critical. *At times, the patient's reason for taking the medication may, in fact, be very different from the clinician's.* If the clinician has made a thorough assessment and supports the use of psychotropic medication for a patient, any reason may be a good enough reason to start. Ultimately it is not essential that the patient and the clinician have the *same* rationale for taking the medication, but it is essential that there must be *a* rationale for taking the medication.

Box 4.4 Talking to patients

The practitioner may believe that an overweight female patient is depressed and assumes that she concurs. She may be willing to take antidepressant medication in part because she feels badly, but inwardly she may hope it will make her lose weight, and then she will be more attractive. If asked whether the medicine will help her to lose weight, the clinician can reply, *"It may or may not have a direct effect on your weight, but I do expect that, if you are feeling less down and more in control, you will be better able to stick with a healthy diet and exercise plan that would help control your weight."*

Last, there may be some non-reality-based (psychotic) reasons for taking medication that develop in patients with true psychotic conditions. Even when their rationale appears delusional, if medication is needed, there may be no need to correct the delusion in order for medication to be taken and to be effective. What is important is to have a workable relationship between clinician and patient.

An interesting example of this latter scenario comes from an English psychiatrist[1] who was treating a patient who was obviously delusional. She felt her neighbors were talking about her and saying derogatory things behind her back. When she eventually came into the psychiatrist's office, he persuaded her to start antipsychotic medication, hoping that it would diminish her hallucinations and delusions. The patient did not believe she had delusions, but did have confidence in this psychiatrist. She agreed to take the medications on a trial basis, and, in fact, came back in several weeks with the report that people were no longer talking about her. Although the psychiatrist believed this was because of the antipsychotic effect of the medication, the patient verbalized this improvement as having occurred because the psychiatrist was secretly talking to the neighbors and advising them to stop the malicious gossip. Although not true, it was not crucial that the psychiatrist correct this mistaken belief. As long as there was a consensus that coming to see the psychiatrist and taking the medication was helpful, they could agree on a medication treatment plan.

The use of metaphor

Many of the concepts of mental health and illness as well as the use of psychotropic drugs in treatment are often mysterious for many patients, and, as discussed earlier, are filled with prejudice. A very useful way for practitioners to discuss with patients the process of using psychotropics to treat their emotional illness is to use common metaphors. By analogizing mental health conditions and the effects psychotropic medication can bring, as in the following examples, the clinician can often enlighten the patient in a way that promotes adherence and agreement.

In depression

The clinician can discuss the effects of depression as being like looking at life through very dark sunglasses. Everything looks dim, indistinct, ominous and, at times, scary. When the glasses are dark enough, patients may have difficulty finding their way and making decisions, and may feel lost and apprehensive. Antidepressant medications will help them gradually to remove the dark glasses so that life may be seen in the light, showing its clarity and joy.

For patients with dysthymic disorder, a chronic low-grade depression, the clinician can discuss how they are living life at "snorkel depth." They are expending great energy to tread water to keep themselves from sinking. They do not sink to the bottom and drown, but feel they are working very hard just to minimally stay afloat. They are often just below the surface of the water, unable to see the clouds and the sunshine that life has to offer. Medication can provide support analogous to a raft on which they can sit; without having to work so hard to keep from sinking, they will be able to see the clouds, sunshine and the beauty above the surface of the water.

In bipolar disorder

Bipolar disorder can be analogized to being on a small boat in the middle of the ocean during a furious storm. Giant waves will raise patients to great heights, then send them crashing down. They are often hanging on for dear life, afraid of being overturned and swamped. They may often have very little energy left for doing anything but pure surviving. Mood stabilizing medication can help calm the waves so that patients can sit comfortably on the boat and begin to observe their surroundings. Things that may not have been apparent before will emerge, and new choices will be present. They can now see a pier to which they may wish to go, or a new island that they may wish to explore. Once the sea is calmer, they may even be able to start out on a distant journey to places they previously could only imagine.

In panic attacks

Following the concept that a panic attack is a "biological false alarm," the clinician can use the analogy of a smoke detector. A smoke detector on the wall of an office has a useful purpose; it is there to warn of danger. If there were a fire, it would emit loud sounds and light to warn people that they need to take action. If the clinician were to light a fire in a wastebasket, it would set off the smoke detector, telling people to leave the building. A panic attack is like a smoke detector with an electrical short circuit. It will trigger and sound alarm when there is no fire or minimal danger. It will be just as loud and, perhaps, even more scary than usual, since it comes on suddenly when no danger is apparent. Typically, when a smoke detector goes off, people exit the building very quickly and call for professional help. This is similar to patients going for emergency medical care because of the alarm that their body is sending them during a panic attack, even when no obvious danger is present. If the smoke detector continues to be triggered, patients may continue to seek reassurance or medical care when there is no fire. Use of medication to treat panic attacks is analogous to fixing the electrical problem so that the alarm triggers only when true danger is apparent. In the initial stages, however, patients may be considerably anxious and be on guard for any alarm, even if the circuitry has been fixed (analogous to the anticipatory anxiety of panic disorder).

Reference

1   John Doran MD, personal communication during Stratford-on-Avon Conference on Nurse Prescribing, July 2001.

5   Starting medication

- Monotherapy   54
- Overlap and "indications"   54
- What is the target of the medication?   56
- Choosing a starting dose   56
- Loading doses   57
- The art of choosing a medication   58
- Selecting medication in the previously treated patient   61
- The liver-impaired patient   62
- The kidney-impaired patient   63
- How many pills to prescribe?   64
- Polypharmacy – from the doghouse to the penthouse   64
- Typically helpful combinations with best combinations   66
- The five points of education about psychotropics   67
- Other issues to be discussed   69
- Special consideration when prescribing an antipsychotic   70
- Informed consent   70
- Involuntary medication   71
- Education as treatment   72
- The use of placebo   72
- References   73

There are multiple factors for the clinician to consider in choosing and starting medication. Ideally, medication should be selected using evidence-based data, confirmed efficacy, documented safety, known dosage range and likely response rates. Also, it would be helpful if all data, including studies with negative results, were available. Head-to-head comparisons of other medications used to treat the same illness would be particularly useful.

The gold standard for such data is the double-blind, placebo-controlled study of effectiveness. While such studies are available for some mental health medications and some clinical conditions, there are many situations in which well-defined, double-blind placebo-controlled studies do not exist, or give contradictory results. In other cases, studies of newer medicines are compared to outdated treatments and not to other more popular, currently used medications.

Data used in support of using medications are often confounded by a number of other issues:

- Placebo response rates in psychotropic medication trials are very high; therefore, many patients in these studies would improve without the presence of active medication and this makes the exact amount of positive change difficult to assess.
- Many studies documenting medication effectiveness are open-label studies, in which both clinicians and patients know whether the patients are receiving active medication or placebo. Such studies are notoriously inaccurate, and may show a positive bias toward the medication being utilized.
- Many medications are used for broad indications, including non-FDA-approved indications. Their usage is supported by word of mouth, "curb stone consultations" or non-evidence-based beliefs.
- Pharmaceutical companies fund much of the research on medications. They have a vested interest in manufacturing and selling their products. Studies with a positive result, showing that the active medication is beneficial, will almost certainly be published and promoted to the practitioner. Negative studies, or ones in which the active ingredient is shown to be less effective than other medications, may or may not reach publication. This is sometimes referred to as the "file drawer effect" as these negative studies are "filed away" not to be seen. Some companies have signed agreements to make all studies available to practitioners, regardless of the outcome. This is a step in the right direction but not uniformly followed by all manufacturers.

While clinicians study scientific data and constantly strive to obtain further information, prescribing decisions must be made daily when definitive, evidence-based studies are unavailable or conflicting. There are, however, useful general strategies in helping a clinician to move ahead when scientific data are unavailable. These principles become part of the art of mental health prescribing, and are summarized in the sections below.

Monotherapy

For any condition, the use of a single medication, monotherapy, is always the simplest and safest treatment. When effective, it is the treatment of choice. In many mental health conditions, however, medication monotherapy is unsuccessful or only partially successful. While successive trials of monotherapies may ultimately identify one medication that satisfactorily controls most or all target symptoms, it is increasingly common to use polypharmacy in mental health prescribing. Multiple medications from one category, or medications from different categories, may be necessary to treat the patient's condition satisfactorily. Possible medication combinations that are safe and relatively useful are described later in this text

Overlap and "indications"

Over the last 15 years, one of the most dramatic changes in day-to-day practice has been a broadening range of usage for many medications and classes. While the names of medication categories have persisted (e.g., "antidepressants," "antipsychotics" and "mood stabilizers"), many medications within each category are used for much broader symptom profiles or other diagnoses. Antidepressants are used not only for depression, but also for anxiety disorders, bulimia, impulse control disorders, chronic pain and a long list of other conditions. Similarly, both traditional and atypical antipsychotic medications are used for bipolar disorder in addition to psychosis. Newer atypical antipsychotics are also now used as add-ons in the management of treatment-resistant depression, obsessive–compulsive disorder (OCD) and eating disorders. Although not a complete list, the spectrum of mental health uses of various commonly used mental health medications (as of 2021) is summarized in Table 5.1.

Table 5.1 Other common mental health uses of FDA-approved drugs

Medication	Common mental health uses – some "non-approved"
Antidepressants	
Bupropion	Depression, attention deficit disorder (ADD), smoking cessation, medication-induced sexual dysfunction
Citalopram	Depression, obsessive–compulsive disorder (OCD)
Doxepin	Sleep
Fluoxetine	Adult, adolescent and pediatric depression, bulimia, autistic disorder, panic disorder, OCD, premenstrual dysphoric disorder (PMDD), bulimia
Fluvoxamine	OCD, pediatric OCD, depression
Mirtazapine	Depression
Paroxetine	Depression, OCD, PTSD, panic disorder, social anxiety disorder, generalized anxiety disorder (GAD)
Sertraline	Depression, OCD, PTSD, PMDD, panic disorder
Trazodone	Sleep
Venlafaxine	Depression, GAD
Mood stabilizers	
Carbamazepine	Bipolar disorder, "organic" psychosis, borderline personality disorder, aggression, alcohol withdrawal, schizophrenia, restless legs syndrome, PTSD
Lithium	Bipolar disorder in children and adults, rage reactions, PMDD, treatment-refractory depression
Valproic acid	Bipolar disorder, schizophrenia, panic disorder, hypnotic sedation, agitation in dementia, PTSD
Anti-seizure medication	
Clonazepam	Bipolar disorder, panic disorder, OCD
Lamotrigine	Bipolar disorder, treatment-refractory depression
Oxcarbazepine	Mania, bipolar disorder, aggression disorder
Topiramate	Bipolar disorder, appetite suppression/weight control when using other psychotropics
Antipsychotics	
Atypical antipsychotics	Psychosis, schizophrenia, bipolar disorder, treatment-resistant depression, OCD, bulimia
Quetiapine	Sleep
Traditional antipsychotics	Bipolar disorder, schizophrenia

(*continued*)

Table 5.1 Cont.

Medication	Common mental health uses – some "non-approved"
Other medications	
Clonidine	PTSD, ADD, sedative/hypnotic
Verapamil	Bipolar disorder
Cholinesterase inhibitors	
Donepezil	Dementia, memory difficulties secondary to psychotropic usage, remedy for anticholinergic side effects
Galantamine	Dementia, memory difficulties secondary to psychotropic usage, remedy for anticholinergic side effects
Rivastigmine	Dementia, memory difficulties secondary to psychotropic usage, remedy for anticholinergic side effects
Anti-anxiety agents	
Benzodiazepines	Anxiety, panic disorder, GAD, OCD, sedative/hypnotic, phobias, treatment-resistant bipolar disorder, adjunctive treatment for psychosis, social anxiety disorder, PMDD
Buspirone	GAD

Sources: Pharmaceutical company product labeling; *The Maudsley Prescribing Guidelines* (2013), 13th edn., Informa Healthcare; Jamcak PG *et al.* (2006) *Principles and Practice of Psychopharmacotherapy*, 4th edn., Williams & Wilkins.

What is the target of the medication?

While the presence of a diagnosis is helpful and desirable, precise diagnosis in mental health may be elusive and there may be multiple co-morbid diagnoses. Although every effort should be made to arrive at a precise diagnosis, the generation of a differential diagnosis may be the optimal level of specificity possible for a particular patient. It is quite permissible to treat target symptoms without a precise diagnosis. As noted in Chapter 3, identification of these target symptoms is an important part of the initial evaluation. It is possible to modulate or correct certain symptoms while an ultimate diagnosis is being considered and evaluated. Sometimes a more precise diagnosis emerges with time and more targeted medication treatment can follow; in other cases, a diagnosis remains elusive indefinitely. If the prescription of psychotropic medications adequately treats significant symptoms, and is tolerated by the patient without adverse consequences, ongoing medication treatment is justified even if an exact diagnostic label is not discovered.

Choosing a starting dose

Overall, initial dosing strategies may be summarized in the following statements:

1   Standard dosing is useful for many patients.
2   Start with half doses for several days, when possible.
3   Use high-level dosing only if necessary, in cases of intense or incapacitating symptoms.

The Physicians' Desk Reference, The Maudsley Prescribing Guidelines, individual drug package inserts, pharmacological textbooks and Appendices 2, 3, 4 and 5 of this text list typical starting doses for various psychotropics. In the uncomplicated non-hospitalized patient with moderate symptoms, the doses found in these sources are reasonable initial doses. For the mild to moderately symptomatic outpatient, however, there is little to lose, and potentially something to gain, by starting with half the standard dose for the first day or two. By using less than a usual starting dose for the first several days, patients are often spared significant side effects if they are particularly sensitive to the medication. Although rare, in the event of acute drug allergy, half dosage also minimizes the amount of allergic response. If patients are started on a half dosage, the full typical starting dose should be attained rapidly – no later than by day 3.

Other situations when initial half dosing is recommended include:

1 geriatric patients
2 anxious "medication averse" patients
3 patients who perceive themselves as "medication sensitive."

When treating *outpatients* with mild to moderate symptoms, increase the medication dose by 25–50 percent every 4 days as tolerated by the patient. For *inpatients* and/or those with severe symptoms, increase medication by 50–100 percent every 2–4 days depending on symptom severity and side-effect tolerance.

In an *inpatient setting*, with a patient who has intense symptomatology, larger initial doses may be necessary. The possibility of increased side effects is counterbalanced by the need for rapid symptom control. Psychotic patients, deeply depressed and suicidal patients, patients with intense mood swings and extremely anxious patients usually need higher initial doses and in an inpatient setting, their status can be monitored continuously.

If rapid dosage titration is attempted, ensure there is frequent oversight, support and monitoring by inpatient staff or, when outside the hospital, by the family. With larger dosing, more frequent direct observation and/or telephone contact between clinician and patient is necessary. When using larger doses of medication with an outpatient, follow up should be no less frequent than every 2–7 days as the patient's clinical condition warrants.

Always use blood levels to adjust dosage for TCAs, lithium, valproic acid, carbamazepine and clozapine (see Chapter 25).

Loading doses

The vast majority of psychotropic medications are taken orally as pills, capsules or liquid concentrates. As described earlier, gradually increasing doses of psychotropic medication is generally the preferred dosing strategy to minimize side effects and allow the patient to accommodate to the medication. There has been limited research into giving patients larger than normal amounts of medication as a "loading dose" in order to facilitate behavioral management and rapid symptom control of agitated, psychotic or manic patients in an emergency room setting or on an inpatient unit. The majority of evidence relating to loading doses of medication refers to the use of valproic acid for manic patients, or oral and intramuscular antipsychotics and benzodiazepines (alone or in combination).

Over the last 20 years, a number of studies have looked at the use of intramuscular antipsychotic medications alone, intramuscular benzodiazepines alone and the combination of these medications for the rapid tranquilization of severely agitated patients. Obviously, when a patient is willing to take oral medications, the use of pills and liquid concentrate is desirable. However, when an agitated, psychotic patient is unable or unwilling to take oral medications, some form of intramuscular medication is necessary. A commonly used combination of medication in this clinical scenario is 5–10 mg of intramuscular haloperidol plus 2 mg of intramuscular lorazepam.[1-2]

Haloperidol 10 mg plus 25–50 mg of promethazine is also a mixture that has literature support for its effectiveness and tolerability.[3-4] Intramuscular aripiprazole, olanzapine and ziprasidone have been approved by the American Food and Drug Administration, and the first two of these are available in the UK. The most recent large-scale data suggest that intramuscular second-generation antipsychotics are as effective, but no more effective, than intramuscular haloperidol.[5] They are, however, more expensive, require more frequent re-injection to control symptoms and do not result in shorter lengths of stay in emergency settings. It is expected that further evidence will emerge that evaluates various combinations of medication in the urgent treatment of severely agitated patients. Most data to date supporting the use of atypicals are related to oral doses of medication, not intramuscular uses.[6-8]

The other compound that has evidence to support the use of rapid loading doses is valproic acid. There have been several studies showing that oral valproic acid in doses of 30 mg/kg of body weight per day for the first 2 days of treatment of acute mania followed by 20 mg/kg per day is effective and well tolerated.[9-11]

Loading dose strategies for lithium have been attempted where a single dose of 600–1200 mg is given initially and then the stabilization dose of lithium is calculated based on a serum lithium level drawn 24 hours later.[12] Although possible, this strategy is little used and has not been studied extensively, especially regarding whether this method achieves more rapid clinical outcomes than standard lithium dosing. Carbamazepine has been loaded in patients at risk for seizures, but has generally not been used in loading strategies for psychiatric purposes. Oral olanzapine loading has been reported in which a loading dose of 40 mg per day is given for 2 days, followed by 20–30 mg per day for the ensuing 2 days, then reducing to 15 mg per day.[13] This small sample tolerated the procedure well, although the number of patients was minimal. In general, other psychotropics (including all antidepressants, stimulants, anticholinergics and anti-anxiety medications) have not been studied with loading dose strategies.

The art of choosing a medication

For purposes of example, this section discusses choosing an antidepressant. However, similar logic applies to mood stabilizers, antipsychotics and other medication groups.

Since overall efficacy is approximately equal among antidepressants[14] there are several good medicines from which to choose without one clear, consistent first choice for all patients. For a patient who has never taken antidepressants, and for whom there is no previous treatment history, several factors may be of use, and these are summarized in Table 5.2. Any or all of these indicators may be important to a clinician in choosing a particular medication.

Table 5.2 The art of choosing a medication

In a patient who has not previously been treated, you may choose a particular medication because it:

- Will also treat co-morbid conditions present
- Avoids a particular side effect
- Avoids complicating a medical condition
- Avoids an interaction with another medication
- Has side effects that may be to the patient's advantage
- Is preferred by the patient
- Has been helpful to a close blood relative of the patient
- Is affordable for this patient

The presence of a *co-morbid condition* may dictate the optimum first medication choice. A medication used successfully for several conditions can "kill two birds with one stone." For example:

- A patient with panic disorder and episodes of depression may get relief for both conditions from using an antidepressant rather than a benzodiazepine. The benzodiazepine could work well for the panic, but is likely to do little for the depressive component.
- A person with schizophrenia who has a strong component of depressive affect is likely to receive more benefit from an atypical antipsychotic (which often has some antidepressant activity) than from a traditional antipsychotic (which is likely to have little).
- A person suffering from attention deficit disorder and depression could have both illnesses improved by the use of bupropion or a stimulant.

In choosing a medication, a clinician may try to *avoid a particular side effect* that would be of significant concern or risk to the patient. Ziprasidone may create less weight gain than olanzapine for an already obese psychotic patient. Bupropion, or mirtazapine will likely cause less sexual interference than an SSRI for a depressed patient who is significantly concerned about sexual performance. (See Chapter 19 for a more detailed discussion of these issues.)

Concurrent medical conditions, if any, may affect the choice of medication. A clinician will want to use medications that minimally affect the stability of concurrent medical illnesses. For example, patients with an elevated white sugar and cholesterol might preferentially not be started on an atypical antipsychotic, since many of these are associated with further increase in blood sugar or blood lipids. It is also possible to use medications that may have a positive beneficial effect on the concurrent medical condition. A depressed patient with migraine headaches might benefit from an SSRI, a class of medication that has been shown to be useful in the treatment of migraine.[12–13,15–16]

Medications currently used by a patient can also point toward one psychotropic medication rather than another. If, for example, the addition of an antidepressant will result in an altered blood level of a currently taken medication (perhaps via a P-450 interaction), medical management becomes more complicated. An example of this is a patient who is being treated with cyclosporine for rheumatoid arthritis. Such a patient will have cyclosporine levels altered by the addition of nefazodone or fluvoxamine, both of which alter the P-450 enzymes 3A/3 and 3A/4 that metabolize cyclosporine. Therefore, these drugs may not be the first choice of antidepressant for this patient. A patient who is taking a TCA for pain control could have the blood level of the TCA changed if fluoxetine or paroxetine is added because of P-450 enzyme 2D6 blockade. Therefore, an initial choice of antidepressant such as venlafaxine or mirtazapine without this potential interaction would be simpler. Such interactions seldom rule out choosing a particular antidepressant medication. Even if an interaction could occur, a particular medication can be an effective, safe choice if the interaction is known. When possible, serum blood levels of the substrate are followed, and with or without serum level monitoring, it may be appropriate to adjust the dose of any substrate substance when adding the new psychotropic.

Utilizing the intrinsic side effects of a particular medication may incline a clinician toward a particular choice. For example, a depressed patient with a sleep disorder might be started on a more sedating antidepressant such as mirtazapine, or doxepin, where the sedative effect would be useful in improving sleep problems. Likewise, a patient who has psychomotor retardation and is oversleeping might benefit from an activating medication such as desipramine, bupropion or reboxetine. A depressed patient with low appetite might benefit from a medication that potentially stimulates appetite such as mirtazapine or amitriptyline whereas a patient with excessive appetite might benefit from a medication that, as a side effect, has the potential to lower appetite, such as bupropion.

Patient preference is another possible factor in medication choice. While a clinician should not choose a particular medicine solely on the basis of patient preference (unless it is clinically reasonable and appropriate), it is often much easier to convince patients to try a particular medication toward which they are favorably predisposed. Patients may have heard positive reports about a specific medication from friends, relatives or co-workers. They may have read about the positive aspects of a particular drug in the media or on the Internet, which inclines them favorably to that medication choice. Sometimes, however, with the blizzard of television advertisements about mental health medicine, patients can be unnecessarily swayed toward a medicine which may be inappropriate for them, and the clinician will need to educate them about the reasons why a different medicine would be more helpful or less dangerous.

The reverse is also true. A patient may be negatively predisposed to one particular medication for exactly the same reasons. The clinician can have a difficult time prescribing a medication if a patient has heard significant negative feedback regarding the drug. If the patient's beliefs are based on misinformation, corrective education may be helpful and necessary. If there are two equally effective choices, however, and the patient feels strongly for or against one of them, the clinician will have more success prescribing that medication which the patient already believes will help and/or be well tolerated.

Of some value is a history of *positive response in a close blood relative*. When there has been a positive medication response in a first-degree relative, the identified patient may also benefit from this medication. The current patient may also be favorably predisposed to trying a particular medication if a family member has responded well to it. This method, however, is far from an absolute predictor, and the clinician should not hesitate to try other medications. Clinical lore is replete with family trees in which various family members have responded well to different medications.

Lastly, *cost* must always be considered. No matter how elegant a clinician's thinking, a prescription for a medication is useless if the patient cannot afford to fill it. Knowing (or asking about) the patient's financial resources, insurance coverage and/or willingness to pay out of pocket are important issues when there are equally effective medication choices that vary in cost. If a generic medication is cheaper and, in the clinician's mind, a reasonable choice, there is little reason not to use it (see Chapter 26 on generic medicines). Even when a particular medication is a decided second choice, a clinician may choose a less expensive medication if a patient cannot afford the first choice. Being able to purchase and comply with a second choice is much better for the patient than offering a first-choice prescription that never gets filled.

Selecting medication in the previously treated patient

Again using depression for purposes of illustration, when a patient presents having had previous trials on antidepressants, it is useful to ponder several other clinical factors in addition to the issues in the above section. Clearly, the most important and overriding factor is a *previous positive response* to a particular medication. If a patient has had a good response to a particular medication, completed treatment and stopped medication, a strong first choice to treat recurrence would be to use the same medication.[17] *Patients who have episodic illness with symptom-free intervals will often respond to the same medication during a recurrence.* It is neither necessary nor prudent for the clinician to prescribe a newer medication just because it is new, or because it happens to be one of the clinician's current favorites. Additionally, patients are positively predisposed to retrying a medicine that they know from experience is effective and tolerable.

This general principle can be modified in two ways:

1   The patient did respond to medication, but had considerable side effects while taking it.
2   The patient has relapsed despite taking the medication.

The first principle is illustrated by the use of tricyclic antidepressants. While shown to be no less effective than newer antidepressants, TCAs have a side effect profile that, for most patients, is much more burdensome than that of newer antidepressants. If a patient suffered significant side effects while taking a TCA, a trial of a newer medication would be indicated. Another example would be a depressed patient who responded well to an SSRI, but had significant sexual dysfunction. Such a patient might benefit from the use of a medication with less propensity for sexual dysfunction, such as bupropion, mirtazapine or nefazodone.

The second exception to retrying a previously used medication involves the patient who has relapsed while on the medication. An example would be a patient who initially did well on a medication, but lost the antidepressant effect quickly thereafter. Such a patient does not usually respond to the re-institution of the same medication, and a change to another medication within the class or to another class of antidepressants is much more likely to be helpful. (See Chapter 9 for more information about this issue.)

The liver-impaired patient

Patients with impaired hepatic functioning, from whatever cause, create special issues for the mental health clinician when prescribing psychotropic medication. Because of their impaired hepatic function, these patients may be more susceptible to side effects from hepatically metabolized medications, and serum blood concentrations may be altered significantly. In general, it is the *severity of the liver disease rather than its cause* that most directly affects serum blood concentrations. Therefore, assessment of the severity of problems with liver function should be undertaken with a panel of liver function tests before beginning psychotropic medication in liver-impaired patients. In general, the more abnormal the liver function test, the more severe the impairment and the lower the initial psychotropic dose should be. Unfortunately, the test values do not always precisely correlate with the level of impairment of drug metabolism.

Other considerations for hepatically compromised patients include the following:

Box 5.1 Clinical tip

Almost all psychotropics are primarily metabolized by the liver. The notable exceptions are lithium, topirimate, amisulpride (UK only) and sulpiride (UK only), which undergo minimal hepatic metabolism and are primarily excreted through the kidney.

---

1   Whenever possible, *consider using medications* that have minimal liver metabolism and/or are *excreted primarily through the kidney*.
2   Patients with hepatic dysfunction are more sensitive to the routine side effects of hepatically metabolized drugs, even at levels which are technically "therapeutic."
3   When using a hepatically metabolized medication in a hepatically compromised patient, the following strategies should be employed:
  • start at a lower dosage than normal
  • make any dosage increase slowly
  • watch for side effects from medication build-up
  • if a medication has valid serum blood-level testing, monitor these levels frequently.
4   The ultimate target dose of the medication will generally be lower than in non-hepatically impaired patients.
5   Severe liver disease, which may be characterized by marked elevation of liver function tests, jaundice, ascites and encephalopathy, can require particularly delicate clinical management. For patients with severe liver disease:
  • Begin any psychotropic at the lowest possible dose.
  • Avoid compounds with a long half-life.
  • Observe carefully for sedation and cognitive interference.
  • Psychotropics with a strong history of possible hepatic dysfunction are contraindicated. Therefore, avoid nefazodone, MAOIs, carbamazepine, valproate, lamotrigine and sertindole (UK only).

Table 5.3 Preferred choices of psychotropics for the hepatically impaired patient

Psychotropic classification	Recommended drugs
Antidepressants	SSRIs Imipramine (in low dose)
Antipsychotics	Haloperidol Aripiprazole Olanzapine Paliperidone Amisulpride (UK only)
Mood stabilizers	Lithium
Anxiolytics	Lorazepam and oxazepam (in small doses)

Source: Adapted from *The Maudsley Prescribing Guidelines* (2009), 10th edn., Informa Healthcare, pp. 381–384.

- Sedatives or anxiolytics should be used with great caution, at a low dose, because of the potential of precipitating further encephalopathy or falls.
- *The Maudsley Prescribing Guidelines*[18] should be seen for a summary of current research on individual psychotropics and parameters of use in hepatically compromised patients.

Preferred medications to be used in the hepatically impaired patient are listed in Table 5.3.

The kidney-impaired patient

A parallel situation occurs for patients who have renal impairment. Whenever possible with these patients, psychotropics that have primary *hepatic* metabolism should be considered as first-line drugs. When possible, the renally excreted medications mentioned above, including lithium, gabapentin, topirimate, amisulpride (UK only) and sulpiride (UK only), should be avoided. Prior to beginning psychotropic medications with a renally impaired patient, an assessment of the severity of renal impairment should be undertaken, remembering that renal function will decline with age and that some level of renal impairment will occur even if serum creatinine is not elevated. Principles of medicating the renally impaired patient include:

- Start any medication at the lowest tolerable dose. It may be necessary to divide doses to maintain tolerability.
- Make any dosage increases slowly.
- Watch for side effects from medication build-up.
- If the medication has valid serum blood levels, monitor them frequently.
- Observe for side effects of sedation, postural hypotension and confusion.

Information on specific recommendations for individual psychotropics is, again, documented in *The Maudsley Prescribing Guidelines*.

Preferred psychotropic medications for the renally impaired patient are shown in Table 5.4.

Table 5.4 Recommended medications for the renally impaired patient

Psychotropic classification	Recommended drugs
Antidepressants	SSRIs (most experience is with fluoxetine and paroxetine)
Antipsychotics	Atypical antipsychotics, including olanzapine, aripiprazole and ziprasidone. Quetiapine and risperidone may be started in smaller than usual doses. Haloperidol
Mood stabilizers	Carbamazepine, lamotrigine and valproic acid
Anxiolytics	Lorazepam

Source: Adapted from *The Maudsley Prescribing Guidelines* (2009), 10th edn., Informa Healthcare, pp. 369–377.

How many pills to prescribe?

The general rule of thumb for the number of pills to prescribe to a patient is enough to last until their next scheduled follow-up visit plus a few more. At the initial evaluation this principle should be adhered to firmly, such that the patient has enough medication to last only until he or she can be seen again, but not significantly in excess of that. At this first visit, the clinician does not know the patient well and cannot be sure about the patient's ability to take the medication in a safe and responsible manner as prescribed. By prescribing only sufficient medication to reach the next visit, one also emphasizes the necessity of the follow-up visit for reassessment in order to obtain further medication. As the clinician gets to know a patient better, and finds that he or she is responsible, more latitude can be given regarding how many pills are dispensed. It is particularly important to avoid giving large quantities of pills to suicidal or medication-abusing patients. If there is concern about the patient's suicidal ideation and the possibility of overdose, it may be reasonable to prescribe only 3 or 4 days' worth of medication, requiring frequent refills, so that the patient does not have access to a large number of pills until he or she is more stable. While this is inconvenient for the patient, it is safer, particularly if prescribed medications are ones that are dangerous in overdose (e.g., tricyclic antidepressants, lithium and MAO inhibitors). Another strategy at an initial interview of a potentially suicidal patient is to give a 10-day or 2-week supply of medication, but insist that the prescription be handed to, filled by and administered by a family member or other responsible party. It is always unwise and poor practicing habit to prescribe a large number of pills and/or multiple refills to a patient whom the clinician does not know well. Long-term patients on a stable medication regimen, well known to the clinician, can be prescribed a 30-day supply of medications with an appropriate number of refills to reach the next visit, or even a 90-day supply for chronic medications.

Polypharmacy – from the doghouse to the penthouse

Polypharmacy of psychotropic medication is an area in which there has been a major shift in philosophy. As recently as the early 1990s, it was believed by most prescribers that one medication was invariably preferable to a combination of medications. Within the medical community there was an implicit or expressed assumption that a patient taking several medications was being inappropriately treated with polypharmacy. This was particularly the case when two medications from the same class were used. This practice was generally regarded as being representative of sloppy prescribing, potentially harmful to the patient, and poor clinical practice. As the knowledge of psychotropics has progressed, and patient expectations of full relief have increased, it is clear that many patients not only benefit from multiple medications, but also that a multiple medication regimen may be essential to achieving and maintaining their recovery.

In the twenty-first century it is now not uncommon,[19] to have a patient on several antidepressants simultaneously, particularly if they have different mechanisms of action. Similarly, with mood stabilizers, some bipolar patients simply cannot be stabilized on one medication alone, but improve considerably on a combination of mood stabilizers from different medication families.[20]

For example, a patient may experience panic attacks and depression. On an antidepressant alone the patient may be overstimulated, or have partial control over anxiety symptoms; while on a benzodiazepine alone, the patient may have breakthrough depressive symptoms or breakthrough panic attacks. On the two classes of medications together, the patient feels in control – neither depressed nor anxious.

Another common example of the patient helped by polypharmacy is the bipolar, depressed patient who – when on a mood stabilizer alone – has breakthrough depressions, but – when on an antidepressant alone – has lack of response, hypomanic overstimulation or erratic, unpredictable response. When the two medicines are given together, however, the patient remains mood-stable and free from depression.

Polypharmacy is also becoming more common in treatment-resistant psychosis and schizophrenia.[21] And multiple antipsychotics or an antipsychotic plus another class of medication is not unusual practice.

Synergy

Another factor supporting polypharmacy is the additive response of patients taking two medications from the same class simultaneously. There can be an additive, synergistic effect between two medicines such that the overall benefit is greater than that achieved by either of the medicines alone – in common terms, "one plus one equals three."

The use of combined mood stabilizers in treatment of bipolar patients demonstrates this principle. On lithium or valproic acid alone, the patient may have a partial but limited response. When lithium and valproic acid are used together, the patient is significantly improved and has fewer relapses.[22] If patients were asked to rate themselves on a score of 0 to 100 (see Box 6.2 in the next chapter), they might rate themselves at 35 on lithium alone, 40 on valproic acid alone, but 90 on the combination.

The best clinicians – those sought out as tertiary referral sources, or experts used for consultation – often practice polypharmacy. Those who do it expertly are leaders in their field. Polypharmacy has gone from the "doghouse" to the "penthouse."

Inadvertent polypharmacy

While planned, rational polypharmacy can be quite helpful to patients, there are several circumstances that result in inadvertent, non-therapeutic polypharmacy. Such polypharmacy is not helpful, may reflect clinician inexperience, and may lead to increased side effects, drug interaction and cost. Chapter 6 discusses the circumstance when the clinician gets "caught in the middle" during a cross-taper of two medications. In this scenario the patient takes two medications, one of which may not be needed.

A second common scenario leading to unintentional and unwise polypharmacy involves a patient who has been stable over a long period of time on medication A alone. Symptoms flare up or a breakthrough occurs. To deal with breakthrough symptoms (e.g., psychotic symptoms in a schizophrenic patient, manic symptoms in a bipolar patient, panic symptoms in a panic disorder patient), a second medication B is added. If the patient responds, the clinician may fail to assess whether the second medication (B) can be stopped once the crisis has passed. Even if the addition of medicine B was necessary and beneficial during the crisis, can the patient be managed on medicine A alone after the crisis remits? If medication B makes a substantial improvement, could medication A now be eliminated? Newly added medicine B alone may be sufficient.

Some patients who experience multiple relapses over time may develop a very complicated medication regimen and inadvertent polypharmacy. The group most vulnerable to non-therapeutic polypharmacy is the elderly population. Older patients who have been treated over much of their lives for mental health conditions may be taking an impressively large number of various medications in different classes. It is not uncommon to be confronted with a new elderly patient who has been taking four, five, six or more psychotropics for many years. This accumulation of medications may lead to excessive complexity of regimen, increased side effects, interactions with other non-psychotropic medications, and unnecessary cost. Since geriatric patients are particularly sensitive to medication side effects and dosages, it is very important to re-evaluate their regimen frequently and to check to see whether all medications are still necessary.

It goes without saying that monotherapy should be instituted first to see if it results in a satisfactory response. It is quite unusual to begin polypharmacy from the start unless monotherapies of several different medications have already been tried and been found to be less than useful. Whenever multiple medications are prescribed for any condition, the clinician must be cognizant of the possibility of an increased number of side effects. It is also possible that a medication combination will increase the severity of one particular side effect such as sleepiness, dizziness or sexual dysfunction.

Typically helpful combinations with best combinations***

In the treatment of depression[23]

    SSRI or SNRI with aripiprazole***
    SSRI or SNRI with bupropion
    SSRI or SNRI with mirtazepine
    SSRI or SNRI with bupropion and mirtazepine
    SSRI or SNRI with lithium***
    SSRI or SNRI with T3
    SSRI or SNRI (for depressed peri-menopausal or postmenopausal women)
    Perphenazine and amitriptyline (for psychotic/delusional MDD)
    SSRI or SNRI with stimulant (depressed patients with ADHD, binge eating disorder or sleep apnea)
    SSRI or SNRI with trazodone at bedtime (depressed patient with insomnia not responding to SSDRI/SNRI alone)
    SSRI or SNRI with quetiapine at bedtime (depressed patient with insomnia not responding to SSDRI/SNRI alone)

SSRI or SNRI with benzodiazepine (depressed patient with anxiety or panic not
responding to SSDRI/SNRI alone)
SSRI/SNRI plus light box (seasonally depressed patients, but also useful for other
depressed patients)
Tricyclic with ketamine
SSRI or SNRI with ketamine***

In the treatment of anxiety

SSRI or SNRI with benzodiazepine***
SSRI or SNRI with buspirone
Tricyclic with benzodiazepine
Tricyclic with buspirone

In the treatment of psychosis[19–22, 24–25]

Atypical antipsychotic with typical antipsychotic
Atypical antipsychotic (especially aripiprazole) plus clozapine***
Typical antipsychotic plus clozapine
Atypical antipsychotic plus SSRI or SNRI (especially for schizoaffective disorder
depressed type***

For mood stabilization

Any combination of lithium, carbamazepine, lamotrigine and/or valproic acid
Any of the above four medications with second-generation antipsychotic
Any of the above four medications with a typical antipsychotic
Any of the above four medications with clozapine
Any of the above four medications with a benzodiazepine

Sleep disordered patients of various diagnoses

SSRI or SNRI with trazodone at bedtime (depressed patient with insomnia)
SSRI or SNRI with quetiapine at bedtime (depressed patient with insomnia)
SSRI/SNRI with benzodiazepine (depressed patient with insomnia)
Any antipsychotic or mood stabilizer with zolpidem, zaleplon or eszopiclone
(psychotic and/or mood unstable patient)

The five points of education about psychotropics

There are five principles that should be emphasized to every patient who is beginning a
psychotropic medication. They are simple and may, for some clinicians, seem obvious.
Patients, however, are not intuitively aware of these principles, and they should always be
presented directly to any patient during the first session when medication is prescribed.
A written list of these principles which can be given to the patient is often a time-saver.

1   *Take the medication as prescribed every day.* Patients need to understand that
regular dosing is central to obtaining and maintaining response. Antidepressants,

antipsychotics and mood stabilizers are generally not to be taken on an "as needed" basis (often abbreviated in medical orders as "PRN" from the Latin *pro re nata*). With medication for mood, taking more medication when feeling worse on a particular day is also of relatively little use. If patients are not consistently doing well on a particular regimen, it may be necessary to increase the dose on a regular basis; however, this is a decision that should be made on the advice of the clinician. The patient must understand that missing doses, or changing the dose day-to-day depending on one's mood, is contraindicated.

2   *It may take time to see a response.* Many patients, anticipating instant relief, expect a response quickly and, if this does not occur, will stop the medication.

3   *Don't stop the medication without contacting me.* Particularly early on in treatment, patients who are not immediately responding, or who may be experiencing side effects, need to be cautioned against stopping medication without the clinician's input. Often a simple dosage adjustment or medication change can rectify a problem. In other cases, the clinician may decide to encourage the patient to continue to take the medication for a longer period to adapt. It is important to instruct the patient to call before deciding that the current situation is intolerable.

4   *Don't stop the medication just because you're starting to feel better.* Patients are often prone to discontinuing their medication after starting to feel better, unless they are given specific instructions to continue medication for the purposes of maintaining response.

5   *Call with any concerns or questions.* Patients should not only be given permission, but be encouraged to contact the clinician if they are not doing well or have questions. Patients should be advised to stay in contact with the clinician, particularly during the early stages of treatment.

Box 5.2 Talking to patients

To present the timeframe for response in a valid but optimistic way, a clinician can say: *"You may notice some positive benefit within a few days, but it often takes several weeks for medication levels to rise in your system and for you to begin to notice feeling better."*

Box 5.3 Talking to patients

"As you begin to feel better, I want you to continue the medication until, together, we decide to stop. If you stop too quickly, there is a good chance your symptoms will return. By continuing the medication, even after you begin to respond, we give you a better chance to stay well. In time, we will discuss a plan to discontinue your medication successfully."

Other issues to be discussed

Whenever a new medication is started, other specific areas must be discussed with the patient, including:

- medication interactions and/or medications to be avoided with this prescription
- activity restrictions
- dietary restrictions
- laboratory screening tests, including serum blood levels, when necessary (discussed in Chapter 25)
- common side effects (discussed in Chapter 19).

With most psychotropics, there are minimal activity restrictions. Particularly if medications are begun at a low dosage and increased gradually, patients can drive a vehicle, operate machinery and engage in other physical activity, including vigorous exercise. If a medication is considerably sedative, is started at a high dose or the patient appears to be experiencing significant side effects in the initial stages of starting a new medication, the prescriber can advise the patient to avoid these activities temporarily. This condition either passes quickly, or the patient may be changed to a different medication. When significant side effects have occurred when starting the drug, the clinician should be especially vigilant with future dosage increases.

There are, however, some situations in which extra caution must be maintained and, in certain cases, driving proficiency evaluated. These include:

- symptoms of sedation, psychomotor impairment, dizziness or blurred vision which do not improve and the patient wishes to or needs to continue driving (these are the same symptoms which predispose patients to an increased fall risk)
- the clinician notices any of the above symptoms in the patient's presentation
- the patient or the patient's family show concern about the ability to walk or drive safely.

If these situations occur or if there is doubt about a patient's ability to perform these activities safely, it is best to recommend a temporary cessation of the medication and ask for family/caretaker input about the patient's level of alertness and coordination at the first follow-up visit. In some instances, the prescriber may need to advise the patient to walk with assistance and/or not to drive until the situation resolves. Such advisement should be noted in the patient's chart. In situations of significant concern where the patient is likely to require the medication for an extended period but the problems persist, the prescriber may request that the patient pass a driving road test at a commercial driving school, although this is unusual.

With the exception of lithium (salt and fluid considerations) and MAO inhibitors (significant dietary restrictions), there are virtually no psychotropics that require dietary restrictions. In general, patients may eat a normal balanced diet without constraints. If weight gain becomes an issue, however, calorie restriction may be necessary. (See Chapter 19 for issues on weight gain, and Chapter 20 for further information on lithium toxicity and MAO inhibitor diets.)

Special consideration when prescribing an antipsychotic

When antipsychotic medication is prescribed for acutely and/or seriously psychotic patients, limited explanation about the nature of the medication is required. Describing the target symptoms of the medication is usually sufficient and the word "antipsychotic" need not even be mentioned. For example, the clinician might say:

> "This medication will help decrease the voices in your head."
> "This medication will help you feel less confused."
> "This medication will help you feel less anxious and worried that people are trying to harm you."

Especially with the advent of atypical antipsychotics, antipsychotic medication is commonly prescribed both on-label and off-label for patients who are not psychotic (e.g., for mood stabilization, for augmentation in treatment-resistant depression or with serious anxiety disorders). With the advent of the Internet, it is to be expected that many patients will research a medication shortly after leaving the prescriber's office. Rather than have the patient receive an unpleasant surprise and become concerned, the wise clinician will discuss the nature of the medication at the outset.

Box 5.4 Clinical tip

When prescribing an antipsychotic-class medication to a non-psychotic patient, the prescriber can say: *"Mrs. Parker, as always, I want you to be informed about any medication that I prescribe. I am suggesting a prescription of … This is from a class of medications that has been called 'antipsychotic.' This is because it does have usefulness with people who have that problem. You have no symptoms of psychosis and are not psychotic. To some people, though, the name sounds frightening. I wanted you to know that this medication also has a broad range of other uses and can be quite beneficial for a variety of other symptoms. There is considerable research to support its use for the symptoms you have, specifically… It is safe and in common usage. Most importantly, I did not want you to be surprised or upset by any information that you might read about this medication. Do you have any questions or concerns that I can answer now?"*

Informed consent

For years, lawyers, legal scholars and healthcare professionals have debated the issue of what constitutes informed consent for taking medication. There is no single agreed-upon assessment of what constitutes a patient being fully informed and what constitutes true "consent." When working in an institutional setting, rules may be established by the institution for written, informed consent prior to use of any medications. In an out-patient office, there is wide variability as to how clinicians implement informed consent.

Some clinicians do obtain written, informed consent for each medication prescribed in an outpatient office, particularly if it is being used for a non-FDA approved indication.

While this may have some benefit, it is not uniformly deemed medico-legally necessary. A significant number of clinicians will document a discussion of expected benefits of the medication, possible side effects, possible alternatives to this medication and overall risks. This is then documented in the written record with a phrase such as "outcomes, side effects, alternatives and risks discussed."

At the first session, clinicians should obtain a written "Consent to Treatment" that may include the use of recommended medication. This document should remain a permanent document within the patient's record. Such consent could be worded:

> I consent for [name of clinician] to assess and treat me. This treatment may include psychotherapy, medication, and/or other recommended therapy for mental health problems which is administered within current community standards.
>
> Signature
> Date

The issue of informed consent becomes more complicated for the incompetent patient and for non-emancipated minors. Patients declared legally incompetent, and for whom a guardian has been appointed, should have consent for medications signed by the legal guardian. Except in emergency situations, no medication should be started until this consent is obtained. Minors under the age of 18, unless fully emancipated from their families, should also have written informed consent from the parent or legal guardian prior to beginning medication.

Emergency situations (usually present in an emergency department or on an inpatient unit) can supersede the necessity of obtaining written informed consent for both incompetent patients and minors. In such cases, the clinician should document the nature of the emergency, the medication prescribed and the dosage. Every attempt should be made to obtain consent from the appropriate party as soon as possible. If repeated emergency dosing is necessary, the necessity of continued emergency medication should be noted and documented in the chart.

Involuntary medication

Involuntary medication (medicating patients against their will) with an adult patient is a totally distinct issue, and is different from medicating the incompetent patient or minor as discussed above. Adult patients who are being treated involuntarily retain their right to accept or refuse medication unless they are deemed legally incompetent. It is generally necessary for a court or judge to determine that an involuntary patient can be medicated against his or her will. *Except in emergency circumstances*, which should be documented as such, *a written court order must generally be obtained prior to medicating an involuntary patient.* There are variations of law from state to state, and country to country, regarding involuntary medication procedures. These should be consulted to determine the appropriate procedure in any given locale.

Involuntary medication is an area of law that is fraught with complications and medico-legal pitfalls. Except in emergency situations, clinicians will frequently find it helpful to consult knowledgeable colleagues, legal counsel or administrators within an institution in which they practice, prior to medicating an involuntary patient.

Education as treatment

When starting medication, do not underestimate the power and therapeutic benefit of patient education. Instructing the patient on why the medication is being prescribed, how it is being prescribed, a simple description of its method of action and its intended effects, and describing any possible side effects, has powerful therapeutic benefit. Informed, knowledgeable patients are, in general, more adherent with treatment and more likely to follow through with their treatment plan.

The use of placebo

There are several reasons why clinicians consider using a placebo – a "sugar" or "dummy" pill which has no active ingredient.

- Some clinicians, and/or patients' families, believe that a patient's mental health symptoms are "all in their head," implying that the symptoms are a mental construct which the patient creates or "uses" to their advantage. Under this assumption, these clinicians advocate administering a placebo to "prove" that the symptoms are "imaginary" or fool the patient into getting better.
- Some prescribers are familiar with the high frequency of "placebo effects" in psychotropic medication clinical trials and seek to use a dummy pill to their therapeutic advantage.
- Still other prescribers feel stymied by difficult and/or non-responsive patients and are pressed to "do something" for the patient when other remedies have failed.

In Latin, "placebo" means "I will please" and the driving force behind the use of placebos in medical practice is usually a strong wish on the part of the clinician to please the patient regardless of the wisdom of the intervention. Prescribing a substance which the clinician knows has no therapeutic activity serves the convenience of the physician more than it promotes the patient's welfare. While it may appear that there is justification to prescribe a dummy pill, *use of a placebo creates problems and risk to the therapeutic relationship*.

The American Medical Association[26] is clear on its prohibition that a placebo cannot be given simply to soothe a difficult patient. *Unless patients are enrolled in a documented research study* (in which they are clearly informed that they may be taking a placebo), *there is no place for the use of a placebo in general medication management*. Even if some short-term benefits might occur, they are rarely long-lasting. Symptoms of underlying biological illness almost always quickly recur, and little has been gained by the use of the placebo. Any use of a placebo also creates a "secret" for the clinician, the patient's family and/or the unit staff, which becomes an increasing burden to all concerned. If the patient becomes aware of the deception, all trust with the clinician is lost and the therapeutic alliance is broken, usually irrevocably.

A clinician who feels that he/she has nothing left to therapeutically offer a patient must say so gently but directly. Those who may be tempted to use a placebo should instead ask themselves, "What am I going to do 30 days from now when the placebo effect wears off?"

References

1 Currier GW and Simpson GS (2001) Risperidone liquid concentrate and oral lorazepam versus intramuscular haloperidol and intramuscular lorazepam for treatment of psychotic agitation. *Journal of Clinical Psychiatry* 62: 153–157.

2 Hillard JR (2002) Choosing antipsychotics for rapid tranquilization in the ER. *Current Psychiatry* 1(4): 22–29.

3 Alexander J *et al.* (2004) Rapid tranquillisation of violent or agitated patients in a psychiatric emergency setting. *British Journal of Psychiatry* 185: 63–69.

4 Huf G *et al.* (2007) Rapid tranquilization in psychiatric emergency settings in Brazil. *British Medical Journal* 335: 869.

5 Leung JG *et al.* (2011) Comparison of short-acting intramuscular antipsychotic medication: impact on length of stay and cost. *American Journal of Therapeutics* 18(4): 300–304.

6 Tohen M *et al.* (2000) Efficacy of olanzapine in acute bipolar mania: a double-blind placebo-controlled study. *Archives of General Psychiatry* 57: 841–849.

7 Zarate CA *et al.* (2000) Clinical predictors of acute response with quetiapine in psychotic mood disorders. *Journal of Clinical Psychiatry* 61: 185–189.

8 Fukutaki K and Allen M (2002) Rapid stabilization of acute mania. *Primary Psychiatry* 9(1): 60–62.

9 Martinez JM *et al.* (1998) Tolerability of oral loading of divalproic sodium in the treatment of acute mania. *Depression and Anxiety* 7: 83–86.

10 Hirschfeld RM *et al.* (1999) Safety and tolerability of oral loading divalproic sodium in acutely manic bipolar patients. *Journal of Clinical Psychiatry* 60: 815–818.

11 McElroy SL and Keck PE (1996) A randomized comparison of divalproex oral loading versus haloperidol in the initial treatment of acute psychotic mania. *Journal of Clinical Psychiatry* 57: 142–146.

12 Carroll BT *et al.* (2001) Loading strategies in acute mania. *CNS Spectrums* 6(11): 919–930.

13 Byrne P (2007) Managing the acute psychotic episode. *British Medical Journal* 334(7595): 686–692. doi: 10.1136/bmj.39148.668160.80

14 American Psychiatric Association (2010) Major depressive disorder, available at: www.psychiatry.org/psychiatrists/practice/clinical-practice-guidelines

15 Marcus D (1993) Serotonin and its role in headache pathogenesis and treatment. *The Clinician Journal of Pain* 9: 159–167.

16 O'Carroll P (2001) Serotonin and the mind–body dilemma. *TEN* 3(3): 56–59.

17 Fava M *et al.* (2002) Treatment approaches to major depressive disorder relapse, Pt 2. *Psychotherapy and Psychosomatics* 71(4): 195–199.

18 The Maudsley Prescribing Guidelines (2009) 10th edn., Informa Healthcare, pp. 380–385.

19 Treatment-resistant depression, available at: www.webmd.com/depression/guide/treatment-resistant-depression-what-is-treatment-resistant-depression#1

20 Kirk DD *et al.* (1997) Comparative prophylactic efficacy of lithium carbamazepine and the combination in bipolar disorder. *Journal of Clinical Psychiatry* 58: 470–478.

21 Tiihonen J *et al.* (2019) Association of antipsychotic polypharmacy vs monotherapy with psychiatric rehospitalization among adults with schizophrenia. *JAMA Psychiatry* 76(5): 499–507. doi: 10.1001/jamapsychiatry.2018.4320

22 Solomon DA *et al.* (1997) A pilot study of lithium carbonate plus divalproex sodium for the continuation and maintenance treatment of patients with bipolar I disorder. *Journal of Clinical Psychiatry* 58: 95–99.

23 Thase, ME. Top 10 drug combinations in MDD: past, current and future. Presented at: Psych Congress, October 3–6, 2019, San Diego.

24　Ortiz-Orendain J *et al.* (2017) Antipsychotic combinations for schizophrenia. *Cochrane Database Systematic Review* 2017(6): CD009005.

25　Dunner D (2014) Combining antidepressants. *Shanghai Archives of Psychiatry* 26(6): 363–364. doi: 10.11919/j.issn.1002-0829.214177

26　Use of placebo in clinical practice, available at: www.ama-assn.org/delivering-care/ethics/use-placebo-clinical-practice

6   Follow-up appointments and strategies

- When do I schedule follow up?   75
- How long does it take?   76
- Inpatient medication follow up   77
- Preparing for a follow up   77
- Goals of a follow up   78
- Two simple, powerful questions   79
- Mental health prescriber and/or primary care provider   83
- The power of positive comments   85
- What is an adequate trial?   86
- Switching medication and side effects   87
- Feedback from others   89
- Helping a patient stay on medication – the adherence dilemma   91
- Antipsychotics and movement disorders at follow up   95
- For primary care providers – how and when to refer to a mental health
  specialist   95
- Missed doses   97
- Parenteral medications   99
- Information and tips for prescribing practice   99
- References   101

After the initial evaluation, the next most important element of medication management is the follow-up session. Having a structure in mind for this meeting is crucial to successful management. Follow-up sessions are likely to be repeated many times, and it is wise to spend time early in one's prescribing career defining and refining what is essential for a thorough, medically complete and time-efficient session. This chapter sets out the key elements of an effective follow-up session, and highlights some exceptions to the general rules.

When do I schedule follow up?

The timeframe for a follow-up session will be determined by the severity of the patient's condition and whether the patient is in the hospital or seen as an outpatient.

In an outpatient setting, the first follow-up session usually takes place from 1 to 2 weeks after the initial evaluation. This 7–14-day interval allows for medication to begin taking effect, for the patient to accommodate to minor side effects, and for you, the clinician, to have valid information about whether the medication is working. At the initial evaluation session, the patient was encouraged to contact you by telephone if significant problems emerged.

You would likely choose to schedule a follow up *sooner than 1 week* if one of the following conditions is present:

1 If the patient is in a serious mental health crisis, it may be important to schedule follow up at any point within the first 7 days, depending on how worried you are about the patient's clinical condition.
2 If the patient has serious medical problems that may be affected by the use of psychotropic medication, or if you are concerned about the medical status of the patient.
3 Anxious, needy patients may wish to be seen sooner because they are uncomfortable with the concept of not having professional contact. Beginning what they perceive as a medicine that may be problematic for them, they will perhaps need reassurance and support to remain adherent.

At times, the practitioner's schedule, availability, or the mandate of the clinic may solely determine the timing of a follow-up visit even when this is not ideal.

Box 6.1 Primary care

Unfortunately in some primary care offices, it is not uncommon to schedule follow-up medication appointments many weeks after the initial appointment. In some cases, a follow-up appointment is not scheduled at all – advising the patient to "call if you have any problems." When dealing with mental health medication, this model is inappropriate, dangerous and will lead to frequent non-response or non-adherence. Lack of timely follow-up visits can lead many patients to stop medications prematurely because of minor side effects, or not to understand how or when the medication is supposed to work. When an initial prescription runs out and the patient is not seen, medication may not be renewed appropriately. Always schedule a face-to-face follow-up evaluation 10–14 days after the initial visit. During the period of the COVID-19 pandemic, telemedicine appointments will suffice and are often safer, particularly for those patients who might be at higher risk for virus transmission.

How long does it take?

Ideally, the length of time devoted to a follow-up medication visit would be dictated by the needs of the patient. For primary mental health practitioners, a 30-minute follow-up exam will allow adequate time to evaluate the effectiveness of medication, adjust dosage, remedy side effects, make any medication changes, and review significant issues in the patient's life. Especially after a patient becomes known to a clinician, a surprising amount of counseling and psychotherapy can be accomplished during a session that is ostensibly for medication follow up. Some patients spend only a few minutes receiving a refill prescription and spend the majority of a session in "talk therapy." Primary care providers and mental health practitioners whose time is tightly managed can usually complete the medication portion alone in 15–20 minutes.

Inpatient medication follow up

In inpatient settings, monitoring of medication will often occur at an entirely different frequency and level of intensity. It is not unusual for patients to be seen by their prescribers every day, particularly just after arrival at the hospital. It is not, however, unreasonable to evaluate medications every second or third day if the patient is improving without significant side effects and is not labile. Once a patient is stable on medication, weekly follow-up visits are typical. For a long-term chronically hospitalized patient, monthly visits for the first year followed by a visit every 3 months is usual. The elements of the evaluation in the hospital are essentially similar to those of the outpatient follow-up visit, with the addition of feedback from the unit staff concerning the patient's condition.

Preparing for a follow up

Detailed, lengthy preparation is generally not needed prior to meeting with a patient for a follow-up visit. However, some brief re-familiarization with the patient's chart, clinical course, current medications and any occurrences that have transpired since the last visit can be done quickly. Whenever possible, a similar brief review should be done prior to returning a patient's clinically related telephone call.

Just prior to seeing the patient, take a minute to look at the patient's medical record, and specifically at the following three items:

1   the last progress note of face-to-face contact, noting any intervening telephone calls, crises or input from other sources
2   the patient's current medication list
3   the laboratory results/physical exam/allergy sections of the chart, noting any needed laboratory tests, current allergies, changing physical condition or reports/data from other healthcare providers.

This review usually takes no more than a minute or two but accomplishes several crucial tasks, especially for the busy clinician seeing many patients. It clears the clinician's mind from any previous patient activity and focuses him or her on the patient at hand. It prepares the clinician to present to the patient refreshed, refocused and knowledgeable about the current patient's issues, strengths, dilemmas, progress and medication issues. It also minimizes the likelihood that the practitioner will commit any of a series of embarrassing or potentially careless errors that could occur when past history, treatment or medical issues are not noted or remembered. The prepared practitioner is viewed by the patient as professional, unhurried and attentive to their needs, and as someone in whom they can have confidence.

Conversely, the unprepared clinician comes across to the patient as disorganized, rushed and less likely to be focused on a patient's individual needs. Busy practitioners are tempted to rush in to meet the patient as they open the medical record, trying to save time by talking to the patient, thinking, evaluating and trying to read the chart at the same time. This is to be discouraged, since it inevitably leads to spotty perform-ance on the five most important tasks that the clinician must accomplish during the follow ups:

1   know accurately what has transpired with this patient up to this point
2   evaluate the patient's current state
3   logically think through the data gathered to make clinical decisions
4   modify the treatment plan
5   communicate directly and clearly to the patient.

No matter how organized, intelligent or knowledgeable a clinician is, the above five tasks simply cannot be accomplished simultaneously.

Goals of a follow up

Specific goals in a follow-up session are to:

- check target symptoms
- quantify response
- underscore progress
- address side effects
- assess any pertinent medical changes
- use the input of significant others.

The key questions to be answered with respect to medication are:

- Is the medication effective?
- Is the dose appropriate?
- Is the patient adhering to the treatment?
- Is the patient experiencing side effects that might interfere with adherence?
- Is any addition or change to medication necessary?
- How are any non-medication therapies progressing and working with the medication?

The assessment of medication effectiveness has two principal elements:

- evaluation of the target symptoms identified in the initial evaluation
- quantification of response.

Target symptom assessment

In a follow-up session, the target symptoms that were identified and highlighted in the initial evaluation should be inquired about specifically and individually. For example:

- Has the patient's sleep pattern changed?
- How is the patient's concentration in settings where mental focus may be needed?
- Has the patient's eating, appetite or weight changed?
- Have there been any panic attacks?

- How often has the patient heard voices?
- What is the frequency and/or intensity of any other identified target symptoms?

It is useful to ask if any new symptoms have emerged since the initial visit. At the first follow up, it is also important to check if there were any specific items of history or symptomatology that the patient did not discuss in the initial evaluation.

Quantification of response

A crucial part of the follow-up session is helping patients and the practitioner to quantify symptom response to medication. This quantification will help clarify the otherwise subjective nature of their responses to questions such as "How are you feeling?" The patient will often respond "good," "fair," "okay," "not very good," "better," or something similar. Different patients use these words quite differently. In order to make precise decisions about medication dosage, it is necessary to probe the meaning of these responses. If a patient's words are taken at face value, without the assessment of specific data, inherent inaccuracies will occur in clinical decisions made about dose, or this may result in an unnecessary change of regimen.

When patients say they are "good" or "better," they should be asked, "What specifically is improved since the last time I saw you?" This will usually lead into a discussion of target symptoms. The clinician should also ask about any target symptoms the patient does not spontaneously report as different. Because patients are almost always interested in pleasing the clinician, many will say that things are "going better" or they are "well" just because they think it is what the clinician wants to hear. When the target symptoms are probed, it can turn out that there have been minimal changes in the symptoms you have targeted to treat.

Patients who say "no change," "I'm no better," or "this stuff isn't working" can, when their target symptoms are evaluated, discover that some symptoms have improved, but they failed to notice the improvement. In some cases, target symptoms are better but the patient has attributed the reason for the improvement to other causes.

Similarly, when patients say that a medication is working "fairly well" or "so-so," the clinician is often left in a quandary as to what to do with the dosage unless he or she pursues the meaning of those words. Quantification of the patient's response is essential to decisions about dosage.

Two simple, powerful questions

Two simple questions allow the clinician to quantify the patient's response and provide significant data that will help decide whether or not the medication dose needs to be changed.

Box 6.2 Talking to patients

1 *"Rate yourself on a scale from 0 to 100 – with 0 being the worst you've ever felt with your [depression, anxiety, etc.] and 95–100 as feeling comfortable, well, and balanced. No one is at 100 all the time. Give me two numbers. Where were you before starting medication, and where are you now?"*

After the patient gives you the two numbers, take the second of these responses and ask: *"What would need to be different for you to get from this number to 95?"*

Beyond the information it provides to the clinician, many patients find this brief exercise engaging and useful. It helps them to think more precisely about how they are responding to medication. Some patients will say that it is hard to quantify, although most can and do make this assessment quite readily. Interpretation of these numbers also gives you a clear framework on how to proceed with medication dosage.

Generally, there are two types of answers that emerge from the second question (what needs to change to get to 95?) that provide perspective. Some patients refer to target symptoms that have not improved, or have improved only partially. A second type of response will describe environmental issues, for example:

- Now I need to change jobs.
- All I need now is a new boss.
- Now if my wife and I would stop fighting.
- If only I had time for a vacation.
- If my parents would stop criticizing me.

If the patient refers to target symptoms and is not close to the target figure of 95, it is clear that the illness is only partially treated and generally an increase in dosage is indicated. On the other hand, the second type of response, referring to the patient's environment or lifestyle, is unlikely to be affected by medication changes and it may be that a dosage change is not indicated.

These two questions can, and should, be asked at each succeeding follow-up session until patients consistently rate themselves at 90 or above.

Know what is changing medically

Prescription of psychotropic medication is a process that cannot be taken out of the context of the patient's overall health and medical treatment. It is imperative that, at every follow-up session, the clinician inquires about other medical changes, including other non-psychotropic medication additions that may have occurred since the last session.

While some illnesses, medications or treatment may have little impact on the mental health prescription, others may have a critical or life-threatening impact and knowledge of other medical treatment is essential.

Illnesses or non-psychotropic medication changes can:

- worsen or improve the mental health condition
- affect the blood levels of the psychotropic via P-450 interactions or by other mechanisms (e.g., decreased GI absorption), requiring dosage adjustment
- account for new or intensified side effects that might otherwise be attributed to the psychotropic
- lead to changes in adherence with the psychotropic.

Inquiry into what medications are being prescribed by other providers may also uncover circumstances in which two or more practitioners are providing the same or multiple psychotropics. If the practitioner does not become aware of this, it can lead to possible medication interaction or undiscovered abuse.

Inquiry about medical problems and medications does not imply that the prescriber should treat these medical problems, unless trained and credentialed to do so. In general, except for primary care providers, most mental health prescribers will not treat the patient's medical conditions. (See Chapter 9 for further information about this issue.)

Side effects at follow up

Further goals of the follow-up session include side-effect assessment and management. The key point to remember here is that the patient should be asked specifically "Are you having any side effects or unwanted symptoms from the medication?" The patient should assess the frequency, intensity and amount of interference with functioning caused by these side effects. When they are minor, reassurance may be all that is needed. If they are more significant, the clinician must decide whether to modify dosage, reassure and wait, add a remediative factor, or change medication. This topic is crucially important and is discussed in detail separately in Chapter 19.

Adjunctive medical or laboratory evaluation

In addition to obtaining a verbal report of progress or lack thereof, possible medication side effects, new medications from other providers and the onset of any new medical conditions, the prescriber should assess the need for any laboratory monitoring. When appropriate, serum blood levels of the psychotropics should be obtained (this topic is discussed in detail in Chapter 25). At each visit, the prescriber should also assess whether any other laboratory tests are needed. Competent clinical practice requires that the clinician consider any potential effects that the psychotropic medication may have on other bodily systems by performing appropriate examinations and/ or laboratory tests. Based on normal results, only further observation will be necessary. In other cases, however, if there are significant abnormalities, change of dosage, change of medication, or change to a different medication class may be indicated. Other appropriate monitoring schedules for specific medications and groups are listed in Table 6.1.

> Antipsychotics: recommended physical monitoring in Severe Mental Illness (SMI) health checks results/outcomes to be shared between healthcare providers.
> Baseline monitoring: to be done by the initiating organization – urea and electrolytes (U&Es); full blood count (FBC); liver function tests (LFTs); thyroid function tests (TFTs); prolactin; fasting/random glucose/HbA1C (hemoglobin A1C); lipids/cardiovascular disease (CVD) risk calculation, blood pressure (BP) and pulse; weight/BMI (waist circumference, diet, physical activity); electrocardiogram (ECG) – where mandated for specific antipsychotics (e.g., haloperidol), identified CV risk, family history, additive risk with concurrent medication; smoking (number of cigarettes or packs/day). Monitoring in the first 6 weeks – to be done by the prescribing practitioner or organization.

Table 6.1 Recommended laboratory monitoring for psychotropic medication for antipsychotics

---

For antipsychotics

1 Observe for possible movement disorder symptoms. AIMS examination done at least every 6 months.
2 Weight/BMI: measured at baseline, at every visit for 9 months, then every 3 months thereafter.
3 Prolactin (for clients on risperidone or first-generation antipsychotics): measured at baseline, at 6 months, then annually.
4 Electrocardiogram (for clients on thioridazine or ziprasidone): obtain baseline ECG only in clients at risk for QTc prolongation. (See Chapter 20.) Periodic monitoring would be dependent on changes in electrolyte status (hypokalemia or hypomagnesemia) as a result of diuretic therapy, diarrhea, etc.
5 BUN, creatinine and liver functions should be performed yearly.
6 Blood pressure should be measured frequently during dose titration or if symptoms of hypotension emerge.

For antidepressants

1 Routine laboratory tests are generally not necessary although yearly liver function tests can be drawn in patients thought to be at high risk for liver dysfunction.
2 Maintenance liver function tests every 6 months during continuation of nefazodone (in addition to monitoring for clinical signs and symptoms of hepatic dysfunction in medical progress notes).

For mood stabilizers

Lithium	Electrolytes, BUN/ creatinine, CBC, TSH, U/A, ECG (if > 35 years old), pregnancy test.	While titrating, check drug level 8–12 hours after last dose within 7 days of any dosage increase until desired level is reached.	Check drug level (8–12 hours after last dose) every 3 months with BUN/creatinine and electrolytes; check TSH every 6 months; follow BMI/weight.
Valproic acid	CBC with differential, LFTs, pregnancy test.	Within 7 days of dosage increase until desired level and/or clinical stability is reached.	LFTs, CBC every 6 months. Once stable, the drug level can be checked for compliance with dose, emergence of side effects or loss of therapeutic effect; follow BMI/weight.
Carbamazepine	Na, CBC with differential, BUN/ creatinine, LFTs, TSH, pregnancy test.	Na, CBC, LFTs, drug level within 7 days of dosage increase. Because of enzyme auto-induction, once desired level is reached, recheck 2–4 weeks later to ensure that serum level has been maintained.	Na, CBC, BUN/ creatinine, LFTs at 6 months; check serum level if loss of therapeutic effect; follow BMI/weight.
Lamotrigine	The use of lamotrigine does not require routine monitoring of any clinical laboratory parameters, although the patient's skin condition should be inquired about and/or evaluated regularly because of the known occurrence of serious skin reactions.		

Table 6.1 Cont.

For stimulants

1 Height and weight every 6 months (in children and adolescents).
2 Pulse every 3 months, and blood pressure every 6 months (in patients > 12 years old).

Sources: Adapted from Antipsychotics – recommended physical monitoring in severe mental illness (SMI) health check results/outcomes to be shared between healthcare providers, available at: www.derbyshiremedicinesmanagement.nhs.uk/assets/Clinical_Guidelines/Formulary_by_BNF_chapter_prescribing_guidelines/BNF_chapter_4/Antipsychotics_physical_monitoring.pdf (accessed 1/4/2020); Riddle MA *et al.* (2011) *Pediatric Psychopharmacology for Primary Care*, 2nd edn., Center for Mental Health Services in Pediatric Primary Care, Johns Hopkins School of Public Health, available at: www.derbyshiremedicinesmanagement.nhs.uk/assets/Clinical_Guidelines/Formulary_by_BNF_chapter_prescribing_guidelines/BNF_chapter_4/Antipsychotics_physical_monitoring.pdf (accessed 1/4/2020).

Annual monitoring in primary care: general physical and cardio metabolic health; national screening programs; medicine reconciliation and monitoring:

1 inquire about smoking, alcohol and drug use
2 inquire about diet and activity levels
3 check blood pressure and pulse
4 cv risk assessment
5 measurement of body mass index (BMI)
6 check for the development of diabetes
7 check renal function
8 follow up national screening where appropriate (e.g., breast/cervical/bowel)
9 sexual health screening, contraception, etc.
10 check the accuracy of the record of medication prescribed by the general practitioner and the psychiatrist
11 if new medicines or changes to physical health have increased the risk of prolonged QTc, arrange ECG.

Collaborate with specialist services where there is:

- poor response to treatment
- non-adherence to medication
- intolerable side effects of medication
- co-morbid substance misuse
- physical health effect on insulin function, independent of weight gain. Metabolic effects are also seen in patients prescribed typical antipsychotics.

Mental health prescriber and/or primary care provider

Corrected QT interval (QTc): antipsychotics may prolong the QTc interval – a rising QTc should be monitored and a QTc of >499mSec is a *red flag* and should be acted upon.

1 Check the machine has worked it out correctly by doing the calculation yourself.
2 Review other QTc lengthening medications (www.crediblemeds.org) and get potassium magnesium and calcium blood test and correct if necessary.

3   Consider reducing dose of antipsychotic immediately (and then thinking what to do next and repeat ECG in a week).

4   Consult cardiologist if in doubt.

Observe for possible movement disorder symptoms. AIMS examination done at least every 6 months.

Weight/BMI: measured at baseline, at every visit for 9 months, then every 3 months thereafter.

Prolactin level (for clients on risperidone or first-generation antipsychotics): measured at baseline, at 6 months, then annually.

Electrocardiogram (for clients on thioridazine or ziprasidone): obtain baseline ECG only in clients at risk for QTc prolongation. Periodic monitoring would be dependent on changes in electrolyte status (hypokalemia or hypomagnesemia) as a result of diuretic therapy, diarrhea, etc.

BUN (blood urea nitrogen), creatinine and liver functions should be performed yearly

Blood pressure should be measured frequently during dose titration or if symptoms of hypotension emerge.

Follow-up schedules for monitoring of fasting blood sugar levels and lipid profiles are documented in Chapter 9 and will not be repeated here.

For antidepressants

Routine laboratory tests are generally not necessary for antidepressants except TCAs, yearly liver function tests can be drawn in patients thought to be at high risk for liver dysfunction.

Maintenance liver function tests are needed every 6 months during continuation of nefazodone (in addition to monitoring for clinical signs and symptoms of hepatic dysfunction in medical progress notes).

Anti-anxiety medications likewise do need routine blood level monitoring although features of common anxiolytics are listed in Table 6.1.

Smoking

Cigarette smoke is a potent inducer of the liver enzyme known as cytochrome P-450 1A2 (CYP1A2). Drug levels in the blood may be increased if a patient stops smoking tobacco. Increased psychotropic levels will also occur if smoking is replaced by Nicotine Replacement Therapy (NRT). Mental health practitioners will also need to consider the potential for fluctuation in effect when tobacco use is not consistent. Significant effects have been reported in patients who change smoking habits while prescribed clozapine. Attempts to stop smoking should be planned in conjunction with the psychiatrist.

Family medication response

If the clinician has asked the patient to investigate the use of psychotropics by family blood relations, ask what information has been uncovered.

Maintaining the bond with the patient

Another (often unspoken) goal of the follow-up session is to maintain and strengthen the alliance between clinician and patient. The relationship you maintain with the patient can be as important as the prescription you write. In some clinical situations, it is more important. A solid alliance with a patient will not overcome medication that is ineffective or poorly tolerated, but it will foster the trust necessary to keep the patient adherent with your prescription. When patients feel listened to, respected, empathized with and made partners in medication decisions, they will often gather the courage to try a medication about which they are anxious, and to persist even if they are uncomfortable. Although serious adverse consequences of psychotropics are uncommon (see Chapter 19), when they do occur, the quality of the relationship with the prescriber will often significantly influence the patient behavior and in some cases the propensity for the patient to blame the prescriber. On occasion, the quality of the bond between the prescriber and patient can prevent a lawsuit.

The very fact that the follow-up session is scheduled and carried out indicates that the clinician is interested in how the patient is progressing, and what role the medication is taking in that progress. It also indicates willingness to answer questions about the medication, and to help the patient manage any bothersome side effects.

At follow-up sessions, the clinician has an opportunity to reinforce the treatment plan outlined in the initial session and to identify the patient's position on the timeline toward recovery. If the patient is not fully recovered at the first follow-up session – which he or she most often is not – it is important to state that full recovery is not expected immediately. If there are promising signs and improvement in some symptoms, this indicates that the medication and therapy programs are "on the right track" and this should be underscored. At this session, it is also possible to see if the patient has followed through with any talking therapy that may have been suggested during the initial treatment plan.

The power of positive comments

Patients taking mental health medication are anxious, depressed, confused and demoralized, and some have lost hope of ever feeling better. As part of their illness, often they have received negative comments, disparaging remarks and overt criticism from family and friends, as well as poor work evaluations. They may have perceived that others think little of them or look down on them. Many patients, in fact, look negatively on themselves. It is crucially important that the clinician remains upbeat, positive and enthusiastic, and shows measured hopefulness about the potential benefits of psychotropic medication treatment. This cannot be stressed strongly enough. *There can never be too many encouraging statements, compliments, or too much praise for the patient's behavior and improvement.*

When possible, use phrases such as:

* You did well to...
* I am impressed by...
* I can see all the effort you put into...
* You showed good judgment when...

- Wow, it is impressive that…
- You obviously gave a lot of thought in coming up with that decision.
- You showed a lot of strength to endure…
- That must have taken a lot of strength to…
- Your lab tests look great.
- I appreciate that you stayed with our plan despite…
- Given what you have had to face, you have done better than a lot of people would have.
- You have been really patient with…
- You did just what I would have wanted you to do.
- I see why you did what you did, and I think you did the best you could with the situation you faced.
- Well done!
- Great job!
- Congratulations!
- Very nice!
- Keep up the good work!

Finding positive ways to discuss the patient's actions, decision-making and adherence provides powerful reinforcers to the treatment plan. The alliance with the clinician is greatly strengthened by these brief but meaningful statements, which can often mean continuation and eventual success with your recommendations in the face of medication non-response, side effects, or a stressful personal life crisis.

If the clinician has a mindset to consciously support and reinforce the patient in some way at each visit, it is usually not hard to find an area of discussion around which to make these affirmations, even in the most regressed, negativistic or non-compliant patient.

What is an adequate trial?

The length of time on which you keep a patient on a specific medication is a clinical decision based on the assessment of several factors, including:

- Is the patient showing any response? Is the response increasing with time?
- How intense were the patient's symptoms? Is the patient's condition deteriorating during the current trial of medication?
- How well is the patient tolerating the medication (severity of side effects)?
- Are the side effects lessening or intensifying with time?
- Has the patient reached (or come close to reaching) a therapeutic dose of the drug, and maintained the therapeutic dose for a period of time?
- What other promising medication alternatives do you have if you switch?
- How willing is the patient to pursue a continuation of the current trial?

Although some patients will only respond fully to a drug at 30 to 60 days after beginning medication, most patients will have begun to show some initial sign of response by 30 days. Further gradual improvement can appear later. *It is unlikely that a patient who shows no change in symptoms at 30 days will suddenly (or gradually) show significant improvement at a later date.* Therefore, clinically useful timeframes for medication trials of an individual medication are as follows:

- For a mildly to moderately symptomatic outpatient, continue a medication for 30 days before switching. During this period the dose of the drug is likely to be increased using the quantification of response data noted earlier in this chapter.
- For an inpatient or severely symptomatic outpatient, continue a medication for 15 days before switching. With these individuals, particularly on an inpatient unit, the use of multiple medications on a daily or an as-needed basis is common and often necessary for acute behavioral control and management during this first 2 weeks.

These general time guidelines can be modified by several circumstances. For example, a patient's medication trial may be shortened owing to significant medication side effects or intolerance. It does not, however, usually make clinical sense to change a patient's antidepressant, mood stabilizer or antipsychotic every several days for "non-response," since a valid, expectable response is simply unlikely to occur in that period.

Conversely, a patient's medication trial may be lengthened if partial response is occurring, and full therapeutic dosing has not been reached. An outpatient who has shown some improvement but has not achieved full response may become substantially asymptomatic with a longer period on medication. A patient who has required low initial dosages with very gradual increases (because of side effects, concurrent medical condition or advanced age, for example) may not have reached full therapeutic levels in 30 days. If the patient is tolerating the drug, continuation of a medication may extend for 60 to 90 days before a valid assessment of its usefulness can be made. Therapeutic blood levels, when appropriate, can also guide this process, assuming patient tolerance. Maintain a drug for at least 30 days after adequate therapeutic blood levels have been reached to assess response.

 Box 6.3 Clinical tip

Significant drug effect is unlikely unless at least modest gains have been seen in the first month. Continuing a medication for 6–12 months with an expectation (and message to the patient) that *"you will feel better in a while – just keep taking it"* is not good medicine, and is seldom true. Either decide that medication is not useful for this patient or change medications, but do not simply continue the drug and wait for response. This practice occurs most frequently in primary care offices or institutional settings.

Switching medication and side effects

Table 6.2 gives some practical advice about switching medication, based on the amount of response and the intensity of side effects.

A measure of experience helps in knowing whether a certain side effect is likely to pass with time or, once present, is unlikely to go away. If side effects are serious, interfering with functioning and/or increasing in intensity, it is usually necessary to change

Table 6.2 When to change antidepressants

Side effect	Intensity	Level of improvement
Little or none	*Partial*	*Significant or full*
None or mild	Change	Increase dose
Maintain dose	Moderate but tolerable	Increase dose slowly
Increase dose slowly	Maintain dose	Significant or serious
Change	Change	Decrease dose or change

medications, sometimes as soon as the initial follow-up visit. If side effects are lessening and have minimal interference with the patient's day-to-day life, it may be quite appropriate to wait until at least the second follow-up visit to see if symptoms pass fully or become more tolerable. Chapter 19 gives detailed advice on strategies for managing side effects without necessarily needing to change drugs.

When changing, gradual is best

With most psychotropics, once a decision has been made to change medications, there should be a *gradual cross-taper* from one medication to the other – that is, the first medication can be gradually decreased in dosage at the same time as the second medication is being started. In general, if the dosage is moderate or high, this is a better strategy than stopping the first medication totally before starting a second medication. Stopping totally can leave the patient "uncovered" and symptomatic for a period before the second medication begins to take effect. This principle applies to virtually all medicines in all classes, including antidepressants (except MAOIs), antipsychotics, mood stabilizers and anti-anxiety medications. If the patient takes a small dose of medicine, no taper is necessary.

 Box 6.4 Clinical tip

When changing medication, a cross-taper of medications is almost always safer.

A notable exception to the principle of cross-tapering is when the medication to be stopped or started is a monoamine oxidase inhibitor (MAOI). If the MAOI is being stopped, the patient must be totally off it for at least 2 weeks prior to starting another antidepressant. If the medicine to be started is an MAOI, the safe starting point is determined by the time to full elimination of any current medication with which the MAOI could interact. Generally, it is safe to begin an MAOI 1 week after stopping the previous medication. (The commonly used psychotropic that needs a much longer interval before starting an MAOI is fluoxetine, which has a long-acting metabolite, norfluoxetine, that is not excreted for up to 4 weeks.)

During a cross-taper the clinician may see that the patient is beginning to feel better with the addition of a second medication, and decide to continue with both medications. By assuming that both medications are necessary to the patient's response, however, the

Table 6.3 Medication changeover sheet

Day	(Medication A)	(Medication B)
1		
2		
3		
4		
5		
6		
7		
8		
9		
10		
11		
12		
13		
14		

clinician may get "caught in the middle" of a changeover. In general, in the change from medicine A to medicine B, it is best to continue a cross-taper until medicine A is fully stopped, and maintain the patient solely on medicine B before deciding that both medications are necessary. If the patient begins to backslide on medicine B alone, it is simple to return to the combination. Using two medications can at times be beneficial, but this should only be decided in hindsight, rather than stopping in the middle and assuming it to be so.

When changing medications, especially via a gradual taper, a written instruction sheet is crucial. Patients can easily mishear, misunderstand or forget orally given schedules under the best of clinical circumstances. As shown in Table 6.3, a "changeover sheet" with blanks to be filled in by the clinician with specific dosage amounts is a valuable educational office tool. An example of such a sheet filled in by the clinician is shown in Table 6.4. Some clinicians may prefer to use numbers of pills rather than milligrams, as in Table 6.5.

Feedback from others

Input from a caretaker, adult child, parent or other person who may be knowledgeable about the patient's condition is especially helpful in making appropriate assessments at the follow-up session. This is particularly so if a patient is not a good observer of his/her own behavior. If a caretaker, relative or friend accompanies the patient to the office, it is generally helpful to briefly ask this person about his or her perception of the patient's response. Early in treatment, severely ill patients, geriatric patients or persons

Table 6.4 Completed medication changeover sheet (dosage)

Day	*(Medication A)*	*(Medication B)*
1	300 mg	10 mg
2	300 mg	10 mg
3	250 mg	10 mg
4	250 mg	10 mg
5	200 mg	20 mg
6	200 mg	20 mg
7	150 mg	20 mg
8	150 mg	30 mg
9	100 mg	30 mg
10	100 mg	30 mg
11	50 mg	30 mg
12	50 mg	30 mg
13		Call me

Table 6.5 Completed medication changeover sheet (number of pills)

Day	*Medication A (100 mg)*	*Medication B (10 mg)*
1	3 pills	1 pill
2	3 pills	1 pill
3	2 pills	1 pill
4	2 pills	1 pill
5	2 pills	2 pills
6	2 pills	2 pills
7	1 pill	2 pills
8	1 pill	3 pills
9	1 pill	3 pills
10	1 pill	3 pills
11	0 pills	3 pills
12	0 pills	3 pills
13	—	Call me
14		

who are not good self-observers will often return to the clinician saying that nothing has changed or nothing is better. When input from the family member is obtained, it reveals that significant benefits have started to occur. While the patient may not be fully responsive, many times family members will begin to see positive changes before patients themselves identify progress.

Helping a patient stay on medication – the adherence dilemma

As with medications in general, non-adherence with psychotropic medication is a major public health problem.[1-3] Patients often do not take all their prescribed medication, or frequently miss doses. Some patients cut down on their medication doses because they are concerned about side effects or cost. Others, for a variety of reasons, stop medication altogether without informing the clinician. Unbeknownst to the clinician, some patients throw the prescription away and never start the medication. How then can the clinician raise the odds for successful adherence? Some factors are listed in Table 6.6.

Forming a strong initial contract with patients is the cornerstone to adherence. This contract should include the clinician's assessment or diagnosis, why the medication is indicated, what symptoms the medication is intended to help and an outline for duration of usage. It is important to make sure that patients understand the plan and agree to it. Such an approach ensures that the patient becomes an active participant in the process, and raises the likelihood of adherence.

One of the most important elements to eliminating missed medication doses is to establish a simple regimen with the fewest daily doses possible.[4] Repeated medication studies have shown that the higher the number of doses per day, the more likely it is that patients will miss one or more doses. Many psychotropics can be dosed once daily, and do not require multiple doses to be effective. Simplicity of dosing (e.g., the same strength and number of pills at each dose) also helps. Avoid every other day, twice weekly, or otherwise complicated schedules unless a patient's clinical situation and response demand it.

Early, frequent contact with patients will also increase the odds of adherence. The longer the time until the first follow-up session, the more likely it is that patients will not comply or will have taken the medication in an inappropriate way. Over the first 4–6 weeks, at least two follow-up sessions should be undertaken, to reinforce the medications and the treatment plan, as well as to assess for any side effects.

Availability of the clinician by telephone will also improve adherence. If patients know that they can call the clinician, simple issues can be clarified immediately, allowing them to continue the medication appropriately until the next visit. Telephone reassurance and

Table 6.6 Factors that can increase adherence with psychotropic medication

---

- An openly discussed and reinforced agreement with the patient as to why the medication is to be taken, in what doses, and for how long
- A simple medication regimen with the fewest daily doses possible
- Written directions for taking the medication
- Regular follow-up visits
- Assessing adherence at follow-up visits
- Evaluating and remediating side effects of the medication
- Assessing patient resistance to taking medication
- Prompt telephone availability between office sessions

---

education about what they are experiencing can prevent patients from discontinuing medication prematurely.

Another extremely important item in improving adherence is to ask about, listen for and remediate side effects. While there are many explanations for patient discontinuation of medication, the single largest reason is that the medication produces a side effect that patients find intolerable.[5-7] Because of their discomfort, patients do not comply. (See Chapter 19 for an in-depth discussion of side-effect management.)

The clinician should also, in the first several follow-up sessions, ask about and evaluate signs of resistance. If patients are hesitant about increasing a dose or continuing on the medication, the clinician needs to inquire specifically about the hesitation. Often it is an issue that can be handled quickly and expediently. If a patient has serious resistance, it may be better to halt the medication trial or delay the dosage increase and deal with the resistance first. In a mildly/moderately symptomatic patient, if the resistance is addressed, the medication can be retried when the patient is more cooperative and understands the rationale for the treatment plan.

It is also useful for the clinician to assess how many pills a patient has been taking daily. How much medication does the patient have left? Does that match the patient's records? If the patient has far too much medication left over it is a clear sign that the medication has not been taken consistently, and the reason for this needs to be evaluated.

If patients do improve, but stop medication prematurely or intermittently, encourage them to step back and look at the "big picture." Use specific dates, holidays and life events as markers or identifiers to reinforce your assessment of the positive results that the patient has experienced.

Box 6.5 Talking to patients

"Let's remember where you were last Christmas. You weren't working and you were living at your parents' home. You were feeling so anxious that you were fearful of going to the store by yourself. After you had taken the medication for 3 months, you were able to go out to the mall alone, apply for a job, and were thinking about moving into your own apartment. After you stopped medication in March, you felt too anxious to go to the job interview and spent most of the day watching television because you didn't want to leave the house. When you started medication in May, you began to look forward to getting out again. Remember, that's when you went to the neighborhood picnic that you enjoyed so much. You even began to think about wanting to visit your cousin in Springfield. When you stopped medication in August, that's when you canceled the trip to see your cousin and started lying on the couch again for hours each day. I think there is a direct connection between your taking the medication and being able to do many of the things you want to do."

A final factor that will help to increase adherence is flexibility about the decision as to when and how to discontinue medication. If patients have the clear understanding that the clinician will not maintain a rigid, inflexible approach to discontinuation, they are usually more willing to tolerate medication for a period of time until a mutually agreed discontinuation date can be determined. Stopping medication will be discussed in more detail in Chapter 8.

Long-acting antipsychotic medication

Patients with serious mental illnesses, including schizophrenia, schizoaffective disorder and serious bipolar disorder are well known to be non-adherent with antipsychotic medications. This can lead to frequent relapses, hospitalizations, and behavioral and social consequences from the re-emergence of psychotic symptoms. The use of long-acting injectable antipsychotic medications has been a continual recommendation to promoting adherence. Since the FDA's approval of the first second-generation long-acting medication – risperidone long-acting injectable (LAI) in 2003 – six additional second-generation LAI As have been approved:

- aripiprazole LAI
- aripiprazole lauroxil LAI
- olanzapine pamoate LAI
- paliperidone palmitate monthly injection
- paliperidone palmitate 3-month LAI
- risperidone LAI for subcutaneous (SQ) injection.

In practical terms, it makes virtually no difference what the official indication was for approval since they all have been used on-label or off-label for a variety of psychotic indications. Important considerations in using long-acting depot preparation traditional neuroleptics are listed in Table 6.7.

Unlike oral formulations of these medications, the long-acting formulations have some significant differences in approved indications and their practical use in clinical situations. The reader is referred to an excellent up-to-date, practical guide on their use[8] for specific details and from which Table 6.8 is taken.

In general, because of the flexibility in adjusting initial doses of medications, most clinicians prefer to utilize oral formulations at first, eventually changing to long-acting preparations once a stable final dose is reached. Depending on which medication is used, a period of overlap between the oral dosing and the initiation of the long-acting medication may be necessary. Using long-acting preparations at first complicates finding the most effective doses since the evaluation of clinical response would often take weeks or even months. In some less frequent situations where future non-adherence is strongly suspected, a clinician might utilize a long-acting preparation at first, assuming that using an oral formulation would result in non-adherence very quickly. In this case, the clinician will make an educated guess as to the best starting dose of the LAI. Figure 6.1 gives the approximate equivalents of a long-acting preparation to oral doses.

Table 6.7 Using long-acting depot preparations of traditional neuroleptics

---

1 Preferably stabilize the patient on the oral medication first.
2 When switching to depot preparations, use the lowest effective dose.
3 Use the longest possible recommended dosing intervals between injections.
4 Are you what you do? Allow adequate time (at least 1 month) to assess adequacy of symptom response.
5 For breakthrough symptoms, which may occur when depot preparations are first used, supplement the depot preparation with oral doses of medication and adjust the depot dosage at the next injection. Do not attempt to manage breakthrough symptoms initially with further injections of depot medication.

Table 6.8 Second-generation long-acting injectable antipsychotics: a practical guide

Medication	Clinical pearls
Aripiprazole LAI	If patient experiences adverse reactions to 400-mg dose, consider reduction to 300-mg
Aripiprazole lauroxil LAI	Not interchangeable with aripiprazole lauroxil 675-mg LAI
Aripiprazole lauroxil 675-mg LAI	Not interchangeable with aripiprazole lauroxil LAI
Olanzapine pamoate LAI	REMS program: patients must be observed for 3 hours after receiving dose due to risk of PDSS
Paliperidone palmitate monthly injection	Administering the two starting doses in the deltoid muscle helps attain therapeutic concentrations rapidly
Paliperidone palmitate 3-month injection	Patients should be stable on paliperidone palmitate monthly injection for 4 months prior to starting 3-month LAI
Risperidone LAI	When increasing dose, clinical effects of new dose should not be expected earlier than 3 weeks after the higher dose
Risperidone LAI for SQ	Patients stable on oral risperidone dose of <3 or >4mg/d may not be candidates

Source: Parmentier BL (2020) Second-generation long-acting injectables: a practical guide. *Current Psychiatry* 19(3): 24–32.

Note: LAI – long-acting injectable; PDSS – post-injection delirium/sedation syndrome; REMS – Risk Evaluation and Mitigation Strategy.

Table 2

Oral-to-LAI dose equivalency recommendations

Medication	Aripiprazole lauroxil LAI			Paliperidone palmitate monthly injection				Olanzapine pamoate LAI			Risperidone LAI for SQ	
Oral daily dose	10 mg	15 mg	≥20 mg	3 mg	6 mg	9 mg	12 mg	10 mg	15 mg	≥20 mg	3 mg	4 mg
LAI equivalency	441 mg every 4 weeks	662 mg every 4 weeks OR 882 mg every 6 weeks OR 1064 mg every 8 weeks	882 mg every 4 weeks	39 to 78 mg	117 mg	156 mg	234 mg	During the first 8 weeks of treatment: 219 mg every 2 weeks OR 405 mg every 4 weeks. After 8 weeks of treatment: 150 mg every 2 weeks OR 300 mg every 4 weeks	During the first 8 weeks of treatment: 300 mg every 2 weeks. After 8 weeks of treatment: 210 mg every 2 weeks OR 405 mg every 4 weeks	During the first 8 weeks of treatment: 300 mg every 2 weeks. After 8 weeks of treatment: 300 mg every 2 weeks	90 mg	120 mg

LAI: long-acting injectable; SQ: subcutaneous

Figure 6.1 Oral-to-LAI dose equivalency recommendation.

Source: Meyer JM (2018) Converting oral to long-acting injectable antipsychotics: a guide for the perplexed – Corrigendum. *CNS Spectrums* 23(2): 186.

The author of the above-mentioned guide lists "clinical pearls" regarding each specific medication and these are shown in Table 6.8.

Antipsychotics and movement disorders at follow up

The emergence of a movement disorder must be considered during any follow-up evaluation of a patient being prescribed an antipsychotic medication. These possible side effects are discussed in more detail in Chapter 19. Extrapyramidal symptoms and tardive dyskinesia, in particular, are known and potentially serious complications of antipsychotic medication therapy. Fortunately much less common with atypical antipsychotics than traditional antipsychotics, these movement problems are appearing at a lower rate in recent years, but do still occur. Failure to assess for these side effects may constitute an area of liability for the clinician in antipsychotic prescription. It is wise to ask a few targeted questions and document the response at each follow-up session.

- Have you noticed any joint stiffness?
- Have you noticed any changes in your gait or walking?
- Have you had any difficulty speaking words?
- Have you noticed any new or unusual movements of your face, tongue or extremities?

Some clinicians prefer to perform a full AIMS test at each follow-up session, and some agencies require it. Not all prescribers feel a need to perform this exam on each visit, however, if the above questions are answered negatively and no unusual movements are seen on direct observation. Depending on the medication prescribed, an AIMS examination should be performed and documented every 3 to 6 months. The procedure for an AIMS test is detailed in Appendix 6.

For primary care providers – how and when to refer to a mental health specialist

Both specialist providers and primary care providers (PCPs) will benefit from cultivating contacts with those experienced in psychotropic prescribing. This may be a psychiatrist who works with adults or children, or a mental health nurse practitioner with specialty training. Having a tertiary referral source available (a university-based psychopharmacologist or an especially knowledgeable practitioner in the community) is also helpful, but is not always possible in all communities. The reality of medical practice in many areas is that mental health prescribing specialists are in short supply, and often have a long waiting period for appointments.

Emergency, same-day evaluations for psychotropics are often only available through an emergency department or psychiatric hospital. Because of these realities, a PCP will often have to make urgent decisions about psychotropic medication with a limited comfort level.

In general, a patient is appropriate for referral to an available mental health specialist when:

- the patient is acutely and highly suicidal
- the patient is psychotic

- bipolar symptoms are present, or emerge during treatment
- the patient has been minimally responsive to the PCP's prescriptions
- the patient experiences multiple disabling side effects from psychotropics
- the diagnosis is uncertain and the appropriate course of medication is unclear
- the PCP needs assistance with a "difficult" patient (see Chapter 23 for more on this topic)
- the PCP wants clarification/confirmation of the need for ongoing habit-forming psychotropic medications
- the patient's medical condition is seriously adversely affected by a mental health problem requiring medication
- the patient has a complex psychopharmacological combination of medications
- the PCP is uncomfortable managing this particular patient or a specific class of medications
- repeated relapse occurs when medication is withdrawn
- there is patient frustration with the process of repeated medication trials.

Box 6.6 Talking to patients

Making the referral to a mental health specialist is not always simple. Some patients resist the referral, and never follow through. There is no single way to ensure that the patient will accept the referral, although some of the following approaches are helpful:

- Emphasize that it is you, the PCP, who needs assistance, not the patient: *"Mrs. Gordon, I have tried several antidepressants with you for your depression and I need some consultation and help. I would like you to see Gloria Boyle. She works regularly with these types of medications and can help me decide what is best for you."*
- If the referral is for medication, specifically using the term *"psychopharmacologist"* or *"practitioner with expertise in mental health medication"* may carry less stigma than referral to a *"psychiatrist"* or *"therapist."*
- Describe the initial visit as a *"consultation,"* with the possibility of return to your care when the situation is appropriate: *"Miss Porter, I would like to get a consultation from Dr. Pindar. He is a specialist in this area of medication. Once he has evaluated your situation, he, you, and I can decide how best to follow up. Regardless, I would like to stay involved, and if it is appropriate for me to continue to prescribe, I will do so. Most of all, I want to ensure that you get the help you need."*
- If you are not willing to continue to prescribe a particular medication without a confirmatory evaluation, say so clearly but not punitively: *"Mr. Edwards, we have been prescribing [name of medication] for your anxiety. When we stopped the medication your anxiety returned, and recently you have requested additional refills in increasing frequency. Before I am willing to continue prescribing, I want a second opinion about your condition to see if we are on the right track. Greg Boyle is a nurse*

practitioner who deals with anxiety medications regularly, and I would like you to see him."

- If the patient has expressed reluctance regarding the referral, recognize the patient's ambivalence and your inability to provide what he or she needs. Focus on these needs: *"Mr. Vincent, I can see that you are not pleased with the idea of my referring you to a mental health specialist. I am concerned about the intensity of your depressive symptoms. You have been 'hanging on by your fingernails,' sleeping poorly, losing weight, and you have begun thinking that the world would be better off without you around. We have tried several antidepressants. You have been very diligent in taking the medication as I have asked, but have minimally improved and experienced side effects that really bother you. Despite your strength in following through with my recommendation, I see you wearing down and tiring out. The most important thing is to get you well as quickly as possible. I know you would prefer to do this another way, but I am worried about you. I need some assistance, and I want you to see Dr. Wong. I have worked with her several times before, and she has been extremely helpful. Will you keep an appointment if my staff helps to arrange it?"*
- Involve the family. For example, in any of the above dialogues, if the patient still refuses referral you could request to talk to the patient's family. *"Mrs. Donovan, I believe you are at serious risk for worsening of your depression. Things are not better despite both our best efforts. I need to talk with your daughter to discuss my concerns, since I cannot continue to prescribe for you when your condition is worsening as it is. I feel I need some assistance."* If the patient agrees, call a responsible family member.
- Utilize one of the individualized "patient levers" discussed in Chapter 4.

Missed doses

No matter how conscientious a patient may be, missing an occasional dose of medication is understandable and a fact of clinical practice.

The instruction given here regarding missed doses is generally applicable for most patients and most oral mental health medications.

 Box 6.7 Talking to patients

"If you miss a dose of medication, take it when you remember, unless it is 4 or less hours until your next scheduled dose. If your regular dose will occur within 4 hours, skip the missed dose and resume your normal dose at the regularly scheduled time. Do not double up on your medication to 'make up' for the missed dose."

Exceptions to this principle include:

1 Short half-life serotonergic antidepressants such as paroxetine and venlafaxine that are particularly sensitive to serotonergic rebound withdrawal (see Chapter 8).

Because of the propensity of such short half-life medications to produce unpleasant rebound symptoms (including dizziness, nausea, agitation and sleeplessness) when a dose is missed, patients should take the missed dose whenever they remember it, particularly if they are experiencing some measure of serotonergic rebound withdrawal.

2   Sedative medicines taken once daily at bedtime. If patients remember such a medication in the morning, they may or may not find this medication too sedative for daytime activities. For those who cannot risk any sedation, it may be safer to wait until their next bedtime dose before taking any further medication. A second alternative is for the patient to take a smaller amount (one-fourth to one-half of their regular dose) in the morning and then take a full dose at bedtime as prescribed.

How patients respond to missed doses

The clinical results of missing a dose vary markedly from patient to patient. Some patients are significantly sensitive to even a single missed dose of their psychotropic, and will notice symptoms within hours of missing it. Other patients seem impervious to such missed doses and, unless there are frequent missed doses resulting in significantly lower serum blood levels, they note very little difference in their clinical condition.

The clinical reaction to missing a dose of medication is composed of two elements:

1   any physiological reaction caused by the sudden absence of the medication
2   the return of target symptoms that the medication is attempting to treat (e.g., anxiety, depression, psychosis, etc.).

Our level of scientific understanding of what happens when a dose is missed is almost solely related to the first of these factors. We do understand clearly the serotonergic withdrawal syndrome that occurs with strongly serotonergic antidepressants, and the withdrawal syndrome from benzodiazepines. Our clinical experience supports our knowledge that patients taking short half-life compounds are much more vulnerable to withdrawal phenomena than those taking long half-life compounds. Short half-life antidepressants such as paroxetine and venlafaxine cause many more serotonergic withdrawal symptoms than long half-life compounds such as fluoxetine. When stopped quickly, short half-life benzodiazepines such as alprazolam cause more withdrawal symptomatology than longer half-life compounds such as chlordiazepoxide, diazepam or chlorazepate. This scientific evidence is solid, and knowledge of a compound's half-life is necessary in order to assess whether a patient's reaction to a missed dose is likely to be withdrawal-related.

Where our science is limited is in relation to the second element – the propensity for a particular patient to have a return of symptoms quickly when a medication is missed. Some patients are quite vulnerable to symptomatic return, and will become anxious, depressed or psychotic quickly, sometimes even after just one missed dose. Other patients can go several days or even weeks without obvious reaction to missing regular dosing. What biological (or psychological) underpinnings cause one patient to react this way and another not, are unclear. Only past clinical experience with a particular patient can help the clinician to decide how vulnerable that patient is likely to be. While each clinician should encourage patients to be conscientious and diligent about taking their medication regularly, what happens in reality with a specific patient is quite variable.

Parenteral medications

The vast majority of psychotropic medications are dispensed in oral form – pills, capsules, liquid preparations, or, for some medication, as dissolving lozenges. Intramuscular dispensing of medication is used in the following circumstances:

1   For immediate behavioral control in acutely psychotic or manic patients. This usually involves the use of an antipsychotic, a benzodiazepine, or both.
2   For the acute treatment of extrapyramidal side effects (usually from traditional antipsychotics), anticholinergic medication such as benztropine, an antihistamine such as diphenhydramine, or a benzodiazepine may be used intramuscularly.

Box 6.8 Clinical tip

At this time, there are no intramuscular or intravenous preparations of antidepressants or stimulants. Intramuscular dosing is seldom used in an outpatient setting except for the depot antipsychotics. The practical use of intravenous medication in mental health treatment is rare, since those patients who are agitated enough theoretically to benefit from the direct intravenous injection are often physically too disruptive to permit intravenous access to be established.

Information and tips for prescribing practice

Knowledge about size, expiration dates and other pill facts can often allay a patient's fears or answer questions during follow-up sessions.

Pill size

The amount of medication in a typical pill or capsule will fit on the head of a pin. Most of the substance of a pill or capsule is composed of inactive elements, including filler and the capsule used to contain the granules or powder. The manufacturer can, therefore, determine the size of the pill rather arbitrarily. The size of the pill has no relationship to its potency or the amount of medication contained within. Larger pills or capsules are larger so that they are easier to handle. Their size does not necessarily reflect strength or the number of milligrams in the dose.

Milligrams of medicine

Patients often confuse the number of milligrams in a pill with its potency, assuming that a 500-mg pill is considerably stronger than a 1-mg pill. The clinician may wish to explain that with psychotropics, as with many other medications, the number of milligrams in two *different medicines* is not usually comparable. Many psychotropics have a dosage range that is a fraction of 1 mg to several mg, while other medications have typical therapeutic dosages measured in thousands of milligrams. The effective range of dosage is unique to each medication, and has no bearing on its strength. When comparing capsules of *the same medication*, however, higher milligram doses are proportional to strength; that is, 100 mg of medicine A is twice as strong as 50 mg of medicine A.

Expiration dates

Patients often ask how long their medications will stay "good," particularly if they use a medication only infrequently, and may have it on hand for a lengthy period of time. A drug's expiration date is generally 2 years after it has been sealed in the container by the manufacturer. The projection of continued stability to this date is based on a closed and protected environment, and no longer applies once the original container is opened. As long as the medication has not come into contact with water, been partially dissolved, or been exposed to excessive heat or the sun (for example, left on a car dashboard or in a glove compartment for a prolonged period), medications remain active. Most medications, however, will become less potent with time. The rate of declining activity correlates with many factors, but most tablets or capsules retain most of their potency for at least 1 year after the expiration date, even after the container has been opened. The clinician can reassure patients that office samples or prescription pills will retain the majority of their potency for at least 1 year beyond the expiration date. However, any pills exposed to water or excessive sunlight, or not kept in brown-shaded pharmacy pill containers, run the risk of earlier deterioration. Pills that have become wet have extremely variable potencies. When a pill is exposed to water or other liquids, it often becomes impossible to know how much of the active medication ingredient remains in a partially dissolved pill, and such items should generally be thrown away. Psychotropic medications do not "go bad," transform into other chemicals or become toxic with time.

Traveling when on psychotropic medications

Patients traveling away from home, particularly if they are at a distance or in developing countries, benefit from a simple precaution: tell them to pack two separate stores of medication, each containing enough medication to last for the entire trip. One set is to be packed in the luggage, and one to be kept on the person. In the event that the personal supply is lost, there is a second supply in the luggage; in the event that the luggage does not reach the intended destination, the patient has a full supply on their person. Having a second supply drastically simplifies the situation when the patient's supply of medicine is lost, stolen, knocked into the toilet by the hotel maid, or meets some other fate.

While many psychotropic medications are commonly available in most parts of the developed world, there are some countries where specific medications will not be available or will be significantly difficult to obtain. Since patients can have significant symptom breakthrough or rebound physical symptomatology when they stop their medication abruptly, the simple double-packing precaution virtually ensures that they will not need to undergo needless discomfort while traveling. This precaution will turn out to be unnecessary 98 percent of the time, but in the event it does become necessary, it can be extremely helpful.

Traveling with psychotropic medications, even in less developed countries, is generally not a problem at customs or immigration. It may be helpful, however, to carry psychotropic medications in the original, pharmacy-labeled containers, rather than putting a large number of pills in an unmarked container with no identification. This is a simple precaution that further reinforces that the medication is a validly prescribed medication rather than some other substance.

References

1 Semouh A *et al.* (2018) Psychotropic medication non-adherence and associated factors among adult patients with major psychiatric disorders: a protocol for a systematic review. *Systematic Reviews* 7: 10. doi: 10.1186/s13643-018-0676-y

2 Gebeyehu D *et al.* (2019) Psychotropic medication non-adherence among patients with severe mental disorder. *BMC Research Notes* 12: article number: 102.

3 Bulloch A *et al.* (2010) Non-adherence with psychotropic medications in the general population. *Social Psychiatry* 45(1): 47–56. doi: 10.1007/s00127-009-0041-5

4 Parks J (2019) *Key Substance Use and Mental Health Indicators in the United States: Results from the 2019 National Survey on Drug Use and Health*, available at: www.samhsa.gov/data/sites/default/files/reports/rpt29393/2019NSDUHFFRPDFWHTML/2019NSDUHFFR1PDFW090120.pdf

5 American Medical Association (2015) 8 reasons patients don't take their medications, available at: www.ama-assn.org/delivering-care/patient-support-advocacy/8-reasons-patients-dont-take-their-medications

6 CentralLogic (2017) Medication noncompliance: why won't patients take their meds?, available at: www.ensocare.com/knowledge-center/medication-noncompliance-why-wont-patients-take-their-meds

7 Hugtenburg J *et al.* (2013) Definitions, variants, and causes of nonadherence with medication: a challenge for tailored interventions. *Patient Preference and Adherence* 7: 675–682. doi: 10.2147/PPA.S29549

8 Parmentier BL (2019) Second-generation long-acting injectable antipsychotics: a practical guide. *Current Psychiatry* 19(3): 24–32.

7 Medication, psychotherapy and "What else helps?"

- The first session dilemma   103
- Patient's preference   104
- What can medication do?   105
- Who prescribes psychotropic medication?   105
- Other adjunctive therapies   107
- Beyond medication and helping the patient stay well   107
- Work–life balance   109
- References   111

With the introduction of psychoactive medications in the 1950s, and with their increasing usage over the subsequent decades, several issues have emerged regarding the interrelationship of psychotropic medications and psychotherapy ("talking" therapy with any of a variety of formats and orientations). These include theoretical issues about the value of medication in the overall treatment of a patient, as well as the practical issues of whether a psychotherapist can also be a medication provider.

During the 1960s and 1970s a battle raged between the "talking therapy" supporters and the "biological" school as to which method would best treat a person with psychological problems. Psychotherapists in the "therapy only" camp saw medications as intrusive, unnecessary and even harmful. Their belief was that relief was provided by talking with patients, understanding their problems and assisting in resolving developmental conflicts and early life traumas. Within this view, medications were at best marginally tolerated Band-Aids that missed the true nature of treatment and cure.

Some biologically oriented mental health professionals, on the other hand, began to assume that medication was the way to change brain functioning and that biological change was the only method leading to symptom relief. If the right combination of medication and/or medications could be found, the patient could eventually be "cured." In this framework, verbal therapy was superfluous and of relatively little value. Such clinicians also began to discount the importance of the prescriber–patient relationship, feeling that the only important mechanism was the chemical effect of the medication.

While vestiges of this debate remain, most clinicians now see value for both medication and psychotherapy. Both have importance, and both can result in symptom relief. Often the combination of medication and verbal therapy is the most efficient route to rapid symptom relief.[1–4]

The first session dilemma

Even if a patient is first screened over the telephone, an initial evaluative session can present the mental health clinician with a clinical decision. Is this to be a psychotherapy or medication evaluation? In general, this dilemma should be resolved in favor of evaluating for and prescribing medication at the earliest opportunity. While there is always a possibility that initial psychotherapeutic interventions may have a significant impact, even targeted verbal psychotherapy typically takes several sessions or longer to be significantly useful. On the other hand, medication can, for many patients, make significant and rapid inroads into symptomatology. Anti-anxiety, mood-stabilizing and antipsychotic medications can often be effective within a matter of days. As medication levels are slowly raised, psychotherapeutic interventions can then also be undertaken.

Another factor favoring early medication intervention is that psychological distress is often accompanied by (or has as an intrinsic feature) difficulty with concentration, attention and other cognitive functions. Full cognitive focus is often necessary to participate in and profit fully from verbal interventions. Therefore, if medication can positively affect the patient's cognitive focus, attention and energy level, patients can better utilize psychotherapy and be more involved in their own treatment.

In the course of the initial evaluation, if it appears that the patient is suffering from a condition that is likely to respond to medication and the patient is agreeable, the evaluation session should be structured as described in Chapter 3 to obtain the necessary information that can lead to medication prescription. If the clinician is in doubt or senses resistance on the patient's part regarding medication, it may be helpful to engage the patient in the decision and together negotiate how the process should proceed.

Box 7.1 Talking to patients

After you begin to hear the patient's initial complaints, one way to engage the patient in being an active part of this medication/psychotherapy decision is to say: *"I am hearing that you are experiencing … [list the target symptoms] and having trouble with your [job, marriage, friendships, etc.]. I believe your symptoms may be helped with medication. In order to safely choose medication and begin it today, I need to gather some medical information. This will mean we won't be able to spend as much time talking about the problematic environmental issues in your life today. I know these issues are important to you, but we will not have time to focus on both. What do you think would be most helpful?"*

If the patient agrees to evaluation for medication, proceed with the elements described in Chapter 3. If the patient opts for discussing family/environmental/interpersonal issues, it is seldom helpful to insist on medication until the patient has had the opportunity to deal with these concerns even if it requires several visits to do so. If you feel strongly about the probable positive benefit of medication, an agreement can be made to follow the patient's preference during this visit. At the end of the session, state that you would like to discuss the medication issue at the next session and mention the reasons why you believe this might be helpful. This allows the patient to have an opportunity to mull over the idea in the interim.

Patient's preference

At times, patients come to the clinician with a clear agenda in mind for the type of treatment they desire – medication alone or psychotherapy alone. In this case, it is not unreasonable initially to accede to the patient's wishes, even if combination therapy may ultimately be seen as desirable. Patients who have verbal therapy as a goal may show considerable resistance to starting medication. If the clinician automatically launches into the medication evaluation and prescription, the patient will feel that important issues are being ignored or overlooked. Once psychotherapy has begun and a trusting relationship has been established, and if symptoms persist, the suggestion of medication may be better received.

Likewise, patients who present requesting medication may be reluctant to undertake psychotherapy until they have evaluated the benefit of medication alone. Patients who believe in the primary value of medication are often resistant to, and apprehensive about, entering into a verbal therapy relationship and revealing personal history. If the medication management relationship with the prescribing clinician proceeds well, patients may be open to entering into a more in-depth psychotherapy. Alternatively, if the clinician is able to spend 20–30 minutes in medication follow-up sessions with the patient, often the treatment evolves into talking therapy over time without ever being identified overtly. When the clinician is non-judgmental, accepting and supportive, patients begin to trust and confide as important conflictual issues emerge for discussion.

It is a fundamental premise of this book that a combination of both forms of treatment – psychotropic medication and psychotherapy of various kinds – will not only be helpful, but also should be instituted for many patients. While not all patients will opt for both therapies, it is the task of the clinician to reinforce that a combination of verbal and medication therapy is the preferred treatment. If, in fact, the patient will only accept a recommendation for one of the two modalities, it is generally easier to accept the patient's request and institute either medication or psychotherapy as a beginning point for treatment. In this case, *it is essential that the patient be re-evaluated in 4 to 6 weeks to assess whether this single modality (i.e., medication alone or psychotherapy alone) is making significant progress.* If so, it is not unreasonable to continue this program. If the patient is not significantly improved or may even be worse, the practitioner should insist on beginning the previously unused form of treatment

While it is the duty of the clinician to recommend combined therapy when appropriate, little is lost in the treatment of most outpatients with mild to moderate symptoms by taking a "wait and re-evaluate" approach while beginning the type of therapy the patient prefers.

The introduction of medication therapy may become necessary for a patient involved in ongoing psychotherapy who experiences a sudden life crisis. Crises such as a death, job change, serious illness, financial reversal, separation or divorce can significantly upset the equilibrium of the patient's life, and verbal therapy alone may be insufficient. The introduction of medication at that time may be a useful and welcome intervention. The reverse can also be true. A successfully treated "medication only" patient may find, in the face of a crisis, that more frequent active verbal intervention and support is needed at such a time. Individual, couples or family therapy can provide the necessary help to stabilize the crisis situation for a time-limited period.

What can medication do?

A continuing and evolving area of research is the question of what can, or cannot, be treated with medication. While illness symptoms involving behavior, affect, anxiety and mood can often be positively modified by medication, some symptoms remain stubbornly resistive to medication effect. Also there are many aspects of what we label as "personality" that cannot be changed or modified significantly with medication. Even among psychopharmacologists, there is significant debate as to whether it would be useful or desirable to alter personality structure. It is the premise of this book that the major mental illnesses – depression, bipolar disorder, anxiety disorders and psychosis – involve symptoms that profoundly and negatively affect the way people feel and function. As practitioners, we can and should treat the symptoms of these illnesses in an attempt to help the patient. The borderline between treating these symptoms and treating underlying personality remains blurred. Although some may fear that we will soon cross (or have already crossed) the line into areas of the human mind that we should not be modifying, we are still far from being able satisfactorily to treat many of the symptoms that are clearly disabling to our patients. To fail to continue to treat illness as we refine the borderline between illness and personality ignores our calling as healthcare professionals, to heal.

Who prescribes psychotropic medication?

When psychotropic medication emerged into clinical practice during the 1950s and 1960s, it was the province of the psychiatrist to prescribe. Many changes in the medical and mental health landscape have occurred which alter the way psychotropic medication is provided. These include:

- growing demand for mental health prescription
- fewer psychiatrists to meet this demand, particularly in underserved locations and populations
- increasing safety and ease of prescribing newer psychotropics
- emerging comfort of primary care providers in prescribing psychotropics
- growth in the number of advanced practice nurse prescribers, both in primary care and in mental health
- financial pressure to provide mental health care in the most cost-effective manner.

There are now three common delivery systems for provision of psychotropic medication and mental health therapies:

1 a single person (psychiatrist or advanced practice mental health nurse with prescriptive authority) who provides both mental health therapy and medication
2 a non-medical psychotherapist (psychologist, social worker, counselor or other mental health professional) who provides mental health counseling and therapy, with medication provided by a mental health specialist (psychiatrist or advanced practice mental health nurse)
3 a non-medical psychotherapist providing psychotherapy with a primary care provider (family practice physician/advanced practice nurse, internist, OB/GYN or other medical specialist) prescribing the psychotropic medication.

Each modality has advantages and disadvantages, and these are listed in Tables 7.1, 7.2 and 7.3.

While much philosophical debate remains as to the desirability of who should prescribe, some communities simply do not have sufficient numbers of mental health prescribers to provide this service, even if that is desired. In other communities, multiple variations of the above three delivery systems co-exist.

Table 7.1 One-stop shopping – psychiatrist or advanced practice mental health nurse only

Advantages	Disadvantages
Simple, efficient for patient	Most expensive method of delivering medication and psychotherapy
Unified treatment approach	
Works well for patients with a complicated psychotropic medication regimen	Mental health specialists may be less expert in the evaluation/treatment of other medical conditions

Table 7.2 Non-medical psychotherapist with mental health specialist prescribing (psychiatrist or advanced practitioner nurse)

Advantages	Disadvantages
Less expensive than "one-stop shopping"	Requires good communication between the two parties, or mixed messages to the patient may result
Allows specialists to do what they do best	May be inconvenient for patient to see two different practitioners
Better than psychotherapist plus primary care provider (PCP) for complicated mental health problems, poorly responding patients or a frequently changing medication regimen	

Table 7.3 Non-medical psychotherapist with primary care provider prescribing psychotropics

Advantages	Disadvantages
Allows for smoother integration of mental healthcare for a patient with multiple medical complaints	Requires frequent communication between the providers to ensure unified treatment
Less costly prescription method than using a mental health specialist prescriber	PCP may not have most expert psychotropic knowledge about complicated mental health conditions, combination treatments, unresponsive patients or a regimen that requires frequent adjustment
Easy access to serum levels/laboratory tests	
Useful for patients on a stable medication regimen with minimal side effects	
Can permit simpler access to insurance formularies	May be inconvenient for the patient to see two different practitioners

Other adjunctive therapies

The majority of this chapter has focused on the two primary mental health treatment modalities – psychotropic medication and psychotherapy. Over the past 50 years, multiple other treatments have emerged as useful modalities in general or with specific clinical diagnoses. While discussion of the indications, evidence-based effectiveness and side effects of each of these modalities is beyond the goals of this text, prescribers will wish to consider whether their use may be beneficial alone or in combination with medication. Medications could be safely combined with any of the treatments listed alphabetically in Table 7.4, although each instance should be evaluated individually.

Beyond medication and helping the patient stay well

When psychotropic medications are prescribed, patients often ask, "What else can I do, besides take the medication"[5-6] – that is to say, are there any lifestyle changes that may promote recovery and maintain wellness?

While it would be helpful if a specific dietary regimen were beneficial in mental health treatment, numerous studies over several decades have failed to demonstrate that specific diets, or specific dietary elements, have a major primary role to play in psychiatric wellness positively or negatively. That being said, the Mediterranean Diet (see Table 7.5 below)[5] has been associated consistently with improved general health and improved mental health in particular.[6]

Studies of the beneficial effects of *exercise* are numerous and results are generally consistent.[7-9] In children,[10] adults,[11] seniors,[12] men[13] and women,[14] moderate amounts of vigorous exercise can improve mood and anxiety. Physical activity can increase strength and endurance, maintain bone density, improve cardiovascular capacity, lower blood pressure and heighten the patient's sense of well-being. Clinician attention to the patient's lifestyle, with a focus on physical activity, is therefore clearly warranted.

Table 7.4 Mental health treatments and modalities that might be combined with medication

- Acupuncture
- Assertiveness training
- Aversive conditioning
- Behavioral deconditioning
- Behavioral dialectical therapy
- Transcranial magnetic stimulation (TMS)
- Deep muscle relaxation
- Electroconvulsive therapy (ECT)
- Exposure therapy
- Eye movement desensitization and reprocessing (EMDR)
- Family therapy
- Gestalt therapy
- Group therapy
- Light box usage
- Mindfulness meditation
- Music, art, drama therapy
- Psychoanalysis
- Social skills training
- Stress management techniques
- Vagus nerve stimulation

Table 7.5 Mediterranean Diet

- Starches should consist of whole grains and legumes
- Fruits and vegetables can be eaten without limit
- Focus on eating fatty fish, like salmon or albacore tuna, in place of red meat
- Add in healthy fats, like raw nuts and olive oil
- Enjoy sweets and wine in moderation

Source: Mediterranean diet: a heart-healthy eating plan, available at: www.mayoclinic.org/healthy-lifestyle/nutrition-and-healthy-eating/in-depth/mediterranean-diet/art-20047801

Table 7.6 General Dietary Recommendations

- *Eat more fruits and vegetables.* Aim for 7 to 10 servings a day of fruit and vegetables.
- *Opt for whole grains.* Switch to whole-grain bread, cereal and pasta. Experiment with other whole grains, such as bulgur and farro.
- *Use healthy fats.* Try olive oil as a replacement for butter when cooking. Instead of putting butter or margarine on bread, try dipping it in flavored olive oil. Raw nuts.
- *Eat more seafood.* Eat fish twice a week. Fresh or water-packed tuna, salmon, trout, mackerel and herring are healthy choices. Grilled fish tastes good and requires little cleanup. Avoid deep-fried fish.
- *Reduce red meat.* Substitute fish, poultry or beans for meat. If you eat meat, make sure it's lean and keep portions small.
- *Enjoy some dairy.* Eat low-fat Greek or plain yogurt and small amounts of a variety of cheeses.
- *Spice it up.* Herbs and spices boost flavor and lessen the need for salt.
- *Red wine in moderation*

In general, avoid:[5]
- refined grains, such as white bread, white pasta, and pizza dough containing white flour
- refined oils, which include canola oil and soybean oil
- foods with added sugars, such as pastries, sodas and candies
- deli meats, hot dogs and other processed meats
- processed or packaged foods

Most patients will benefit from a recommendation to increase the amount and frequency of their physical activity no matter what their baseline is. However, contrary to popular opinion, it has not been demonstrated that even vigorous physical exercise, alone or in combination with diet, can successfully treat severely mentally ill patients. While there are a multitude of benefits to including exercise as part of an overall regimen for general good health, it should not be assumed that exercise alone can substitute for more specific treatments such as psychotherapy and/or medication. Recommendations for increasing exercise should include doing so gradually, rather than suddenly, to avoid injury in the previously sedentary patient. Suggest that the patient work up to a goal of an exercise regimen of 30 minutes per day three times per week.[15]

Other than these factors, in our current state of knowledge, diet plays a relatively small role in mental health treatment other than in maintaining balanced health and nutrition, with emphasis on elements of the Mediterranean Diet as shown in Table 7.6. Vitamin supplements have failed to be shown as a primary treatment for mental illness. Except for vitamin supplements prescribed for the alcoholic patient, the significantly malnourished patient and the pregnant woman, most psychiatric patients do not require additional vitamins. Many of the preparations sold by health-food stores claiming to be helpful for depression, anxiety or stress have little solid evidence to support their use, and can be quite costly (see also Chapter 11).

Work–life balance

Helping patients to assess and, when necessary, manage their workload, job expectations and *work schedule* can also help them get well and stay well.[16–17] Appropriate diagnosis and targeted medication cannot overcome excessive work hours, failure to take breaks during the workday, postponing or eliminating vacations, or trying to please an overly demanding boss. It may be useful to discuss priorities with patients such that they can realistically meet their financial needs while balancing their work lives. Although assessment of the patient's schedule and work environment may be time-consuming, the beneficial results are great. Failure to do so may result in the difference between successful and failed treatment.

Practical suggestions from the practitioner can include the following elements:[18]

Married to your work? Consider the cost

It can be tempting to rack up hours at work, especially if you're trying to earn a promotion or manage an ever-increasing workload or simply keep your head above water. If you're spending most of your time working, though, your home life will suffer. Consider the consequences of poor work–life balance:

- *Fatigue.* When you're tired, your ability to work productively and think clearly might decrease, which could take a toll on your professional reputation or lead to dangerous or costly mistakes.
- *Poor health.* Stress is associated with adverse effects on the immune system and can worsen the symptoms you experience from any medical condition. Stress also puts you at risk of substance abuse.
- *Lost time with friends and loved ones.* If you're working too much, you might miss important family events or milestones. This can leave you feeling left out and might harm relationships with your loved ones. It's also difficult to nurture friendships if you're always working.
- *Increased expectations.* If you regularly work extra hours, you might be given even more responsibility which could lead to additional concerns and challenges.

Strike a better work–life balance

As long as you're working, juggling the demands of career and personal life will probably be an ongoing challenge. But if you can learn both to set limits and look after yourself, you can achieve the work–life balance that's best for you.

Setting limits

You can't manufacture time. If you don't set limits, then work or other obligations can leave you with no time for the activities and relationships you enjoy. Consider these ideas:

- *Manage your time.* Cut or delegate activities you don't enjoy or can't handle – or share your concerns and possible solutions with your employer or others. Organize household tasks efficiently, such as running errands in batches or doing a load of laundry every day; don't save all the laundry for your day off. Do what needs to be done and let the rest go.
- *Make a list.* Put family events on a weekly calendar, and keep a daily to-do list at home and at work. Having a plan helps you maintain focus. When you don't have a plan, it's easy to be enveloped by the plans and priorities of others.
- *Learn to say no.* Whether it's a co-worker asking you to spearhead an extra project or your child's teacher asking you to organize a class party, remember that it's OK to respectfully say no. When you stop accepting tasks out of guilt or a false sense of obligation, you'll have more time for activities that are meaningful to you.
- *Leave work at work.* With the technology to connect to anyone at any time from virtually anywhere, there might be no boundary between work and home unless you create it. Make a conscious decision to separate work time from personal time, and if necessary, discuss this with your supervisor.
- *Reduce e-mail access.* Check e-mails no more than three times a day – late morning, early afternoon and late in the day. If you access e-mail first thing in the morning, you tend to focus on and respond to other people's issues rather than being pro-active about your own needs.
- *Take advantage of your options.* Ask your employer about flex hours, a compressed work week, job sharing, telecommuting or other scheduling flexibility. The more control you have over your hours, the less stressed you're likely to be.
- *Try to shorten commitments and minimize interruptions.* Most people can sustain a maximum level of concentration for no more than 90 minutes. After that, the ability to retain information decreases dramatically. When interrupted during a task, you need double or triple the time of the interruption to regain full concentration on your task.

Caring for yourself

A healthy lifestyle is essential to coping with stress and to achieving work–life balance. Try to:

- *Eat a healthy diet.* The Mediterranean Diet – which emphasizes fresh fruits and vegetables and lean protein – enhances the ability to retain knowledge as well as improving stamina and well-being.
- *Get enough sleep.* Lack of sleep increases stress. It's also important to avoid using personal electronic devices, such as tablets, just before bedtime. The blue light emitted by these devices decreases your level of melatonin, the hormone associated with sleep.
- *Make time for fun and relaxation.* Set aside time each day for an activity that you enjoy, such as practicing yoga or reading. Better yet, discover activities you can do with your partner, family or friends – such as hiking, dancing or taking cooking classes.
- *Volunteer.* It's important not to over-schedule yourself. But research indicates that volunteering can contribute to a greater sense of work–life balance. Selective

volunteering might lower your levels of burnout and stress and boost your emotional and social well-being.

- *Bolster your support system.* At work, join forces with co-workers who can cover for you – and vice versa – when family conflicts arise. At home, enlist trusted friends and loved ones to pitch in with child care or household responsibilities when you need to work overtime or travel.

If your employer offers an employee assistance program, take advantage of available services.

Remember, striking a healthy work–life balance isn't a one-off project. Creating a work–life balance is a continuous process as your family, interests and work life change. Periodically examine your priorities and make changes, if necessary, to make sure you're keeping on track.

References

1 Sammons M (2015) Combining psychotropic medications and psychotherapy generally leads to improved outcomes and therefore reduces the overall cost of care, available at: www.apadivisions.org/division-55/publications/tablet/2015/04/combininations
2 Cuijpers P (2014) Adding psychotherapy to antidepressant medication in depression and anxiety disorders: a meta-analysis. *World Psychiatry* 13(1): 56–67. doi: 10.1002/wps.20089
3 Friedman MA *et al.* (2006) Combined psychotherapy and pharmacotherapy for the treatment of major depressive disorder, available at: https://pdfs.semanticscholar.org/1245/ff1a6f8b089 26e51a3caad528372dbadcd95.pdf
4 Otto MW *et al.* (2008) Combined psychotherapy and pharmacotherapy for mood and anxiety disorders in adults: review and analysis. *Clinical Psychology: Science and Practice* 12(1): 72–86, available at: https://doi.org/10.1093/clipsy.bpi009
5 Schultz R (2018) These women treated their anxiety with food: here's what they ate, available at: www.healthline.com/health/best-diets-for-mental-health#3
6 Lassale C *et al.* (2018) Healthy dietary indices and risk of depressive outcomes: a systematic review and meta-analysis of observational studies. *Molecular Psychiatry* 24(7): 965–986. doi: 10.1038/s41380-018-0237-8
7 Salmon P (2001) Effects of physical exercise on anxiety, depression and sensitivity to stress: a unifying theory. *Clinical Psychology Review* 21(1): 33–61.
8 Sexton H *et al.* (2001) How are mood and exercise related? Results from the Finnmark study. *Social Psychiatry and Psychiatric Epidemiology* 236(7): 348–353.
9 Dimeo F *et al.* (2001) Benefits from aerobic exercise in patients with major depression: a pilot study. *British Journal of Sports Medicine* 35(2): 114–117.
10 Williamson D *et al.* (2001) Mood change through physical exercise in nine- to ten-year-old children. *Perceptual and Motor Skills* 93(1): 311–316.
11 Toskovic NN (2001) Alterations in selected measure of mood with a single bout of dynamic Taekwondo exercise in college-age students. *Perceptual and Motor Skills* 92(3 Pt. 2): 1031–1038.
12 George BJ and Goldberg N (2001) The benefits of exercise in geriatric women. *American Journal of Geriatric Cardiology* 10(5): 260–263.
13 Kiernan M *et al.* (2001) Men gain additional psychological benefits by adding exercise to a weight-loss program. *Obesity Research* 9(12): 770–777.
14 Lee RE *et al.* (2001) A prospective analysis of the relationship between walking and mood in sedentary ethnic minority women. *Women & Health* 32(4): 1–15. doi: 10.1300/J013v32n04_01

15 Hassmen P *et al.* (2000) Physical exercise and psychological well-being: a population study in Finland. *Preventive Medicine* 30(1): 17–25.

16 Mental Health Foundation (n.d.) Work–life balance, available at: www.mentalhealth.org.uk/a-to-z/w/work-life-bal

17 Mental Health America (2021) Work life balance, available at: www.mhanational.org/work-life-balance

18 Work–life balance: tips to regain control, available at: www.mayoclinic.org/healthy-lifestyle/adult-health/in-depth/work-life-balance/art-20048134

8   Stopping medication

- When to stop a psychotropic   114
- Tapering medications   116
- "When I stopped, I got worse"   116
- Benzodiazepine withdrawal   118
- Management of discontinuation syndromes   122
- Relapse versus discontinuation syndrome   122
- When to stop medication more quickly   123
- New episode or relapse?   124
- Side effects pass quickly   124
- Unplanned stoppages of medication   124
- Complex discontinuation   126
- Reference   126

One of the first questions patients ask, often before they even begin medication, is "How long do I have to take this?" Beyond a straightforward request for information, the patient may be asking what the clinician's viewpoint is on the commonly held myth that once a person starts on a psychotropic medication, it must be continued for life. At other times, the question may be based on the assumption that there will be a number of side effects to "bear with," and the patient wants to know how long the period of discomfort will be. These questions are an opportunity for the prescriber to begin to discuss the "game plan" for medication treatment.

There are relatively few patients who are started on medication and continue indefinitely without at least one medication-free trial to observe for relapse. While, in fact, a percentage of patients do need medication on a chronic or life-long basis, this is recommended only when the clinician is armed with the results of at least one trial off the medication. *During a first trial of starting medication, there are almost no historical or response data that will accurately predict whether or not a patient will need to stay on medication indefinitely.* Severity of illness, length of symptoms prior to treatment, length of time needed for response to medication or family history of emotional illness cannot accurately foretell whether a patient will require long-term medication. However, *during a first medication trial it is not sound clinical practice to automatically assume that chronic, long-term medication will be necessary.* The number of previously documented illness episodes may suggest that relapse is likely at some point, but not always *when* this will occur.

The one useful predictor available to the clinician during a second or subsequent trial of medication is the result of previous trials off medication. If a patient has been on medication for this condition, tried being off medication on several occasions and relapsed quickly into similar symptomatology with each stoppage, there is a strong likelihood that it will happen again.

Box 8.1 Talking to patients

When a patient, during a first medicine trial, asks "Will I be on this forever?" the answer is invariably: *"We do not know yet and I assume not. Here is how we will find out…"* followed by discussing the regimen outlined here and in Chapter 5. Knowing that he or she will be taken off medicine at a certain time in the future will usually satisfy the patient so that the trial can be started.

The clinician can and should *involve the patient in the decision of when discontinuation of medication is attempted.* Some measure of knowledge that the clinician has flexibility as to when this trial will occur goes a long way toward initially securing the patient's adherence.

A significant number of patients who come to the treatment setting resistant and skeptical about medication may change their mind when they notice the positive results that the medicine achieves. When the issue of stopping the medication is ultimately raised, they may actually be quite apprehensive and hesitant about stopping. In such patients, the principle of a medication discontinuation is not abandoned, but a short delay is not unreasonable, if necessary, to help them deal with their apprehension.

When to stop a psychotropic

If possible, do not attempt to stop a psychotropic medication in the midst of a major life event (see Table 8.1). Stopping at the same time as a job change, final exams, marriage, divorce, changing residences, moving to a different town, taking a promotion or undergoing other significant life stress leaves both the patient and the clinician uncertain as to the cause if relapse does occur. Did the symptoms recur from stopping the medication, or from this significant life stress? In general, it is much better to find a relative lull in the patient's life to attempt medication stoppage. Then, if any symptoms do recur, these can be more clearly related to stopping the medication. If the patient is in simultaneous psychotherapy while taking medication, it is also preferable not to stop psychotherapy and medication at the same time for similar reasons. Faced with major life stressors, it is preferable to err on the side of continuing a few months "too long" and perhaps finding out that the patient could have done without medication, rather than discontinuing medication "too soon" and creating a significant crisis in a patient's life, which is already altered by the current stressor.

In today's society, there are patients for whom a comfortable "smooth spot" in their life cannot be found. Even after several delays, their lives continue to be busy and hectic. Eventually, for these patients, the patient and clinician must decide on an appropriate stopping time even if it is not ideal. On occasion, this can be as long as several years from the initiation of medication.

Table 8.1 Issues related to stopping medication

When?

- Usually after 6–12 months of *remission*
- No simultaneous big life changes
- Include the patient in the decision

How?

- Gradual taper
- Speed of the taper depends on current dose, and the length of administration
- Assess the patient's feelings

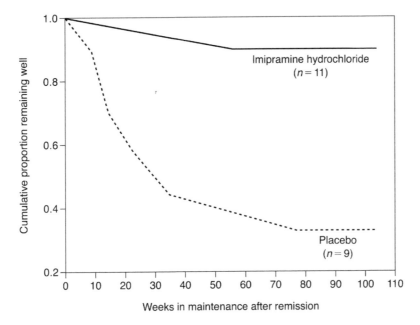

Figure 8.1 Survival analysis for maintenance therapies in the recurrent depression extended study.

Source: Berwian IM (2017) Predicting relapse after antidepressant withdrawal – a systematic review. *Psychological Medicine* 47(3): 426–437. doi: 10.1017/S0033291716002580

Note: Difference between the two groups, $p = 0.006$ by the Mantel-Cox test.

With depression, there is statistical evidence[1] to help us decide the earliest possible time to stop medication. The rate of relapse curve (i.e., the percentage of patients who relapse when medication is stopped) flattens out 32 weeks (about 8 months) after remission (see Figure 8.1).

As can be seen, the rate of relapse is minimally greater at 10 months or 12 months than it is at 8 months. This suggests that for mild to moderate depression, "the earliest opportunity" when a decision to stop medication could be made is 6 months from the time of remission. If a patient has had a significant major depression or prolonged response time to full recovery, a longer time on medication is desirable. Continuing medication for 9–12 months *from the time of remission* (not the time of starting medication) will allow the patient sufficient opportunity for his or her life to recover from the disruption of a significant depressive episode. These timeframes likewise apply to panic disorder, generalized anxiety disorder and social anxiety disorder. Although the statistical evidence is far less complete, medications for a first episode of bipolar disorder and psychosis conditions, which tend to be quite disruptive to the patient's life generally, should be continued for a minimum of 9–12 months.

Tapering medications

The brain is sensitive to changes in blood levels of psychotropic medications. With a few exceptions (see below), medication should always be gradually tapered rather than discontinued suddenly. The speed of such a taper will depend on the patient's *dose* and *duration* of medication administration (see Table 8.2). When faced with a choice, a slower taper is almost always preferable to and safer than a rapid one.

In general, the higher the dose of medication and the longer the patient has been on the medication, the more gradual the taper. For someone who has been on a small dose of medication for a short period of time, a taper may not be necessary.

While this overall recommendation is appropriate in the vast majority of patients, it can be modified depending on the special circumstances of an individual patient. These can include patient feelings about, and reaction to, the initial taper. A very hesitant patient or one who shows a greater than expected reaction to the initial lowering of doses may benefit from a slower taper.

"When I stopped, I got worse"

Most psychotropics are not habit forming, and do not cause "withdrawal" in the traditional sense. Some medications, particularly some antidepressants, do cause a discontinuation syndrome (which is a set of primarily physical symptoms) if the medicine is stopped suddenly. It is important to recognize this syndrome, both to educate and reassure the patient, and to treat it when necessary. Particularly when they occur without warning, the symptoms of discontinuation syndrome can be significantly distressing to patients. The medications that do, and do not, cause a discontinuation syndrome are listed in Tables 8.3 and 8.4, respectively. Clues that a discontinuation syndrome is occurring are listed in Table 8.5.

Table 8.2 Discontinuing medications

Low to moderate dose/short administration (less than 6 months)
- Decrease by 25–50% of maintenance dose
- Every 1–2 weeks

High dose/long administration (greater than 6 months)
- Decrease by 10–25% of maintenance dose
- Every 2–4 weeks

Table 8.3 Psychotropics that may cause discontinuation syndromes

---

- SSRIs, particularly short half-life compounds such as paroxetine and venlafaxine
- Benzodiazepines
- TCAs
- MAOIs ("REM Rebound" with vivid dreaming)

Table 8.4 Psychotropics that do **not** cause discontinuation syndromes

- Mood stabilizers, including lithium, lamotrigine, valproic acid and carbamazepine
- Antipsychotics, both traditional and atypical

Table 8.5 Tip-offs that a discontinuation syndrome may be occurring

- A recent stoppage of a medication has preceded the symptoms, especially if it was done suddenly and rapidly. Discontinuation syndrome occasionally happens *during* a taper of medication when the dose is decreased significantly.
- Patient has been on the medication for at least 5 weeks.
- Onset of symptoms within 1–3 days of dose decrease or stoppage.
- Symptoms go away, or are substantially improved, in 7–10 days.
- Symptoms remit if the medication is restarted or increased in dose.

Table 8.6 Symptoms of an SSRI discontinuation syndrome

- A Agitation, anxiety, dizziness, light-headedness, disequilibrium
- B Balance problems, bad dreams
- C Concentration problems
- D Dizziness, diarrhea, nausea, vomiting
- E Electric shock-like sensations
- F Flu-like symptoms

Source: Haddad P (1998) The SSRI discontinuation syndrome. *Journal of Psychopharmacology* 12(3): 305–313.

The following sections will discuss discontinuation syndromes as they occur in specific medication groups.

SSRI discontinuation syndrome

The most common SSRI discontinuation symptoms are dizziness, nausea, lethargy and headaches. The dizziness and lack of equilibrium are often the most bothersome symptoms to patients, and are most noticeable when patients rotate their head quickly. They may feel that they will lose their balance, although they seldom do. A useful mnemonic for remembering the symptoms of SSRI discontinuation is the "ABCDEF" list in Table 8.6.

TCA discontinuation syndrome, as shown in Table 8.7, includes the symptoms mentioned above for SSRIs, but the disequilibrium and the sensory, "electric shock" and "flu-like" symptoms occur far less often.

Antipsychotics and mood stabilizers

Although antipsychotic medications and mood stabilizers do not cause a discontinuation syndrome, they should still be tapered as gradually as possible for other reasons. Because of the intense and potentially life-disrupting symptoms of bipolar disorder and psychosis, gradual, lengthy tapers are preferred. This gives both the clinician and the patient an opportunity to see any return of symptomatology at a low level, long before

Table 8.7 Symptoms of a TCA discontinuation syndrome

- Nausea, vomiting, diarrhea, stomach upset
- Agitation/irritability
- Difficulty sleeping
- Depression/low mood
- Flushing, sweating, tremors

Table 8.8 Symptoms of stimulant withdrawal

- Intense cravings for stimulants
- Sleep difficulties
- Decreased cognitive function
- Extreme mood swings
- Chills
- Body aches
- Tremors and shakiness
- Fatigue
- Exhaustion
- Difficulty concentrating
- Depression
- Anxiety

full-blown mania or psychosis occurs. The clinician may then quickly raise the dose if psychotic or manic symptoms appear, before a serious episode emerges. Although it would be pharmacologically safe to taper the medication over a period of several weeks, it is often clinically more helpful to taper over several months, with intermittent visits, appointments and evaluations by the clinician to observe for potential relapse. *Stopping antipsychotic medications and mood stabilizers does not cause a discontinuation syndrome.*

Stimulants

Stopping the chronic use of a stimulant medication, particularly if large doses have been taken for more than several weeks, can result in a withdrawal syndrome that presents a clinical picture quite different from the antidepressant and benzodiazepine withdrawal syndromes described above and below. Since stimulants promote wakefulness, decreased appetite and increased energy, and are antidepressant; sudden withdrawal of these compounds results in transient reversal of these effects. Stimulant withdrawal is characterized by the symptoms listed in Table 8.8.

With the exception of the depressed mood that, when severe, may be accompanied by significant suicidal ideation (a "crash"), the physical signs of stimulant withdrawal are annoying to the patient but are not intrinsically dangerous. They generally pass in 3–7 days.

Benzodiazepine withdrawal

Because of their frequency of use as well as their propensity for abuse, dependence and withdrawal, stopping medications from the benzodiazepine group deserves special mention. For more than half a century, beginning with chlordiazepoxide, benzodiazepines have been prescribed in large quantities for a wide variety of conditions by practitioners of all specialties. Alprazolam, lorazepam, clonazepam and diazepam consistently populate the list of the most frequently prescribed mental health medications. A comparison of benzodiazepines is given in Table 8.9. For a variety of reasons, including patient overuse, inattentive prescriber oversight, patients obtaining medicines from multiple prescribers and, more recently, the availability of non-prescribed benzodiazepines over the Internet, there is a high frequency of patients who utilize large doses of benzodiazepines for extended periods of time. Withdrawal from benzodiazepines when they have been taken extensively requires oversight by a healthcare professional. Other important considerations to consider in benzodiazepine withdrawal are discussed below and in Chapter 10.

Benzodiazepine discontinuation

Tapering benzodiazepine medication used to treat anxiety may also lead to some confusion on the part of the clinician. When benzodiazepines are stopped suddenly from moderate doses, there can be symptoms of true physiological withdrawal that can include those listed in Table 8.10.

Table 8.9 Benzodiazepine comparison chart

Benzodiazepines	Half-life of parent compound in hours [half-life of primary active metabolite]	Approximately equivalent oral dosages of various medications in mg
Alprazolam (Xanax, Xanax-XR)	6–12	0.5
Chlordiazepoxide (Librium)	5–30 [36–200]	25
Clobazam (Frisium, Urbanyl, Mystan)	12–60	20
Clonazepam (Klonopin, Rivotril)	18–50	0.5
Clorazepate (Tranxene)	[36–200]	15
Diazepam (Valium)	20–100 [36–200]	10
Estazolam (ProSom)	10–24	1–2
Flunitrazepam (Rohypnol)	18–26 [36–200]	1
Flurazepam (Dalmane)	[40–250]	15–30
Halazepam (Paxipam)	[30–100]	20
Loprazolam (Dormonoct)	6–12	1–2
Lorazepam (Ativan)	10–20	1
Lormetazepam (Noctamid)	10–12	1–2
Nitrazepam (Mogadon)	15–38	10
Nordazepam (Nordaz, Calmday)	36–200	10
Oxazepam (Serax, Serenid, Serepax)	4–15	20
Prazepam (Centrax)	[36–200]	10–20
Quazepam (Doral)	25–100	20
Temazepam (Restoril, Normison, Euhypnos)	8–22	20
Triazolam (Halcion)	2	0.5

Sources: Adapted from Benzodiazepines, Johns Hopkins Psychiatry Guide, available at: www.hopkinsguides. com/hopkins/view/Johns_Hopkins_Psychiatry_Guide/787140/all/Benzodiazepines; Benzodiazepine equivalency table, available at: www.benzo.org.uk/bzequiv.htm; Griffin CE *et al.* (2013) Benzodiazepine pharmacology and central nervous system-mediated effects. *The Ochsner Journal* 13(2): 214–223, available at: www. ncbi.nlm.nih.gov/pmc/articles/PMC3684331/

Table 8.10 Symptoms of benzodiazepine withdrawal

- Sweating
- Tremors
- Agitation
- Nausea
- Rapid pulse

These symptoms can overlap with, and may be confused with, relapse of the initial anxiety condition for which the patient was being treated. Therefore, a gradual taper of benzodiazepines is useful and gives the clinician and patient the best chance to distinguish any mild withdrawal symptoms from relapse of the anxiety disorder. Rapid, sudden stoppage of very high doses of benzodiazepines can cause seizures; therefore, patients on large amounts of benzodiazepines should always be tapered slowly.

In the highly motivated patient, benzodiazepine withdrawal can be accomplished as an outpatient, although at times, particularly if multiple or complex mixtures of medications have been taken, an inpatient withdrawal may be necessary, at least initially.

- General, semi-structured strategies for benzodiazepine withdrawal can be accomplished as outlined below. In actual practice, withdrawal is tailored by a number of factors including the patient's overall psychological and medical status, their motivation, their personality, their lifestyle, as well as current and past stressors. Although a fixed timetable for withdrawal is a basis on which to begin, successful discontinuation is usually best managed through flexible patient–clinician negotiation, based on the patient's progress.
- Patients taking high doses for longer periods of time will have significant difficulty with a rapid taper and have a high failure rate. Discontinuation in such patients is much more likely to be successful if done very slowly. As shown in Table 8.11, such a taper for a patient taking 6 mg of alprazolam consistently for an extended period might require up to a year to accomplish.
- Patients taking irregular or erratic doses of benzodiazepines (e.g., 4 mg one day, 15 mg the next day, 10 mg the day after that, and so forth) can usually be withdrawn starting at a smaller dose than the chronic user who has been taking a consistently high dose.
- Benzodiazepines with a short half-life (for example, alprazolam, lorazepam or oxazepam) are difficult to withdraw from using the original compound since the short half-life results in frequent peaks and valleys of serum blood level. Such medications are more successfully withdrawn when the equivalent dose of diazepam is substituted for the parent compound at the outset. Diazepam itself has a half-life of 43–55 hours. However, when the active metabolite is included, the figure may be extended to over 8 days. Thus, it is more smoothly excreted from the body than short half-life compounds. The withdrawal is then accomplished by gradually tapering the dose of diazepam. Some clinicians utilize the same principle by substituting clonazepam (half-life between 18 and 50 hours) for the original medication. A representative example of a diazepam-substitution taper is shown in Table 8.11.
- Inevitably there will be one or more periods during a withdrawal that will prove difficult for the patient. Although it may be useful to temporarily cease further decreases in dosage for a period of time to allow for accommodation, it is important not to

Table 8.11 Slow benzodiazepine taper from high dose

	Morning	Midday/afternoon	Evening/night	Daily diazepam equivalent
Starting dosage	alprazolam 2 mg	alprazolam 2 mg	alprazolam 2 mg	120 mg
For 1 week	alprazolam 2 mg	alprazolam 2 mg	alprazolam 1.5 mg diazepam 10mg	120 mg
For 1 week	alprazolam 1.5 mg	alprazolam 2 mg	alprazolam 1 mg diazepam 10mg	120 mg
For 1 week	alprazolam 1 mg diazepam 20 mg	alprazolam 2 mg	alprazolam 1 mg diazepam 20 mg	120 mg
For 1–2 weeks	alprazolam 1 mg diazepam 20 mg	alprazolam 1 mg diazepam 10 mg	alprazolam 1 mg diazepam 20 mg	110 mg
For 1–2 weeks	alprazolam 1 mg diazepam 20 mg	alprazolam 1 mg diazepam 10 mg	alprazolam 0.5 mg diazepam 20 mg	100 mg
For 1–2 weeks	alprazolam 1 mg diazepam 20 mg	alprazolam 1 mg diazepam 10 mg	Stop alprazolam diazepam 20 mg	90 mg
For 1–2 weeks	alprazolam 0.5 mg diazepam 20 mg	alprazolam 1 mg diazepam 10 mg	diazepam 20 mg	80 mg
For 1–2 weeks	alprazolam 0.5 mg diazepam 20 mg	alprazolam 0.5 mg diazepam 10 mg	diazepam 20 mg	80 mg
For 1–2 weeks	alprazolam 0.5 mg diazepam 20 mg	Stop alprazolam diazepam 10 mg	diazepam 20 mg	60 mg
For 1–2 weeks	Stop alprazolam diazepam 20 mg	diazepam 10 mg	diazepam 20 mg	50 mg
For 1–2 weeks	diazepam 25 mg	Stop midday dose; divert 5 mg each to morning and night doses	diazepam 25 mg	50 mg
For 1–2 weeks	diazepam 20 mg	-	diazepam 25 mg	45 mg
For 1–2 weeks	diazepam 20 mg	-	diazepam 20 mg	40 mg
For 1–2 weeks	diazepam 18 mg	diazepam 20 mg	diazepam 38 mg	-
For 1–2 weeks	diazepam 18 mg	diazepam 18 mg	diazepam 36 mg	-
For 1–2 weeks	diazepam 16 mg	diazepam 18 mg	diazepam 34 mg	-
For 1–2 weeks	diazepam 16 mg	diazepam 16 mg	diazepam 32 mg	-
For 1–2 weeks	diazepam 14 mg	diazepam 16 mg	diazepam 30 mg	-
For 1–2 weeks	diazepam 14 mg	diazepam 14 mg	diazepam 28 mg	-
For 1–2 weeks	diazepam 12 mg	diazepam 14 mg	diazepam 26 mg	-
For 1–2 weeks	diazepam 12 mg	diazepam 12 mg	diazepam 24 mg	-
For 1–2 weeks	diazepam 10 mg	diazepam 12 mg	diazepam 22 mg	-
For 1–2 weeks	diazepam 10 mg	diazepam 10 mg	diazepam 20 mg	-
For 1–2 weeks	diazepam 8 mg	diazepam 10 mg	diazepam 18 mg	-
For 1–2 weeks	diazepam 8 mg	diazepam 8 mg	diazepam 16 mg	-
For 1–2 weeks	diazepam 6 mg	diazepam 8 mg	diazepam 14 mg	-
For 1–2 weeks	diazepam 5 mg	diazepam 8 mg	diazepam 13 mg	-
For 1–2 weeks	diazepam 4 mg	diazepam 8 mg	diazepam 12 mg	-
For 1–2 weeks	diazepam 3 mg	diazepam 8 mg	diazepam 11 mg	-
For 1–2 weeks	diazepam 2 mg	diazepam 8 mg	diazepam 10 mg	-
For 1–2 weeks	diazepam 1 mg	diazepam 8 mg	diazepam 9 mg	-
For 1–2 weeks	-	diazepam 8 mg	diazepam 8 mg	-
For 1–2 weeks	-	diazepam 7 mg	diazepam 7 mg	-
For 1–2 weeks	-	diazepam 6 mg	diazepam 6 mg	-
For 1–2 weeks	-	diazepam 5 mg	diazepam 5 mg	-
For 1–2 weeks	-	diazepam 4 mg	diazepam 4 mg	-

(*continued*)

Table 8.11 Cont.

	Morning	Midday/afternoon	Evening/night	Daily diazepam equivalent
For 1–2 weeks	-	diazepam 3 mg	diazepam 3 mg	-
For 1–2 weeks	-	diazepam 2 mg	diazepam 2 mg	-
For 1–2 weeks	-	diazepam 1 mg	diazepam 1 mg	-

Source: Adapted from Ashton CH (2002) *The Ashton Manual*, available at: www.benzo.org.uk/

Note: An example of a slow benzodiazepine taper for high dosage/lengthy and consistent usage – in this instance from alprazolam 6 mg per day. Note that initially, the diazepam is gradually substituted without a decrease in the total equivalent benzodiazepine dose for the first 4 weeks.

backslide and revert to earlier higher doses. Usually, with appropriate support and time, the patient will subsequently be able to resume the taper.

- Most patients who have used a benzodiazepine for anxiety control will need other methodologies to control their anxiety once the medication is stopped. The clinician should institute other helpful techniques for anxiety management, including deep muscle relaxation, breathing exercises, biofeedback, meditation, visualization and exposure therapy to phobic situations as the taper is proceeding.
- Based on an appropriate assessment of the patient, the clinician should have a plan on when and if other non-habituating medication will be provided to the patient for symptom control. Ideally, the patient should be managed with non-pharmacological means; however, if the use of a non-habituating medication becomes necessary, antidepressants, buspirone, antihistamines and beta blockers each may prove useful.
- Common discontinuance symptoms occurring during withdrawal and benzodiazepine taper include anxiety, irritability, agitation, restlessness, insomnia, muscle aches and tension, nausea, depression, lethargy, diaphoresis, nightmares and blurred vision.

Management of discontinuation syndromes

Once mild discontinuation symptoms have been identified and the time-limited nature of their occurrence outlined, most patients can tolerate them satisfactorily without treatment. If reassurance and support are not sufficient to make the situation tolerable, or the symptoms are severe, active management may be necessary as shown in Table 8.12.

Common examples of the final strategy shown in Table 8.12 include substituting fluoxetine (a long half-life compound) for paroxetine (a short half-life compound). Fluoxetine plus nortriptyline can substitute for venlafaxine. These longer half-life products, or combinations, can often be tapered more comfortably with fewer symptoms of discontinuation.

Relapse versus discontinuation syndrome

With antidepressants the symptoms of discontinuation may overlap, in part, with the symptoms of the original condition being treated with the antidepressant. It is

Table 8.12 Management strategies for discontinuation syndromes

- Slow the taper
- Return to a previous comfortable dose to accommodate a more gradual subsequent taper (when an extra or higher dose is prescribed and the symptoms remit, it is a useful indicator that discontinuation syndrome is active and is the likely cause of the symptoms)
- Substitute longer half-life medications for short half-life compounds, and then taper the long half-life medications

important to make the distinction between these two phenomena. *The most important criterion to differentiate relapse (return of original depressed symptoms) from a discontinuation syndrome (physical symptoms caused by stopping the medication) is the time in which symptoms progress or disappear.*

Discontinuation syndrome symptoms almost invariably go away within 10 days. If symptoms have not gone away, or have not substantially improved, by the seventh day, the possibility of relapse is more likely.

Other signs suggestive of relapse are:

- increasing intensity, rather than decreasing intensity, over time
- a repetition of the signs and symptoms of the original illness (rather than new symptoms)
- gradual occurrence rather than sudden onset (which is more likely with discontinuation syndrome).

If a patient experiences significant symptoms of relapse during a taper, it is usually of little value to continue the taper. Once relapse is definitively diagnosed and distinguished from a discontinuation syndrome, "getting over the hump" does not occur. If the taper is continued, the clinician is usually forced to restart the medication later, but with a more severely depressed patient.

Most patients "know" when they are having a relapse of symptomatology, and their report can generally be trusted. It bears repeating that antidepressants are not, in general, habit forming, and are not abused by patients. There is, in general, no street market for SSRIs, tricyclics or other newer antidepressants. Therefore, when patients say, "I need the medicine again," they are usually right.

When to stop medication more quickly

The exceptions to the "gradual taper" rule are few but important. They include when the patient becomes *pregnant*, develops *an allergy*, or suffers *serious side effects*.

Most patients when they become pregnant will want to discontinue medication as rapidly as possible. If, after a discussion of the risks and/or benefits of stopping medication, it is decided to discontinue medication, do so quickly. While it is possible that this may lead to some discontinuation phenomena with antidepressants or benzodiazepines, it is medico-legally preferable, and often fits with the patient's wishes. Many women would rather take the risk that rebound symptoms may occur than extend the medication period significantly into the first trimester of pregnancy. This is discussed more in depth in Chapter 13.

If the patient develops an allergy to the medication, it is better to stop the medicine quickly, precipitously if necessary, than risk the intensification of allergic symptoms that themselves may be life-threatening.

Rare, serious side effects (including seizure, fainting episodes, dramatic decreases in white blood cell count, severe vomiting, documented heart rhythm irregularity or gastrointestinal bleeding) are other reasons to stop medication at once. While the statistical likelihood of each of these side effects is low (see Chapter 19), when they occur in a particular patient, they become a crisis. It is much easier to justify stopping the medication and dealing with any rebound symptomatology than to continue the medication that may perpetuate these intense and life-threatening side effects.

New episode or relapse?

For purposes of documenting whether returning symptoms are part of a new episode of illness or part of a relapse from a current episode of illness, it is arbitrarily assumed that if patients have not experienced any similar symptoms within a 2-month period following stoppage of the medication, they have recovered from this particular episode. If the symptoms do recur within that 2-month period, it is again (rather arbitrarily) assumed that this is a relapse of the initial episode. This distinction may be important at a later time when the clinician and patient discuss the possibilities of chronic, long-term medication treatment (see Chapter 9).

Side effects pass quickly

When medications are stopped, *side effects often disappear before therapeutic effects*. If a patient decides prematurely to stop medications, and some objectionable side effects resolve, the patient may believe that he or she is better off not taking the medication. This may be true in terms of the objectionable side effects, and the patient, if initially feeling well emotionally, may be resistant to restart the medication. In this circumstance, both clinician and patient need to observe carefully for signs of relapse over the next 1–6 weeks. If such relapse occurs, a return to medication should be suggested. If the objectionable side effects were sufficiently uncomfortable and the patient is resistant to restarting the original medication, a change of medication may be more favorably received.

Unplanned stoppages of medication

The above sections of this chapter refer to planned stoppages of medication. Patients may, however, stop medication on their own without contacting the clinician. When this occurs, the clinician should not automatically assume that this is a significant problem. The situation can be a useful opportunity to assess the outcome, renegotiate a contract and form a more workable agreement with the patient. These unplanned stoppages can occur in a number of ways, as shown in Table 8.13.

Commonly, a patient who has made a unilateral decision to stop medication fails to follow through with an appointment. If there is a missed appointment and no contact from the patient, the clinician should always call to discover the reason for the absence. The clinician needs to find out if the patient has just forgotten the appointment, has decided to stop medication, has decided to see another clinician or has not come for

Table 8.13 Possible causes of unplanned stoppages

• The patient fails to show up for an appointment and has no more medication
• The patient makes a conscious unilateral decision to stop medication
• The patient is experiencing side effects
• The patient thinks he or she is well and no longer needs medication
• The patient cannot afford to purchase the medication

---

another reason. If the medication has been prematurely stopped, written documentation of the patient's decision should be made in the chart.

At other times, patients will come for their assigned follow-up session, but will indicate to the clinician that they have unilaterally decided to stop one or more of the medications they have been taking. This is often cloaked in the notion that they "forgot" a dose of medicine for several days, and decided to use this as an opportunity to see what would happen when they were medication-free. In other cases, patients may have been experiencing a particularly problematic side effect, decided they could not tolerate the medication and stopped it without contacting the clinician.

Some patients may present for an appointment and insist on stopping the medication, even though they have not yet done so. Despite a recommendation from the clinician that they stay on the medication longer, patients may insist that they cannot, or will not, continue medication.

In any of these scenarios, patients' decisions may represent an open, overt wish to stop medication or at other times there will be a hidden agenda in stopping the medication, such as:

• They are having a side effect they have not told you about (e.g., sexual problems).
• They may be receiving resistance from someone important to them. A spouse, partner, parent or adult child may have been giving them information that counters what you have been telling them, and convinced them that being off medication is the better course of action. Occasionally, this other person may be another healthcare professional who has told them that the medication may be harmful or that they "don't need it."
• They perceive an unspoken downside to "successful" medication treatment (for example, manic patients may not want to give up the ability to work long hours in a day because it keeps their income high or raises their stature in the eyes of a supervisor).

Regardless of the reason, when patients stop medication prematurely, it does not mean that the clinician must stop contact and involvement with them. It can be a useful opportunity to reassess the status of the current treatment and, if necessary, revise the plan in a mutually agreed fashion. Some patients will wish to continue contact with the clinician even if they are not taking medication. They will continue using the clinician for support, guidance, clarification and help with their life problems, even though they stopped taking their pills. A clinician can stay in contact with a patient, and continue to be a support, without agreeing that stoppage of the medication was a good thing. It may be quite appropriate to take a "wait and see" approach to medication stoppage, while both clinician and patient watch for any significant change.

When patients stop medication prematurely, the clinician may be surprised to find that these individuals do reasonably well when they are off medication. Even experienced clinicians have had the experience of thinking that a patient needed medication, and was likely to seriously relapse without it, only to find that the patient stopped medicine safely and satisfactorily without relapse. We are far from omniscient in knowing how medication will affect patients.

Ambivalent patients who have stopped medication and then do relapse may become much more cooperative than they were initially in terms of retrying the same or another medication. Many reticent patients need to prove to themselves that they are going to relapse before continuing medication. Only when they do relapse are they willing to become more engaged in the treatment process, and to take medications on a regular basis.

After stopping medication, some patients experience a limited relapse, but decide that limited symptoms are tolerable. The clinician may have no choice but to go along with this, even if this level of symptomatology leaves the patient partially handicapped in the clinician's eyes. Although some patients will see relatively quickly that they are not doing well and need to be back on medication, others may take months or years to make that decision. Sometimes, only at this later date when a patient returns does the clinician hear about a hidden agenda that was not discussed when the patient initially stopped medication.

Complex discontinuation

In some clinical instances, a patient may have stopped high doses of multiple medications from different medication classes simultaneously, thus precipitating a mix of psychiatric and discontinuation symptoms. In other situations, medication stoppage can be complicated by alcohol and/or recreational drug intoxication or withdrawal. At times, the effects of one drug may temporarily minimize or block symptoms of another substance (e.g., alcohol ingestion can mask symptoms of cocaine withdrawal). Such situations can result in a multitude of signs and symptoms presenting to the clinician, and can be exceedingly complex and evolve over a period of several days. In general, an inpatient hospital stay will be necessary to evaluate and safely manage these clinical occurrences.

Reference

1 Kupfer D *et al.* (1992) Five-year outcome for maintenance therapies in recurrent depression. *Archives of General Psychiatry* 49: 769–773.

9 The long-term patient

* Who should receive long-term treatment?   128
* A symptomatic crisis in a stable patient – general principles   129
* "The medicine stopped working" – getting back on TRAACCC   130
* Inappropriate requests   134
* Is newer medication better?   135
* Periodic reassessment   137
* Concurrence for a change of medication   137
* Conflicting advice from others   138
* References   139

Chapter 8 described the issues involved in stopping medication. Once discontinued, many patients do well off medication without recurrence of symptoms. While it is incorrect to assume initially that all patients will need long-term or life-long medication for their mental health problems, a percentage of patients do relapse when they discontinue medication. If relapses are frequent or occur quickly after medication is stopped, especially when these relapses are repetitive, the clinician and patient together should consider the possibility of maintenance, longer-term medications to block further relapses and/or minimize their extent. As with many issues regarding mental health medication, it is important to include the patient in the decision regarding if and when a maintenance medication program is begun.

For some patients, the decision to continue on medication "for the foreseeable future" can be relieving and reassuring. When medication serves to prevent or minimize future illness, patients' lives are considerably smoother and more comfortable, and have a consistency that allows them to grow personally, maximize work potential and have greater satisfaction in relationships. For other patients, the decision to stay on medication is an extraordinarily difficult one that will be resisted, sometimes strongly. For these patients, staying on medication in the long term raises many of the same issues they felt when starting medication: "Am I weak?" "Shouldn't I be able to control my symptoms with my mind and will?" "Am I a constitutionally inferior person?" "Why does this keep happening to me?" Concerns about side effects of long-term medication usage, medication interactions, pregnancy or menopause can also arise.

Even some persons who consent to take medication chronically do so with resistance, reluctance and a feeling of having "failed." Internally, such patients may never feel that this is a positive decision, and consent only because of a feeling that there is no other choice.

Some patients who do not follow the clinician's suggestion for a maintenance medication regimen will relapse, sometimes seriously. Despite repeated relapses, some patients remain doggedly resistant to the concept of taking medication over the long term.

Who should receive long-term treatment?

Several factors are important in deciding when to suggest long-term medication treatment to a patient. This decision is seldom made after the initial (index) symptom episode, except in unusual and high-risk situations. More likely, a plan for maintenance will occur after one or several relapses off medication.

Factors that the clinician should consider in recommending maintenance medication include:

1   Relapse characteristics
   - the *speed* with which relapse occurs
   - the *number of relapse episodes*
   - the *intensity and strength* of each relapse episode
   - the *length of time that it takes to return to health and full functioning* after restarting medication.
2   The patient's condition while on medication
   - assessment of *the intensity and interference from medication side effects*, if any, that a patient experiences while on medications
   - the *level of symptom control* when taking medication. Is the improvement mild, modest or virtually complete?
3   Personal characteristics and preferences
   - the *patient's level of insight and awareness* regarding his or her own psychological state
   - the *patient's ability to recognize signs of relapse*
   - the *patient's wishes.*
4   Support system
   - the extent and consistency of *family or other support*
   - sometimes, the *wishes of the patient's family.*

In general, patients with mild to moderate depression, anxiety disease or symptoms of bipolar disorder will have had a minimum of two relapses after the initial index episode before chronic medication is likely to be considered. For some patients, this principle may be shortened to one relapse following the initial index episode. If the first relapse after the index episode is particularly serious, long-lasting or slow to recover from, the clinician may decide to suggest maintenance treatment with medication without waiting for a third episode. A first relapse of psychosis will generally require strong consideration of prophylactic long-term medication.

Other indications that may prompt a clinician to suggest an earlier use of long-term medication are relapse episodes that include symptoms of:

- significant deficits of functioning
- severe loss of work productivity
- deep marital discord
- threats or episodes of self-harm, or harm to others.

Since patients vary greatly in their feelings about taking medication long term, it is important to assess such feelings and take them into account when deciding whether or not to use medication chronically. Patients who have been intensely dysphoric or have had significant lifestyle interruptions because of their illness are often justifiably frightened about further relapses. These patients may request chronic medication even before the clinician's recommendation. When patients raise this issue, it becomes an important point of negotiation, and one that should be openly discussed with them and, if indicated, with their family.

At other times, patients may be resistant to maintenance medication even when the clinician feels it would be desirable. Assuming that they are legally competent, patients may need to experience relapses and the consequences of the relapses more often than the clinician feels is helpful. While clinicians may advise and recommend maintenance medication, patients remain masters of their own domain and may choose medication-free intervals, even if the likely results in the clinician's judgment are future relapses.

A situation which occurs with some frequency is that of the family wishing to have the identified patient remain on maintenance medication when the patient does not agree. The patient may be overtly opposed to this medication plan, does not see the need for it, or feels that the side effects of the medication are unacceptable. Patients who become angry, disagreeable, less productive, socially isolated or substance abusers when they relapse can be a significant irritation or worry to their families. Unless the patient has become an acute danger to self or others, however, families may need to accept relapses and persistent symptoms when a legally competent patient refuses chronic medication. Except in the case of an incompetent patient with a legal guardian, it is the identified patient, not the family, who will make the final decision. The clinician may see the problem and recommend, or even suggest strongly, that medication could be useful, but the final decision rests with the patient and not with the family. When a patient has a guardian authorized by the court, he or she has the authority to require the patient to adhere to a longer-term medication protocol.

At times, the family may use incentives or disincentives to induce the patient to take medication. These incentives may include willingness to offer housing, financial support or transportation that are provided only on the agreement that the patient complies with long-term medication treatment. A spouse or partner may only agree to stay in a relationship with the patient if medication is continued. Patients may complain about such arrangements, but ultimately have the choice of whether or not to participate.

A symptomatic crisis in a stable patient – general principles

Long-term patients, who may be doing well on medication maintenance with minimal symptomatology, can present to the clinician at any point describing a new onset of depressive, anxiety, manic or psychotic symptoms. The challenge then facing the clinician is assessing these breakthrough symptoms. The most difficult issue, but also the most important, is determining whether or not the new symptoms represent a true relapse (and hence a medication failure), for which additional medication intervention is likely to help. A relapse indicative of medication failure needs to be differentiated from new or transient symptoms that might respond best to psychotherapy, lifestyle alteration or other interventions and do not require medication change. Sometimes utilizing both pharmacological and non-pharmacological methods is necessary.

In order to assess this important but sometimes complicated question, issues regarding both medications and lifestyle need to be addressed by the clinician. It is often necessary to revisit areas of evaluation that have been initially assessed during the early stages of treatment. A specific guideline for this process is outlined in the next section of this chapter.

When the issues below are evaluated, it may be quite clear to the clinician what is most likely to account for the patient's new symptoms. In some cases, non-adherence to the prescribed regimen, underdosing, changes in regimen or independent medical causes have altered the physiological blood level of the patient's psychotropic medication. If so, patient education along with a change of psychotropic dosage may re-establish equilibrium fairly rapidly.

In other circumstances, medication issues have little to do with the new symptoms. Major life stressors alone may have precipitated symptom emergence. It is remarkable how often patients do not see or understand the connection between major issues in their life, and the triggering of symptoms or relapse. It is only after the clinician has raised such a possibility that the patient begins to see the connection. When this is the case, making the connection may be sufficient for the patient to understand and endure the symptoms and/or make appropriate changes to improve the situation. At other times, it may be necessary to recommend new or increased psychotherapy sessions, or some other behavioral intervention to deal with the patient's stressors. For occupational stressors, a change of work hours, intervention with a supervisor or a leave of absence may be necessary to allow the symptoms to remit. On those occasions when behavioral stressors are time-limited and likely to be concluded within a short period, observation and waiting may be all that is necessary. To deal with personal stressors, individual, marital or family treatment may be indicated.

As with the initial decision to start medication, *the most important criterion to determine whether more or different medication is necessary is the amount of functional disruption that is occurring because of the symptoms.* When functional disruption is significant, in spite of a seemingly adequate medication regimen or environmental stressors that may need to be amended, a change of medication is often warranted. When possible, a change to another medication within the same classification can be useful. If monotherapy is ineffective, the addition of a second or even a third medication may be necessary (see the section in Chapter 5 on polypharmacy). For some conditions, medications within one classification (e.g., antipsychotics or mood stabilizers) may achieve a satisfactory response and renewed equilibrium. Combining different classifications of medication – such as adding an antidepressant to a mood stabilizer, adding an anti-anxiety medication to an antidepressant or adding an antidepressant or anti-anxiety medicine to an antipsychotic medication – may also yield positive results. Each patient must be individually evaluated to determine the medication formula to be adopted.

"The medicine stopped working" – getting back on TRAACCC

For a patient who has experienced relapse or has breakthrough symptoms after a long period of stability on medication, a useful acronym for the clinician is "getting the patient back on TRAACCC" (see Table 9.1). This acronym guides the clinician to those elements that should be addressed in evaluating significant breakthrough symptoms. The acronym is a useful memory device, although in real-world clinical

Table 9.1 Getting back on TRAACCC (RAATCCC)

- **T**alking therapy
- **R**e-evaluation
- **A**lcohol and drugs
- **A**dherence
- **C**hange medication
- **C**ombination therapy
- **C**onsultation

---

situations, the practitioner applies these items in a slightly different order – RAATCCC (**R**e-evaluation, **A**lcohol, **A**dherence, **T**alking therapy and **C**hanging medication followed by **C**ombination therapy and **C**onsultation) – which will be the order that is presented here.

Re-evaluation

When breakthrough symptoms occur, the clinician should consider a diagnostic and symptomatic *re-evaluation*. A re-evaluation is the cornerstone of assessing relapse and should cover five different areas:

1 diagnosis
2 medication choice
3 lifestyle
4 alcohol and drugs
5 compliance.

Diagnosis

If a patient has developed new or returning symptoms, it is sometimes because the clinician's initial assessment was only partially correct, or was incorrect. A depressed patient may, in fact, have bipolar disorder. A patient diagnosed with panic attacks may develop a depressive episode. A schizophrenic patient may develop a substance abuse problem. A patient with a mood disorder may develop significant anxiety – in the form of either generalized anxiety or panic attacks. Any of these may not have been recognized in the initial assessment. Particularly if it has been a long time since the initial evaluation, it is useful to conduct a fresh assessment of symptoms, even when the patient may have given negative responses in the past to questions about specific symptoms. It is surprising how often new and previously unrevealed information can be elicited in a re-evaluation done years after the initial assessment.

There are many reasons why additional or new information may be elicited:

- Patients may have developed new symptoms that were not present originally.
- Patients have begun to reformulate certain behaviors or feelings as "symptoms" that were not seen as symptoms at the time they were originally seen.
- Patients may have been embarrassed to admit to certain symptoms on an initial visit to a new clinician for fear the clinician would refuse to treat them or look negatively on them because of their symptoms or behavior.

Medication

- Is the patient getting proper amounts of medication? Exactly how much, how often and when is the patient taking psychotropic medications? (Sometimes what the clinician is prescribing is not what the patient has been taking!) Without initially mentioning the correct regimen, ask the patient how many pills of what size or color he/she is taking at what times.
- Have any medical conditions arisen that may account for the patient's complaints? Some of these may be related to the medication prescribed, and others may not. For example, has the patient developed an unrelated medical condition that is altering his or her mental health status, such as diabetes mellitus, hypertension, mononucleosis or hepatitis C?
- Is the medication prescribed causing a medical complication? For example, if the patient is taking lithium, has he or she developed low thyroid function as a side effect? Have abnormalities of liver function begun as a reaction to the prescription given?

Box 9.1 Clinical tip

Appropriate medical screening laboratory tests are indicated for any sudden symptomatic crisis in an otherwise stable patient. This usually includes chemical tests of liver and kidney function, fasting blood sugar, TSH, CBC and serum psychotropic levels, where appropriate.

- What non-psychiatric prescription medications is the patient taking? Are any of these new? Is there any other prescriber working with the patient who has altered the regimen?
- Is the patient taking any new over-the-counter preparations? Has the patient begun a new generic preparation or had another psychotropic preparation recently that could account for the new symptoms?

Symptoms and lifestyle

- When did these breakthrough symptoms begin?
- Was the onset sudden or gradual?
- Are these symptoms similar to the previous episode, or new?
- What specific symptoms have occurred?
- Is the onset of these symptoms associated with any life events?
- Has the patient had any recent significant life stressors? (At times, significant stressors have occurred, but the patient has not associated these with the symptoms.)

Alcohol and drugs

A re-evaluation of the patient's substance use is necessary even when the patient has claimed limited or no substance use in the past. Alcohol or drug usage is one of the most common behaviors that patients may have minimized or not been willing to admit when initially seen. At other times, the patient was, in fact, not using substances at the time of the initial diagnosis but has begun to do so now. If such usage is present, the clinician will need to reaffirm that it may interfere with the medication's ability to control symptoms and may have a substantial negative bearing on the patient's response. If the clinician's suspicion remains high, a blood screen for toxicology, a blood alcohol level or a serum GGT can be warranted (see Chapter 25).

Adherence

As mentioned at other times in this text, patient non-adherence with medication is often a significant cause of incomplete response or loss of response. The clinician should evaluate the patient's adherence with the regimen that has been prescribed. It is often best to evaluate this with open-ended questions, such as: *"Tell me exactly which medications you are taking and when you are taking them?"* This way the clinician is more likely to get an accurate sense of what the patient is actually doing at home. This open-ended question is preferable to the clinician repeating the presumed regimen and then asking if the patient is following that regimen, which makes it far too easy for the patient to say "Yes," whether or not the medicine is actually being taken as prescribed.

Talking therapy

Many patients who are managed on medication alone and develop a symptomatic crisis may need the initiation of psychotherapy or *talking therapy*. Patients who have developed new stressors in life may find it considerably useful to have a short course of individual therapy, cognitive therapy, couples' treatment or family therapy to deal with new or worsened stressors in their life. Patients who may have been resistant to psychotherapy when medication was first begun can be more amenable to such therapy when a symptomatic crisis emerges. For patients who have been on a "medication only" regimen, the clinician may wish to be more insistent on the necessity of psychotherapy. In doing so, the clinician reinforces the known benefits of the combination of psychotherapy and medication in the treatment of most emotional illnesses.

Change medication

When it is determined that lack of medication effect is likely, changing medication is usually the most common and first remedy that most clinicians consider. It can be helpful in many situations but is not the only option and should not be automatically assumed to be the best remedy. Steps 1–4 of this RAATCCC approach should always be performed before a medication change is assumed to be necessary.

Combination therapy

Combination medication therapy has become a common practice in psychopharmacology to treat breakthrough symptomatology. As has been covered in detail in Chapter 5, addition of another medicine from the same class or medications from different classes may return the patient to symptomatic stability. The synergy generated by two medications taken together can restore symptomatic control. See Chapter 5 for information regarding helpful combinations.

Consultation

A consultation is almost always of benefit with a patient who is losing symptomatic response, particularly if a clinician has tried a number of remedies or therapies with minimal or no response. A primary care provider, as well as a mental health specialist, can benefit from consultation with a psychopharmacologist as to possible medication changes or additions. The simple act of having another practitioner evaluate the patient provides a "fresh look" at the patient's problems. Sometimes the prescribing clinician may have fallen into "blind spots" as to the patient's diagnosis or treatment, and these may be discovered by a practitioner with another viewpoint. Such consultation can also be of significant benefit to a patient who has been through a number of medications with limited success. Such patients become discouraged and frustrated, and begin doubting whether the primary clinician can help them. By obtaining a consultation, they are often renewed in their willingness to continue efforts toward symptomatic control.

If a patient asks for evaluation services for a spouse, parent or child with whom they are in significant conflict, however, this can create clinical dilemmas. Confidentiality and practicality may dictate that these new evaluations be performed by other clinicians.

Inappropriate requests

The relationship between the provider of mental health medication and the patient may also, over time, lead to inappropriate requests for clinician services. When trust is built and judgment respected, patients, often in an unintended way, may ask for additional medical services beyond mental health medication. *Unless the clinician is trained, credentialed and comfortable with providing other medical services, it is generally not appropriate for the psychotropic provider to attempt to be a general medical provider to mental health patients.* It is not uncommon for patients to ask for prescription of non-mental health medications, either as a "one time" prescription or, in some cases, as ongoing medication. Requests for pain medication, headache remedies, cough and cold medications, blood pressure medications, cardiac, respiratory and diabetic medications should, in general, be referred to the patient's family physician, family nurse practitioner or general health provider. Patients may also ask, "while they are here," to get a refill for ongoing prescriptions usually obtained from their general medical provider, or ask for treatment of conditions that may require further medical assessment.

Unless the clinician is trained in and routinely provides general medical care, this is an area that may create medico-legal problems and/or be outside the scope of practice for the clinician. When patients request treatment for headaches, backache, respiratory infections, sore throats or other complaints, they should be referred to their primary care provider. Refills of ongoing non-psychotropic medications should generally be provided by the original prescriber or that person's coverage group.

Another problematic area involves the request for medication refills without appropriate face-to-face contact and follow up. This practice is often overtly proclaimed or covertly assumed by the patient to be justified under the assumption that "since you have seen me for so long, you know me. You shouldn't have to continue to see me face-to-face to prescribe my medications." Patients who are doing well, and not having side effects or relapses, may begin to assume that their psychotropic medication can just be renewed without active management, and resist follow-up appointments. The problem of minimal-contact patients is covered in more detail in Chapter 23.

Is newer medication better?

Given the pace of change in treating the biological aspects of mental illness, and in medication research and development, new psychotropic medications are continually being introduced. The challenge facing the professional is assessing the value of any new medication in the care of a particular patient. Pharmaceutical companies vigorously promote each new medication, extolling its benefits compared to older medications and competing products. The task for the clinician is to sort out which of these medications offers genuine advantages in therapeutic efficacy, convenience or possible price.

Of most interest and significance is when a new class of medicine is introduced that may offer a novel or improved biological approach to treatment. New mechanisms of action may offer the patient the opportunity for more targeted and effective treatment, with potentially fewer side effects. Once a class of medications is established, however, it is not uncommon for competitors to produce "sister medications" with similar mechanisms of action and overall efficacy. While these medications are promoted vigorously as superior products, they may in actuality offer minimal therapeutic advantage. There may be some advantages in flexibility of dosing, routes of administration or cost to the patient, but the new product often does not offer fundamental substantive improvements. All parameters of new medications should be carefully evaluated. There may be no substantial reason to alter the patient's medication regimen just because a new medication becomes available.

If a clinician chooses to consider prescribing a new medication based on limited positive response to or problematic side effects from the patient's current medication, clear clinical goals need to be established. When a trial of new medication is undertaken, both patient and clinician should evaluate the expected results and agree on a timeframe for such evaluation. A return to the older (often cheaper) regimen may be desirable if substantial clinical improvement is not seen within the allotted time.

Pharmaceutical companies will periodically "rebrand" an older medication under a new name. Although touted as "new" medications, they are often an existing medication marketed for a new therapeutic indication (e.g., Prozac [fluoxetine] was rebranded as Serafem for premenstrual dysphoric disorder; Wellbutrin [bupropion] was reintroduced as Zyban for smoking cessation; and Sinequan [doxepin] was remarketed as Silenor for sleep). In these cases, the underlying chemical compound is not changed, only the pill description and packaging. If the practitioner wishes to use that compound for the new purpose, there is usually little reason not to prescribe the established, often generic and cheaper version of the drug.

At other times, the same chemical medication will be marketed under a new name with a new formulation or preparation. Examples include: valproic acid which was manufactured in a time-release preparation and marketed as Depakote and Depakote-ER; Wellbutrin (bupropion) was developed in a time-release preparation and marketed as Wellbutrin XL and Wellbutrin SR; Seroquel SR is a "new" time-release formulation of Seroquel (quetiapine); Adderall XR was introduced with the same mixture of psychostimulants as Adderall, but in a time-release format (America only). Each of these "new" medications in a different formulation must be evaluated on its own merits. In some cases, the time-release formulation provides significant convenience and the possibility of once-daily dosing which is likely to increase patient adherence. With other medications, the "newer" and likely more expensive brand preparation offers little advantage over the existing preparations.

What do the terms "atypical" and "second generation" mean?

Confounding to the prescriber can be terminology applied to new medications. Most recently applied to the groupings of antipsychotic medications, the term "atypical" has been applied to newer medications or groups of medications. The intent of its use is to identify that the "atypical" medication is different from the previously or currently used medicines and groups. The term often develops if the newer medication is new or different in chemical structure, clinical usefulness and/or side-effect profile. Unfortunately, it is a term that can be confusing and misleading. Within a short period of time, if an "atypical" medication or group of medications has significant benefits over the existing treatments, it rapidly comes into common acceptance and use. Thus, "atypical" medications may become the norm, and in fact, become "typical" in clinical practice. Later, when even newer medications of a third differing type emerge, "atypical atypicals" (or similarly confusing terms) come into use.

The heterogeneity of this "atypical antipsychotic" group can be seen from the evolution of the term.[1] It was initially proposed in 1993 by Dr. J Lieberman to describe drugs that:

- showed efficacy in antipsychotic screening paradigms
- did not induce catalepsy
- did not up-regulate D2 receptors
- did not induce tolerance
- showed no, or markedly reduced, induction of acute extrapyramidal symptoms and tardive dyskinesia
- did not elevate prolactin levels (risperidone, although it elevates prolactin, is considered an atypical).

Stahl[2] has suggested further criteria, specifically that atypical antipsychotics:

- show greater improvement in negative symptoms of psychosis than haloperidol
- are effective for symptoms that have been refractory to treatment with conventional antipsychotics.

A similar problem exists with the use of "second-generation" as opposed to "first-generation" medications. Again, this has been used to describe a group of medications that are considered different in chemical structure, clinical usefulness and/or side- effect profile from a previous group. The problem arises when the group is not truly homogeneous and/or some authors, researchers or companies prefer to describe certain medications as "third generation" without universal acceptance or agreement. (For example, aripiprazole has been labeled by some as a "third generation" antipsychotic based on D2 receptor partial agonism or D2 functional selectivity, but this label is not universally accepted.)

Still others suggest that antipsychotics could be organized in a less confusing way by specifying the receptors which they affect; e.g., "dopamine antagonists" (first generation), "dopamine-serotonin antagonists" (some second generation), "multi-targeted" (other second generation) and "dopamine-functionally selective" (third generation).

These overlapping and at times controversial terms persist simultaneously in the current nomenclature. In this text, the term "atypical" is solely used for the latest generation of antipsychotic medications, including olanzapine, quetiapine, risperidone, ziprasidone, asenapine, vilazodone, lurasidone, iloperidone, paliperidone and aripiprazole. Because the term is so widely accepted, it has been used here despite its time-limited usefulness and potentially confusing aspect. Thus, members of this group are "atypical" in the sense that they are new and chemically different from traditional antipsychotics (often referred to as traditional antipsychotics, phenothiazines, first-generation or traditional neuroleptics). With a more benign side-effect profile and wider clinical utility (purportedly due to increased serotonergic activity and differing amounts of dopamine receptor blockade), this "atypical" group of antipsychotic medications has become a frequent first choice in treating psychosis. In this text, the label of "second-generation" antipsychotic could generally be substituted for "atypical" antipsychotic.

Periodic reassessment

If patients do not fully recover from their initial presenting mental health episode and continue to have moderate or significant functional impairment, restricted work productivity or residual social impairment, periodic reassessment of the diagnosis and treatment plan is indicated.

Long-term medication-management patients, particularly those who have not reached optimum response, should have a diagnostic and therapeutic reassessment periodically, even if they do not have a full-fledged "relapse" or symptomatic crisis. If the primary clinician's assessment does not reveal significant positive results, consultation with a colleague, supervisor or psychopharmacologist may yield useful information for possible therapeutic changes.

When reassessment is performed, the following questions highlight the areas to be investigated:

- Is the original diagnostic assessment correct?
- Has the patient developed any new medical or psychiatric conditions since the original assessment?
- If the patient's medical state has changed, how does this affect the overall mental health or medication treatment plan?
- Are target symptoms being adequately treated?
- Are there any new treatments or combinations of treatments that might reasonably improve the patient's situation?
- Have side effects emerged over time?

Concurrence for a change of medication

If the decision to alter a long-standing therapeutic regimen is made, it should not automatically be a unilateral decision on the part of the clinician. Because of the sheer quantity of newer psychiatric products being introduced, there will be many times when a newer medicine might be considered for a patient who has been relatively stable. If the clinician sees no likely therapeutic advantage of the new product, there is no reason even to raise the possibility. When, however, there may be some possible benefit, it is essential to partner with the patient regarding any possible change.

For the patient, changes in a long-standing medication program may have significant psychological consequences or raise anxiety, even if there are potential gains to be made. A change to a new medication may result in partial response or loss of response before beneficial changes occur. Although this is mediated, one would hope, by cross-tapering (slowly decreasing the current medication while gradually adding the new preparation), there is the potential for disruption in the patient's functioning. The timing of such a change should be negotiated with the patient and every attempt be made to avoid performing the changeover at times of significant stressful events in the patient's life. As with the decision to stop medication altogether (discussed in Chapter 8), it is generally better that medication changes be tried outside periods of major life stress such as marriage, divorce, job change, buying or selling a house, or a geographical move.

As has been discussed at other points in this book, concurrences and agreement about a change are desirable. This should not be taken to mean that the clinician should cede all discussion to the patient. The clinician is the professional and the person whose expertise and judgment are required.

While the practitioner can be soft and suggestive with recommendations, at times an indecisive patient will need or directly ask for the clinician's assessment. "What would you do?" requires a direct and clear response. If two choices are truly of equal value and safety, the perceived positives and negatives of a potential change of medication should be spelled out by the practitioner.

Conflicting advice from others

Every patient, even those who maintain a good therapeutic alliance with the clinician and comply with medication recommendations, may be presented with conflicting advice and differing opinions from other people in his or her life. Well-intended, but possibly misguided, friends or relatives may offer simple or extensive advice and/or pressure about taking psychotropic medication. There may be those individuals in the patient's life who do not value (or openly oppose) the use of mental health medication. The patient may experience direct and at times strong suggestions to discontinue medications, disregard treatment or terminate the relationship with the mental health provider. These urgings can come from a variety of sources:

- the patient's spouse
- the patient's family, including parents or adult children
- the patient's friends, neighbors or confidants
- the patient's employer
- self-help groups
- Internet chat rooms
- the patient's primary care provider
- other healthcare providers or specialists
- the patient's psychotherapist.

The latter three sources may seem surprising, but even seasoned healthcare providers sometimes have preconceived notions about psychotropics. The medication-management provider should always be aware of input from such sources, which may emerge at any time. It is useful for the clinician periodically to assess how the patient is feeling about the medication regimen and overall treatment. It is useful to invite the patient to discuss any input he or she has heard, and any articles or other sources of information he or she has read that may call into question the current treatment plan. If uncertainty has arisen, clarification of the plan and reassurance about the wisdom of the treatment is usually sufficient to allay patient anxiety.

If the resistance or conflicting advice is coming from a spouse or close family member, ask the patient about scheduling a three-way meeting involving the clinician, the patient and the relative. This session can allow the relative to ask questions about the patient's diagnosis and treatment, medication prescribed and side effects, the length of treatment and any other issues about the overall anticipated treatment plan. It will also offer the opportunity for the clinician to get additional feedback about the patient's medication response (or lack thereof) and functioning on a day-to-day basis outside the treatment setting. Concerns or worries that this third person may have about the use of psychotropic medications can be addressed. After receiving solid factual information from the clinician and feeling that they have had input into the patient's care, such hitherto resistive family relatives will often feel included in the treatment plan and their resistance usually diminishes. If, by the end of this session, a relative still remains quite opposed to the use of psychotropic medications but medication prescription will continue, the clinician can recognize the relative's right to a personal opinion and request that he or she keeps such opinions to him-/herself so as not to make the patient confused, hesitant or anxious.

Occasionally the clinician must take more active steps if patients indicate that they are getting conflicting advice from other medical or mental health providers. If needed, and with a patient's consent, the medication prescriber should contact such persons and discuss the overall treatment plan. A simple telephone call to a primary care provider, a psychotherapist, a nurse practitioner or other healthcare provider who is involved in the patient's care can often clarify whether, in fact, conflicting information is being given. Even if there has been misinterpretation on the patient's part and there is no active disagreement about the use of psychotropic medications, this presents as an opportunity for the prescriber to strengthen the overall treatment team's position, and ensures that the patient is not caught between prescribers with differing viewpoints.

On rare occasions, the prescriber will need to be forthright and direct with another healthcare provider about the necessity for ongoing psychotropic medications. If the other provider feels that such treatment is unnecessary or inappropriate, he or she must be asked to defer to the prescriber in managing the patient's mental health care. While this is unusual, a direct discussion of the case will usually simplify the situation and allow the patient to continue without confusing input.

References

1 Lieberman JA (1993) Understanding the mechanism of action of atypical antipsychotic drugs: a review of compounds in use and development. *British Journal of Psychiatry* 163(Suppl. 22): 7–18.
2 Stahl S (1999) *Psychopharmacology of Antipsychotics*, Informa Healthcare.

10 Benzodiazepines and stimulants – useful, but controversial

• History of benzodiazepines	140
• Uses and side effects of benzodiazepines	141
• Stimulant medication and its appropriate uses	144
• Other uses of stimulant medication	145
• Why so many? The "me too" concept of medication development	145
• Dosing of stimulants	146
• Side effects of stimulants	147
• Abuse of stimulants	147
• Notes and references	150

While the prescription antidepressants, mood stabilizers and antipsychotics are discussed in other parts of this text, there are two medicine classes – benzodiazepines and stimulants – which are in common usage, but have significant controversial issues about their prescription which can influence prescribing decisions. Therefore, these two medication groups will be discussed in greater detail here for the prescribers' convenience.

History of benzodiazepines

As we now know, anxiety disorders are the most common and among the most disabling of mental disorders in adults and adolescents.[1] It has been estimated by the Epidemiological Catchment Area (RCA) study[2] that approximately one quarter of people will experience severe symptoms, disability and handicap as a consequence of anxiety disorders at some time during their lifetime. Therefore, it is not surprising that with the onset of mental health medication prescription, there has been a desire for useful treatments for anxiety. As the prescriptions of barbiturates and meprobamate were diminished in the 1960s and the 1970s because of problematic side effects and habituation, the search for a more effective and safer anxiety medication intensified.

The first benzodiazepine, chlordiazepoxide, was synthesized in 1955 by Leo Sternbach, while he was working at Hoffman-La Roche on the development of tranquilizers. The compound showed very strong sedative, anticonvulsant and muscle relaxant effects in animal tests. These impressive clinical findings led to its speedy introduction throughout the world in 1960 under the brand name Librium. This was soon followed in 1963 by the

Table 10.1 Benzodiazepines available in the United States and their half-lives

Generic name	Brand name	Half-life* (hours)
alprazolam	Niravam (brand discontinued), Xanax, Xanax XR	half-life 6–26 hours (short-acting)
chlordiazepoxide	Librax	half-life 30–100 hours (long-acting)
clobazam	Onfi	half-life 71–82 hours (long-acting)
clonazepam	Klonopin	half-life 20–50 hours (long-acting)
clorazepate	Tranxene	half-life 20–100 hours (long-acting)
diazepam	Valium	half-life 20–100 hours (long-acting)
estazolam	ProSom (brand discontinued)	half-life 10–24 hours (medium-acting)
flurazepam	Dalmane (brand discontinued)	half-life 40–100 hours (long-acting)
lorazepam	Ativan	half-life 10–20 hours (medium-acting)
midazolam	Versed (brand discontinued)	half-life 2.5 hours (short-acting)
oxazepam	Serax (brand discontinued)	half-life 5–15 hours (short-acting)
temazepam	Restoril	half-life 10–20 hours (medium-acting)
triazolam	Halcion	half-life 2–5 hours (short-acting)

Source: Adapted from Benzodiazepines: overview and use, available at: www.drugs.com/article/benzodiazepines.html

*Note: The time it takes for the amount of a drug's active substance in your body to reduce by half.

synthesis of diazepam which was marketed by Hoffmann-La Roche under the brand name Valium.

Uses and side effects of benzodiazepines

The benefits of benzodiazepines and the apparent lack of discouraging factors led to an alarming rise in benzodiazepine prescriptions. In the late 1970s, benzodiazepines became the most commonly prescribed of all drugs in the world.[1] In1980, Tyrer reported[3] that each day about 40 billion doses of benzodiazepine drugs are consumed throughout the world.

Benzodiazepines (often referred to as benzos) as a class have now been in common use as anti-anxiety/sedative/hypnotics medication for decades. They continue to be among the most commonly prescribed medications for sleep and anxiety in primary care and mental health patients alike with over 92 million prescriptions written in 2019. As many as 11.5 percent of Americans report using a benzodiazepine at least once in a 1-year period and 1.5 percent use a benzodiazepine on a nightly or regular basis. A benzodiazepine is prescribed in over 66 million physician appointments per year. These astounding statements must be balanced with the data in 2018 which show that roughly 5.4 million people in the United States aged 12 years and older abused or misused a benzodiazepine in the previous year.[1] Also of concern is that over the 7 years from 2010 to 2017, there was an increase of more than 787 percent of overdose deaths which included benzodiazepines. The vast majority of these deaths involved benzodiazepines taken with prescription opioids. Unless a person has a reason for decreased pulmonary function, an overdose of benzodiazepines alone (without other drugs, medications or alcohol) is highly unusual.

These compounds are listed in Tables 10.1, their common uses in Table 10.2 and their common side effects in Table 10.3

Table 10.2 Common uses for benzodiazepines

Anxiety reduction/panic attacks
Sleep induction
Adjunctive in mania/schizophrenia and acute behavioral disturbance
Muscle relaxation (back sprain–diazepam)
Tremors/akathisia
Alcohol withdrawal (clonazepam and diazepam)
Tension-related conditions (e.g., headaches)

Table 10.3 Common side effects of benzodiazepines

Common but less dangerous side effects of benzodiazepines include:
- Drowsiness/fatigue
- Ataxia/decreased motor response
- Dry mouth
- Confusion
- Disinhibition

Source: Benzodiazepines: overview and use, available at: www.drugs.com/article/benzodiazepines.html

The high usage of these compounds reflects a predictable anti-anxiety effect at low doses and sleep-inducing effects at moderate doses with relatively few serious side effects as noted above.[4] Although abuse, dependence, discontinuation syndrome and oversedation are well-known possible complications, these compounds are remarkably useful and safe when prescribed intelligently and used in moderation. Despite their common prescription by many practitioners, there are those prescribers or clinical settings where benzodiazepine prescriptions are unnecessarily avoided. Prescribers fear that the patient will become addicted, or that the clinician's willingness to prescribe tranquilizers will be taken advantage of.

A commonly used phrase is "A benzo is a benzo is a benzo…", meaning the drug class is relatively homogeneous in indications and uses. In addition, side effects are virtually identical or are very similar. In general, there is no safety advantage to one benzodiazepine over another, other than the issues created by long half-life compounds noted in Table 10.1. These can cause possible "hangover effects" or amnesia in the morning. Their habituating properties are also generally similar although shorter-acting benzos have a somewhat higher risk of habituation and physical tolerance.

It is of crucial importance in choosing a benzodiazepine or other sedative hypnotic to match the half-life of the compound chosen with the type of difficulty the patient is having. For example, a patient with a consistent level of anxiety throughout the day would benefit from longer-acting medication (such as clonazepam) which might only need to be given twice a day. A shorter-acting medication (such as alprazolam) might require up to four doses a day.

Similarly, a patient who is having difficulty in falling asleep, but stays asleep once asleep, would benefit from a short-acting benzo as a hypnotic that would induce sleep but would likely be metabolized and excreted prior to awakening, leaving minimal morning medication hangover. Such a short-acting compound would not be used in a patient with sleep continuity disturbance, since the patient needs help in the middle of the night, not shortly after taking the medication. A short-acting compound would be metabolized and excreted, and be of minimal help when the patient needs it most. Patients with early morning awakening would be better treated with an intermediate-acting compound, which, it is hoped, would be present in sufficient amounts to sustain longer sleep until their normal awakening time. In general, long-acting sedative/hypnotics such as flurazepam (with a half-life of 2–5 days) are problematic for many patients since they give a significant sedative effect during the day, and make it difficult for the patient to rise without a morning medication hangover. Older patients in particular are at risk for drug accumulation and drug hangover, leading to increased risk of falls or accidents.

Except in patients with a history of substance abuse, who often may require – from the patient's point of view – an increasing dose of medication, most individuals will maintain an anti-anxiety effect over the long term without dosage escalation. Used as a hypnotic, however, a benzodiazepine may lose the hypnotic effect over time with repeated usage. Other individuals can comfortably utilize the medication safely for sleep induction over the long term, particularly if taken less than every night.

Those who take benzodiazepines nightly for several months can experience some rebound insomnia, lasting 1–7 days, when the medication is stopped.

Benzodiazepines and dementia – a false correlation

For several years there has been an Internet buzz about the possibility that the use of benzodiazepines caused an increase in dementia. This has been predominantly fueled by rumor, innuendo and non-fact-based Internet sites. There has now been a comprehensive large-scale review on a nationwide basis looking at this concept.[5] In over 235,000 patients, the authors confidently state that this large cohort study "did not reveal associations between the use of benzodiazepines ... and subsequent dementia." There were even some limited results which supported a protective effect against dementia.

It is possible that this false association began because of the large numbers of individuals who have used benzodiazepines and a similarly large group who have also developed dementia. Therefore, there is significant overlap with the two large cohorts. However, a statistical overlap does not indicate a causative effect and the above study clearly refutes any causation. This study also looked at the use of non-benzodiazepine, benzodiazepine-like sleeping medications, often called the Z drugs – eszopiclone (Lunesta), zaleplon (Sonata) and zolpidem (Ambien, Ambien CR Edluar, and Zolpimist). Similarly, there was no causal effect between the use of these medications and dementia.

Benzodiazepine withdrawal

With very high doses of benzodiazepines taken over extended periods of time, frank physical withdrawal and seizures may result from sudden discontinuation. Benzodiazepine withdrawal symptoms include:

- muscular twitches/tremors
- anxiety
- insomnia
- irritability
- mild delirium
- if severe withdrawal, seizures and paranoia.

This is seldom a problem if the clinician actively monitors the patient's condition and progress, limits the quantities prescribed and gradually lowers the dosage when stopping the medication. This issue is covered in more depth in Chapter 8.

Geography, politics and benzodiazepines

Geography and politics have altered the availability of high-potency benzodiazepines in different countries. Triazolam has been withdrawn from the UK market because of its ability to cause retrograde amnesia (loss of memory for events that occurred in the several hours <u>before</u> the medication was taken). Triazolam remains fully available in the United States, with recommendations to use smaller doses (0.25 mg) to avoid this complication. Rohypnol (flunitrazepam), in contrast, is available in the UK by private prescription, as well as in some other countries including Mexico and India. It has, however, never been available in the United States, having gained the label of a "date rape" drug, thus being too dangerous to use.

The commonality to these two preparations is that both compounds are high-potency benzodiazepines that may cause increased side effects at higher doses in sensitive individuals, or when combined with alcohol. Used in smaller doses, under appropriate medical oversight, neither drug is likely the dangerous compound portrayed, but they are both medications that should be prescribed with caution in modest doses.

New labeling

In 2020, the American Food and Drug Administration requested revisions to boxed warnings for this group as well as in patient medication guides. These warnings are not really new information, they are simply underscoring what we have known for many years and attempting to reinforce the potential risks for prescribers and patients. The FDA Commissioner has stated: "While benzodiazepines are important therapies for many Americans, they are also commonly abused and misused, often together with opioid pain relievers and other medicines, alcohol, and illicit drugs."[6] Although the precise risk of benzodiazepine addiction remains unclear, population data clearly indicate that both primary benzodiazepine use disorders and polysubstance addiction involving benzodiazepines do occur. Data from the national survey on drug use and health for 2015–2016[7] suggest that half a million community-dwelling U.S. adults were estimated to have a benzodiazepine use disorder for 2015–2016.

Stimulant medication and its appropriate uses

The general term "stimulant" refers to properties of certain drugs or medications which "stimulate" or enhance a particular body system, such as cardiac stimulants or respiratory stimulants. In mental health, however, the term is used specifically to identify a group of medications – especially norepinephrine and dopamine – which have a variety of neurological and physical effects and are postulated to act by affecting brain catecholamine neurotransmitters.

First used for behaviorally disturbed children, benzedrine began to be used in 1937. Eleven years later, dexedrine was introduced, with the advantage of having equal efficacy at half the dose. Methylphenidate (marketed as Ritalin) was introduced in 1954 with the hope that it would have fewer side effects and less abuse potential.

Table 10.4 List of available stimulants grouped by underlying active ingredient

Amphetamine	Adderall, Adderall XR, Evekeo
Methylphenidate	Concerta, Daytrana, Desoxyn, Metadate, Metadate CD, Methylin, Ritalin, Ritalin SR, Ritalin LA, Aptensio, Contempla XR, Jornay PM, Quillchew, Quillivant XR, Adhansia XR, CoTempla, Adzenys, Desoxyn
Dexmethylphenidate	Focalin, Focalin XR
Mixed salts	Mysdaysis
Dextroamphetamine	ProCentra, Dextrostat, Zenzedi, Dexedrine
Lisdexamfetamine	Vyvanse

Proliferation of both branded and generic stimulants has escalated rapidly. Currently, there are a staggering array of branded stimulants as shown in Table 10.4. The underlying chemicals contained in these brands, however, are closely related and/or stereoisomers of the parent compounds such as amphetamine and dextroamphetamine, or lisdexamphetamine, methylphenidate and dexmethylphenidate. Other than the speed with which the medication enters the system (immediately or time release) and the modality of preparation (pills, capsules, liquid or patch), these medications have generally similar effects, uses, side effects and prescriptive patterns. Although, as with all psychotropics, there is individual variability of response to any particular drug in this medication class, there is little statistical therapeutic advantage for one medication over another. It is often useful for the beginning clinician initially to learn well one or two preparations/medications and be less concerned with the remainder of the list. With experience, other preparations can be learned.

Other uses of stimulant medication

Because of stimulants' wide effects in the central and peripheral nervous systems (such as increased alertness, wakefulness and arousal; enhanced endurance, productivity and motivation; increased motor activity, heart rate and blood pressure), they have been used in mental health practice in a variety of additional clinical situations. These include:

- to counteract lethargy and fatigue
- to reduce sleepiness and increase wakefulness
- to decrease appetite and promote weight loss
- to treat narcolepsy
- off-label as a third- or fourth-line treatment for clinical depression
- as a remedy for the side effect of dizziness due to lowered blood pressure.

Why so many? The "me too" concept of medication development

A prescriber might, and probably should ask why there are so many medications in this class with virtually the same or similar ingredients and preparations. Five of the medications in Table 10.4 have been introduced in the last 5 years, despite the fact that there already were multiple preparations of stimulants on the market and that this class of medications has been utilized successfully since the 1950s. Other than the development of a skin patch which does not require swallowing a pill, none of these medications is significantly "new" compared to what was already available. As has happened with antidepressants and antipsychotics, when a new therapeutic indication is discovered, pharmaceutical companies will often test and market medications which are very similar in actions and side effects. There are multiple reasons for a company to formulate and sell "me too" medications, virtually all of which have to do with limiting expense and maximizing profitability.

It is very expensive for a company to discover, test and ultimately obtain approval from regulatory bodies regarding safety and efficacy for a new product. One way of limiting these costs is to develop a medication which has an already proven mechanism of action in other products. This greatly increases the likelihood that the company's "new" medication will be effective and have relatively few side effects. Second, medications taken for mental health problems are often taken regularly for long periods of time or are re-instituted after a clinical relapse when the medication is stopped, resulting in substantial sales. Third, a branded "me too" medication may be covered and paid for by medical insurance. Thus, the company has a medication which will have a large potential for profit.

Although this is not the only consideration, a prescriber must consider cost to the patient as one element of the prescriber's medication choice. An older generic medication may be just as effective as a newer brand-name preparation at a considerably lower cost. A prescriber therefore must make every effort to ascertain whether a "new" medication is truly different and/or has significant advantages. If so, the prescription of a branded medication which inevitably is more expensive than available generic preparations may be wise. If not, with the "new" medication being essentially a "me too" clone, prescription of a generic or an older tried and true medication, with which the practitioner has considerable familiarity, may be the better choice.

Pharmaceutical representatives will always tout the company's rationale for a recently introduced branded product which may or may not actually provide significant advantage taking into account the increased costs. Colorful advertisements in medical journals or the provision of samples to the practitioner should not greatly influence the prescriber's decision-making if clinical advantage is minimal or not present (see also Chapter 26 on generic medications).

Dosing of stimulants

The initial dosing of stimulants in immediate-release and sustained-release preparations can be seen for each specific medication in Appendices 4 and 5. For *children and adolescents*, for example, the American Academy of Child and Adolescent Psychiatry recommends[8] starting doses of 2.5 mg of mixed salt amphetamines (Adderall) or 5 mg of methylphenidate (Ritalin and others). If symptom control is not achieved, the dose generally should be increased in weekly increments of 2.5–5 mg for mixed salt amphetamines or 5–10 mg per dose for methylphenidate. Full symptom control may require multiple doses during the day. In general, patients are started on immediate-release preparations. When symptom control is achieved, long-acting preparations may be substituted. For individuals who are deemed to be at higher risk for abuse of medication, long-acting preparations are preferred because they may minimize the potential for abuse.

When long-acting preparations are used, their effect may not carry over into the late afternoon or early evening. If concentration and attention is needed at those times of day (for homework or other activities), it may be useful to provide a small "tail" dose of an immediate-release preparation later in the day. When doing so, the clinician must be aware that such a "tail" may produce a delay in sleep onset.

Dosing strategies in *adults* vary, although one common practice is to start at modest doses (2.5–5 mg of an immediate-release product) and increase after a week, aiming for target doses of 0.5 mg per kilogram of body weight.[9]

Side effects of stimulants

Because of the stimulatory effect of this class of medication on norepinephrine and dopamine, the common side effects of stimulants are relatively easy to predict. They include:

- decreased appetite
- weight loss
- difficulty initiating or maintaining sleep
- irritability
- headache
- jitteriness and palpitations
- feeling flushed or sweating
- behavioral tics.

While clinicians and researchers have long been concerned about the cardiovascular effects of stimulants, recent studies have been reassuring. Children followed over a 10-year period showed no increase in blood pressure or heart rate when treated with stimulants[10] and cardiovascular events were rare.[11–13]

Abuse of stimulants

As outlined above, the process for prescribing stimulant medications is generally straight-forward and not difficult. There is, however, one significant area relevant to stimulant prescription that can potentially create significant problems – medication misuse, abuse and diversion. Each of these terms is defined differently, but all three apply to the inappropriate usage of stimulants. "Misuse" is a generalized term in which a medication is utilized for a purpose or dose that is not consistent with medical guidelines. With stimulants, this can involve unauthorized escalation of the dose by the patient or utilizing the medication primarily to obtain a drug "high."

Drug "abuse" has been defined by the APA's *Diagnostic and Statistical Manual* as repeated, recurrent use of a substance despite adverse consequences of its use. Some individuals, particularly those with chemical dependency or substance use disorder, are prone to abuse stimulants, and such patients require careful monitoring. Both of these issues, as well as guidelines to clinicians for minimizing these possibilities, are covered in more depth in Chapter 22 on the misuse of medication.

"Diversion" of medication is a third clinical entity which is unfortunately common with stimulant prescription. Diversion occurs when medication prescribed for one individual is given to another for whom it is not prescribed. This happens with frequency in high schools, on college and university campuses, or in other group settings where teens and young adults spend considerable time together. Medications are "shared," traded for other medications/goods/services or sold for money.

Research surveys have documented the pervasive extent of medication diversion. In a 10-year longitudinal study of youth to whom stimulants were prescribed for ADHD, it was found that 22 percent misused their medication and 11 percent diverted it.[14] A survey of 11,000 college students at over 100 university campuses in the United States calculated that 7 percent of students had misused their stimulants for non-medical purposes during their lifetime and 4 percent of them had done so in the past year.[15] Stimulants in the higher education arena are seen as "study aids" and therefore as valuable commodities to increase concentration, wakefulness, study skills and exam performance. Two different Internet surveys reported the incidence of stimulant misuse for the purpose of increased concentration at 6.0 percent and 5.4 percent, respectively.[16–17]

The clinician, then, is caught in a bind. Stimulant medications are helpful, targeted treatments which improve patient clarity, organization and attention to detail in those patients who have the diagnosed mental condition ADHD. Yet at the same time, there is the widely documented possibility for medication misuse and diversion. These are useful agents and it would be inappropriate for a clinician to avoid starting stimulant prescriptions altogether solely because of possible abuse by some patients. In certain situations, a prescriber may "inherit" a patient from another prescriber or setting who has benefited from stimulant use and has utilized them responsibly. To *pro forma* stop such a prescription would also not be prudent. Therefore, most prescribers do prescribe stimulants, but maintain vigilance to the signs and behaviors of potential misuse. These warning signs are listed in Table 10.5.

Several points are important to note in reading Table 10.5:

* Virtually all of the statistical data collected on stimulant misuse shows that immediate-release stimulants are abused almost exclusively in comparison to long-acting, time-release preparations. While it might seem that limiting stimulant prescriptions solely to long-acting preparations would solve the misuse problem, this is not a practical solution. There are clearly some patients who do not respond sufficiently well to long-acting preparations, and get full symptom relief only with

Table 10.5 Warning signs of possible stimulant misuse

* Frequent or continuous requests for increased dosage levels
* Missed appointments and inconsistent attendance at follow-up appointments
* Repeated lost prescriptions or requests for an early refill
* Calls for an emergency supply of medication
* Symptoms of psychosis (especially hallucinations which can occur at high doses of stimulants)
* Syncope, shortness of breath and palpitations (all of which can occur at elevated stimulant doses)
* Insistent demands for immediate-release stimulants as opposed to time-release preparations
* Other behavioral signs of substance abuse (see Chapter 22)

Source: Signs and symptoms of amphetamine abuse, available at: www.narconon.org/drug-abuse/amphetamine-signs-symptoms.html

immediate-release preparations. It is also easier to raise dosage and assess therapeutic effect with immediate-release preparations and switch later to time-release products.

- In the statistical studies cited above, the vast majority of individuals who misuse and abuse stimulants had a history of chemical dependency and/or a substance use disorder. Therefore, screening for these disorders is a critical part of initial ADHD treatment and the use of stimulants for other purposes. For those patients who have active signs of substance abuse and/or a strong history of abusing psychostimulants or other drugs, treatment for these issues must be undertaken first prior to any prescription of stimulants. When stimulant prescription is deemed appropriate for these individuals, it would be wise to avoid the use of immediate-release preparations and begin treatment with time-release preparations only.
- No clinician, no matter how diligent, can totally eliminate the possibility of medication misuse and diversion in her/his prescribing practice. There are a number of strategies that a clinician should undertake to minimize and counteract medication misuse. These are discussed in detail in Chapter 22 and it would be beneficial for the reader to proceed to that chapter before starting the next chapter of this text in sequence.

Some clinicians, particularly those in institutional settings, advocate the use of patient "Contracts" or "Advisories" when prescribing stimulants. These documents usually contain specifics about the necessity of adherence to prescribed medication dosing and the consequences for medication misuse or its diversion. The effectiveness of such contracts is unclear. In all likelihood the sociopathic, personality-disordered or drug-abusing patient would not be dissuaded from inappropriate use of medication by having signed a contract. Nevertheless, such documents do alert patients to the clinician's response for such behavior.

When used, usually two areas are covered in the contractual agreement:

- The clinician states how *patient* behaviors such as lost, stolen or otherwise misplaced prescriptions and doses will be managed. With stimulants, the appropriate response is that no additional medications will be provided and no early renewals of the prescription will occur. Unlike other abusable prescription medications (for example, benzodiazepines), abrupt stoppage of stimulants may be uncomfortable for the patient, but does not represent a serious health or safety concern. Going without stimulant medication for a period of time may also serve to reinforce to the patient that they need to be more careful in the future.
- A second area discussed in such contracts is especially useful in an institutional setting. This section can describe how *the clinician* will respond to any documented occurrence of diversion or misuse. The appropriate response in this situation is prompt and permanent discontinuation of stimulant prescription. The prescriber should also report the incident to the institutional authorities for whatever further action is appropriate. To make this policy effective, of course, the clinician must follow through on his/her policy quickly and consistently to establish an institutional climate of appropriate control. If the clinician fails to do so with the thought of being "lenient," it only serves to increase the likelihood of future misbehavior on the part of the identified patient or others at the facility.

Notes and references

1 Brooks M (2020) Despite dangers, docs continue to co-prescribe benzos, opiods, available at: www.medscape.com/viewarticle/923935

2 Eaton WW *et al.* (1981) The Epidemiologic Catchment Area Program of the National Institute of Mental Health. *Public Health Reports* 96(4): 319–325.

3 Tyrer P (1980) Dependence on benzodiazepines. *British Journal of Psychiatry* 137: 576–577; see also Mehdi T (2012) Benzodiazepines revisited. *British Journal of Medical Practitioners* 5(1): a501.

4 McGee M and Pres R (2002) Benzodiazepines in primary practice: risks and benefits. *Resident Staff Physician* 48 (4): 42–49.

5 Osler M and Jørgensen MB (2020) Associations of benzodiazepines, Z-drugs, and other anxiolytics with subsequent dementia in patients with affective disorders: a nationwide cohort and nested case-control study. *American Journal of Psychiatry* 177(6): 497–505.

6 Statement from Stephen M Hahn, MD, Commissioner of the U.S. Food and Drug Administration.

7 Substance Abuse and Mental Health Services Administration (2017) *Results from the 2016 National Survey on Drug Use and Health: Detailed Tables*, Center for Behavioral Health Statistics and Quality Rockville, MD.

8 Greenhill LL *et al.* (2002) Practice parameter for the use of stimulant medications in the treatment of children, adolescents, and adults. *AACAP Official Action* 41(2) (Suppl.): 26S–49S, available at: www.jaacap.org/article/S0890-8567(09)60553-0/abstract

9 Aashish P (2012) Diagnosis and treatment of ADHD in adults. *Carlat Psychiatry Report* 10(*2*): 4–5.

10 Vitiello B *et al.* (2011) Blood pressure and heart rate over 10 years in the multimodal treatment study of children with ADHD. *American Journal of Psychiatry* 10: 1176.

11 Perrin JM (2008) Cardiovascular monitoring and stimulant drugs for attention-deficit/hyperactivity disorder. *Pediatrics* 122(2): 451–453.

12 Schelleman H *et al.* (2011) Cardiovascular events and death in children exposed and unexposed to ADHD agents. *Pediatrics* 127(6): 1102–1110.

13 Cooper WO *et al.* (2011) ADHD drugs and serious cardiovascular events in children and young adults. *New England Journal of Medicine* 365(20): 1896–1904.

14 Wilens T *et al.* (2006) Characteristics of adolescents and young adults with ADHD who divert or misuse their prescribed medications. *Journal of the American Academy of Child and Adolescent Psychiatry* 45: 408–414.

15 McCabe SE *et al.* (2005) Non-medical use of prescription stimulants among US college students: prevalence and correlates from a national survey. *Addiction* 100: 96–106.

16 Teter CJ *et al.* (2005) Prevalence and motives for illicit use of prescription stimulants in an undergraduate student sample. *Journal of American College Health* 53: 253–262.

17 Sussman S *et al.* (2006) Misuse of "study drugs": prevalence, consequences, and implications for policy. *Substance Abuse Treatment, Prevention, and Policy* 1: 15.

11 "Natural" substances – do they help?

• Are natural substances superior to prescription medicines?	152
• The shopping bag presentation	152
• Potentially helpful natural substances	154
• Potentially harmful natural substances	159
• Notes and references	160

A natural product is a chemical compound or substance produced by a living organism – that is, found in nature. In the broadest sense, natural products include any substance produced by life. In discussing the substances as they may relate to psychotropic medication, other texts may refer to them as complementary, alternative and integrative treatments; dietary supplements, homeopathic remedies, vitamins, minerals, nutraceuticals, "foods," herbs or metabolites. This book will use the broad term "natural substances."

For the mental health prescriber, it is less important what name is given to the class than to know which are potentially useful as add-ons and which may have no place in the prescriber's toolbox. On occasion, it is important to recognize which of the substances can, in fact, be dangerous, to be avoided at all costs. Therefore, this chapter will be divided into helpful natural medicines, neutral substances which have no proven benefit but are deemed harmless, and harmful natural substances. Before doing so, however, some general comments are necessary to show why this knowledge is essential for every practitioner.

For many, the word "chemical" has come to mean synthetic, man-made or laboratory-produced substances that are, for some individuals, things to be avoided.[1] Some patients have an overwhelming belief that "natural" substances are safer and more useful than synthesized medications. The practitioner may not be aware until the patient is in the office of his/her belief about natural substances, as many patients will arrive at the office for an evaluation carrying an entire bag of various substances that they had been taking. Particularly with the advent of the Internet, patients will often ask practitioners about the benefit or risks of certain natural products about which they have read or started to take.

The use of natural substances for prevention or treatment of a wide variety of medical conditions is a large and growing field. Without too much difficulty, a reader may find vast numbers of articles, journals, advertisements and recommendations for the use of natural products for conditions such as sleep problems, anxiety, depression, diabetes, boosting of the immune system, weight loss, as well as protection from and/ or cure of cancer. It is well beyond the scope of this text to evaluate many of these claims and products. Nonetheless, it becomes important to discuss some of the more commonly used preparations that have been suggested to improve mental health or treat mental conditions. No matter whether the practitioner utilizes and/or believes in the effectiveness of these substances, he/she cannot avoid dealing with the issue because:

- Some natural substances are, in fact, helpful.
- Some natural substances are patently dangerous.
- Some patients have already utilized a few or many natural substances in their attempt at self-help and will ask the practitioner about the wisdom of their use.
- For some patients, natural substances are the best or only treatments they will accept.

Are natural substances superior to prescription medicines?

This question cannot be answered in broad-brush fashion. Each compound must be looked at specifically to assess its possible benefit and/or risks. It is reasonable, however, to state that the vast majority of vitamins, minerals, spices and foods are neither significantly beneficial nor harmful. The practitioner cannot assume that all "natural medicine" is fraudulent or automatically will not have any benefit, since a handful of natural compounds have reasonable scientific evidence to support their use. Some of these compounds have been used for centuries even though a mechanism of action is not yet understood.

Although infrequent, at times it is possible to utilize natural substances as a first alternative in some mental illnesses. Patients with a strong predisposition toward these products may find it much more palatable to accept one of these "natural" treatments, at least as a first alternative. Such an approach by a practitioner allows time for the bond between prescriber and patient to become stronger. If the natural substance has benefits, it is not inconceivable that it could be continued as a primary treatment. If this "natural" treatment is ineffective, which may only become apparent after 4–6 weeks, the patient may have enough faith in the practitioner to be willing to try prescription medications

There are a small number of patients who are almost fanatical about using vitamins, minerals, herbs, etc., as treatment. In this case when this becomes apparent, the practitioner may find it more beneficial to make an early referral to a homeopathic practitioner or another medical practitioner knowledgeable about the use of natural products.

The shopping bag presentation

In this situation, the well-meaning patient brings in a large number of vials, bottles or envelopes filled with a wide variety of natural substances. As has already been mentioned in Chapter 3, early on in the prescriptive process the practitioner will want to know what prescription and non-prescription substances the patient may already be taking. After the prescriber says that he/she needs to know all the substances that the patient is taking, the shopping bag appears at the second visit.

While time-consuming, the prescriber should at least look at the label of each of these substances for the medical record as well as to advise the patient authoritatively. As has been mentioned, the vast majority of these substances are neither helpful nor harmful. When appropriate, each one should be verbally labeled as such for the patient. In general, it is not helpful to rapidly state that all of these substances are useless or unnecessary. In doing so, the practitioner will send a signal that he/she thinks the patient is ignorant or has made mistakes.

Box 11.1 Talking to patients

When a prescriber is presented with a small or large number of natural products, each bottle or package should be at least cursorily seen. Obviously if the patient is taking something that is harmful, this needs to be mentioned, although this tends to be uncommon. A visual technique, particularly for those patients who have many such substances is to begin three piles, one pile of helpful products, one of those which may be harmful and a third pile which is "neutral." It is not unusual to find some substances with which the practitioner is not familiar. If there is time, such a substance can be researched on the computer during the session. At other times, there is pressure to complete the evaluation and it would be too time-consuming to do this with multiple different compounds. In this case, the practitioner should note the names of these substances and research them briefly after the appointment, between the first and second visits. There can be a temptation to simply assure the patient that everything he or she is taking is OK even though the practitioner may not know that for sure. This should be avoided so that useful preparations can be utilized and supported. For neutral substances, the practitioner may state: *"I am familiar with these substances and I do not believe there is any valid scientific evidence to support their use in the treatment of your condition, but I do not necessarily recommend that they be stopped. It will be up to you whether you continue them or not, although I suspect you are spending a significant amount of money on these products for which science has not shown benefit. In the future, if you decide to take a new supplement, please inform me before you do so, so I can advise you."*

In dealing with these patients, the practitioner may wish, if possible, to include a recommendation for at least one natural substance where scientific evidence for its usefulness has been documented even when the practitioner's aim is to write a medication prescription. By doing so, the practitioner can recognize the patient's belief in the use of natural products and state *"these two prescriptions will work together to treat you in the fastest and most effective manner."*

Potentially helpful natural substances

Folate

Folate, also known as folic acid or Vitamin B9, is an important nutrient, present in leafy green vegetables and in fortified grain products, which is required for the human body to perform many essential processes on a day-to-day basis. Folate deficiency is one of the most common nutritional deficiencies in the world and has often been associated with many neuropsychiatric disorders. Low folate levels have been specifically associated with depression and dementia in some studies.[2] In general, folate level should be tested before using supplementation for depression or mild cognitive impairment. It has been used as a supplement in the treatment of depression but *does not work as a standalone treatment for depression*.[3] Some sources have suggested that supplementation is useful even in the absence of folate deficiency, although this practice has not been uniformly supported by evidence. Several older studies found that up to 35 percent of depressed patients are folate deficient. In seniors, the incidence of deficiency was even more marked and might still be as high as 90 percent. However, at least in the United States, FDA-required folate supplementation of grain products since 1998 and higher public awareness of the need for B-vitamin consumption and supplementation have reduced the relevance of these studies. Notwithstanding some promising studies and the 2007 meta-analysis and 2009 review, Mischoulon and Rosenbaum conclude that the data are still too preliminary to recommend consumer action beyond supplementation of folate deficiencies at this point. Two hundred to 500 μg per day have been used for adjunct treatment.[4–5] Folate is generally well tolerated in standard doses although stomach upset, skin inflammation, skin itching, nausea, flatulence, diarrhea and anemias have been reported.[6–7] Genetic variations in the MTHFR gene may reduce the ability to benefit fully from oral folate supplements, may be related to folate deficiency and/or account for the variation of response to the addition of folate.[8]

At the current time, the FDA has approved only one form of folate – l-methylfolate (Deplin) for use in the treatment of depression and schizophrenia. It has not been approved as a primary treatment, but rather as an additive form of treatment.[9]

SAM-e (S adenosyl Methionine)

SAM-e is an endogenous, intracellular *amino acid metabolite* and enzyme co-substrate involved in multiple crucial biochemical pathways, including biosynthesis of hormones and neurotransmitters. Used in a dosage range between 400 mg and 1600 mg this amino acid has shown usefulness in the treatment of major depressive disorder.[10] More similar to a vitamin than a drug, SAM-e is a natural metabolite that the body needs more of as we age or if we become ill. SAM-e is generally safe and evidence-based in the treatment of depression. It is also a promising neuroprotectant. SAM-e has been approved as a prescription drug for depression in Germany, Italy, Spain and Russia, and has been in use in Europe for over three decades. In the United States, it is available over the counter and is typically used as an adjunct to the prescription of another antidepressant. Its advantages are that it does not cause sexual dysfunction and may actually lessen the sexual dysfunction that comes with serotonergic antidepressants. It also does not interfere with cognition or memory. Its most common side effects are nausea, diarrhea, vomiting and abdominal distress.[11] Rarely, it causes serotonin syndrome – a potentially deadly complication that causes agitation, anxiety, confusion, nausea, vomiting and palpitations (see Chapter 20 on serious side effects). As with any compound that has some measure of antidepressant activity, it may precipitate hypomanic or manic symptoms in a bipolar patient.[12]

Ginkgo biloba

Ginkgo biloba is an ancient Chinese herbal remedy that has been shown to have significant neuroprotective effects; until recently, this was confirmed by all sources.[13–14] Two recent major studies, however, and a Cochrane review cast doubt on the validity of the prior, smaller and shorter studies, and determined that in the aggregate, the data do not support the use of ginkgo in the prevention of Alzheimer's disease. The recent evidence is mostly negative, though the studies are still inconsistent. Although ginkgo has a small effect in protecting against mild cognitive impairment/dementia, it probably does not prevent it. Given ginkgo's relatively low cost and benign risk profile, providers may support its use in these conditions.[15]

Ginkgo's effect on memory enhancement has had conflicting results. While some evidence suggests that ginkgo extract might modestly improve memory in healthy adults, most studies indicate that ginkgo doesn't improve memory, attention or brain function. This herbal supplement derived from the leaves of the ginkgo tree has also been used to counteract antidepressant-related sexual problems.[16]

When used orally in moderate amounts (80–240 mg per day in divided doses), ginkgo appears to be safe for most healthy adults. It can cause: headache, dizziness, heart palpitations, upset stomach and constipation. Ginkgo has the potential to reduce the effectiveness of alprazolam, fluoxetine and imipramine. Its use with ibuprofen or anticoagulants may reduce blood clotting and increase one's risk of bleeding

Melatonin

Melatonin, whose chemical structure is N-acetyl-5-methoxytryptophan, is a neurohormone that has been shown to be effective in treating jet lag and shift-work adjustment. There is some evidence that it is a promising treatment for other sleep problems, including sleep latency insomnia and sleep enhancement, although the research in these areas remains limited. Many other mental health conditions have purportedly been improved by the use of melatonin, but this remains unproven.

Melatonin is classified by the FDA as "generally regarded as safe" for short-term use. It can readily be found in pharmacies and supermarkets in capsules or tablets containing 1 mg and 3 mg. Because the metabolism of the drug varies considerably from person to person and is decreased with advancing age, it is generally recommended that the patient be started on a small dose such as 1 mg per day, gradually working up to 3 mg. If the issue is to counteract the effect of jet lag heading west to east, 1 to 3 mg at the local bedtime is recommended. When traveling east to west, one half of the above dose immediately following a night or an early morning awakening is the recommended first dose.[17]

A special situation which bears mentioning is the use of melatonin during pregnancy for disrupted sleep. Many patients perceive melatonin as being safe and produced by the body and therefore of less risk during pregnancy. While this hormone is, in fact, produced normally by the body, it occurs in very small amounts. The typical dose of melatonin (1–3 mg) elevates blood melatonin levels up to 20 times higher than normal. We know very little about the impact of high levels of melatonin on the developing fetus. Thus, it is typically advised for pregnant women with sleep problems to use medications with a better characterized reproductive safety profile, such as doxylamine (brand name Bonjesta). Each tablet contains 20 mg of doxylamine succinate, an antihistamine, and 20 mg of pyridoxine HCl (a vitamin B6 analog); benzodiazepines may also be used with effectiveness and relative safety.[18–19]

The compound itself does not have significant toxic effects, but commonly reported side effects include mild fatigue, dizziness, headache, irritability and sleepiness. There are known interactions with zolpidem, benzodiazepines, a wide variety of antidepressants, warfarin, beta blockers and glaucoma medication. If the melatonin is to be used in the same patient with any of these medications, it is best to look for the specific interaction and possible complications in a text focused on natural remedies and their side effects such as Mischoulan and Rosenbaum's *Natural Medications for Psychiatric Disorders*;[20] or Richard Brown's *How to Use Herbs, Nutrients and Yoga in Mental Health Care*.[21]

Omega-3 polyunsaturated fatty acids (fish oil)

Omega-3 polyunsaturated fatty acids are some of the most studied natural compounds in the treatment and prophylaxis of mental health conditions. This has come in part from observations that cultures whose diet is high in fish, such as the Japanese, have lower rates of depression.[22] Expert dietary recommendations include eating oily fish at least twice a week, but even when this is followed, additional supplementation with fish oil capsules appears to have benefit in the treatment and prophylaxis of mood disorders. Approximately 60 percent of the current placebo-controlled studies show a benefit[23]as an adjunctive medicine in the treatment of depression[24-25] and the stabilization of bipolar disorder.[26] There is also valid data that regular amounts of omega-3s should be included in a heart-healthy diet. Multiple other claims for its usefulness in a wide variety of mental health conditions have been made, but the evidence is slim and unconvincing as yet.

Side effects are essentially the same as those for eating fish and appear minimal. The most common side effect is indigestion and flatulence. Since predatory fish including tuna, salmon, perch, pike and swordfish are used in its preparation, there may also be contaminants which include mercury and PCBs (polychlorinated biphenyls). While measurable, there are not enough of these contaminants to prevent the recommendation of omega-3s as an *adjunctive* treatment in depression and bipolar disorder. While fish oil may be helpful in delaying or preventing first or subsequent depressive episodes, there is limited evidence that it can be used as a primary treatment without the additional prescription of another psychotropic agent. In spite of this, omega-3s may provide a standalone treatment option for people concerned about side effects, such as the elderly, people with multiple medical conditions, and women who are pregnant or breastfeeding.[27] There is some evidence of omega-3s serving as a neuroprotective agent, although the research proving this trait is still evolving.

Part of the confusion about efficacy studies of omega-3s is that fish oil contains various amounts of EPA (eicosapentaenoic acid) and DHA (docosahexaenoic acid). Although most fish oil capsules contain 1000 mg of fish oil, the proportion of EPA to DHA and the total amount of fish oil in each capsule varies considerably. It has now been shown that a high EPA to DHA formula is best for mental health uses. Since a significant amount of the research has not utilized this ratio, negative study outcomes may be due to testing with an ineffective formula. For the prescription and patient use therefore, when choosing an omega-3 preparation, an EPA to DHA ratio should be at least 3:2, and if possible 2:1. Instruct the patient to read and compare labels carefully prior to purchase and use. For major depression, 1–2 g/day of an EPA+DHA combination, with at least 60 percent EPA, is recommended.[28] Caution is needed in prescribing fish oil with bipolar depression, because the omega-3s may bring on mania, as can most antidepressants.[29]

St. John's Wort (Hypericum perforatem)

St. John's Wort is another natural compound that has been studied and widely used throughout Europe and the United States. Considered as a blooming flower plant or a weed, there are numerous studies confirming its effectiveness in depression.[30] Although virtually all the studies were short-term in nature (24–26 weeks at most), there are multiple studies that support the use of St John's Wort in mild to moderate depression.[31–32] There is some indication that it could also be useful in severe depression.[33]

Taken in standard doses (300 mg three times a day) St. John's Wort is relatively safe with relatively few side effects, although phototoxicity does occur in susceptible individuals. There is a long list of potential interactions with other medications, especially medications which affect liver and intestinal enzyme function. It is beyond the scope of this text to identify all the potential interactions and Mischoulan and Rosenbaum's *Natural Medications for Psychiatric Disorders*[34] or Richard Brown's *How to Use Herbs, Nutrients & Yoga in Mental Health Care*[35] should be consulted for detailed information on these interactions. It is important to mention one common potential interaction: St. John's Wort should not be combined with other non-prescription or prescription antidepressants in order to prevent serotonin syndrome.

It is a common recommendation for patients who prefer natural treatments to be given St. John's Wort as an initial treatment for mild to moderate depression. If it is not effective in 4–6 weeks, it should be stopped before substituting another agent, particularly an SSRI or SNRI. Brown *et al.* opine[36] that 35 double-blind randomized trials found that the dropout rate and adverse effect ratio for patients taking St. John's Wort were similar to placebo and slightly lower than SSRI.

Valerian root

Valerian is the root of a grassland plant. There are multiple varieties of valerian, although only one strain (Valeriana Officinalis), has been studied. It is the most commonly used herbal sleep medication in both the United States and Europe.[37] There have been many studies of its use in inducing sleep and improving the quality of sleep. Based on a meta-analysis performed by Bent *et al.*[38] there is approximately an 80 percent positivity rate for improved sleep. These studies, however, had numerous methodological deficits and some had commercial bias. Therefore, their results should be looked at with some skepticism.

The dosage of valerian varies widely in the studies from 75 mg to 3000 mg, taken one half hour before sleep. It may take several weeks of regular dosing to notice an effect. Side effects were mild and generally not serious, but included an increased risk of diarrhea.[39] Precautions include not using it in persons who have liver disease or children under the age of three. An advantage to this preparation of valerian is that there is virtually no hangover effect in the morning.

CBD (cannabidiol)

Cannabidiol (CBD) is the second-most prevalent of the active ingredients of cannabis (marijuana). While CBD is an essential component of medical marijuana, it is derived directly from the hemp plant, which is a cousin of the marijuana plant. While CBD is a component of marijuana (one of hundreds), taken alone it does not cause a "high." According to a report from the World Health Organization, cited by Black *et al.*, in humans, CBD exhibits no effects indicative of any abuse or dependence potential and to date, there is no evidence of public health-related problems associated with the use of pure CBD.[40]

The antipsychotic, neuroprotective, anxiolytic and sedating properties suggest a potential therapeutic role for CBD and other nabiximols (the group to which CBD belongs) to treat various psychiatric disorders. The use of CBD at higher doses (above 1200 mg per day) showed some promising results in case studies of schizophrenia and psychosis occurring in patients with Parkinson's disease. Regarding the use of CBD to treat anxiety disorders, its anxiolytic effect can help patients with PTSD-related and social performance-related anxiety, and nabiximols can reduce the anxiety associated with the onset of tics. Of all the cases examined,[41] the strongest evidence was found for the treatment of cannabis-related disorders. The use of nabiximols yielded positive results in multiple studies of moderate to severe cannabis use disorder

Although touted for treatment uses in anxiety, sleep disturbance and chronic pain, there is currently limited evidence regarding the safety and efficacy of CBD for the treatment of psychiatric disorders.[42] However, available trials reported potential therapeutic effects for specific psychopathological conditions, such as substance use disorders, and chronic psychosis. There is also some favorable evidence in patients with Autism Spectrum Disorder for reducing hyperactivity, self-injurious behaviors, anxiety and insomnia. Nabiximols showed *no credible effect in the treatment of ADHD, while CBD was also found to be ineffective for bipolar disorder*. There is scarce evidence to suggest that cannabinoids improve depressive disorders and symptoms, Tourette syndrome or PTSD[43] without sufficient high-quality evidence in human studies pinpointing effective doses for treatment. Because CBD is currently predominantly available as an unregulated supplement, it's difficult to know exactly what amount of active ingredient a person is getting. Advice to patients should be, "If you decide to try CBD, talk with your primary care doctor – if for no other reason than to make sure it won't affect other medications you are taking."[44]

How to dose CBD is a common question among practitioners. Indeed, preclinical and clinical research indicates an extremely wide range of doses that have been used. More often than not, studies use the terms "low-dose" patients and "high-dose" patients. In the research, at least one author has defined "high dose" as between 150 and 600 mg of CBD.[45] Given the inconsistency in evidence-based dosing suggestions, the best advice is to "start low and go slow," with gradually increasing doses over a minimum of 2 weeks in which the clinician titrates to the desired effect.

CBD is becoming established in U.S. medicine, not just in terms of developing an evidence basis but also in its increased legalization, availability and clinical use. CBD is safer and more uniform in its composition than "medical marijuana," and it is associated with less variability in response. However, it is clear that further large-scale randomized controlled trials are required to better evaluate the efficacy of CBD in both acute and chronic illnesses.[46]

Potentially harmful natural substances

Kava

Kava or *Piper methysticum* (sometimes referred to as Kava Kava) is native to the islands of the South Pacific and is a member of the pepper family. Kava has been used as a ceremonial beverage in the South Pacific for centuries. It has been used in the West primarily for insomnia and anxiety. Currently it is used in a dosage of 150–400 mg per day, prepared in extracts, capsules, tablets and beverages. The reason that it is included in the potentially harmful section of this text is because it has a rare but serious danger of liver damage/failure, which can lead to death.[47] Given that there is only a modest benefit and a potentially life-threatening side effect, it is not generally recommended for use.[48]

DHEA

DHEA (5-Dehydroepiandrosterone) is a natural steroid produced in the adrenal glands, the gonads and the brain. It is the most abundant circulating steroid in humans. DHEA supplementation may help with depression, but it has a long list of potential hormonal side effects and drug interactions.[49] With the current state of knowledge and research, most authorities caution against use of DHEA for any mental health reason.[50]

Ma Huang (ephedra)

Primarily used for weight loss/obesity and to enhance athletic performance, ephedra has many serious side effects. It is also touted for hay fever, nasal congestion, asthma, bronchitis, colds and flu. The research-supported data for purported benefits are seriously outweighed by its side-effect profile which includes high blood pressure, heart attacks, muscle disorders, seizures, strokes, irregular heartbeat, loss of consciousness and death. Ephedra is banned in the United States and many other countries. Ephedrine and pseudoephedrine (both contained in ephedra) are legal depending on the particular U.S. state. These compounds are sold as ingredients of a popular decongestant (Sudafed)[51] under special regulatory procedures. They are also ingredients used in making methamphetamine.

Kratom

Kratom (*Mitragyna speciose*)[52] is a tropical evergreen tree native to Southeast Asia. Although there is much controversy as to its benefits, safety and risk, it is listed within the potentially dangerous section in this text because there has been a continuous drumbeat about its safety.

Indigenous populations have historically chewed the leaves or brewed them as a tea to improve endurance and reduce fatigue. Chemically within the opioid family, this natural but potentially problematic substance can be a stimulant in small doses, but a sedative and producer of euphoria in larger doses.[53] In the Western world, Kratom has been used as an energy booster, to relieve pain, to reduce symptoms of opioid withdrawal and is touted to treat a wide range of physical and mood problems including depression.[54] As with any opioid, there are potentially serious adverse effects including the possibility of addiction, withdrawal and overdose leading to death.[55] The use and potential abuse of this compound has continually been widely debated to the point that the FDA attempted to ban its use.[56] Subsequently due to public pressure, this potential ban was withdrawn.[57] Virtually no research has addressed the interaction between psychotropic medications and this herbal compound.[58]

Summary

The above section of the text is not intended in any way to list or describe all the plant-based or other natural substances which are harmful to the human body. Those listed here are only those that have been commonly reported to be risky, but have also been purported to be of benefit for mental health conditions or behavioral problems by other sources. Readers desiring a more thorough list should consult two of the references at the end of the chapter.[59-60]

In general, substances not mentioned in this chapter are benign in their safety profile and/or have not been promoted to be useful in the treatment of mental health conditions. It is probably best, however, to research a particular compound when and if a patient comes to the office having taken it or desiring your expert opinion since the number of potential natural substances is an ever-changing and growing list

Notes and references

1   Natural doesn't necessarily mean safer, or better, available at: https://nccih.nih.gov/health/know-science/natural-doesnt-mean-better

2   Fava M and Mischoulon D (2009) Folate in depression: efficacy, safety, differences in formulations, and clinical issues. *Journal of Clinical Psychiatry* 70 (Suppl. 5): 12–17.

3   Bottiglieri T (2005) Homocysteine and folate metabolism in depression. *Progress in Neuropsychopharmacology and Biological Psychiatry* 29(7): 1103–1112.

4   Mischoulon D and Rosenbaum JF (2008) *Natural Medications for Psychiatric Disorders: Considering the Alternatives*, Lippincott, Williams & Wilkins.

5   Bottiglieri T (1996) Folate, vitamin B-12 and neuropsychiatric disorders. *Nutrition Review* 54(12): 382–390. See also the more comprehensive discussion in Bottiglieri T. (2005) Homocysteine and folate metabolism in depression. *Progress in Neuropsychopharmacology and Biological Psychiatry* 29(7): 1103–1112.

6   Fava M and Mischoulon D (2009) Folate in depression: efficacy, safety, differences in formulations, and clinical issues. *Journal of Clinical Psychiatry* 70 (Suppl. 5): 12–17.

7   Fava M *et al.* (1997) Folate, vitamin B12, and homocysteine in major depressive disorder. *American Journal of Psychiatry* 154(3): 426–428.

8   Lake JA and Spiegel D (2007) *Complementary and Alternative Treatments in Mental Health Care*, American Psychiatric Publishing, Inc., p. 123.

9   Fava M *et al.* (1997) Folate, vitamin B12, and homocysteine in major depressive disorder. *American Journal of Psychiatry* 154(3): 426–428.

10   Lake JA and Spiegel D (2007) *Complementary and Alternative Treatments in Mental Health Care*, American Psychiatric Publishing, Inc.

11   SAMe: overview, available at: www.webmd.com/vitamins/ai/ingredientmono-786/same

12   Sharma A *et al.* (2017) S-Adenosylmethionine (SAMe) for neuropsychiatric disorders: a clinician-oriented review of research. *Journal of Clinical Psychiatry* 78(6): e656–e667, available at: www.ncbi.nlm.nih.gov/pmc/articles/PMC5501081/

13   Mental Health America (2016) *Complementary & Alternative Medicine for Mental Health*, available at: www.mhanational.org/sites/default/files/MHA_CAM.pdf

14   Ahlemeyer B and Kriegelstein J (2003) Neuroprotective effects of *Gingko biloba* extract. *Cellular and Molecular Life Sciences* 60: 1779–1792. doi: 10.1007/s00018-003-3080-1

15   Mischoulon D and Rosenbaum JF (2008) *Natural Medications for Psychiatric Disorders*, 2nd edn., Lippincott, Williams and Wilkins.

16   Brown RP *et al.* (2009) *How to Use Herbs, Nutrients & Yoga in Mental Health Care*, W. W. Norton and Company.

17   Ibid.; Mental Health America (2016) *Complementary & Alternative Medicine for Mental Health*, available at: www.mhanational.org/sites/default/files/MHA_CAM.pdf

18   MGH Center for Women's Mental Health (2016) Another medication for pregnancy-related nausea and vomiting, available at: https://womensmentalhealth.org/posts/another-medication-pregnancy-related-nausea-vomiting/

19   Mental Health America (2016) *Complementary & Alternative Medicine for Mental Health*, available at: www.mhanational.org/sites/default/files/MHA_CAM.pdf

20   Mischoulon D and Rosenbaum JF (2008) *Natural Medications for Psychiatric Disorders*, 2nd edn., Lippincott, Williams and Wilkins.

21   Brown RP *et al.* (2009) *How to Use Herbs, Nutrients & Yoga in Mental Health Care*, W. W. Norton and Company.

22   Parker G *et al.* (2006) Omega-3 fatty acids and mood disorders. *American Journal of Psychiatry* 163(6): 969–978.

23   Ibid.

24   Ibid.

25   Muskin PR *et al.* (eds.) (2013) Complementary and integrative therapies for psychiatric disorders. *Psychiatric Clinics of North America* 36(1) (Special Issue), p. 19.

26   Stoll AL *et al.* (1999) Omega-3 fatty acids in bipolar disorder: a preliminary double-blind, placebo-controlled trial. *Archives of General Psychiatry* 56: 380–381.

27   Muskin PR *et al.* (eds.) (2013) Complementary and integrative therapies for psychiatric disorders. *Psychiatric Clinics of North America* 36(1) (Special Issue), p. 19.

28   Muskin PR *et al.* (eds.) (2013) Complementary and integrative therapies for psychiatric disorders. *Psychiatric Clinics of North America* 36(1) (Special Issue), p. 19.

29   Stoll AL *et al.* (1999) Omega-3 fatty acids in bipolar disorder: a preliminary double-blind, placebo-controlled trial. *Archives of General Psychiatry* 56: 380–381.

30   National Center for Complementary and Integrative Health (2017, December) St. John's wort and depression: in depth, available at www.nccih.nih.gov/health/st-johns-wort-and-depression-in-depth (accessed February 22, 2019).

31   Ibid.

32   Ng QX *et al.* (2017, March 1) Clinical use of Hypericum perforatum (St John's wort) in depression: a meta-analysis. *Journal of Affective Disorders* 210: 211–221.

33   Ibid.

34   Mischoulon D and Rosenbaum JF (2008) *Natural Medications for Psychiatric Disorders*, 2nd edn., Lippincott, Williams and Wilkins.

35   Brown RP *et al.* (2009) *How to Use Herbs, Nutrients & Yoga in Mental Health Care*, W. W. Norton and Company.

36   Ibid.

37   Houghton PJ (1999) The scientific basis for the reputed activity of valerian. *Journal of Pharmacy and Pharmacology* 51: 505–512.

38   Bent S *et al.* (2006) Valerian for sleep: a systematic review and meta-analysis. *American Journal of Medicine* 119(12): 1005–1012.

39   Ibid.

40   Black N *et al.* (2019) Cannabinioids for the treatment of mental disorders and symptoms of mental disorders: a systematic review and meta-analysis, available at: www.thelancet.com/pdfs/journals/lanpsy/PIIS2215-0366(19)30401-8.pdf

41   Ibid.

42   Grinspoon P (2018) Cannabidiol (CBD) – what we know and what we don't, available at: www.health.harvard.edu/blog/cannabidiol-cbd-what-we-know-and-what-we-dont-2018082414476

43   Zhornitsky S and Potvin S (2012) Cannabidiol in humans: the quest for therapeutic targets. *Pharmaceuticals* 5: 529–552.

44   Grinspoon P (2018) Cannabidiol (CBD) – what we know and what we don't, available at: www.health.harvard.edu/blog/cannabidiol-cbd-what-we-know-and-what-we-dont-2018082414476

45   Zhornitsky S and Potvin S (2012) Cannabidiol in humans: the quest for therapeutic targets. *Pharmaceuticals* 5: 529–552.

46   Bonaccorso S *et al.* (2019) Cannabidiol (CBD) use in psychiatric disorders: a systematic review. *Neurotoxicology* 74: 282–298, available at: www.ncbi.nlm.nih.gov/pubmed/31412258

47   FDA (2002) Kava-containing dietary supplements may be associated with severe liver injury, available at: www.thebodypro.com/article/kava-containing-dietary-supplements-may-associated-severe-liver-i

48   What is Kava Kava?, available at: www.webmd.com/vitamins-and-supplements/what-is-kava-kava#1

49   Mayo Clinic Staff (2021) DHEA, available at: www.mayoclinic.org/drugs-supplements-dhea/art-20364199

50   Dehydroepiandrosterone. Facts & Comparisons eAnswers, available at: www.wolterskluwercdi.com/facts-comparisons-online/ (accessed August 17, 2017).

51   Ephedra: overview, available at: www.webmd.com/vitamins/ai/ingredientmono-847/ephedra

52   What is Kratom?, available at: www.drugabuse.gov/publications/drugfacts/kratom

53   Veltri C and Grundmann O (2019) Current perspectives on the impact of Kratom use. *Substance Abuse and Rehabilitation* 10: 23–31. doi: 10.2147/SAR.S164261

54   Collman JP (2001) *Naturally Dangerous: Surprising Facts about Food, Health and the Environment*, University Science Books.

55   Ten natural products that kill, available at: www.smithsonianmag.com/science-nature/ten-natural-products-that-kill-38268113/

56   Henningfield JE *et al.* (2018) The abuse potential of kratom according to the 8 factors of the Controlled Substances Act: implications for regulation and research. *Psychopharmacology* 235(2): 573–589.

57   Veltri C and Grundmann O (2019) Current perspectives on the impact of Kratom use. *Substance Abuse and Rehabilitation* 10: 23–31. doi: 10.2147/SAR.S164261

58   Ibid.

59   Ten natural products that kill, available at: www.smithsonianmag.com/science-nature/ten-natural-products-that-kill-38268113/

60   Collman JP (2001) *Naturally Dangerous: Surprising Facts about Food, Health and the Environment*, University Science Books.

Part III
Medicating special populations

12 Using medication with children and adolescents

• Outdated views of pediatric mental health prescription	166
• The scope of pediatric psychopharmacology	167
• Principles of psychotropic prescription with children and adolescents	167
• Diagnostic and conceptual issues in the pediatric prescriptive process	169
• A child's goals differ from those of adults	173
• Parental power struggles over medication	173
• The medical work-up prior to psychotropics	174
• Practical issues in child/adolescent prescription	174
• Notes and references	177

It is estimated that in America almost 21 percent of children aged 9–17 have a diagnosable mental or addictive disorder associated with at least minimum impairment (see Table 12.1). Although a formal nationwide study of American epidemiology continues not to be completed, even older studies[1-2] show staggering percentages of children and adolescents who suffer from mental health conditions.[3-4] Using World Health Organization data, the estimated lifetime prevalence of having one or more mental disorders varies widely across the World Mental Health surveys, from 47.4 percent in the United States to 12.0 percent in Nigeria. In any given year, 5–9 percent of youths aged 9–17 have a serious emotional disturbance that causes substantial impairment in how they function at home, at school or in the community.[1,5] Fifty percent of adults with mental illness will have an onset before the age of 14.[6]

Although the use of psychotropic medications in children and adolescents has been less frequent than in adult patients, there has been a dramatic increase in pediatric psychotropic prescriptions over the past several decades.[8-10] Prescriptions for amphetamines for children increased 120-fold between 1994 and 2009, according to statistics from the United Kingdom's National Health Service. In the United States, prescriptions for childhood antipsychotic drugs prescribed to treat conditions such as bipolar disorder and schizophrenia increased six-fold between 1993 and 2002. According to a study published in the *Archives of General Psychiatry* in June 2006,[11] there continues to be controversy about the wisdom of psychotropic prescription for children. In addition to worries about short- and long-term consequences, particular concern focuses on

Table 12.1 Children and adolescents aged 9–17 with mental or addictive disorders, combined MECA sample, 6-month (current) prevalence* from 2005 to 2011–2012

	%
Anxiety disorders	13.0
Mood disorders	6.2
Disruptive disorders	10.3
Substance use disorders	2.0
Any disorder	20.9

Those with *significant* functional impairment total 11 percent. This estimate translates into a total of 4 million youth who suffer from a major mental illness which results in significant impairments at home, at school and with peers. When extreme functional impairment is the criterion, the estimates suggest that 5 percent of children suffer. Of these, 50 percent of the children receive medication and 80 percent of those medicated found medication helpful.[7]

Sources: Centers for Disease Control and Prevention (2021) Data and statistics on children's mental health, available at: www.cdc.gov/childrensmentalhealth/data.html

*Note: The prevalence of major depressive episodes in adolescents increased from 8.7% in 2005 to 11.3% in 2016.

the possibility of medication prescription as a substitution for other forms of therapy and intervention. This text neither attempts to encourage or discourage the dramatic increase in childhood prescriptions. It is simply fact, however, that this medication practice has been accompanied by relatively limited evidence-based data. Prescribers are often forced to make prescribing decisions without the information on which we would normally like to depend. Societal, parental and school pressures, combined with medical and behavioral intensity, require prescribers to make decisions about psychotropic medication for children. Many of the principles stated elsewhere in this book also apply to pediatric patients, although there are a number of specific facts and techniques that are uniquely useful in child and adolescent psychopharmacological practice. This chapter seeks to provide guidelines for making intelligent decisions in this crucial area.

Outdated views of pediatric mental health prescription

During the latter half of the twentieth century, generalized blanket beliefs by parents, practitioners and society at large about the use of psychotropics in pediatric patients have unfortunately colored their use and acceptance. Up until the last two to three decades, a common belief of many practitioners was that psychotropic medications had strong potential for damaging brain function or interfering with developing physiology and growth in children. Within this view, psychotropics would only be used as a last resort.

More recently, some practitioners who use psychotropics frequently have taken the opposite (but equally untrue) stance that psychotropic medications should be used liberally and automatically to treat almost every child and adolescent behavioral abnormality. Some parents, families and school authorities still adhere to either of these anachronistic views about using psychotropics. Corollaries of these two opposing extremes describe pediatric behavioral problems as "just a phase" that a child will likely outgrow, or that pills/medications are a "quick fix" for virtually any behavior found objectionable or undesirable. Neither of these beliefs is categorically true. Each child should be individually assessed, diagnosed and evaluated for the possible role of psychotropic medications in treating specific behavioral or emotional symptoms.

Psychotropic prescription in children is a balance between any real risks of taking psychotropic medication versus "prescribing before it is time." Earlier fears that all psychotropic medications would be damaging to children were not well grounded, nor have they been borne out to be true. In fact, appropriate targeted prescription of psychotropic medications for properly diagnosed psychiatric conditions can often facilitate the achievement of normal development milestones, increase social interaction and appropriate cognitive development, and improve family dynamics. When left untreated, mental illnesses can cause major disruption in one or more of these areas. The prescriber cannot rationally adhere to a black-or-white, all-or-nothing posture toward prescription in the pediatric population since there are risks to either extreme position.

Risks of premature prescription in children and adolescents include:

- embarking on a long-term therapy without addressing family dynamics
- exposing the patient to unnecessary side effects
- unnecessary labeling of the patient
- unnecessary damage to the child's self-esteem.

On the other hand, the downsides of excessive waiting for patients to "grow out" of the symptoms of a significant mental illness include:

- failed or delayed developmental steps
- poor peer relationships
- lack of appropriate family interactions
- poor academic progress
- shaky self-esteem.

The scope of pediatric psychopharmacology

Pediatric psychopharmacology has gone far beyond the usage of stimulants for attention deficit disorder, which in some countries still dominates the conception of pediatric psychopharmacology. Psychotropic medications are routinely used to treat a wide variety of psychiatric conditions, including psychosis, mood disorders, anxiety disorders, obsessive–compulsive disorders and eating disorders.

Virtually all of the psychiatric illnesses revealed in adults are also present in children, although the clinical presentation may vary in the pediatric patient. Some conditions for which medication pharmacotherapy has been used in children and adolescents are summarized in Table 12.2.[12–16] The wide range of uses for psychotropics in children is changing frequently, and this list is not intended to be comprehensive.

Principles of psychotropic prescription with children and adolescents

Table 12.3 lists some of the important items to be considered when prescribing for children and adolescents.

Table 12.2 Some psychiatric disorders in children and adolescents for which pharmacotherapy has been used*

DSM-V classifications	Medications
Intellectual disability (intellectual development disorder)	Conventional antipsychotics, lithium, naltrexone, buspirone
Pervasive developmental disorders: autism, autistic disorder	Buspirone, conventional antipsychotics, methylphenidate, atypical antipsychotics, selective serotonin-reuptake inhibitors, clomipramine
Attention deficit and disruptive behavior disorders	Amphetamine, dexedrine, bupropion, clonidine, methylphenidate, lisdexamphetamine, atomoxetine, pemoline, selegiline, clonidine, tricyclic antidepressants
Tic disorders: Tourette's disorder	Pimozide, clonidine, atypical antipsychotics
Elimination disorders: Enuresis	Imipramine
Other disorders of infancy, childhood or adolescence: separation anxiety disorder	Alprazolam, buspirone, tricyclic antidepressants, SSRIs
Schizophrenia	Conventional antipsychotics, atypical antipsychotics
Mood disorders: major depressive disorder, Bipolar disorder	SSRIs, SNRIs, tricyclic antidepressants, Carbamazepine, divalproex sodium, lithium, atypical antipsychotics
Anxiety disorders: obsessive–compulsive disorder	SSRIs, clomipramine
Post-traumatic stress disorder (acute)	Benzodiazepines
Eating disorders: anorexia nervosa,	Cyproheptadine
Bulimia nervosa	Selective serotonin-reuptake inhibitors
Primary sleep disorders	Benzodiazepines, imipramine, clonidine

*Note: Although commonly used by practitioners, efficacy has not been firmly established for many of these indications, and literature documentation may be sparse for their use in children. Most medications in this list do not have official FDA approval for the indication listed and depend on the clinician's judgment for use in pediatric populations.

Table 12.3 Child and adolescent prescriptive issues

- The clinician must be as precise as possible in assessment, and in use of standardized codification of diagnoses. Accurate diagnosis is essential to targeted prescription.
- Always evaluate children in their social, family, psychological, developmental, genetic and biological contexts. There may be many factors besides biological illness that strongly contribute to an individual child's psychiatric disorder.
- Information should be gathered from sources other than the identified patient.
- Children are not "little adults." Specific pediatric pharmacokinetic changes may affect blood levels of medications in child and adolescent patients.
- In general, medications should be used only for serious disruptive behavior or symptoms. Ensure that the prescription is for the benefit of the child, not primarily for the benefit of others (parents, teachers, guardians, etc.).
- The child is the patient, but alliance with the parent(s) is crucial to effective prescription.
- Evidence of medication effectiveness in adults does not necessarily predict effectiveness in children, although it has been common practice to prescribe medication to young patients without comprehensive documented evidence of benefit in this population.
- Maintain informed consent from responsible parties. Attempt to obtain consent from the child at the level of the child's understanding.
- Address the child's fears and resistances to medication.
- Medication alone is seldom "the answer."
- If a clinician does not have child pharmacology training, maintain access to a qualified child consultant.

Diagnostic and conceptual issues in the pediatric prescriptive process

A careful, multifactorial assessment is crucial to psychotropic prescription to children and adolescents, particularly in clinical circumstances where prescriptions are being written by non-child psychiatrists or non-psychiatric practitioners. There can be a tendency, particularly in primary care settings, to medicate quickly and in an imprecise fashion for perceived behavioral difficulties. The clinician should utilize not only the identified patient, but also the parents and others to gather information about the child's behavior and emotions. Children are often not the most accurate or detailed historians, and they may be poor observers of their own behavior. Although a child's view of the problem is crucially important, interviews with parents, teachers and other caretakers also provide valuable perspective and data.

Use the family history of emotional illness, if any, to assist the diagnostic assessment. For example, hyperactive or overactive children with a strong family history of bipolar disorder are more likely to be bipolar than to have attention deficit disorder (ADD). Likewise, a family history of anxiety disorder may point to a childhood anxiety disorder rather than ADD as the cause of agitation symptoms. Psychotropic prescription can be complicated by lack of obtainable family history or developmental history in certain patients who have been maintained in custodial settings. It is often difficult or impossible to secure this history from foster care, detention or jails, and even then it may only arrive after a long delay.

Box 12.1 Primary care

Primary care providers may or may not have the time and resources to perform a thorough initial evaluation personally. Large pediatric medical settings may benefit from contractual use of a pediatric or adult/pediatric mental health specialist to help with initial assessment and follow up.

If the child cannot be evaluated by a child psychiatrist or other practitioner with pediatric psychopharmacological expertise, there are a number of standardized diagnostic tools that are useful in increasing the precision of diagnosis for the busy primary care practitioner. During a first evaluation, these include:

- the Kiddie SADS[17]
- the Child and Adolescent Psychiatric Assessment (CAPA)[18]
- the Preschool Age Psychiatric Assessment (PAPA)[19]
- the Behavior Assessment System for Children, 3rd edn. (BASC-3)[20]

During follow-up sessions, helpful tools and measurement scales include:

- the improved Clinical Global Impressions Scale[21]
- the Youth Self-Report[22] and the Child Behavior Checklist[23]

During the evaluation process, whenever possible, time should be spent *alone with the child or adolescent* and then *alone with the parent(s)*. Important diagnostic information is often obtained in separate interviews that would not be brought up if the parent/s and child are only seen together.

Examples of this include:

- a parent who might not discuss a family history of mental illness
- a parent who might not discuss his/her own psychiatric or medication history
- a young patient who will not discuss drug/alcohol usage, sexual activity or possibility of pregnancy.

When possible, use specific diagnostic codes from the *Diagnostic and Statistical Manual* or from the ICD-10-CM (*International Classification of Diseases*, 10th Revision) of the World Health Authority. Avoid prescribing for vague or unspecified problems.

When considering medication prescription, evaluate the seriousness, frequency and consequences of the behavior or symptoms, and not just the inconvenience or nuisance factor. Some child patients are thrust into the "need" for medication in order to "control" their behavior, which is reinforced or insisted upon by parents, custodians or institutional staff. It is particularly important when prescribing to ensure that the medications are also for the benefit of the child, and not solely for the benefit of the parents, teachers or staff. A useful criterion that supports the possible need for medication is *when the symptoms or behavior are a problem/worry to the child personally*. While this criterion is useful, medication may still be indicated even if the child is not keenly aware of the effects of the symptoms.

While many psychotropic medications used in adults are also useful in children, it should not be assumed that studies documenting effectiveness in adults can automatically be used to provide evidence for childhood prescription. While there are some short-term studies of usefulness of medications in child and adolescent populations, there are few long-term studies assessing a medication's effectiveness and/or side effects over time. Since decisions about psychotropics in children may need to be made without the benefit of valid information in the pediatric age group, this issue must be discussed with parents/guardians in the process of obtaining informed consent. This lack of data is usually an issue that younger children may not understand, and is usually omitted from direct discussions with the child patient.

A prime example of this confusion in psychopharmacological prescription for children has been the use of tricyclic antidepressants (TCAs). This group of medications was prescribed for a number of years to children for mood disorders, based on positive-outcome research studies with adults. Although there is some evidence for effectiveness in the treatment of enuresis, OCD and ADHD, efficacy in major depression was never proven. When childhood studies were eventually conducted, the research did not support an antidepressant effect for TCAs in children.[24] On closer study, there was also an increased risk of cardiac arrhythmias with one TCA, desipramine.[25] This lack of effectiveness of TCAs has been speculated to be secondary to the lack of development of the norepinephrine system in children – i.e., a child's brain is not physiologically the same as an adult's brain. Major prescription patterns of several decades were ultimately found to have been guided by assumptions that were simply incorrect.

Similarly, the use of lamotrigine (Lamictal) which is used with significant success in adult bipolar disorder should not be prescribed to patients under the age of 16. It has now been shown that younger patients are more susceptible to a serious skin rash (Stevens-Johnson syndrome or Toxic Epidermal Necrolysis) when lamotrigine is used in this patient population.[26]

Alliances with both the child patient and the parent(s) are crucial to adherence and safe prescriptive practice. The parents must have a clear picture from the clinician regarding the assessment/diagnosis and the role of medications in the treatment of the diagnosed condition. Many parents, unfortunately, may have either overly optimistic or overly negativistic beliefs about the role of medications in treatment. Some are overly concerned about risk and safety, while others are quick to search for a pill to remove any amount of behavioral disruption or distress being experienced.

It is important to manage expectations – on the part of both the parent and the child. Part of the initial prescriptive interview is to provide realistic information on what medications can do, and how long it will take for medications to act. At times, it is as important to describe which symptoms medications are *not* likely to change.

Box 12.2 Talking to patients

To get at this issue, a useful question to ask the parents is: *"What would you wish that medication will accomplish?"*

Box 12.3 Talking to patients

Analogous to the above question, the clinician can ask the child: *"If you could make a medication to do exactly what you would want it to do for you, what would it do?"*

Some parents are prone to see even dramatic signs of significant emotional illness as "just a phase." When significant emotional illness is diagnosed, the clinician must explain possible important sequelae and risks in allowing the illness to remain untreated. Such consequences could include suicidal behavior, accidents, late attainment of developmental milestones, poor self-esteem and disordered relationships with peers. At times, sharing morbidity and mortality data with parents is useful in emphasizing the seriousness of the condition and the necessity for treatment. An example of this type of data is the suicide rate in childhood depression. Suicide is the second leading cause of death for children, adolescents and young adults aged 15–24.[27] Untreated patients with major depression are at twice the risk for suicide as children and adolescents without diagnosed depression.[28] Children with untreated mental illness also have significantly higher use of alcohol and recreational drugs.[29]

If there is significant parental resistance to the use of medication for their child, it may be useful to try other non-medication remedies first unless there is an urgent or crisis situation. This approach offers time for parents to read about medications or get information from other sources. As the child is treated non-pharmacologically, it is also easier to be more precise in targeting symptoms that may be better treated with medication. Reassurance as to the non-addictive nature of most psychotropics should also be emphasized. With resistive parents, it may be useful to specify a reasonable time period for a medication trial (e.g., 4–8 weeks), after which point a reassessment of the benefits will be done before any further action is taken.

A useful strategy for approaching older children or adolescents who may be ambivalent or resistive to medication is to engage patients in a discussion of *why others (parents, teachers) might want them to take medication.* If patients can identify some appropriate reasons, the clinician can explore if any of the potential effects of medicines would be helpful. Some young patients may be willing to try medication for a set, defined period of time to get their parents "off their back."

Special attention must be paid to informed consent issues before medicating children. Except on an emergency basis, written informed consent must be obtained from parents or legal guardians before medication is instituted. This may be particularly complicated when the parents are separated or divorced. When possible, it is wise to obtain informed consent from both parents. When this is not possible, or when one parent is not involved in parenting duties, informed consent must be obtained from the custodial parent and any efforts made to reach the non-custodial parent should be documented.

The clinician should be alert to patient resistances that are particularly common in youthful patients. These can include:

- the fear that their mind will be "controlled" by the medication and that they will "lose free will"
- worries that they will be labeled – either in the family, at school or by their peers – as sick or disabled
- their own belief that they are "bad" for taking medication or that emotional illness is their "fault"
- adolescent patients will often stop medications prematurely because they feel they have "outgrown" them
- adolescents may stop the medication in order to drink alcohol or use recreational drugs.

There are few large-scale, controlled child/adolescent comparisons of medication alone, psychotherapy/family therapy alone and medication combined with psychotherapy.[30] There is one significant study looking at a comparison of various treatment modalities for ADHD which found that targeted medication treatment plus behavioral treatment was superior to psychosocial treatment or community treatment alone.[31] It is the premise of this book that medication treatment, when indicated, should be combined with psychotherapy (and family therapy, when appropriate) to maximize results. Psychotropic medications need to be part of a comprehensive treatment program involving psychotherapeutic interventions, educational interventions, family intervention and milieu management. *Medications alone are seldom curative.* However, when appropriately prescribed, medication response can allow for healing and adjustment to occur, with distinctly lessened interference from the symptoms of emotional disease. As with adults, the beneficial symptom reduction from medication may facilitate and increase the effect of psychotherapy or family therapy.

Persons trained in child psychopharmacology are in short supply in most communities, and are particularly scarce in rural areas. Adult psychiatrists with little child training or family physicians/pediatricians/family nurse practitioners who are not mental health specialists will, therefore, make many psychopharmacological decisions for children. Whenever this is the case, the practitioner should seek access to a *child psychopharmacology consultant* or someone trained in child psychiatry to discuss difficult or non-responsive patients. The lack of child-trained practitioners in rural areas can also unfortunately lead to infrequent or almost non-existent follow up of the psychotropic medications once prescribed. As with adults, children must be seen face-to-face to evaluate medication response.

After appropriate time intervals and stabilization, consideration should be given to a trial of medication discontinuation. Timeframes and practical matters of how/when to do this follow the same principles outlined for adults in Chapter 8. When a trial off medications is indicated, it is often wise to undertake this during summer vacation or school breaks such that, if there is a relapse, the effects are less likely to disrupt academic performance and school functioning.

A child's goals differ from those of adults

In the same way that a practitioner attempts to find common goals with resistive adult patients, the child prescriber should attempt to find reasons for medication usage that children themselves see to be in their best interest.

Some examples of personal motivations that children can see for taking psychotropic medications are:

- increased compatibility with peers and schoolmates
- the ability to control their anger, resisting the impulse to throw out their toys or destroy toys that they value
- by being in more emotional control, adolescents may be less likely to upset their friends and better able to maintain their social relationships
- an irritable adolescent can value decreased anger to maintain a specific connection to a boyfriend/girlfriend
- some adolescents will value the increased self-control and mental focus that will allow their parents to permit them to get a driver's license or have access to a car
- some young patients will take medication to increase concentration and focus, improve academic performance and shed the label of "dummy"
- sad, depressed or anxious adolescents can value a decrease in symptoms to the point where they can obtain and keep a job to earn spending money.

Parental power struggles over medication

Taking medication can become one part of a larger power struggle between children and parents. In an outpatient setting, if children are fundamentally resistant to and actively refusing medication it is seldom useful for parents to force it, since a child has the ultimate veto power by refusing or "cheeking it" and spitting out medication later. Except in crisis or emergency situations (which are usually in institutional settings), it is preferable to work with children's resistances and obtain at least temporary agreement on the use of medication before it is begun.

The use of medication can also be a cause of disagreement between parents. They may have legitimate differences of opinion, or medication may become one of a series of contentions between two arguing parents. The clinician should be attuned to sabotage issues between two parents who may not agree on the cause of the symptoms of the mental health condition and the use of medication in its treatment. The parent who opposes medication use can refuse to administer it when the child is with him or her. Disparaging or derogatory messages about the child's need for medication can be subtly or overtly given. When the clinician becomes aware of this interference, a telephone call or meeting with this parent can be helpful.

The medical work-up prior to psychotropics

The necessary medical evaluation of a pediatric patient for whom a clinician is going to be prescribing a psychotropic will depend on the child's medical history, the length of time since their last physical exam, the presence of somatic complaints and the medication to be prescribed. In general, a physical exam is recommended if:

- it has been more than 6 months since the child's last physical exam
- the child has somatic complaints
- toxins, alcohol or street drugs are being used or their use is suspected
- high-dose medication is anticipated
- the child has a co-morbid medical condition.

Laboratory screening would include:

- a comprehensive metabolic panel, including blood sugar, electrolytes, kidney functions and liver functions
- CBC
- thyroid stimulating hormone level
- urinalysis.

If a high-dose stimulant or desipramine is to be prescribed, or if there is any history of long QTc interval in the family (see Chapter 20), an electrocardiogram (EKG) should also be obtained.

Practical issues in child/adolescent prescription

Physiological differences between children and adults include increased liver mass compared to body weight, a relatively high proportion of body fat and a high volume of extracellular water. In children, these differences can result in a significantly altered ability to distribute and metabolize medication. Typically, metabolic pathways for drugs function at a low level during the perinatal period, become mature by 6–12 months of age and peak between 1 and 5 years. Children's ability to metabolize medication more rapidly persists in childhood, and gradually declines to adult patterns by 15 years of age.[32] The net effect of these pharmacokinetic changes is that, in general, *children and adolescents require larger doses on a milligram per kilogram basis of weight than adults*, to achieve comparable blood levels and therapeutic effects.[33] There is also a specific study with lithium and children showing that, compared to adults, children and adolescents need a higher maintenance serum lithium concentration to ensure that therapeutic levels are achieved.[34]

While these physiological changes are greater or lesser in an individual child, they may be overridden by changes in pharmacodynamics (i.e., receptor-site responsivity, or lack of responsivity to various medications). These individual response variations can be quite dramatic, and totally overshadow any pharmacokinetic issues. Presumably, as with adults, these individual pharmacodynamic variations are based on genetic differences.

Because of the pharmacokinetic issues mentioned above, which lead to more rapid breakdown and excretion, children may also require split dosing (twice, or even three times daily) in order to maintain consistent blood levels and adequate medication effects around the clock. This is particularly true for short half-life compounds such as paroxetine, venlafaxine and gabapentin. This metabolic issue may override the difficulties often associated with multiple doses per day.

SSRI/TCA discontinuation syndromes (see Chapter 8) can occur in young patients as well as in adults. Because of the rapid elimination of these medications in children and adolescents, they may be more prone to such syndromes *between* doses, or if short half-life drugs are given once daily. Likewise, during the stopping of a course of antidepressants a slow, gradual tapering of dose is necessary to minimize the likelihood of discontinuation syndrome symptoms.

Box 12.4 Clinical tip

Whenever possible, avoid having child patients take medication at school since this increases their fear that they will be labeled as ill or "different" by needing to go to the nurse's office to take the medication. The most common scenario when midday dosing is an issue is with the use of stimulants for ADD/ADHD. To circumvent this issue, consider using long-acting stimulant pill preparations such as Ritalin LA, Adderall XR, Concerta, Focalin XR, Vyvanse and Metadate CD. Daytrana transdermal patches also maintain therapeutic effect throughout the school day. These medications are available only as branded preparations. Most antidepressants, mood stabilizers and antipsychotics can be given once daily or, at most, twice daily, in the morning and at bedtime. The only exception to this general principle is a child enmeshed in a very chaotic family in which the clinician may suspect that medication may be given at home erratically or not at all. In this case, dosing the medication at school may be more predictable and dependable even at the risk of labeling by peers.

The medication regimen should be kept simple. Whenever possible, doses should be given once daily. When multiple daily doses are required, doses can be tied to events easily recognizable for the child, such as meals or bedtime, rather than specific clock times.

The tendency to polypharmacy in order to meet parental expectations for a "quick" cure must be avoided. Dysfunctional families may often see medication as a cure-all to multiple ills. There can be resistance to looking at family dynamics and at mental aftereffects of loss, neglect, abuse or trauma, even though these may be significant causes of the child's symptomatology. In such families, pressure can be brought to bear on the clinician for rapid improvement and the addition of multiple medications to achieve response quickly. Underlying this pressure is the wish to deny or avoid other dysfunctional elements in the family.

Box 12.5 Primary care

Particularly when psychotropic medication is prescribed in a general medical/pediatric office, dispel the "aspirin" expectation. In this framework, many parents (and some children) expect psychotropics to work like an aspirin, with relief and effect within minutes to hours of taking the pill. The clinician should describe regular consistent dosing, the need for gradual build-up of dose and the likelihood of response over several weeks to several months.

Box 12.6 Primary care

P-450 interactions between medications, as in adults, are more common when children take multiple medications or have multiple medical problems. Increased side effects or lack of therapeutic response in these children, especially when other non-psychotropics are present, can be indicators of altered psychotropic serum blood levels.

It is important to discuss both the *physical* side effects to medication and the *behavioral* side effects of medications that can indicate excessive dosage or toxicity. Most families are aware of physical side effects such as:

*   excessive napping or sleepiness in school
*   nausea, changes in bowel habits
*   changes in vital signs (increased or decreased pulse rate, lightheadedness from decreased blood pressure, headaches from high blood pressure).

However, youthful patients and their parents may not anticipate behavioral side effects in the same way as they do physiological side effects. When appropriate, any behavioral side effects to the medication prescribed should be described. These can include:

*   agitation, nervousness and restlessness, which may occur with SSRIs and benzodiazepines
*   akathisia (internal restlessness), which may occur with antipsychotics
*   disinhibition, which may occur with benzodiazepines
*   mental confusion or "spaciness," which may occur with almost any psychotropic.

Some children may have difficulty in swallowing medications or be fearful of swallowing large pills, so it is useful to ask about this issue prior to writing a prescription. If concern is expressed, it is helpful to show a picture of the pill in the *Physician's Desk Reference* or other drug reference source to see if the child feels it is of a size that can be swallowed. It is better to discover this in the office than to find out later that evening when the child balks at the first dose. When a child is unable to swallow the recommended pill, the parent can crush or break the pills into smaller components that can be given in apple sauce or ice cream. Even if there is loss of the "timed release" element of a pill that is crushed or opened, this may be less of a problem than a symptomatic child who will not take the pill at all. Liquid preparations, when available, are also a useful alternative. As a last resort, consider prescribing an alternative medication with a smaller pill size.

When prescribing in an outpatient setting, the clinician should start at small doses and go slow with any dosage increase. The response to dosage increases can be evaluated, and pressure to escalate dosage rapidly to quickly "fix" the problem resisted.

The clinician should give information about medications to children in age-appropriate phrases, and then ask for questions. Simple phrases, such as *"this will help your brain work better,"* are useful for young children. It is often useful to give the actual paper prescription for the medication to the child to carry out of the office so that he or she "owns it."

The clinician should assess the child or adolescent's ability to manage his/her own medications. Children aged 4 and under will usually accept medication dispensed by parents without difficulty. If older than 4, the child's adherence is strongly desirable, but the pills should still be controlled and dispensed by the parents. In adolescents who are assessed to be dependable, there is value in allowing them to control their own medications. If they are undependable, erratic, likely to be non-compliant or adversely disposed to the medications, however, parents should be involved in observing them take the medication.

Adolescents are notorious for giving away, selling or trading their medication with peers. When medicating adolescents, the clinician should be particularly attuned to the possibility that patients may be underdosing themselves because they have given or sold their medication to others. Adolescent patients may also be taking medication prescribed for other people.

When prescribing mental health medications, the clinician must maintain contact with the patient's general physician or pediatrician. If the pediatrician is providing follow up of psychotropic medication, the mental health prescriber should discuss with him or her specific improvements expected, potential complications or side effects, or other issues that would constitute a reason for re-evaluation by the mental health prescriber.

Details of uses, doses, side effects and other specific medication issues for pediatric patients can be found in textbooks specifically devoted to child and adolescent psychopharmacology.[35-37]

Notes and references

1 Costello E *et al.* (2003) Prevalence and development of psychiatric disorders in childhood and adolescence. *Archives of General Psychiatry* 60: 837.

2 Robert RE *et al.* (2007) Rates of DSM-IV psychiatric disorders among adolescents in a large metropolitan area. *Journal of Psychiatric Research* 41: 959–967.

3 Rosenbaum JF and Pollock RA (2002) *Update on Children's Mental Health*, American Psychiatric Association Meeting, available at: www.medscape.com/viewarticle/436402.

4 *Report of the United States Surgeon General* (2000), available at: www.surgeongeneral.gov/topics/cmh/childreport.html; *National Children's Mental Health Report Card* (2011), available at: https://childmind.org/article/national-childrens-mental-health-report-card/

5 Friedman RM *et al.* (1996) Prevalence of serious emotional disturbances in children and adolescents. In RW Manderscheid and MA Sonnenschein (eds.), *Mental Health, United States* (chapter 6, pp. 71–89), U.S. Department of Health and Human Services, Substance Abuse and Mental Health Services Administration.

6   Kessler RC (2009) The global burden of mental disorders: an update from the WHO World Mental Health (WMH) surveys. *Epidemiology and Psychiatric Sciences* 18(1): 23–33.

7   Rosenbaum JF and Pollock RA (2002) *Update on Children's Mental Health*, American Psychiatric Association Meeting, available at: www.medscape.com/viewarticle/436402

8   Kutcher S (1997) *Child and Adolescent Psychopharmacology*, WB Saunders.

9   Rosenbaum JF and Pollock RA (2002) *Update on Children's Mental Health*, American Psychiatric Association Meeting, available at: www.medscape.com/viewarticle/436402

10 Friedman RM *et al.* (1996) Prevalence of serious emotional disturbances in children and adolescents. In RW Manderscheid and MA Sonnenschein (eds.), *Mental Health, United States* (chapter 6, pp. 71–89), U.S. Department of Health and Human Services, Substance Abuse and Mental Health Services Administration.

11 Olfson M *et al.* (2006) National trends in the outpatient treatment of children and adolescents with antipsychotic drugs. *Archives of General Psychiatry* 63(6): 679–685. doi: 10.1001/archpsyc.63.6.679

12 DeVane CL and Sallee FR (1996) Serotonin selective reuptake inhibitors in child and adolescent psychopharmacology: a review of published experience. *Journal of Clinical Psychiatry* 57: 55–56.

13 Findling RL *et al.* (1996) Antipsychotic medications in children and adolescents. *Journal of Clinical Psychiatry* 45 (Suppl. 9): 19–23.

14 Alessi N *et al.* (1994) Update on lithium carbonate therapy in children and adolescents. *Journal of the American Academy of Child and Adolescent Psychiatry* 33: 291–304.

15 Devane CL (1997) Psychoactive drug–drug interactions in children, adolescents and adults. *Essential Psychopharmacology* 2(1): 33.

16 Theodore Levin, MD, personal communication.

17 *Kiddie SADS*, available at: www.icctc.org/August2013/PMM%20Handouts/Kiddie-SADS.pdf

18 Angold A *et al.* (2000) The Child and Adolescent Psychiatric Assessment (CAPA). *Journal of the American Academy of Child and Adolescent Psychiatry* 39: 39–48.

19 The Preschool Age Psychiatric Assessment (PAPA), available at: https://devepi.duhs.duke.edu/measures/the-preschool-age-psychiatric-assessment-papa/

20 Reynolds CR and Kamphaus RW (2015) *The BASC-3 (Behavior Assessment System for Children,* 3rd edn.), available at: www.pearsonassessments.com/store/usassessments/en/Store/Professional-Assessments/Behavior/Comprehensive/Behavior-Assessment-System-for-Children-%7C-Third-Edition-/p/100001402.html

21 Kadouri A *et al.* (2007) The improved Clinical Global Impression Scale (iCGI): development and validation in depression. *BMC Psychiatry* 7: 7.

22 Achenbach TM and Rescorla LA (2001) *Manual for the ASEBA School-Age Forms & Profiles,* University of Vermont Research Center for Children, Youth, & Families, available at: www.nctsn.org/measures/youth-self-report-11-18

23 Achenbach TM (1991) *Manual for the Child Behavior Checklist/4–18 and 1991 Profile,* University of Vermont Department of Psychiatry.

24 Daly JM and Wilens T (1998) The use of tricyclic antidepressants in children and adolescents. *Pediatric Clinics of North America* 45(5): 1123–1135.

25 Varley CK and McClellan J (1997) Case study: two additional sudden deaths with tricyclic antidepressants. *Journal of the American Academy of Child and Adolescent Psychiatry* 36: 390–394.

26 FDA warns of serious immune system reaction with seizure and mental health medicine lamotrigine (Lamictal), available at: www.fda.gov/media/112401/download

27 AACAP (2018) Suicide in children and teens, available at: www.aacap.org/AACAP/Families_and_Youth/Facts_for_Families/FFF-Guide/Teen-Suicide-010.aspx

28 Isacsson G *et al.* (1996) Epidemiological data suggest antidepressants reduce suicide risk among depressives. *Journal of Affective Disorders* 41: 1–8.

29 Weissman MM *et al.* (1999) Depressed adolescents grown up. *Journal of the American Medical Association* 281: 701–713.

30 Klein RG (2002) Major depression in children and adolescents. *American Society for Clinical Pharmacology Progress Notes* 11(1): 2–4.

31 MTA Cooperative Group (1999) A 14-month randomized clinical trial of treatment strategies for attention deficit/hyperactivity disorder. *Archives of General Psychiatry* 56: 1073–1096.

32 Perel JM (1999) Inhibition of imipramine metabolism by methylphenidate. *Federation Proceedings* 28: 418; Kraus DM *et al.* (1993) Alterations in theophylline metabolism during the first year of life. *Clinical Pharmacology & Therapeutics* 54: 351–359.

33 Kraus DM *et al.* (1993) Alterations in theophylline metabolism during the first year of life. *Clinical Pharmacology & Therapeutics* 54: 351–359; Rosenberg D and Gershon S (2002) *Pharmacotherapy for Child and Adolescent Psychiatric Disorders*, 2nd edn., Informa Healthcare.

34 Rosen MS (2017) Lithium in child and adolescent bipolar disorder. *American Journal of Psychiatry* 12(2): 3–5, available at: https://doi.org/10.1176/appi.ajp-rj.2017.120202

35 Martin A (ed.) (2010) *Pediatric Psychopharmacology: Principles and Practice*, 2nd edn., American Psychological Association.

36 Green WH (ed.) (2006) *Child and Adolescent Clinical Psychopharmacology*, 4th edn., Lippincott, Williams and Wilkins.

37 Werry JS (ed.) (1999) *Practitioners Guide to Psychoactive Drugs for Children and Adolescents*, 2nd edn., Plenum Press.

13 Pregnancy and psychotropics – rewards and risks

- Clinician principles for prescribing to the pregnant woman   181
- The A, B, C, D, X classification of medication in pregnancy and lactation   183
- Working with the fertile woman, pre-pregnancy   185
- When the patient wishes to become pregnant   186
- While the patient is actively trying to become pregnant   187
- When pregnancy occurs   188
- During pregnancy   188
- Medication prescription for symptoms occurring during pregnancy   189
- Specific conditions and medication groups   190
- Postpartum   196
- Lactation and psychotropics   196
- Specific medicines and medication groups in breastfeeding   198
- Data will change; the decision process will not   201
- Notes and references   202

Prescribing medication during pregnancy is an area that raises anxiety for many practitioners, but it is a crucially important time in a patient's life that also can provide great reward for the clinician. Although we are gradually obtaining increased amounts of clinical information that will help us provide evidence-based recommendations to patients, there is still much that we do not know.

The interface between pregnancy and mental health problems is multifaceted and common. The incidence of clinically diagnosable depression and anxiety during pregnancy and the postpartum period may be as high as 20 percent.[1-2] Women with chronic mental health disorders are at significant risk for unplanned pregnancies as well as pregnancy and birth complications. Many pregnant women fail to identify themselves as depressed or anxious, fail to seek help or do so only after a number of months without the benefit of pre-pregnancy planning.[3] Clinicians who treat fertile and pregnant women with medication face the challenge of limiting fetal risk while at the same time minimizing the impact of the mental health condition on the mother and baby. Potential issues associated with medication usage in a pregnant woman include not only teratogenicity, but also obstetrical complications, perinatal effects to the infant and long-term postnatal behavioral complications. All prescribers should become familiar with the issues in this chapter even if, as occurs frequently, the prescriber seeks consultation and assistance from a colleague who commonly deals with pregnant women.

This chapter focuses on the general approaches to medication and pregnancy as well as the specific recommendations for the various reproductive phases including:

- issues for the fertile woman, pre-pregnancy
- when a woman wishes to become pregnant
- while a woman is attempting to become pregnant
- when the patient becomes pregnant
- medication during pregnancy
- medication during the postpartum and breastfeeding periods.

Each of these timeframes creates different medication considerations for the clinician in dealing with patients, and thus will be considered separately.

Clinician principles for prescribing to the pregnant woman

As has been outlined in other chapters in this book, almost all treatment decisions with psychotropic medications are collaborative. Nowhere is this more important than in making decisions about the use of mental health medications during pregnancy. Ultimately, the mentally competent pregnant woman herself, in concert with her partner, makes the decision as to the use or non-use of a medication. These decisions, however, carry a great emotional charge. When a woman takes medication during pregnancy and then delivers a normal, healthy baby, the patient and her partner are relieved, but may be vigilant for years looking for signs that the medication may have caused problems. In the event of a baby with a problem or disability, clinicians may be legally vulnerable if they acted in a way to coerce or strongly influence the patient regarding medication. Therefore, unless the patient is incapacitated or judged legally incompetent, *the clinician cannot make decisions about medication during pregnancy unilaterally or for the patient*.

In the vast majority of situations, it is the role of the clinician to:

- provide up-to-date, balanced information to the patient and her partner about possible risks of medication and/or the possible complications of untreated illness
- help the woman or couple make the best decision for themselves, always emphasizing that the final decision rests with them
- actively support their final choice, once a decision is reached.

Regardless of the classes of medications used and the patient's life circumstances, there are risks from and benefits to virtually every medication decision during pregnancy. All psychotropic medications diffuse across the placenta which therefore exposes the fetus to potential risk.[4] Clinicians should be open and direct as to what the profession does and does not know. They should be informative and non-judgmental, but avoid making the decision for the patient, and share a balanced picture of the potential upsides and downsides to various choices (as best they are known). This picture will include general considerations as well as specific issues for this individual based on her mental health history, current emotional status and previous response to medication. The clinician's role is that of information provider, clarifier and objective observer of the patient's history and current state. The clinician is not an arbiter or decision-maker. Being familiar with current literature, the clinician should initially present a summary of the known data and research in understandable terms familiar to the patient. This *verbal presentation is more helpful than simply referring the patient to journal articles or books*, which are often written in technical jargon and not easily understood. If the patient does request further detailed information beyond the clinician's digest of the current literature, she can be directed to specific patient-centered websites devoted to issues of reproduction and psychotropics, such as Massachusetts General Hospital Center for Women's Health Perinatal Information Resource Center, at www.womensmentalhealth.org/

Although the clinician need not shield the patient from specific professional references and articles, these should be a third-line source of information. If information is requested beyond the above Internet information, the patient can be referred to reputable summary articles on issues of pregnancy, breastfeeding and psychotropics, such as the references at the end of this chapter.[5–6] (Since this is a rapidly evolving data set, there are likely to be useful articles and/or book chapters published routinely.) Regardless of which professional material the patient reads, *the clinician should always ask that she come to the office to discuss her understanding of the facts that she read and the applicability to her specific clinical situation.* It is often helpful to suggest that the patient bring a copy of any material she has read with her to the office for discussion and decision-making.

Even when the clinician has doubts about a patient's choice, in general, *once she reaches a decision about the use or non-use of medication*, it is most helpful if the clinician finds a way to *support the positive elements of her decision*. The patient needs to know that the clinician is "with her" throughout this process. If the patient's decision is not the one the clinician would have preferred, it is important to keep this belief in the background. The clinician should focus on the benefits and positive reasons for which the patient has made her choice, rather than highlight the potential risks.

Box 13.1 Talking to patients

For example, when a patient chooses to stop medication even though there may be a significant risk of relapse, focus on her wish *to give the best possible, medication-free environment to her child even when it means a potential discomfort to herself.*

Similarly, when a patient chooses to continue medication or start medication during a pregnancy, focus on how the mother is *trying to provide the most stable emotional environment for her future baby.* In this situation, the clinician can also recollect with the patient the intensity of the symptoms that she experienced off medication, and how medication has significantly improved her condition.

In either case, empathize with the patient's difficulty in making this decision. Regardless of what she has chosen, underscore how she has given it much thought and consideration. *Once the woman has chosen a well-thought-out course of action, there is virtually no benefit in highlighting risk when she has already made what she believes to be the best decision for herself and her baby.*

When a patient has attempted to go through a pregnancy medication-free, but then finds she must start medication because her symptoms have become too significant or overwhelming, this decision, too, will be a difficult one. The patient will need to go through a grieving process for being unable to provide a medication-free environment for her child. She may have significant mixed feelings about this choice, even as she knows the medication will help her. The clinician must be attuned to this possibility and help the patient with appropriate grief work, mourning the loss of her ability to carry on without medication.

The A, B, C, D, X classification of medication in pregnancy and lactation

For many years medications have been classified by the American Food and Drug Administration within categories A, B, C, D or X with regard to usage in pregnancy. Because of misinterpretations and difficulty for clinicians and for patients in understanding the meaning of these classifications, they were replaced by a newer system – the Pregnancy and Lactation Labeling Rule (PLLR) format – to assist healthcare providers in assessing benefit versus risk, and in subsequent counseling of pregnant women and nursing mothers who need to take medication, thus allowing them to make informed and educated decisions for themselves and their children. The PLLR removes pregnancy letter categories – A, B, C, D and X. The PLLR also requires the label to be updated when information becomes outdated.[7]

The *Pregnancy* subsection (8.1) includes information for a pregnancy exposure registry for the drug, when one is available. Pregnancy exposure registries collect and maintain data on the effects of approved drugs that are prescribed to and used by pregnant women. Information about the existence of any pregnancy registries in drug labeling has been recommended, but not required until now. Information in the Pregnancy subsection includes a Risk Summary, Clinical Considerations, and Data. Information formerly found in the Labor and Delivery subsection is now included in the Pregnancy subsection.

The Nursing Mothers subsection was renamed as the *Lactation* subsection (8.2), and provides information about using the drug while breastfeeding, such as the amount of the drug in breast milk and potential effects on the breastfed infant.

The *Females and Males of Reproductive Potential* subsection (8.3), new to the labeling, includes information, when necessary, about the need for pregnancy testing, contraception recommendations, and information about infertility as it relates to the drug.

The labeling changes went into effect on June 30, 2015. Prescription drugs and biologic products submitted after June 30, 2015 used the new format immediately, while labeling for prescription drugs approved on or after June 30, 2001, will be phased in gradually.

Labeling for over-the-counter (OTC) medicines has not changed; OTC drug products are not affected by the final rule.[8]

The changes are graphically depicted in Figure 13.1.

The following text will describe the old system which still applies to over-the-counter medication:

> *Category A*. Controlled studies in pregnant women fail to demonstrate a risk to the fetus in the first trimester with no evidence of risk in later trimesters. The possibility of harm appears remote.

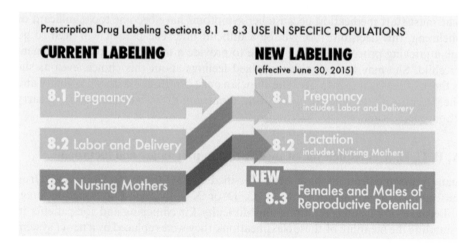

Figure 13.1 Prescription Drug Labeling Sections – use in specific populations.

Source: U.S. Food & Drug Administration (2021) Pregnancy and Lactation Labeling (Drugs) Final Rule, available at: www.fda.gov/drugs/labeling-information-drug-products/pregnancy-and-lactation-labeling-drugs-final-rule

> *Category B*. Presumed safety based on animal studies, with no controlled studies in pregnant women. If animal studies have shown an adverse effect, they were not confirmed in controlled studies in women in the first trimester and there is no evidence of a risk in later trimesters.
>
> *Category C*. Studies in women and animals are not available or studies in animals have revealed adverse effects on the fetus and there are no controlled studies in women. Drugs should be given only if the potential benefits justify the potential risk to the fetus.
>
> *Category D*. There is known evidence of human fetal risk. In some cases, however, the potential risk may be justified if there are no other alternatives.
>
> *Category X*. Highly unsafe: risk of use outweighs any potential benefit. Drugs in this category are contraindicated in women who are or may become pregnant.

While this system is simple and potentially appealing to the clinician, several issues are worthy of note:

- *There are no psychotropic medications in Category A*, and because of the difficulty in performing controlled medication trials in pregnant women, there are unlikely to be any.
- The majority of psychotropic medications are in Category C.
- At times, medications that were initially categorized in Category B were subsequently moved to Category C after further testing and common usage (e.g., bupropion). In other situations, medications started in Category C and were subsequently moved to Category D (e.g., paroxetine).
- Within Categories B, C and D, clinical judgment is necessary in decision-making and no categorization is absolute.

- In general, if medication is going to be prescribed to a pregnant woman and it is appropriate in other aspects, Category C medications should be considered first-line.
- Category D medications are considered second- or third-line, but can be used when the clinical situation dictates and/or other alternatives are unavailable or ineffective.
- Category X medications should not be used.[9]

Working with the fertile woman, pre-pregnancy

If the clinician has followed the suggested initial evaluation guidelines listed in Chapter 3, including questions about pregnancy, last menstrual period and any pregnancy plans, these issues will already have been documented in the patient record.

If a woman presents for her first evaluation for medication and is planning to become pregnant in the near future, this may influence the choice of medication or class of medications toward those with a longer track record of safety during pregnancy. For such women, groups of medications with known teratogenic risk may be less desirable choices than those with minimal known risks. For example, with a depressed patient who is planning to become pregnant shortly, a clinician might choose to use fluoxetine, sertraline, nortriptyline or desipramine (for which there are more documented cases of safe use during pregnancy) and avoid other medications with few evidence-based pregnancy data. Similarly, for a bipolar patient who is planning to become pregnant in the near future, lithium or an antipsychotic are often better choices than carbamazepine or valproic acid, which have known teratogenic effects. The clinician should reinforce the concept that a planned pregnancy is more desirable than an unexpected one, and that planning will simplify decisions about medication. In an initial medication evaluation, issues of family planning and/or birth control should be discussed with all female patients of childbearing age, even if they are not imminently planning on becoming pregnant. This discussion should be documented in the patient record. *For all women of childbearing age where there are any symptoms suggestive of pregnancy, or the possibility of pregnancy cannot be ruled out with certainty, a pregnancy test should be obtained before the patient begins medication.*

When a patient presents for an initial evaluation in the midst of a full-blown mood, anxiety or psychotic episode and yet is actively trying to become pregnant, the clinician should advise the patient to put off such attempts until her mental health episode is treated. Unfortunately, not all patients will follow this advice. To bolster this recommendation, it is helpful to provide a timeframe for which the patient is expected to be on medication. Knowing the length of time that they are expected to take medication, some women will decide to delay their attempt to become pregnant immediately. Because of severe symptoms or chronicity, the clinician may have to revise this initial estimate at a later date. It is to be hoped that, at that time, the patient will be more focused, stable and able to make the most appropriate decision about medication. Even if the clinician suspects that long-term medication treatment will be necessary, a new patient in an agitated state seldom accepts the recommendation for chronic medication early in a patient–clinician relationship. Mention of long-term medication should therefore be put off until the patient is more stable.

Discussion of pregnancy and possible medication complications is particularly important in patients who show impulsive, grandiose, psychotic or confused symptomatology, since these individuals are more likely to experience an unplanned pregnancy.

When the patient wishes to become pregnant

The mildly or moderately symptomatic, cooperative patient

During the medication prescriptive process, when a woman states a specific wish to become pregnant, it allows the clinician together with the patient, to gather information that will help the decision-making process when she ultimately does become pregnant. If it has not already been gathered, obtain information regarding the type, amount and severity of symptomatology during previous pregnancies. Was any treatment used in any previous pregnancies? Was it successful? Approximately how long did it take for the patient to become pregnant?

When the patient brings up the desire to become pregnant, *it may possibly be an appropriate time to stop medication in order to assess her response and watch for any relapse symptoms.* The patient's reaction to a trial off medication prior to attempting to get pregnant may give valuable information to both clinician and patient about whether stopping medication during pregnancy is feasible. If a patient is firmly committed to attempting to become pregnant, the clinician in concert with the patient may choose to taper and stop medication early, even if a full course of therapy has not been completed.

A woman thinking about becoming pregnant may raise several other issues for discussion. Women who are particularly sophisticated about medicine and biological treatments may inquire about the desirability of switching to a very short half-life medication in the hope that the chemical would be entirely excreted in a matter of hours should she become pregnant. Although some patients believe in the intrinsic logic of this action, there is no evidence to date which shows that use of a short half-life compound provides any defined safety benefit. Although a clinician could agree to change medication for this reason, any small advantage is usually outweighed by the uncertainty of response to a new medication. The vast majority of psychotropics are excreted substantially in 2 to 4 days and are virtually fully excreted by 1 week. The notable exception is fluoxetine, whose metabolite, norfluoxetine, may be present in small quantities for up to 4 weeks.

When knowledgeable patients look forward to pregnancy, they will sometimes be interested in switching medications to one that has a longer track record of safety during pregnancy. The clinician may agree to the patient's wishes if she feels strongly about this issue. In general, however, unless the patient is taking a known high-risk medication, most individuals should be continued on medication to which they have responded rather than switching to an untried medication with an uncertain response.

It is important to ensure that *any discussion of the pros and cons of using medication during pregnancy* is *balanced.* In addition to the possible complications of medication usage, which may for some medications include teratogenicity at delivery, neonatal withdrawal, behavioral teratogenicity and increased risk of miscarriage, the *clinician should discuss the possible effects of untreated depression, anxiety, psychosis or other significant mental health symptoms* which are significant.

Studies have shown that mothers who are significantly depressed during pregnancy have a higher risk of pre-term delivery, low birth-weight babies and small gestational-age babies.[10] Additional information has shown that these children born to depressed mothers have poor orientation skills, decreased motor tone, lower activity levels and reduced reflex tone.[11–14] Rondo *et al.* (2003) predicted maternal psychological stress and distress as predictors of low birth weight, prematurity and intrauterine growth retardation.[15]

Although the research is not totally consistent, most studies indicate that significant untreated anxiety states during pregnancy predict poor pregnancy outcomes, shortened gestational age with pre-term birth and lower birth weight.[16–18]

Patients with bipolar disorder are at significant risk both during pregnancy and in the 3–6 months after delivery for relapse and exacerbation of symptoms, especially when mood-stabilizing medication has been stopped.[19–21] Postpartum psychosis, with its potentially devastating consequences, is also closely associated with bipolar disorder.[22–24]

Mothers with schizophrenia or other psychosis show a significant risk for stillbirth, infant death, pre-term delivery and low birth weight. Significant behavioral abnormalities such as refusal of prenatal care, self-mutilation and infanticide are also severe potential complications of untreated psychosis.[25–26] These mothers also have high rates of cigarette smoking, alcohol and drug use and low socio-economic status, all of which further increase the likelihood of poor obstetrical outcomes and neonatal condition.[27–28] Prior to attempting to conceive, it is also reasonable to discuss with the patient decreasing or stopping some of the above-mentioned behaviors that may have additive deleterious effects on pregnancy, such as cigarette smoking, alcohol overuse or recreational drug usage.

The severely symptomatic, mentally compromised patient

If it is the clinician's assessment that the woman wishing to become pregnant is not thinking logically and sanely and/or may be prone to making significantly impaired judgments, it is very helpful to involve the spouse/partner before making decisions about medication use. A more stable partner may be able to influence the opinion of an unstable, impulsive or disorganized patient who may be requesting to stop medication. Before becoming pregnant, if the patient (with or without her partner's agreement) makes a clear choice to stop medication when she becomes pregnant, this decision must be documented along with details of the discussion regarding any anticipated risks.

If a patient has a psychotic or bipolar illness that has resulted in serious psychotic behavior and life-disruptive symptoms, it is generally better to maintain her on antipsychotic and/or mood stabilizing medication for as long as possible prior to attempting pregnancy. If the patient is mentally competent and is insistent on stopping medication despite her history, it may be preferable to wait until the patient becomes pregnant and then stop medication quickly, rather than discontinue medication while she is trying to become pregnant. It may take the patient months or years to become pregnant, during which time a psychotic episode could be devastating.

While the patient is actively trying to become pregnant

By this time in the process with an ongoing patient, if the woman is taking medication, a plan should be documented and agreed upon as to how medications will be handled once she does become pregnant. If the decision is that the patient will be taken off medications as soon as she becomes pregnant, she should be advised to notify the clinician as soon as any signs or symptoms of pregnancy occur, or a positive pregnancy test is obtained. If the patient's medications are discontinued before attempting to get pregnant, the clinician should monitor the patient's condition closely to observe for any clinical worsening. This is particularly important if it takes a long period for the patient to conceive. Some patients who have decided to stop medications while they are trying to get pregnant may find that their symptoms worsen to the point that restarting medications becomes a clinical necessity prior to conception.

If the patient is taking carbamazepine, valproic acid or another anticonvulsant mood stabilizer while trying to conceive, she should be started on folate (minimum of 4 mg a day) to reduce the likelihood of neural tube defects[29] – a known complication of these medications when used during pregnancy.

When pregnancy occurs

Once a patient becomes pregnant, the clinician should document in the medical record when he/she was informed of the possibility of pregnancy, when pregnancy was confirmed by test and the estimated date of delivery. Legally, it is also useful to document any other medications taken at the time of conception in addition to any psychotropic(s) being prescribed. It is quite common for women to be taking various over-the-counter medications and herbal supplements during the early stages of pregnancy – as high as 39.2 percent in one study.[30] Any ongoing use of alcohol or abuse of drugs should also be noted and counsel given to stop these practices. If necessary, the mental health clinician can order a serum pregnancy test to confirm the possibility of pregnancy, and assist the patient in finding an obstetrical or other care provider for prenatal care.

Once the woman is pregnant, the previously agreed plan for stopping or continuing medication is implemented. The clinician should be aware that some patients who may have previously made a plan to continue medications may now have second thoughts, and decide to stop once they actually do become pregnant. If medications are to be stopped, this should occur as quickly as possible once pregnancy is suspected or confirmed. It is better to stop medications quickly rather than maintain a prolonged taper, even if this might be the preferred schedule during circumstances other than those of pregnancy. In general, the patient's wish to be medication-free will usually be stronger than her experience of any discontinuation phenomena.

If medication is to be continued during the pregnancy, it should be decreased to the lowest possible dose that provides reasonable symptom control. In some cases, it may be possible to give medications every second or third day rather than every day. It is particularly important to decrease the medication load during the first trimester when fetal organ development occurs. In general, the time of maximum teratogenic potential is approximately 17–60 days after conception. Therefore, medication dosage should be minimal during that period whenever possible.[31] If the patient has been maintained on a combination of medications, monotherapy may be considered – even if it results in only partial symptom control.

During pregnancy

Although an initial plan of action regarding medication has been established, it is important for the clinician to remain flexible during the pregnancy as clinical circumstances may change. Patients who have decided to remain off medications may worsen to the point that re-institution of medications may become necessary. Within the second or third trimester, when the risk of teratogenicity is less, some patients may decide to re-institute medications that they have avoided during the first trimester. Regardless of whether the patient is on medication or not, her mental health should be monitored frequently for changes. This can be done directly face-to-face, or through a psychotherapist who may be seeing the patient more frequently.

Each patient, and each pregnancy, is unique. Any decisions about medication should be made with careful consideration of *risks of using medications versus the risk of untreated illness for this patient at this time*. Open discussion with the patient (and her partner) about these changing issues should be documented in the patient's chart. Most obstetricians are quite willing to have the mental health prescriber monitor any psychotropics used during pregnancy. Be sure to include any obstetrical provider in the treatment process from the beginning, and at times of any clinical change.

Medication prescription for symptoms occurring during pregnancy

The clinician should follow these basic guidelines when symptoms worsen or emerge during a pregnancy:

- First consider non-pharmacological interventions. These can include cognitive behavioral therapy, individual or group therapy for depression and/or anxiety. Light therapy can be used for depression.[32] For the mildly to moderately symptomatic patient, evaluate life stressors, including job, family and relationship issues, to see if lifestyle interventions may be helpful in decreasing symptomatology.
- With the exception of ECT, non-pharmacological methodologies are usually not sufficiently stabilizing in psychotic patients and, in general, medication will be utilized as the first line of action when such symptoms occur.
- If medication is used, maintain the lowest possible dose that treats the symptoms. Use intermittent dosing, when possible. However, when symptoms are not adequately controlled, increase medication doses to pre-pregnancy doses if necessary.
- Once a decision is made to return to medication, be positive, encouraging and supportive, even if there are known risks.
- For severe symptoms of psychosis, depression or bipolar disorder, make a strong case for starting or continuing medication. In general, *the medication risk to mother and fetus is small in comparison to the sequelae of a major mental breakdown.* Consider hospitalization and/or the use of ECT for treatment and safety.[33–34]
- For the woman who is not thinking clearly, is psychotic, exceptionally anxious or depressed, be sure to include the partner or caretakers to help evaluate the extent of symptomatology and the behavioral risk of the illness. For legally incompetent patients, involve the guardian in any decision about restarting medication.
- Avoid polypharmacy whenever possible.
- In general, unless a medication previously used by the patient is significantly higher in risk than other choices, it is best to return to the medication that was therapeutically effective and tolerated. Pregnancy is not a time to be experimenting with a new regimen.
- Avoid complicated or risky medications such as monoamine oxidase inhibitors during pregnancy.
- Monitor the patient's weight, since excessive increased weight and the presence of gestational diabetes are increased risk factors for fetal neural tube defects.[35] Assist in diet and exercise counseling to maintain reasonable, gradual weight gain during the pregnancy.

- During pregnancy, serum concentrations of medications may change with time because of increase in total body water, decreased protein binding, decreased absorption of drug and increased renal excretion rates. Serum tricyclic levels as well as serum lithium levels can decrease over the course of a pregnancy. When these medications are used, check serum blood concentrations at frequent intervals to maintain consistent, clinically adequate, nontoxic blood levels. These levels should be checked weekly in the third trimester.[36]
- As pregnancy progresses, if a patient remains medication-free, discuss with her any plans for re-instituting medication postpartum. This is especially important if there is a high risk of intensification of symptoms after delivery (e.g., in individuals with bipolar disorder). In some cases, medication doses that have been decreased during the pregnancy will need to be brought back to full dosage shortly after delivery.
- Before delivery, discuss with the patient her plans for breastfeeding and the issues regarding psychotropic medication and lactation (see below).

Specific conditions and medication groups

Evidence-based information about specific medications in a pregnant woman is far from thorough. This section describes recommendations for clinicians regarding specific medications and classes, based on the current information available at the time of publication. These recommendations are not exhaustive, and the reader is referred to excellent summary articles.[37–42]

Depression and antidepressants

When medication is used for mild/moderate depression, consider medications with the most evidence-based information about their use in pregnancy. In general, most commonly used antidepressants appear relatively safe when used during pregnancy, including TCAs and most SSRIs. Tricyclic antidepressants, particularly nortriptyline and desipramine, have not shown teratogenicity. Limited follow-up studies have not revealed any long-term effect on the infant's motor skills or behavioral development. When taken near the time of delivery, TCAs can produce transient perinatal withdrawal symptoms which include hypotonia, lethargy and anticholinergic effects such as tachycardia, urinary retention and constipation.

SSRIs including fluoxetine, sertraline and citalopram have a relatively benign track record when used during pregnancy with no greater risk of major congenital malformations.[43–48] When given in the third trimester, SSRIs have produced a neonatal behavioral syndrome with symptoms of tremor, feeding difficulties, agitation, irritability and rigidity. The syndrome is generally self-limiting and resolves in 1–2 weeks. One follow-up study with fluoxetine used in pregnancy did not show any impairment of language development, cognition, global IQ or behavioral development in early school-aged children. SNRIs and other newer, non-SSRI antidepressants such as duloxetine, trazodone, venlafaxine, desvenlafaxine, milnacipran and bupropion have risks similar in incidence to SSRIs. Experimental work on rats and rabbits did not detect malformations or morphological changes in pups after administration of SSRIs and SNRIs to pregnant females.[49] Dubovicky *et al.* state: "The most recent meta-analyses and reviews suggest that the risks of antidepressant intake during pregnancy for fetal/congenital malformations are small or non-existent, and the risk for poor maternal and fetal outcomes are small to medium."[50] These authors further document the significant risk to mother and fetus from untreated depression and anxiety to include intrauterine growth retardation, low birth weight, and maternal–child relation disturbances.[51] Thus, it is reasonable to say that both treated and untreated depression have some element of risk, and decisions about medication use during pregnancy must be individualized to the severity of the mental health condition, the patient's wishes, the patient's support system and coping skills.[52]

The exception to the general safety of antidepressants in pregnancy is paroxetine. Two major studies, one in the United States and another in Sweden, showed an increased risk of fetal congenital malformations, especially atrial and ventral septal defects following maternal exposure to paroxetine in the first trimester. These two findings led to a revision in the labeling of paroxetine from Category C to Category D suggesting that this compound should not be used as first-line therapy in pregnant women. The American College of Obstetricians and Gynecologists now also recommends fetal echocardiography for women who have been exposed to paroxetine early in pregnancy.[53]

There have been two reports of a potential association between SSRI antidepressant use in pregnant women and the rare, but serious, condition of fetal Primary Pulmonary Hypertension.[54–55] Three follow-up studies did not replicate this finding.[56–58] Based on these conflicting reports, the American Food and Drug Administration issued a statement that the association was unclear, and that clinicians should not alter their current prescribing patterns. Prescribers should continue to prescribe SSRIs for depressed pregnant women when appropriate.[59]

For severe, incapacitating or psychotic depressions, consider hospitalization and/or the use of electroconvulsive therapy (ECT).[60]

Bipolar disorder and mood stabilizers

In contrast to the use of antidepressants described above, which appears to be relatively safe within the scope of our data, the use of mood stabilizers and the treatment of bipolar disorder in pregnancy is considerably more complicated. No mood-stabilizing medication is clearly proven to be risk-free and/or can be conclusively shown to not have a small increase in risk when compared to unmedicated patients. If the patient's course of treatment has been relatively mild and severe episodes have not emerged, it may be reasonable to gradually decrease and stop mood-stabilizing medication so that the patient will be medication-free for 4 weeks prior to conception. Whenever possible, the fetus should not be exposed to mood stabilizers during the first trimester. As with severe epilepsy, with a severe mental health condition such as bipolar disorder and psychosis, there may be no choice but to continue maintenance medication with mood-stabilizing medication during a pregnancy. Of particular concern would be the use of valproic acid, which has had documented teratogenic effects.[61–62] Lamotrigine has had the cleanest record in terms of causing major malformations or other congenital abnormalities in pregnancy. Since each of the major mood stabilizers has a somewhat different risk profile during pregnancy, they will be discussed separately.

Lamotrigine

There has been increasing use of lamotrigine for its mood-stabilizing effect as well as its anticonvulsant effect. Therefore, more data on the use of lamotrigine during pregnancy have been obtained. Of the mood-stabilizing agents, its use appears to be the least likely to cause major malformations or other congenital abnormalities. With the addition of relatively recent studies, the use of lamotrigine seemingly continues to be the safest medication for use during pregnancy.[63] Data supporting this conclusion are:

> Researchers analyzed a total of 21 studies describing pregnancy outcomes and rates of congenital malformations. Compared with disease-matched controls ($n = 1412$) and healthy controls ($n = 774,571$), in utero exposure to lamotrigine (LTG) monotherapy was not associated with an increased risk of major malformations.
>
> Rates of miscarriages, stillbirths, pre-term deliveries and small for gestational age (SGA) neonates were similar in LTG-exposed pregnancies as compared to the general population.[64]
>
> As to the risk of oral facial cleft deformities, the first trimester exposure to lamotrigine does not show an instance different from non-exposed infants.[65]

Lithium carbonate

Lithium remains one of the most effective and well-tolerated mood stabilizers both for acute episodes and episode prophylaxis. It has long been known that exposure to lithium during the first trimester is related to an increased incidence of the cardiovascular malformation Ebstein's anomaly (a downward displacement of the tricuspid valve into the right ventricle, causing backward leakage and weakening of the ventricular outflow to the lungs). Although the risk is known, the incidence of this anomaly with lithium use in pregnancy is relatively small (estimates of 1 additional case in every 100 live births).[66] Recent studies[67–68] also suggest that the incidence may be less than originally thought, although it is still 10–20 times more common in babies exposed to lithium during the first trimester than in the general population. Cardiac fetal ultrasound and fetal echocardiography evaluation performed at 16–19 weeks of pregnancy can reveal the presence of Ebstein's anomaly, and may be useful diagnostic tools in patients who have had first-trimester lithium exposure.

There may be a small but statistically significant increase in the overall risk of major malformations in children prenatally exposed to lithium. When considering the most effective and safest regimen for any specific woman, pregnant women and their providers must take into account the high incidence of relapse of bipolar disorder during pregnancy and/or the postpartum period. Therefore, many authoritative sources suggest that women should *not* discontinue lithium or avoid treatment with lithium during pregnancy.[69]

For women with bipolar disorder, lithium is one of the most effective prophylactic treatments. While some women may desire to discontinue lithium during pregnancy, decisions regarding the use of lithium during pregnancy must take into consideration the high risk of relapse during pregnancy and the postpartum period. Some women may be able to switch to lamotrigine or a combination of atypical antipsychotics and antidepressants, taking into consideration the risks associated with exposure to these medications and the risk for relapse in the setting of a medication change.[70]

If lithium is prescribed, serum levels from consistent oral dosage may drop over the course of pregnancy. Therefore, frequent monitoring of serum blood levels is important and gradually increasing doses may be necessary to maintain adequate blood levels for the first 8.5 months. The *several weeks prior to delivery present something of a conundrum to the clinician.* There have been reports of neonatal toxicity in infants of lithium-treated mothers, including "floppy baby syndrome," hypothyroidism and nephrogenic diabetes insipidus. Based on these data, several groups have recommended decreasing or discontinuing lithium in the several days or weeks before delivery with rapid re-institution of dosage to the mother after delivery.[71-72] This approach, however, destabilizes the lithium level for the mother at the beginning of the postpartum period when the incidence of postpartum depression and psychosis is high for bipolar mothers. In the final analysis, the overall incidence of neonatal toxicity with lithium is low. Also, the limited data on a 3–5-year follow up of infants exposed to lithium are reassuring, with no evidence of significant behavioral difficulties.[73] Therefore most clinicians will maintain the maternal lithium dose or decrease it only minimally prior to delivery.[74] In the latter case, a full dose should be re-instituted rapidly after delivery. Frequent monitoring of serum level is necessary during this time since drastically decreased maternal blood and fluid volumes immediately following childbirth may alter serum concentrations post-delivery compared to recently drawn pre-delivery blood levels.

Despite increasing confidence in the safety of using lithium during pregnancy, the emerging data on the safety of lamotrigine (see above) has prompted some patients who have been taking lithium to wish to change to lamotrigine and discontinue lithium. If the patient is not yet pregnant and has at least several months before attempting to achieve pregnancy, this may be a reasonable strategy. If the patient is already pregnant or plans to become pregnant in the immediate future, the risk of relapse with its own serious complications usually tips the balance in favor of continuing to use lithium throughout the pregnancy unless the patient is strongly opposed.[75]

Topiramate and valproic acid

Both of these anticonvulsants have known risks of minor and major fetal malformations, especially neural tube defects and spina bifida at a rate twice that in the general population. Although the majority of these data were gathered in patients where these drugs were used for seizures, headache and migraine, and not bipolar disorder, subsequent studies have shown that the teratogenic risk is likely due to the compound and not to seizure or headache disorders.

Valproic acid risks are as follows:[76]

1 The absolute risk of major malformations with valproate was 10.93 percent (95 percent confidence interval [CI], 8.91–13.13).
2 In children with in utero exposure to valproate (*n* = 467), relative to children born to women without epilepsy (*n* = 1936), there was a fivefold increase in the risk of congenital malformations (relative risk [RR] = 5.69; 95 percent CI, 3.33–9.73).
3 Valproate use during pregnancy has been associated with a significantly higher risk of neural tube, cardiac, orofacial/craniofacial, and skeletal and limb malformations.
4 The risk of major malformations with valproate is dose-dependent.

Some European countries (France and the UK) have taken steps to limit the use of valproic acid in reproductive-age women.

While topiramate does not appear to carry the extremely high risk of teratogenesis that valproic acid carries, there is a growing body of data which suggests that prenatal exposure to topiramate may be associated with increased risk of oral clefts. Many women appear to be treated with valproate and topiramate despite known teratogenicity risks.[77]

If possible, each of these medications should be avoided during the first trimester. When the risk–benefit ratio is sufficient to prescribe them, there may be some lessened risk of use during the second and third trimesters and at lower doses.[78] When using valproic acid, the principles listed below, as recommended by the European medicine agency's Pharmacovigilance Risk Assessment Committee, should be followed:[79]

- If possible, an alternative to valproic acid should be used in women of reproductive age.
- If valproic acid is the only option, women should use effective contraception and should be closely supervised.
- Doctors who prescribe valproic acid to women of reproductive age must review the reproductive risks associated with this drug and must clearly explain the reason for choosing valproic acid over other options.
- Women taking valproic acid should also take 4 mg of folic acid daily to reduce the risk of birth defects and neurobehavioral sequelae in the context of unplanned pregnancy. (Note: While there are data to indicate that folic acid supplementation reduces the risk of autism/autistic traits in valproate-exposed children, it is unclear if folic acid decreases the risk of malformations in the population.)

For those women who do use anticonvulsants during pregnancy, there is a risk of neonatal hemorrhage after delivery. There is some evidence that its risk can be reduced by giving vitamin K 20 mg daily during the 1–2 months prior to delivery, with 1 mg of vitamin K given intramuscularly to the newborn at birth.[80] Although this cohort study does not support routine use of antenatal vitamin K, prophylaxis might be worth considering when premature delivery is imminent in women using an antiepileptic.[81–82] Weight gain experienced during pregnancy should be monitored, since exceptionally high weight gains have been associated with increased risk for neural tube defects.[83–84] If such weight gain occurs, the clinician should assist the patient in dietary consultation or refer her to a dietician.

Other mood-stabilizing medications

Atypical antipsychotics (which may be used for mood stabilization) are covered in the section below. In clinical practice, higher-potency neuroleptic agents such as haloperidol, perphenazine and trifluoperazine are recommended over the lower-potency agents in managing pregnant women with psychiatric illness. Smaller doses are preferred.[85–86] There is no documented causal link between these medications and teratogenicity. Other treatment modalities for a severely bipolar woman include hospitalization or electroconvulsive therapy.

As noted above, bipolar and depressed individuals are at serious risk for recurrence of their illness in the immediate postpartum period.[87] This risk may be as high as 50 percent. Therefore, any mood-stabilizing medication that had been discontinued before or during pregnancy should be restarted immediately after delivery, and adequate dosage levels should be reached quickly.

Psychosis and antipsychotic medications

Most antipsychotic medications are labeled as FDA Category C. In general, typical antipsychotic medications have been studied much more thoroughly than atypical antipsychotics. If medication is required for psychosis, the clinician might consider better-studied, high-potency, typical first-generation agents such as haloperidol and trifluoperizine, and avoid, if possible, low-potency phenothiazines such as chlorpromazine.

The first and largest published prospective study on the reproductive safety of the atypical antipsychotic agents provided reassuring data regarding the risk of malformations in the first trimester. Investigators prospectively followed a group of 151 women taking olanzapine (Zyprexa), risperidone (Risperdal), quetiapine (Seroquel) or clozapine (Clozaril) and compared outcomes to controls without exposure to known teratogens. There were no differences between the groups in terms of risk for major malformations, or rates of obstetrical or neonatal complications.[88] It should be noted that aripiprazole (Abilify) was not among the medications studied in this research. A subsequent review of research on teratogenesis all shows a relatively benign side-effect profile consistent with other atypical antipsychotics.[89]

Clozapine is the only antipsychotic medication classified in the FDA Category B; however, there are limited data available on which to base an assessment of its safety in pregnancy. The available data do not suggest a significantly increased risk of congenital malformations or spontaneous abortion following exposure, but it is too limited to definitively exclude any increase in risk. The potential for long-term postnatal developmental effects on the fetus is not known.[90] No specific risks for the mother and child can be attributed to the use of clozapine during pregnancy. However, the plasma concentration of clozapine is higher in the fetus compared to the mother; therefore, a minimal dosage should be used.[91]

All antipsychotics have been noted to double the risk of gestational diabetes in mothers exposed during pregnancy, and routine blood sugar monitoring is advised for patients taking antipsychotics.[92]

Routine prophylaxis against extrapyramidal symptoms (EPS) is generally not advised during pregnancy. If such symptoms do emerge, anticholinergic medications should be avoided. When some medication treatment is necessary for EPS, consider diphenhydramine in small doses.

Anxiety and anti-anxiety medications

In general, anxiety, stress and tension during pregnancy should be treated with non-pharmacological methods, including cognitive behavioral techniques, relaxation exercises and psychotherapy to decrease stress in the patient's life.

If medication is necessary, benzodiazepines have been the most studied group. There has been an ongoing debate about the risks of increased cleft lip or palate with first trimester exposure to benzodiazepines. Although initial reports suggested that there may be an increased risk of cleft lip and palate, more recent reports have shown no association between exposure to benzodiazepines and risk for cleft lip or palate. This risk – if it exists — is calculated to be 0.7 percent, approximately a ten-fold increase in risk for oral cleft over that observed in the general population. Nonetheless, the likelihood that a woman exposed to benzodiazepines during the first trimester will give birth to a child with this congenital anomaly, although increased, remains less than 1 percent.[93]

If medication becomes necessary, clonazepam is a reasonable choice in that cord blood levels have been undetectable in most cases if the maternal daily dosage is less than 1 mg a day. Although no maternal or neonatal toxicity has been seen in doses up to 3.5 mg per day, there is increased risk of neonatal toxicity at higher doses (greater than 5 mg a day).[94]

When benzodiazepines are used in the period approaching delivery, discontinuation should be attempted gradually at a rate no greater than 10 percent per day. Such gradual discontinuation is recommended since women taking benzodiazepines at the time of delivery have shown an increased duration of labor and possible withdrawal symptoms in the neonate.[95] The use of buspirone has not been systematically investigated, and there is little information to guide its use during pregnancy.

Postpartum

In a pregnancy where the clinician has been actively involved throughout the process, a plan for medication use or non-use in the postpartum period will have been discussed and documented. In women with histories of bipolar disorder and depression, the clinician should be particularly vigilant for serious postpartum depression or the infrequent, but potentially catastrophic, postpartum psychosis. Those patients with a bipolar history are at significant risk for postpartum worsening of their mood disorder.[96] In those patients with bipolar disorder or psychosis where medication has been stopped or decreased and who will not breastfeed, a rapid institution of full mood-stabilizing medications in the several days postpartum is indicated.

Lactation and psychotropics

The decision to breastfeed while taking psychotropic medications is complicated and involves multiple considerations including:

- the known benefits of breastfeeding to both infant and mother
- the expressed wishes of the mother
- the risk of exposing the infant to medication
- the maintenance of the psychological health of the mother to provide a safe and nurturing environment for the infant.

These issues, which at times conflict, can create a dilemma for both mother and clinician – to safeguard the mental health of the mother while at the same time optimizing the emotional and physical well-being of the infant.

All psychotropic medications enter breast milk and pass into infant circulation to varying degrees, although the relationship between infant serum concentration of these medications and the infant's physiology, behavior and development is unknown. Systematized, evidence-based data on the usage of psychotropics in breastfeeding mothers are virtually absent.

The evidence on which recommendations are made consists primarily of isolated case examples, and retrospective reviews of data from these isolated case examples over time.[97] Such data are further complicated by the fact that not all case examples are documented through physician examination, but may be based solely on maternal report.

One final complication is that older medications used over a longer time often have many more case reports than more recently introduced medications. It is not clear whether an increased frequency of side-effect reports represents a true increased risk for that particular medication, or whether it is only a statistical artifact of the larger number of cases observed over time. It is possible that newer medications may appear safe based on small amounts of data, but would perhaps show equal or a greater number of complications if more case reports were available.

To gather information on which to make recommendations, research has relied on several "objective" data sources. The most easily collectible data are measurements of the concentration of a psychotropic in breast milk. By estimating the consumption of breast milk by the infant during the day, an extrapolation is made as to the amount of medication to which the infant is exposed. Other "objective" measures include comparing the plasma psychotropic concentration in the mother's serum to the concentration in breast milk, resulting in a numerical fraction. If this fraction is less than 1 for a particular medication, it is assumed to be safer than if it is greater than 1 (which could indicate active accumulation of the drug in breast milk or higher rates of passive diffusion into breast milk).

There are relatively few reported cases that involved checking the serum concentration of psychotropic medications in the infant, and most of those reports are measures of parent compound only without measurement of any metabolites. Furthermore, none of these "objective" measures takes into account factors of infant physiology (namely, immature liver function, decreased liver glomerular filtration rate, immature blood/ brain barrier and other infant pharmacokinetic issues).

These data sources are quite inconclusive, and there is little, if any, proof that any of these measures ultimately relates directly to infant/child behavioral or emotional outcome. There are virtually no long-term studies of the effects of neonatal exposure to psychotropics. Because of this dearth of information, women and their partners must be advised that recommendations given by the practitioner have little documented supporting evidence. According to the data available in the literature to date, most psychotropic medications are expected to produce low levels in breast milk with no clinical importance.[98] Those adverse effects from psychotropics seen in infants are generally reversible side effects rather than brain toxicity.[99]

As with decisions about medication during pregnancy, decisions about prescribing psychotropic medications during breastfeeding should be made on an individual basis for each patient and each pregnancy. It is important to take into account what information is known about the medication, as well as the past psychiatric history of the patient, the seriousness of any symptoms during previous episodes as well as the wishes of the patient and her partner.

If the patient does wish to breastfeed her infant and medication use is being considered, the clinician should explain that virtually all psychotropic medications taken by the mother do seep into breast milk in varying concentrations. In general, these concentrations are small, and the effect of these small medication amounts is uncertain over the long term. If the patient is going to be using medications while breastfeeding, several principles are useful:

- Mothers may have a strong predisposition to breastfeed in spite of any medication risk, because there is clear evidence that breastfed infants may have lower rates of gastrointestinal and respiratory ailments, anemia and otitis media. The breastfeeding experience also provides increased opportunity for mother/child bonding.

Factors affecting this decision include:

- Although the exact incidence is not known, in general, currently measured risks to infants from psychotropic medication exposure during breastfeeding are low.[100] Risks of harm or neglect to the infant from a mother who is profoundly depressed, anxious, manic or psychotic can be significant and, at times, catastrophic. In patients with serious symptoms, the treatment should favor the maintenance of the mother's mental health, which may include psychotropic medication at the smallest possible dose that controls the patient's symptoms.
- Consider discarding breast milk product in the 7–10 hours following a dose of medication (the so-called "pump-and-dump" technique). Use formula for feeding during this time period, when concentrations of medication may be high. Utilize only breast milk secreted after the 10-hour window, which is likely to have a lower concentration of psychotropic contained therein.
- Another timing strategy is to breastfeed the child just before his or her longest period of anticipated sleep and then have the mother take the psychotropic just after feeding, which will allow for a lesser concentration of drug in breast milk when the infant awakes and needs to be fed again.
- Premature infants have less well-developed hepatic and kidney function, and therefore may be more at risk to medication exposure effects than full-term infants.
- Have the mother consider weaning the infant sooner than might otherwise be desired, to limit exposure to the medication.
- Monitor the condition of the baby through maternal report and examination by a pediatrician. If symptoms of irritability, somnolence, psychomotor slowing or inappropriate delay in achieving developmental milestones occur, measure the amount of psychotropic medication present in the baby's serum. If the concentration is high, decrease the dosage of psychotropic or discontinue it. If the concentration is low but infant symptoms persist, stop the medication or stop breastfeeding, and obtain a pediatric consultation.
- As with pregnancy itself, the breastfeeding period is not a time to try a new medication previously not utilized. The only time to consider using a new medication is if the patient has had no previous medication trials, or if all previous medications tried have been unsuccessful and/or poorly tolerated.
- With the exception of lithium, which is generally avoided during breastfeeding, no single psychotherapeutic agent seems to be of greater risk than another.
- Use of medication and breastfeeding is an individualized decision based on a risk–benefit analysis for each patient.

Specific medicines and medication groups in breastfeeding

The following recommendations are taken from excellent review articles and these sources should be seen for further details on individual medications.[101–104]

Further information, including additional case reports (or lack thereof) will inevitably emerge in print. The available data on specific medication groups is as follows.

Antidepressants

SSRI antidepressants, which as a group are in common usage, have shown minimal problems during breastfeeding. Sertraline, with no reports of adverse side effects and a relatively short to medium half-life, is a desirable alternative. Fluoxetine, with its long half-life and possible reports of complications, is less desirable during breastfeeding. There is minimal information regarding the use of citalopram, escitalopram, fluvoxamine and vilazodone. Paroxetine, although it has a short half-life, is not recommended for its other properties.[105–106]

Other antidepressants, such as bupropion, venlafaxine, desvenlafaxine, duloxetine, mianserin and trazodone, have minimal data on their use during breastfeeding, and should be considered as alternatives if other medications are ineffective and/or the risk–benefit ratio is favorable.

Collected reports of tricyclic usage during breastfeeding have shown no adverse reports of those infants whose mothers took imipramine, amitriptyline, nortriptyline, desipramine and clomipramine. Doxepin, which has had at least one potential possible adverse effect, is not recommended.[107]

Two medications that are available only in the UK, dothiepin and meclobomide, have not been shown to have adverse effects, but are generally less likely to be recommended, given their potential toxicities.

Although there have been no adverse reactions reported with the use of MAOIs, their prescription during breastfeeding is generally discouraged.[108]

Mood stabilizers

Several of the most commonly used mood stabilizers have limited information as to their safe use during lactation. Since the risk of postpartum exacerbation of bipolar disorder is significant, the use of medication may be highly indicated or mandatory. The clinician may wish to take a stronger-than-usual stance with a patient regarding the use of medications without breastfeeding for these highly vulnerable, at-risk patients.

Overall, the following information from the American Academy of Pediatrics and Neurology provides reasonable recommendations based primarily on the use of mood stabilizers that are also anti-epileptics: According to the Academy, breastfeeding should be undertaken with caution by women undergoing lithium treatment. The breastfed infant should be monitored for serum lithium levels, electrocardiogram and complete blood counts. With regard to valproate and carbamazepine, both the American Academy of Neurology and the American Academy of Pediatrics support breastfeeding if the mother is taking valproate, but the liver function tests and blood counts of the newborn need to be monitored. With regard to lamotrigine, the emerging data suggest that it may be relatively safe during breastfeeding. It should be used during lactation when other safer options are not available. Data for other anticonvulsants are preliminary.[109–111]

Based on current information, as noted below, olanzapine and quetiapine have not shown problematic reactions with breastfed infants. These may be considered as mood-stabilizing alternatives to the above-mentioned medications if the patient insists on breastfeeding during the immediate postpartum period, needs prophylactic anti-psychotic treatment and/or has symptoms necessitating medication.

Antipsychotics

Chlorpromazine, fluphenazine and thiothixine are excreted in breast milk, but have not been associated with definitive problematic outcomes. In general, typical first-generation antipsychotics have been in use for decades and the accumulated data show that they are safe during breastfeeding, although usage is still based on a risk–benefit analysis. As with antipsychotic treatment in general, there has been movement toward using second-generation antipsychotics in preference to first-generation medication. Even though data on the second-generation medications are still limited, olanzapine[112] and quetiapine[113] have the best safety record and should be considered first-line choices.[114] Amisulpride and clozapine are contraindicated based on current information because of accumulation in breast milk.[115–116] Data on the safety of using antipsychotics during breastfeeding and long-term outcomes are essentially absent and need to be a focus of research.

Although many, if not most, young mothers feel considerable pressure to breastfeed, women with a history of psychotic illness are not the best candidates for breastfeeding. It is often recommended that the practitioner advocate for bottle feeding so that the woman can maximize her pharmacologic treatment without worrying about exposing the infant to medication. Bottle feeding also makes it easier for other individuals to participate in caring for the newborn and minimize sleep deprivation, which can be a powerful trigger for psychosis. While breastfeeding is beneficial for both mother and newborn, all of these benefits are lost if the mother becomes psychotically ill during this vulnerable time.[117]

Anti-anxiety medications

Benzodiazepines are excreted in breast milk at a low milk/plasma ratio (0.85). These data support the low incidence of infant toxicity and adverse effects associated with benzodiazepine use during breastfeeding. Lorazepam and clonazepam have been studied more extensively, perhaps have a slightly lower rate of side effects and are the medications of choice. The selection of an anti-anxiety medication is, however, generally made on other factors, most importantly patient responsiveness and the necessity of maintaining maternal well-being.[118–119] The Motherisk program in Canada looked at 124 infants exposed to benzodiazepines (primarily clonazepam and lorazepam). The only side effect noted was sedation in two infants. The mothers of these babies were both taking other psychotropics in addition to the benzodiazepine. Thus, exposed infants should be monitored for sedation, especially if the mother is taking other medications.[120]

If anti-anxiety medication is used, it should be used intermittently. Timing of doses is best when the medication is given to the mother just *after* breastfeeding, to allow for maximum excretion prior to the next feeding.

Data will change; the decision process will not

Two facts about prescribing medication during pregnancy and lactation are inevitable:

- Data on individual medications and classes of medications will change continuously.
- As clinicians, though, we will unfortunately always be using limited and incomplete data for our prescribing decisions.

Significant differences in prescribing patterns may emerge year-to-year, based on increasing amounts of safety or risk data that are collected on an ongoing basis. Medications that enjoy wide prescription and maintain high therapeutic effectiveness will gradually, over time, develop increasing pools of data reflecting their safety or risk during pregnancy and/or breastfeeding. Within the first 3–5 years after the introduction of a medication that is prescribed frequently, a few medication case reports documenting uneventful usage or possible potential problems emerge. Based on these isolated reports, the medication usually moves relatively quickly into a group of medications that *appears* to be relatively safe (and becomes a first- or second-line choice); or shows one or more significant adverse effects (and becomes contraindicated or a less desirable fourth- or fifth-line alternative).

Ten or 20 years from now, we will certainly have more data on medications we currently prescribe, assuming they continue to be used with frequency. Within the first several years of their use, however, newly introduced medications will still have very little data on which to base prescribing decisions about their usage in pregnancy and lactation.

Due to the ethical considerations and the practical obstacles of recruiting research subjects for systematized *prospective* research with pregnant or breastfeeding women, there is a distinct possibility that *we will never see a well-designed study of a medication's safety in pregnancy or during lactation.* Therefore, in all likelihood 20 years from now we will still be using the same *types* of data that we have now – isolated case reports and, eventually, pooled data summaries of these case reports. Because of the rapid evolution of psychopharmacology, the rapid rise in the number of medications we prescribe and the emergence of new classes of medications, we may, in fact, actually have smaller amounts of data on any one particular medication. Unless a new medication is overwhelmingly superior to its prescribing alternatives, and vast numbers of women are prescribed this medication, we will continue to have only small numbers of isolated case reports for any one particular product.

The ongoing and increasing frequency of diagnosable emotional illnesses and the obstacles to prospective, controlled studies will certainly require us to make prescribing decisions with less information than we or our patients are totally comfortable with. During our prescribing lifetimes, therefore, we will continue to:

- present women with evidence-based information, limited as it may be
- include the pregnant woman and her partner in the decision-making process
- help balance the risks of untreated illness versus possible adverse medication effects for each individual woman and each individual pregnancy.

Studies evaluating the emotional, physical and behavioral effects on children born to women taking any particular psychotropic medication can take 7–10 years from the time a medication is introduced. Long-term studies of the behavioral, emotional and physical effects on a child when a mother takes psychotropic medication are logistically very difficult, may never be done or may often become available long after a medication is out of common usage.

The need for clinicians to keep current with research and literature in the prescribing process is nowhere more important than regarding the issue of medication use during pregnancy and lactation. Each new case report of a particular medication used during pregnancy or lactation will bolster our level of confidence when no problems occur, or will increase our concern if potential problems ensue. Whenever a woman presents to us seeking to become pregnant, having become pregnant or desiring to breastfeed, and yet is at risk for emotional illness, we must re-evaluate the current literature so that we can present the most up-to-date information to aid in her decision. There is little doubt, however, that our role in the prescribing process will change little. We must become comfortable with helping a patient to make difficult decisions with less-than-adequate, evidence-based data.

Notes and references

1   Jablensky AV *et al.* (2005) Pregnancy, delivery, and neonatal complications in a population cohort of women with schizophrenia and major affective disorders. *American Journal of Psychiatry* 162(1): 79–91; Stewart DE (2011) Clinical practice: depression during pregnancy. *New England Journal of Medicine* 365(17): 1605–1611.

2   Flynn HA *et al.* (2006) Rates and predictors of depression treatment among pregnant women in hospital-affiliated obstetrics practices. *General Hospital Psychiatry* 28(4): 289–295.

3   Murray L *et al.* (2003) Self-exclusion from health care in women at high risk for postpartum depression. *Journal of Public Health Medicine* 25(2): 131–137.

4   Viquera AC *et al.* (2002) Managing bipolar disorder during pregnancy: weighing the risks and benefits. *Canadian Journal of Psychiatry* 47(5): 426–436.

5   Chisolm MS and Payne JL (2016) Management of psychotropic drugs during pregnancy. *British Medical Journal* 352: h5198, available at: https://doi.org/10.1136/bmj.h5918

6   Liu D *et al.* (2017) The use of psychotropic drugs during pregnancy. *Shanghai Archives of Psychiatry* 29(1): 48–50. doi: 10.11919/j.issn.1002-0829.216115

7   Pregnancy and Lactation Labeling (Drugs) Final Rule, available at: www.fda.gov/drugs/labeling-information-drug-products/pregnancy-and-lactation-labeling-drugs-final-rule

8   Ibid.

9   Ibid.

10 Newport DJ (2001) The neuroendocrinology of maternal depression and stress during pregnancy. *Journal of Gender-Specific Medicine* 16(1) (Suppl. 8): 6–7.

11 Ibid.

12 Rondo PHC *et al.* (2003) Maternal psychological stress and distress as predictors of low birth weight, prematurity, and intrauterine growth retardation. *European Journal of Clinical Nutrition* 57(2): 266–272.

13 Jones NA *et al.* (1998) Newborns of mothers with depressive symptoms are physiologically less developed. *Infant Behavior and Development* 21: 537.

14 Lundy BL *et al.* (1999) Prenatal depression: effects on neonates. *Infant Behavior and Development* 22: 119.

15 Rondo PHC *et al.* (2003) Maternal psychological stress and distress as predictors of low birth weight, prematurity, and intrauterine growth retardation. *European Journal of Clinical Nutrition* 57(2): 266–272.

16 Hosseini SM *et al.* (2009) Trait anxiety in pregnant women predicts offspring birth outcomes. *Paediatric and Perinatal Epidemiology* 23(6): 557–566.

17 Orr ST *et al.* (2007) Maternal prenatal pregnancy related anxiety and spontaneous preterm birth in Baltimore, Maryland. *Psychosomatic Medicine* 69: 566–570.

18 Correia LL and Linhares MB (2007) Maternal anxiety in the pre- and postnatal period: a literature review. *Revista Latino-Americana de Enfermagem* 15: 677–683.

19 Viguera AC *et al.* (2002) Protective effect of pregnancy in women with lithium responsive bipolar disorder. *Journal of Affective Disorders* 72: 107–108.

20 Viguera AC *et al.* (2000) Risk of recurrence of bipolar disorder in pregnant and non-pregnant women after discontinuing lithium maintenance. *American Journal of Psychiatry* 157: 179–184.

21 Finnerty M *et al.* (1996) Acute manic episodes in pregnancy. *American Journal of Psychiatry* 153: 261–263.

22 Blehar M *et al.* (1988) Women with bipolar disorder: findings from the NIMH genetics initiative sample. *Psychopharmacological Bulletin* 34: 239–243.

23 Freeman MP *et al.* (2002) The impact of reproductive events on the course of bipolar disorder in women. *Journal of Clinical Psychiatry* 63: 284–287.

24 ACOG Committee on Practice Bulletins (2008) ACOG practice bulletin: clinical management guidelines for obstetricians-gynecologists. *Obstetrics & Gynecology* 111: 1001–1020.

25 Ibid.

26 Sacker A *et al.* (1996) Obstetrics complications in children born to parents with schizophrenia: a meta-analysis of case control studies. *Psychological Medicine* 26: 279–287.

27 Bennedsen BE (1998) Adverse pregnancy outcome in schizophrenic women: occurrence and risk factors. *Schizophrenia Research* 33: 1–26.

28 Nilsson E *et al.* (2002) Women with schizophrenia: pregnancy outcome and infant death among their offspring. *Schizophrenia Research* 58: 211–229.

29 Koren G (2002) Use of atypical antipsychotics during pregnancy and the risk of neural tube defects in infants. *American Journal of Psychiatry* 159: 136–137.

30 Cleary BJ (2010) Medication use in early pregnancy: prevalence and determinants of use in a prospective cohort of women. *Pharmacoepidemiology and Drug Safety* 19(4): 408–417.

31 *The Maudsley Prescribing Guidelines* (2018), 13th edn., Informa Healthcare.

32 Oren D *et al.* (2002) An open trial of morning light therapy for treatment of antepartum depression. *American Journal of Psychiatry* 159: 666–669.

33 Kasar M *et al.* (2007) Electroconvulsive therapy use in pregnancy. *Journal of ECT* 23(3): 183–184.

34 Miller LJ (1994) Use of electroconvulsive therapy during pregnancy. *Hospital and Community Psychiatry* 45(5): 444–450.

35 Koren G (2002) Use of atypical antipsychotics during pregnancy and the risk of neural tube defects in infants. *American Journal of Psychiatry* 159: 136–137.

36 Poels EMP *et al.* (2018) Lithium during pregnancy and after delivery: a review. *International Journal of Bipolar Disorders* 6: article number 26.

37 Chisolm MS and Payne JL (2016) Management of psychotropic drugs during pregnancy. *British Medical Journal* 352: h5198, available at. https://doi.org/10.1136/bmj.h5918

38 Mayo Clinic Staff (2020) Antidepressants: safe during pregnancy?, available at: www.mayoclinic.org/healthy-lifestyle/pregnancy-week-by-week/in-depth/antidepressants/art-20046420

39 Miller L (1998) Pharmacotherapy during the perinatal period. *Psychopharmacology* 2(3): 263.

40 Altshuler LL *et al.* (1996) Pharmacologic management of psychiatric illness during pregnancy: dilemmas and guidelines. *American Journal of Psychiatry* 153: 592–606.

41 Iqual M *et al.* (2001) Effects of antimanic mood-stabilizing drugs on fetuses, neonates, and nursing infants. *Southern Medical Journal* 94(3): 305–322.

42 Grover S *et al.* (2006) Psychotropics in pregnancy: weighing the risk. *Indian Journal of Medical Research* 123: 497–512.

43 *The Maudsley Prescribing Guidelines* (2018), 13th edn., Informa Healthcare, pp. 348–350.

44 Cohen LS *et al.* (2006) Relapse of major depression during pregnancy in women who maintain or discontinue antidepressant treatment. *Journal of the American Medical Association* 295(5): 499–507.

45 Wisner KL *et al.* (2000) Risk–benefit decision making for treatment of depression during pregnancy. *American Journal of Psychiatry* 157: 1933–1940.

46 Einarson TR and Einerson A (2005) Newer antidepressants in pregnancy and rates of major malformations: a meta-analysis of prospective comparative studies. *Pharmacoepidemiology and Drug Safety* 14(12): 823–827; Ericson A *et al.* (1999) Delivery outcome after the use of antidepressants in early pregnancy. *European Journal of Clinical Pharmacology* 55: 503–508.

47 Nulman I *et al.* (2002) Child development following exposure to tricyclic antidepressants or fluoxetine throughout foetal life: a prospective controlled study. *American Journal of Psychiatry* 159: 1889–1895.

48 ACOG Committee on Obstetric Practice (2006, December) ACOG committee opinion no. 354: treatment with selective serotonin reuptake inhibitors during pregnancy. *Obstetrics & Gynecology* 108(6): 1601–1603.

49 Dubovicky M *et al.* (2017) Risks of using SSRI/SNRI antidepressants during pregnancy and lactation. *Interdisciplinary Toxicology* 10(1): 30–34, available at: www.ncbi.nlm.nih.gov/pmc/articles/PMC6096863/

50 Ibid.

51 Ibid.

52 Liu D (2017) The use of psychotropic drugs during pregnancy. *Shanghai Archives of Psychiatry* 29(1): 48–50.

53 ACOG Committee on Obstetric Practice (2006, December) ACOG committee opinion no. 354: treatment with selective serotonin reuptake inhibitors during pregnancy. *Obstetrics & Gynecology* 108(6): 1601–1603; Källén B and Olausson PO (2008) Maternal use of selective serotonin re-uptake inhibitors and persistent pulmonary hypertension of the newborn. *Pharmacoepidemiol Drug Safety* 17: 801–806.

54 Chambers CD *et al.* (2006) Selective serotonin-reuptake inhibitors and risk of persistent pulmonary hypertension of the newborn. *New England Journal of Medicine* 354(6): 579–587.

55 Källén B and Olausson PO (2008) Maternal use of selective serotonin re-uptake inhibitors and persistent pulmonary hypertension of the newborn. *Pharmacoepidemiol Drug Safety* 17: 801–806.

56 Andrade SE *et al.* (2009) Antidepressant medication use and risk of persistent pulmonary hypertension of the newborn. *Pharmacoepidemiology and Drug Safety* 18: 246–252.

57 Wilson KL *et al.* (2011) Persistent pulmonary hypertension of the newborn is associated with mode of delivery and not with maternal use of selective serotonin reuptake inhibitors. *American Journal of Perinatology* 28(1): 19–24.

58 Wichman CL *et al.* (2009) Congenital heart disease associated with selective serotonin reuptake inhibitor use during pregnancy. *Mayo Clinic Proceedings* 84(1): 23–27.

59 FDA Drug Safety Communication: selective serotonin reuptake inhibitor (SSRI) antidepressant use during pregnancy and reports of a rare heart and lung condition in newborn babies, available at: www.fda.gov/Drugs/DrugSafety/ucm283375.htm

60 Kahn DA *et al.* (2019) Major depression during conception and pregnancy: a guide for patients and families, available at: http://womensmentalhealth.org/wp-content/uploads/2008/04/mdd_guide.pdf

61 Andrade C (2018) Valproate in pregnancy: recent research and regulatory responses, available at: www.psychiatrist.com/JCP/article/Pages/2018/v79n03/18f12351.aspx

62 Prenatal exposure to valproic acid linked to increased risk for autism, ADHD, available at: https://womensmentalhealth.org/posts/valproic-acid-risk/

63 MGH Center for Women's Mental Health (2017) Lamotrigine and pregnancy: meta-analysis shows no increase in risk for malformations, available at: https://womensmentalhealth.org/posts/lamotrigine_pregnancy_no_increased_risk_malformations/

64 Pariente G *et al.* (2017) Pregnancy outcomes following in utero exposure to lamotrigine: a systematic review and meta-analysis. *CNS Drugs* 31(6): 439–450.

65 Dolk H *et al.* (2016) Lamotrigine use in pregnancy and risk of orofacial cleft and other congenital anomalies. *Neurology* 86(18): 1716–1725.

66 Patorno E *et al.* (2017) Lithium use in pregnancy and the risk of cardiac malformations, available at: www.ncbi.nlm.nih.gov/pmc/articles/PMC5667676/

67 Lithium in pregnancy and breastfeeding, available at: www.rcpsych.ac.uk/mental-health/treatments-and-wellbeing/lithium-in-pregnancy-and-breastfeeding

68 Munk-Olsen T *et al.* (2018) Maternal and infant outcomes associated with lithium use in pregnancy: an international collaborative meta-analysis of six cohort studies. *Lancet Psychiatry* 5(8): 644–652.

69 MGH Center for Women's Mental Health (2018) Lithium use during pregnancy: results from an international cohort study, available at: https://womensmentalhealth.org/posts/lithium-international-cohort-study/

70 Ibid.

71 Llewellyn A *et al.* (1998) The use of lithium and management of women with bipolar disorder during pregnancy and lactation. *Journal of Clinical Psychiatry* 59 (Suppl. 6): 57–64.

72 Jacobson SJ *et al.* (1992) Prospective multicentric study of pregnancy outcome after lithium exposure during first trimester. *Lancet* 339: 530–533.

73 Viguera AC *et al.* (2000) Risk of recurrence of bipolar disorder in pregnant vs. nonpregnant women after discontinuing lithium maintenance. *American Journal of Psychiatry* 157: 174–184.

74 MGH Center for Women's Mental Health (2019) Lithium and anticonvulsant mood stabilizers, available at: https://womensmentalhealth.org/posts/lithium

75 Bonari L *et al.* (2004) Perinatal risk of untreated depression during pregnancy. *Canadian Journal of Psychiatry* 49(11): 726–735.

76 Holmes LB *et al.* (2002) Teratogenicity of anticonvulsant drugs. *New England Journal of Medicine* 334: 1132–1138.

77 Kim H *et al.* (2019) Antiepileptic drug treatment patterns in women of childbearing age with epilepsy, available at: www.ncbi.nlm.nih.gov/pubmed/30933252

78 Altshuler LL *et al.* (1996) Pharmacologic management of psychiatric illness during pregnancy: dilemmas and guidelines. *American Journal of Psychiatry* 153: 592–606.

79 Valproate and related substances, available at: www.ema.europa.eu/en/medicines/human/referrals/valproate-related-substances-0

80 Rezvani M (2006) Does vitamin K prophylaxis prevent bleeding in neonates exposed to enzyme-inducing antiepileptic drugs in utero? *Canadian Family Physician* 52(6): 721–722, available at: www.ncbi.nlm.nih.gov/pmc/articles/PMC1780148/

81 Thorp JA *et al.* (1995) Combined antenatal vitamin K and phenobarbital therapy for preventing intracranial hemorrhage in newborns less than 34 weeks' gestation. *Obstetrics & Gynecology* 86(1): 1–8.

82 Rezvani M (2006) Does vitamin K prophylaxis prevent bleeding in neonates exposed to enzyme-inducing antiepileptic drugs in utero? *Canadian Family Physician* 52(6): 721–722, available at: www.ncbi.nlm.nih.gov/pmc/articles/PMC1780148/

83 Goldstein DJ *et al.* (2000) Olanzapine-exposed pregnancies and lactation: early experience. *Journal of Clinical Psychopharmacology* 20: 399–403.

84 Stones SC *et al.* (1997) Clozapine use in two full-term pregnancies. *Journal of Clinical Psychiatry* 58: 364–365.

85 Burt VK *et al.* (2001) The use of psychotropic medications during breastfeeding. *American Journal of Psychiatry* 158: 1001–1009.

86   Austin MV *et al.* (1998) Use of psychotropic medications in breastfeeding women: acute and prophylactic treatment. *Australian and New Zealand Journal of Psychiatry* 32(6): 778–784.

87   Cohen LS *et al.* (1995) Postpartum prophylaxis for women with bipolar disorder. *American Journal of Psychiatry* 152(11): 1641–1644.

88   MGH Center for Women's Mental Health (n.d.) Psychiatric disorders during pregnancy, available at: https://womensmentalhealth.org/specialty-clinics/psychiatric-disorders-during-pregnancy/

89   Cuomo A *et al.* (2018) Aripiprazole use during pregnancy, peripartum and lactation: a systematic literature search and review to inform clinical practice. *Journal of Affective Disorders* 228: 229–237. doi: 10.1016/j.jad.2017.12.021

90   Kar N *et al.* (2016) Clozapine monitoring in clinical practice: beyond the mandatory requirement. *Clinical Psychopharmacology and Neuroscience* 14(4): 323–329. doi: 10.9758/cpn.2016.14.4.323

91   Nguyen HN (2003) Clozapine and pregnancy. [Article in French] *Encephale* 29(2): 119–124.

92   Ibid.

93   MGH Center for Women's Mental Health (n.d.) Psychiatric disorders during pregnancy, available   at: https://womensmentalhealth.org/specialty-clinics/psychiatric-disorders-during-pregnancy/

94   Altshuler LL (1999) The use of medication in bipolar women during pregnancy and postpartum. Presented at the Third International Conference on Bipolar Disorder, June.

95   Iqual MM *et al.* (2002) Effects of commonly used benzodiazepines on the foetus, the neonate and the nursing infant. *Psychiatric Services* 53: 39–49.

96   Munk-Olsen T *et al.* (2012) Psychiatric disorders with postpartum onset: possible early manifestations of bipolar affective disorders. *Archives of General Psychiatry* 69(4): 428–434.

97   Kronenfeld N *et al.* (2017) Use of psychotropic medications in breastfeeding women. *Birth Defects Research* 109(12): 957–997. doi: 10.1002/bdr2.1077

98   Ibid.

99   Ibid.

100   MGH Center for Women's Mental Health (n.d.) Breastfeeding & psychiatric medications, available at: https://womensmentalhealth.org/specialty-clinics/breastfeeding-and-psychiatric-medication/

101   Ibid.

102   Kronenfeld N *et al.* (2017) Use of psychotropic medications in breastfeeding women. *Birth Defects Research* 109(12): 957–997. doi: 10.1002/bdr2.1077

103   ACOG guidelines on psychiatric medication use during pregnancy and lactation, available at: www.aafp.org/afp/2008/0915/p772.html

104   Yager J (2018) Safety of psychotropic medications in breast-feeding, available at: www.jwatch.org/na46826/2018/06/05/safety-psychotropic-medications-breast-feeding

105   Nevels RM (2016) Paroxetine – the antidepressant from hell? Probably not, but caution required. *Psychopharmacology Bulletin* 46(1): 77–104.

106   National Alliance on Mental Illness (2020) Paroxetine (Paxil), available at: www.nami.org/Learn-More/Treatment/Mental-Health-Medications/Types-of-Medication/Paroxetine-(Paxil)

107   Burt VK *et al.* (2001) The use of psychotropic medications during breastfeeding. *American Journal of Psychiatry* 158: 1001–1009.

108   Kohen D (2005) Psychotropic medication and breast-feeding. *Advances in Psychiatric Treatment* 11: 371–379.

109   Mood stabilizers in pregnancy and lactation, available at: www.ncbi.nlm.nih.gov/pmc/articles/PMC4539876/

110   Harden CL *et al.* (2009) Management issues for women with epilepsy – focus on pregnancy (an evidence-based review): vitamin K, folic acid, blood levels, and breastfeeding. Report of the Quality Standards Subcommittee and Therapeutics and Technology Assessment

Subcommittee of the American Academy of Neurology and American Epilepsy Society. *Neurology* 73: 142–149 (Special Article).

111 American Academy of Pediatrics Committee on Drugs (2001) The transfer of drugs and other chemical agents into human milk. *Pediatrics* 108: 776–789.

112 Gardiner SJ *et al.* (2003) Transfer of olanzapine into breast milk, calculation of infant drug dose, and effect on breast-fed infants. *American Journal of Psychiatry* 160: 1428–1431.

113 NCBI (2021) Quetiapine, available at: www.ncbi.nlm.nih.gov/books/NBK501087/

114 Pachiarotti I *et al.* (2016) Mood stabilizers and antipsychotics during breastfeeding: focus on bipolar disorder. *European Neuropsychopharmacology* 26(10): 1562–1578. doi: 10.1016/j.euroneuro.2016.08.008

115 Ibid.

116 Uguz F (2016) Second-generation antipsychotics during the lactation period: a comparative systematic review on infant safety. *Journal of Clinical Psychopharmacology* 36(3): 244–252.

117 MGH Center for Women's Mental Health (2016) Atypical antipsychotics and breastfeeding, available at: https://womensmentalhealth.org/posts/atypical-antipsychotics-breastfeeding/

118 MGH Center for Women's Mental Health (2012) Breastfeeding and benzodia zepines: good news, available at: https://womensmentalhealth.org/posts/breastfeeding-and-benzodiazepines-good-news/

119 Kelly LE *et al.* (2012) Neonatal benzodiazepines exposure during breastfeeding. *Journal of Pediatrics* 161(3): 448–451. doi: 10.1016/j.jpeds.2012.03.003

120 Burt V *et al.* (2001) The use of psychotropic medications during breast-feeding. *American Journal of Psychiatry* 158(7). doi: 10.1176/appi.ajp.158.7.1001

14 Prescribing psychotropics for older patients

- Seniors at risk — 209
- Non-adherence – a major problem — 210
- Principles of psychotropic medication prescription with the elderly — 211
- Regular re-evaluation — 212
- Senior medication problems – general strategies — 212
- Specific psychotropic medication considerations in the elderly — 215
- References — 217

Statistics regarding medication use in older adults are impressive. Although they make up only 16.9 percent of the American population, patients over 65 years account for 30 percent of the use of prescription medications.[1] Depending on whether a community-based or facility-based population is measured, 30–70 percent of the senior age group has been prescribed at least one psychotropic in the prior 90 days.[2] The average individual over the age of 65 fills 13 prescriptions each year, which is almost twice the national average.[3] In the geriatric population, prescription medication is complicated by frequent use of over-the-counter and herbal preparations (often viewed as a way to save money on a limited budget). As many as 10 percent of the elderly use medications prescribed for other people, and 20 percent take medications not currently prescribed by a clinician.[4]

The reasons for increased medication usage in this population are several:

- Compared to a younger person, geriatric patients have more illnesses (both medical and psychiatric) for which medication is used.
- Many elderly patients believe that every problem should have a remedy ("a pill for every ill") and seek medication for relief.
- Particularly in nursing homes, institutional or care settings, patients may not have had a thorough re-evaluation of their medication regimen and can accumulate a long list of medications over the course of their lifetime.

Prescribing psychotropic medications to older individuals presents specific challenges to the clinician. The prescriber must specifically attend to issues regarding the patient's understanding of why the medication is being prescribed, and the ability to cooperate and comply with the treatment regimen.

Seniors at risk

Geriatric patients are physiologically at increased risk for medication problems with the use of psychotropics for several reasons. These include:

- pharmacokinetic changes
- pharmacodynamic changes
- increased frequency of medication interactions
- side effects with lack of compensating physiological mechanisms.

Pharmacokinetic changes

As the body ages, there is a decrease in lean body mass and total body water with a consequent increase in body fat. These changes lead to changes in distribution, half-life and elimination of many psychotropics that are lipophilic and are stored in the body fat. Metabolic breakdown of these lipophilic drugs creates water-soluble forms that can be more readily eliminated, which occurs primarily in the liver. Effects of aging include decreased blood flow to the liver, and decreased liver size and mass.[5-6] Therefore, the drugs that are metabolized from the systemic circulation via first-pass hepatic metabolism are excreted more slowly, have a reduced clearance, and are at risk for accumulation and prolonged half-life. Elimination and excretion, usually through the kidneys, are also affected by aging. As a person ages, there is a decline in the glomerular filtration rate, decreased kidney size, decreased renal blood flow and a decrease in the number of nephrons.[7]

Clinically, the end result of these pharmacokinetic changes is that *older patients may have larger concentrations of medication in their bloodstream when given a "standard" or typical adult dosage*. Medications with a long half-life, that are slow to be eliminated, may accumulate, resulting in exaggerated side effects. Lipophilic medications with long half-lives, such as diazepam, flurazepam and amitriptyline, are particularly poor choices in the geriatric population because their distribution and elimination are altered by several of these mechanisms.[8-9]

Pharmacodynamics

In addition to measurable changes in the blood serum concentration of various psychotropics, elderly patients may have unexpected or unusual pharmacodynamic responses to medications.[10] Within the elderly brain, receptor response can be more sensitive to the action of psychotropic drugs. Therefore, as a patient ages, the therapeutic response and/or excessive response can begin to occur at lower than "normal" therapeutic levels.

Medication interactions

It is well known that the larger the number of medications a patient takes, the more likely it is that the patient will have medication interactions. A patient taking four prescriptions is twice as likely to experience an adverse medication interaction as a patient taking just one medication. If a patient takes seven medications simultaneously, the risk of an adverse reaction increases 14-fold! We also know that the greater the number of diagnoses, the greater the number of medications likely to be prescribed. Because seniors have a greater number of diagnosed illnesses and take a significantly increased number of medications (often of several classes), they are statistically much more likely to have drug interactions with their sequelae than their younger counterparts.

Particularly troublesome side effects for the elderly include sedation, confusion, dizziness and decreased sleep – all of which can be common with psychotropics. Also problematic are anticholinergic effects, including decreased urination, blurred vision and dry mouth.

Elderly persons are less able to compensate for the side effects of many medications.[11] Especially problematic is decreased sensitivity of baroreceptors, which can predispose the senior to postural hypotension, dizziness and the likelihood of falls.

Side effects alone can be severe enough to require hospitalization. One study documented that 16.8 percent of general hospital admissions for the elderly were due to side effects of medication.[12]

Non-adherence – a major problem

Although estimates of non-adherent medication usage in the elderly vary, almost all estimates are high – ranging from 40 to 75 percent. Of a seniors' sample of several hundred patients, only 33.5 percent had "moderate" compliance and almost 20 percent had "poor" compliance.[13] Non-adherent usage may lead to over usage, under usage, sporadic or changing usage of medications. The causes of non-adherence are multiple, but include:

* not understanding the reasons medications are being used, and therefore using them incorrectly
* unintentional non-adherence due to confusion about dosing schedules
* general mental forgetfulness
* intentional non-adherence because of inability to afford the medication and/or omitting doses to "make them last"
* intentional non-adherence because of increased sensitivity to bothersome side effects/toxic reactions to medications.

The geriatric population's tendency toward increasing cognitive changes with advancing age leads to significant forgetfulness and unintentional underdosing, overdosing or missed dosing. Not remembering that they have taken the dose, patients may take a second or third dose unknowingly and unintentionally. Particularly when anticholinergics or sedative hypnotics are included in the regimen, memory interference is common. With impaired memory, patients may forget to take prescribed doses altogether for hours or entire days.

Deliberate overuse of non-prescription drugs (which are usually less costly than prescription medication) is a common occurrence. Patients may use their experience with rapid-acting non-psychotropic medications (e.g., pain pills) as a guide to how they believe psychotropics may act. They will take too much prescribed psychotropic medication in the hope that by taking a larger dose they will get well more rapidly. By being able to improve sooner, they believe they can stop the medication sooner and ultimately save money.

Under usage of medications is a more significant problem in the elderly than in other age groups. Besides the memory problems mentioned above, seniors may take less than prescribed amounts of medication for various other reasons as well. Owing to the high cost of prescription drugs, consistent use of medication may be a major concern for many pensioners who live on a fixed income. Patients will attempt to make their supply of medication last longer by taking doses intermittently to spread them out. Likewise, they may be even more prone than other mental health patients to stopping medications at the earliest opportunity, often as soon as they begin feeling well, believing that they no longer need the psychotropic. Misunderstanding the mechanism of action and the need for continuing doses of psychotropics contributes to a failure to take adequate medication for an adequate period of time. Elderly patients may also stop a prescription medication prematurely and begin an over-the-counter remedy in the hope that it will sustain the effect, be just as useful and be less expensive.

Frequently, side effects common to the use of psychotropics can cause elderly patients to underdose themselves. Anticholinergic, sedative and hypotensive side effects of psychotropics, which are especially bothersome to seniors, can lead geriatric patients to underdose themselves or stop medication early.

Principles of psychotropic medication prescription with the elderly

Two statements can guide the clinician in the prescribing of psychotropic medications to the elderly:

1   *Less is more* with regard to:
    - dosage of medication prescribed
    - number of medications prescribed
    - length of time for which medications are prescribed.

2   *More is better* with regard to:
    - giving instructions
    - vigilance for side effects
    - frequency of follow-up evaluations.

Although many of the principles described in this section are important for all age groups, they are particularly crucial when prescribing psychotropic medications to the geriatric population:

- minimize the number of medications used
- start low and go slow with dosage increases
- remember that the ultimate therapeutic dose of drug may be lower than that used in younger adults
- for the patient taking chronic psychotropics, the amount of drug necessary for therapeutic response can change with advancing age (and usually decreases)
- lengthen the time period between dose changes to allow the patient to adjust to any new or increased side effects, and to observe for response (positive or negative)
- avoid psychotropic medications for minor or non-specific diagnoses
- use medication for agitation and behavioral control only when necessary, and then in minimal doses.

Because of the increased sensitivity to side effects in older patients and the decreased ability to compensate for them, clinicians should always consider whether non-pharmacological means are useful in treating a mental health condition in the elderly (see Chapter 17 for a discussion of these non-pharmacological alternatives). If medication is used, monotherapy is always preferable to polypharmacy. However, despite the downside of using multiple medications, some geriatric patients may require intentional polypharmacy by the clinician to obtain an adequate therapeutic response.

In general, *when starting a medication in a geriatric individual, the clinician should use half the dose typically used for an adult patient.* Further dosage increases should be accomplished more gradually and at greater intervals than those timeframes used in younger adults. This will allow elderly individuals to adapt to both the therapeutic effect and any side effects from the medication. Because lower starting doses are used and dosage increases leading to a final therapeutic dose are spread out, it may take a longer period of time to assess the therapeutic response to a particular medication. A trial of medication may take several months to be performed safely and simultaneously allow for assessment of adequacy of response.

Regular re-evaluation

Particularly in elderly patients who are followed over time, or patients maintained in an institutional care setting, the clinician must regularly re-evaluate the patient's medication regimen. During such an assessment, it is important for a clinician to consider eliminating any unnecessary medications and minimizing the overall medication prescription burden.

Questions to be asked by the prescriber during re-evaluation should include:

- Is each of these psychotropics still necessary to this patient?
- Has the patient had an interval without medication to observe for ongoing clinical necessity?
- Could any medications be discontinued that were added during a crisis that has now passed?
- Would a lowering of dosage accomplish a continuing satisfactory therapeutic result?
- Is the patient experiencing any new or added side effects from the psychotropics?
- Is the patient cognitively and physically still able to manage his or her own medications safely?
- Have the patient's mental, physical or financial circumstances changed such that the medication prescription regimen should be altered?
- Has the patient been adherent to his or her regimen? (e.g., are refills being filled on time, early or late? Are there more pills left over from a previous prescription than there should be if the patient were taking the medication as directed?)
- If non-adherence is suspected, is further education or reinforcement necessary to emphasize why, how and when the medication should be taken?

Senior medication problems – general strategies

During evaluation and initial prescription

At the initial evaluation of any geriatric patient, the clinician should perform a comprehensive review of all prescription, non-prescription and herbal medications that the patient takes. Prior to the actual patient visit, it is often useful to ask the patient or caregivers to prepare a list of medication names, doses, frequency of administration and length of time each one has been taken. This gives patients and/or their caregivers the opportunity to formulate such a list at their leisure in a more organized and complete way, rather than attempting to produce the information on the spur of the moment in the office.

In addition to other considerations of effectiveness and therapeutic benefit for a geriatric patient, the clinician should consider the following information in recommending medication.

- How many prescription medications does the patient take?
- How many non-prescription medications does the patient take?
- How many clinicians does the patient consult?
- Can the patient tolerate the addition of another medication?
- What side effects are likely to occur?
- Does the initial starting dosage need to be modified?
- What medication interactions are likely?
- Is the patient mentally, physically or financially impaired in a way that will affect the choice of medication or its administration?
- Does the patient have sensory or literacy problems that may affect the his or her understanding of instructions or ability to carry them out?
- Does the patient live alone?
- Can the patient self-administer the medication prescribed?
- Is special packaging required?
- What frequency of re-evaluation is necessary to determine if the medication is safely tolerated and effective?
- If the medication is effective, what target date is appropriate to evaluate when it may be stopped?

Communication between the clinician and patient is crucial in obtaining medication adherence. It is vitally important that geriatric patients understand the nature of their mental health condition, the role of medications in treatment and the limitations of the medications' effect. Patients must know what the medications can do and will not do, and the timeframe in which a therapeutic response is expected. The clinician must explain possible drug interactions and side effects. Once explained, it is important to obtain at least a verbal response from patients that they understand the regimen and will adhere to it. For this medicine, is taking extra doses helpful or, in fact, harmful? Whenever possible, PRN dosing (as needed) should be minimized and the patient given a schedule that is consistent day to day. If extra doses are permitted or recommended, at the patient's discretion, how much medication can be taken and how often?

In prescribing a dosage regimen, the clinician should attempt to match the regimen to the particular patient's daily schedule. When possible, dosages should be attached to predictable elements of daily routine such as meals or bedtime, rather than dosing in the middle of the day. It may be necessary to ask about the timing of these daily events in *this* patient's life. Some persons who live alone may have idiosyncratic eating and sleeping times. The drug regimen should be kept simple, using once-daily dosing whenever possible.

Visual or mechanical aids are very helpful to the prescriptive process with the geriatric population. Written instructions as well as charts are useful ways to explain medication dosing. The patient can be advised to obtain a partitioned "pill minder" at the pharmacy to organize dosages for a day or a week, which will minimize unintentional repeat dosing. Color-coded bottles may be helpful in distinguishing one medication from another. Large lettering on any instructions or on pill bottles is also useful. Patients with arthritis or hand pain should have medication bottles without safety caps, which may be difficult to open. The pharmacist should be alerted on the written prescription of the necessity to utilize these aids for a patient. The patient should be encouraged to use one pharmacy for all medications – both psychotropic and non-psychotropic. Computerized pharmacy medication profiles at a single pharmacy can alert the pharmacist to potentially problematic drug interactions of medications prescribed by multiple clinicians.

When discussing medications with geriatric patients, clinicians should realize that they have a decreased attention span and may need repetition in order to understand the nature of their medication regimen. When a patient will self-administer medication, a caregiver or family member can be included at the time of giving prescription and dosing instructions so that the caregiver may repeat and reinforce the instructions at a later time. In the very busy primary care office when time is of the essence, it may be helpful to have one of the clinical office staff review and/or provide these directions to the patient and the caregiver. Whenever possible, all directions should be also given in written form.

Senior patients may need specific direction on what to do if a medication supply runs out and any consequences that can occur if the medication is stopped suddenly (e.g., discontinuation syndrome). If there is risk involved in allowing the supply to run out, the patient needs specific directions to contact the clinician before using the last dose. Patients must be aware that it is not routinely good practice to decrease the dose to try to make the current amount last longer or, worse yet, stop the medication without notifying the clinician.

Especially in the senior population, whenever an antipsychotic medication is to be prescribed, it is important to perform and document a baseline AIMS test, so as to be able to compare the patient's baseline with any movement problems which may occur after a psychotropic is begun (see Chapter 20 and Appendix 6).

During follow-up visits

Patients should bring a list of all medications they are currently taking to each follow-up visit, and update the list with any new medications from other prescribers. At the first follow-up visit, the clinician should ask the patient to explain how many pills of each psychotropic medication he or she is taking and at what time of day. As has been mentioned before, it is better to have the patient and/or caregiver describe when and in what dosage the medication is taken rather than have the clinician read off what is expected. In this latter circumstance, the patient will often say, "Yes, that's what I do," even when it is not so. It is surprising how often the patient is not taking the medication in the amount or frequency that the clinician has prescribed!

Once a year, patients should bring in all pill bottles of medications they are currently taking so the clinician can review with the patient each of the psychotropics, how often they are taken, for what condition they are being taken and any side effects that may have occurred. For long-term patients, the patient's advancing age may justify a dosage decrease, or it may be possible to discontinue one or more medications.

Specific psychotropic medication considerations in the elderly

No psychotropic medication choices are ideal or risk-free in geriatric patients, given the inherent potential fragility of the aging body and mind. Certain psychotropic medications, however, carry added risk for elderly patients, and should be avoided whenever possible. These medications are listed in Table 14.1.

In general, drugs with a narrow therapeutic index, such as lithium carbonate and tricyclic antidepressants are medications where changes in blood level can lead to serious side effects or toxicity in the elderly. In order to minimize risk, more frequent monitoring of serum blood levels is necessary, with vigilance for the addition of any agent that could alter blood level.

Antidepressants

Virtually all SSRIs, SNRIs and other new antidepressants offer advantages over TCAs in the elderly population. Another useful class of medication to treat depression for this group is stimulants that have been shown on multiple occasions to have rapid antidepressant activity with minimal drug interactions and side effects.[14–16] Issues of habituation and abuse are lessened in the geriatric age group, and stimulants can be especially useful in the medically ill, depressed elderly because of their rapid onset of action and minimal medication interactions.

Anti-anxiety agents, sedative hypnotics

If benzodiazepines are necessary, shorter-acting medications, such as alprazolam, oxazepam, triazolam and temazepam, are preferable to longer-acting agents. Benzodiazepines should be used judiciously in small doses, since no benzodiazepine is without some increased sedation/fall risk in the elderly. Anxiety disorders may be better treated with antidepressants or non-medication therapies such as CBT if longer-term medication is necessary.

Any sedative medication from any classification, whether of short or long half-life, can cause excess sleepiness and increase the risk of falls and subsequent hip fractures.[17] Patients can awaken confused or ataxic in the middle of the night as they arise to use the bathroom. The clinician should carefully assess the risk–benefit ratio before prescribing anything as a sedative/hypnotic.

Table 14.1 Psychotropic medications to be used with caution in elderly patients

Class of medication	Medications	Effect
Tricyclic antidepressants	Amitriptyline, doxepin	Strong anticholinergic and sedating properties; may induce arrhythmias
	Desipramine	Sleep interference
Long-acting benzodiazepines	Chlordiazepoxide, diazepam, flurazepam	Long half-life, oversedation, high fall risk
Antihistamines	Diphenhydramine, cyproheptadine	Strong anticholinergic activity and effects
Beta blockers	Propranolol	May worsen respiratory function
Traditional antipsychotics	High doses of any antipsychotic medications	Hypotension, sedation, falls

Antipsychotics

With the exception of clozapine, which has major potential side-effect concerns for the elderly, in general, atypical antipsychotics (olanzapine, quetiapine, risperidone, ziprasidone, asenapine, vilazodone, lurasidone, iloperidone, paliperidone and aripiprazole) have safety and tolerability advantages over traditional antipsychotics.[18] Markedly lower incidence of movement and neurological complications make these agents preferable choices to earlier agents for seniors (see Chapter 19). The one issue of concern with antipsychotic medication use involves the blanket, class-wide warning about the use of these medications in elderly patients with dementia-related psychosis. This area will be further discussed in Chapter 20 on "Danger Zones." Clozapine, with a side-effect profile that includes lowered seizure threshold, blood dyscrasias, strong anticholinergic properties and significant orthostatic hypotension, is generally a fourth or fifth choice after the other atypical antipsychotics for elderly patients.

Mood stabilizers

There are no controlled data studies of mood stabilizer effectiveness specifically in the geriatric population. Safety and side-effect profiles have been more thoroughly collected for the anticonvulsant mood stabilizers in the epileptic population rather than the mental health population. None of the commonly used mood stabilizers is without at least one potential side effect that could be troublesome or hazardous to an elderly patient (see Table 14.2). Therefore, mood stabilizer decisions should be made on a case-by-case basis using a risk–benefit assessment for each patient.

Atypical antipsychotics, such as olanzapine, quetiapine, risperidone, ziprasidone, asenapine, vilazodone, lurasidone, iloperidone, paliperidone and aripiprazole, may have usefulness as mood stabilizers in this population. Further safety and risk issues for these compounds are emerging from the large multicenter trials being conducted by the National Institute of Mental Health (NIMH).[19]

Other considerations

Of particular concern in the elderly is the risk of hypotension, dizziness and falls. Seniors who use psychotropic drugs, particularly benzodiazepines and antidepressants,

Table 14.2 Possible adverse effects of mood stabilizing medications

Drug	Possible adverse effects
Carbamazepine	Ataxia, dizziness, hyponatremia, cardiac conduction disturbance
Valproic acid	Ataxia, dizziness, weight gain, tremors
Gabapentin	Somnolence, dizziness, ataxia
Lamotrigine	Somnolence, dizziness, ataxia, diplopia, rash
Topiramate	Dizziness, ataxia, difficulty concentrating, tremors, word-finding difficulty

Source: Adapted from Bourdet SV *et al.* (2001) Pharmacologic management of epilepsy in the elderly. *Journal of the American Pharmaceutical Association* 41(3): 434.

are at almost twice the risk of hip fracture secondary to a fall than are patients not taking these medications.[20]

Medication-induced cognitive changes are also a major concern in the elderly. The incidence of delirium and dementia increase with age; the addition of medication can further complicate cognitive ability. Even mild cognitive impairment may negatively impact patients' day-to-day functioning and their ability to comply adequately with their overall healthcare medication regimen. This is a particular concern if the patient lives alone.

References

1   Santos-Pérez MI (2019) A cross-sectional study of psychotropic drug use in the elderly: consuming patterns, risk factors and potentially inappropriate use. *European Journal of Hospital Pharmacy* 28(2), available at: https://ejhp.bmj.com/content/early/2019/06/11/ejhpharm-2019-001927

2   Ibid.

3   Lindsey PL (2009) Psychotropic medication use among older adults. *Journal of Gerontological Nursing* 35(9): 28–38, available at: www.ncbi.nlm.nih.gov/pmc/articles/PMC3128509/

4   Lamy PP *et al.* (1992) Drug prescribing patterns, risks, and compliance guidelines. In C Salzman (ed.), *Clinical Geriatric Psychopharmacology*, 2nd edn. (pp. 15–37), Williams & Wilkins.

5   Wynne HA *et al.* (1993) The association of age and frailty with the pharmacokinetics and pharmacodynamics of metoclopramide. *Age and Ageing* 22: 354.

6   Wynne HA *et al.* (1989) The effect of age upon liver volume and apparent liver blood flow in healthy man. *Hepatology* 9: 297.

7   Lindeman RD *et al.* (1985) Longitudinal studies on the rate of decline in renal function with age. *Journal of the American Geriatric Society* 33: 278.

8   Hammerlein A *et al.* (1998) Pharmacokinetic and pharmacodynamic changes in the elderly: clinical implications. *Clinical Pharmacokinetics* 35(1): 49–64.

9   Offerhaus L (ed.) (1997) *Drugs for the Elderly*, 2nd edn., WHO Regional Publications, European Series.

10 Ibid.

11 Ibid.

12 Col N *et al.* (1990) The role of medication noncompliance and adverse drug reactions in hospitalizations of the elderly. *Archives of Internal Medicine* 150: 841–845.

13 Shruthi R *et al.* (2016) A study of medication compliance in geriatric patients with chronic illnesses at a tertiary care hospital. *Journal of Clinical and Diagnostic Research* 10(12): FC40–FC43, available at: www.ncbi.nlm.nih.gov/pmc/articles/PMC5296451/

14 Pickett P *et al.* (1990) Psychostimulant treatment of geriatric depressive disorders secondary to medical illness. *Journal of Geriatric Psychiatry and Neurology* 3(3): 146–151.

15 Emptage RE and Semla TP (1996) Depression in the medically ill elderly: a focus on methylphenidate. *Annals of Pharmacotherapy* 30(2): 151–157.

16 Corp SA *et al.* (2014) A review of the use of stimulants and stimulant alternatives in treating bipolar depression and major depressive disorder. *Journal of Clinical Psychiatry* 75(9): 1010.

17 Leavy B *et al.* (2017) The impact of disease and drugs on hip fracture risk. *Calcified Tissue International* 100(1): 1–12. doi: 10.1007/s00223-016-0194-7

18 Blake L *et al.* (n.d.) Optimal management of psychosis and agitation in the elderly, available at: www.medscape.org/viewarticle/429889

19   Murray R *et al.* (2017) Atypical antipsychotics: recent research findings and applications to clinical practice: proceedings of a symposium presented at the 29th Annual European College of Neuropsychopharmacology Congress, 19 September 2016, Vienna, Austria. *Therapeutic Advances in Psychopharmacology* 7(1) (Suppl.): 1–14. doi: 10.1177/2045125317693200

20   Turnheim K (1998) Drug dosage in the elderly: is it rational? *Drugs and Aging* 13(5): 357–379.

15 Medication of sleep problems

- Facts and definitions   220
- Stages of sleep   220
- Evaluating a sleep problem   221
- Principles of treating sleep disorders   224
- Treatment of sleep problems   225
- Necessity of follow up   229
- Sleep problems in special populations   229
- Notes and references   231

Sleep disorders affect 60 million adults per year in the United States. Fifty percent of adults at some point in their lives are affected by insomnia. The prevalence of short sleep (less than 7 hours) is over 35.4 percent.[1]

Insufficient sleep is associated with a number of medical problems linked to 7 of the 15 leading causes of death in the United States, including cardiovascular disease, malignant neoplasm, cerebrovascular disease, accidents, diabetes, septicemia and hypertension.[2] Many of the people with a sleep problem will approach their medical practitioner for help and request medication.[3]

Difficulty in sleeping is one of the most common presenting requests to a medication clinician. Based on accurate diagnostic assessment, the prescription of medication to aid sleep is generally safe, can be extraordinarily helpful for patients, and can help to speed recovery from a primary mental health disorder. On the other hand, poor prescribing habits and/or over-prescription of sleeping medication can cause daytime sleepiness, accidents, falls, exacerbation of medical illness and possible habituation to medication. Some clinicians, unfortunately, withhold the prescription of sleeping medication unnecessarily, while others prescribe prematurely, lacking sufficient evaluation and follow up. The prescription of sleeping medication is neither an area to be feared and avoided, nor should it be the immediate, automatic response to a patient who is having difficulty sleeping. This chapter will discuss the principles of assessment of sleep problems and the informed prescription of sedative/hypnotic medication.

Facts and definitions

Several key definitions are important in order to discuss the issue of sleep.[4] These include:

- Insomnia – difficulty in initiating or maintaining sleep; or having sleep that is non-restorative.
- Psychophysiological insomnia – a condition in which a patient who begins having difficulty sleeping becomes increasingly anxious and worried that he or she will not sleep, which then makes it more difficult to fall asleep, perpetuating a problematic cycle leading to further insomnia.
- Rebound insomnia – increased difficulty sleeping after a patient who has been taking a sleep medication on a chronic basis stops the medication suddenly.
- Sleep latency – the interval between the time when patients lie down to sleep and the time they actually fall asleep.
- Sleep efficiency – the amount of time that a patient actually sleeps divided by the amount of time a patient spends in bed trying to sleep, expressed as a fraction or percentage (e.g., a patient who is actually asleep for 5 hours while in bed for 8 hours has a sleep efficiency of 5/8, or 62.5 percent).
- Phase-shifted sleep – a situation when persons get adequate hours of sleep, but do so at unusual times or at times that interfere with usual day and evening functioning (e.g., they sleep from 6 p.m. to 3 a.m. – phase advanced sleep; or 4 a.m. until noon – phase delayed sleep).
- Sleep apnea – transient periods of breathing cessation during sleep. Central sleep apnea results from failure of the respiratory centers in the medulla; obstructive sleep apnea (OSA) is caused by collapse or obstruction of the airway during REM (rapid eye movement) sleep.[5] Both types of apnea result in disrupted sleep, non-refreshing sleep and daytime fatigue.
- Restless leg syndrome (RLS) – a common central nervous system disorder characterized by uncomfortable "creepy, crawly, bubbly, or tingling" sensations in the legs, which usually appear at rest, are relieved temporarily by movement, worsen during the evening or night and can interrupt the ability to fall asleep.[6]
- Periodic limb movements of sleep (PLM) – stereotypical flexing motions of the legs that occur in clusters of 20–40 seconds during sleep, which can cause arousal and daytime sleepiness. PLMs occur frequently in persons with restless leg syndrome.
- Insufficient sleep syndrome – a condition that results from persons who recurrently consciously attempt to "get by" with less than their usual amounts of sleep, in order to accommodate shift work, exams, multiple jobs, social or family expectations; this leads to fatigue and irregular sleep patterns.[7]
- Narcolepsy – recurrent, irresistible, brief episodes of sleep during the day accompanied by spells of muscle weakness when emotionally upset (cataplexy), and visions or vivid dreamlike states in the drowsy state just before sleep (hypnogogic hallucinations) or just prior to awakening (hypnopompic hallucinations).[8]

Stages of sleep

Sleep is not a consistent, uniform activity. There are distinctly demarcated stages of sleep that can be easily differentiated on an electroencephalogram (EEG). Broadly, sleep is divided into non-rapid eye movement (non-REM) sleep and rapid eye movement (REM) sleep, which is the stage in which we dream. Non-REM sleep is divided into stages one, two, three and four, with stage one being the lightest stage and stage four the deepest. The vast majority of our sleep is taken up by the non-REM stages, and routinely occurs in a cycle. The cycle begins with stage one, progressing in depth to stages two, three and four. The cycle then reverses itself back to stages three, two and one, followed by a REM period. This cycle repeats itself three to four times per night, and can be seen most clearly in the top graph in Figure 15.1, which shows the typical stages in a child's sleep. The subsequent graphs show sleep patterns for young adults and elderly individuals. The most important element of these comparison graphs is that as we age, we have significantly less deep sleep (stage four) and more of the lighter stages of sleep, with many more frequent awakenings. This becomes particularly important when discussing sleep with elderly individuals, since it is a normal, expectable, physiological phenomenon that their sleep is lighter and more disrupted than it was when they were younger.

Evaluating a sleep problem

The important factors to be addressed in an evaluation of a sleep problem are listed in Table 15.1 and elaborated on in the subsequent text.

When a patient first presents describing difficulty with sleep, the clinician should find out how long this sleep problem has been occurring. Sleep problems are divided into *transient insomnia* (limited to a few nights), *short-term insomnia* (less than 3 weeks) and *long-term insomnia* (of more than 3 weeks' duration).[9]

Generally, transient and short-term insomnia have a different set of causes to chronic (or long-term) insomnia.

Transient and short-term insomnia can often occur owing to:

* periods of emotional distress or bereavement
* initiation or discontinuation of pharmaceuticals
* use/abuse/withdrawal of streets drugs or alcohol
* recent onset of a physical or painful illness, such as musculoskeletal injury or peptic ulcer disease
* work-shift changes
* jet lag.

When evaluating short-term insomnia, it is important to ask about *recent stressors and lifestyle changes*. Patients are not always cognizant of the effect that certain lifestyle changes, such as jet lag, changes in work shift, personal crisis or the initiation of a chemical or pharmaceutical can have on their sleep, even if it may be obvious to the clinician. At times, the patient may be aware of the event(s), but has not made the connection to their insomnia.

A clinician must know *when* during the night patients are having trouble. Are they having difficulty falling asleep, but once asleep stay asleep? Are they having minimal difficulty falling asleep, but awaken in the middle of the night (sleep continuity disturbance)? Or are they having trouble with awakening before they have completed a full

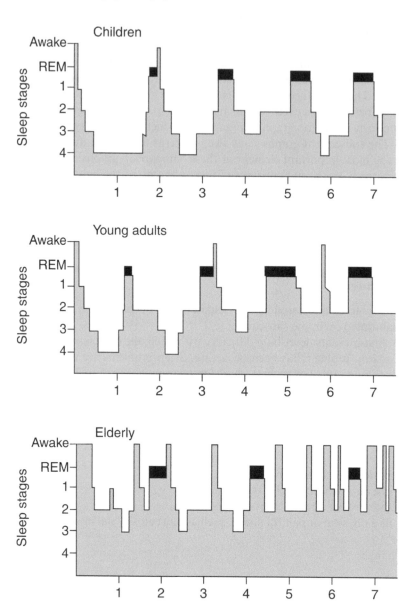

Figure 15.1 Sample sleep graphs of children, young adults and seniors.

Source: Kales A and Kales JD (1974) Sleep disorders: recent findings in the diagnosis and treatment of disturbed sleep. *New England Journal of Medicine* 290: 487.

night's sleep (early morning awakening)? If medication is to be prescribed, these timing factors will strongly affect the choice of medication to be recommended. Is the amount of sleep normal in duration but occurring at the "wrong time" (phase-shifted sleep)? (In this case, sleep medication is unlikely to be the best treatment or may not be prescribed at all [see below].)

Table 15.1 Factors in a sleep evaluation

1 Duration of the sleeping problem (how long has the patient had difficulties with sleep?)
2 When during the night does the problem occur? For example, does the patient have:
   • difficulty falling asleep?
   • sleep continuity disturbance (awakening in the middle of the night)?
   • early morning awakening?
3 Are there recent events that may have precipitated the sleep problem?
4 Evaluation for the various causes of sleep disorders including:
   • medical diseases
   • psychiatric disorders
   • substance abuse and withdrawal
   • prescription medications
   • non-medication substances
   • primary sleep disorders
   • sleep apnea
   • restless leg syndrome
   • periodic limb movements of sleep

In general, insomnia that has lasted for more than 3 weeks (and may have persisted for months or years) has other causes than those listed above for short-term insomnia. Long-term insomnia is much more likely to have at its root significant medical disease, major psychiatric conditions or substance abuse. For some of these patients, a psycho-physiological cycle of insomnia has been established, where worrying about continued inability to sleep produces even more difficulty in falling or staying asleep.

The prescriber should screen for *medical diseases* associated with insomnia, including hypertension, hyperthyroidism, respiratory insufficiency, cardiovascular insufficiency and chronic pain. *Prescription medications* that can be associated with difficulty sleeping include antihypertensives, diuretics, steroids, stimulants, bronchodilators, decongestants, histamine antagonists and xanthines such as theophylline.[10–13]

Many *psychiatric disorders*, including depression, bipolar disorder, a variety of psychotic conditions and anxiety disorders such as PTSD, panic attacks and generalized anxiety disorder can present with difficulty sleeping either as a primary or a secondary complaint.

Onset of insomnia temporarily associated with the recent initiation of any psychotropic medications should be noted, since many antidepressants, stimulants and atypical antipsychotics have been linked with sleep disturbance. In some cases, a recent increase in dosage of one of these medications may also lead to disordered sleep.

Approximately 10–15 percent of patients with insomnia have substance abuse problems.[14] Many patients do not understand that alcohol, although it may help initiate sleep for some individuals, will generally lead to middle-of-the-night awakening and the perception of insomnia. Although alcohol is often referred to as a central nervous system "depressant," in this context it means that *it decreases overall neuron firing and may have a calming or sedative effect*. (It does not mean that it necessarily causes depression or is "depressogenic.") Particularly when the alcohol consumption is heavy, it may initially induce sleep. When the alcohol levels drop owing to metabolism and excretion, however, the CNS rebounds in activity and neuron firing becomes more active, leading to awakening or disrupted, non-restful sleep.

Patients should also be questioned about their daily intake of caffeine and particularly whether caffeine is taken after 3 p.m.

Other useful screening questions of a patient with long-term insomnia that may elicit symptoms suggestive of a *primary sleep disturbance* include:

- In the evening or night, has the patient had any unusual, restless, painful or "creepy, crawling" feelings in their legs that are temporarily relieved by movement? (restless leg syndrome)
- Has anyone told the patient that he or she snores heavily, coughs/chokes repeatedly or has irregular breathing at night? (sleep apnea)
- Is there any history of spells of muscle weakness triggered by emotional upset? (narcolepsy)
- Is there any history of "burning the candle at both ends" and trying to "make your-self get by with less sleep than you need?" (insufficient sleep syndrome)

For those with chronic sleep problems, information from the patient's sleep partner is helpful. Ask the partner specifically about any periods of difficulty in breathing, choking, coughing or apneic spells. It is also helpful to evaluate the *patient's daily routine*. How much exercise does the patient get? How much, and when, does he or she eat? What is the evening routine, particularly in the several hours before bedtime?

For chronic insomnia, a *physical exam* should be performed with specific focus on the presence of nasal obstruction, a low-hanging palate, an unusually small mandible size or an enlarged thyroid, any of which could lead to obstructive sleep apnea. The patient's weight and blood pressure should be recorded. Hypertension and/or obesity are positively correlated with obstructive sleep apnea.

The patient should be referred for polysomnography in a sleep lab if:

- any of the above questions for primary sleep disorder are answered positively
- appropriate therapy for a short-term sleep disorder is unsuccessful and the condition persists
- a patient is exhibiting daytime sleepiness to the point of having difficulty staying alert while driving, or if the patient is experiencing academic/occupational problems secondary to tiredness and fatigue
- a sleeping partner notices distinct apneic periods.

 Box 15.1 Clinical tip

It is well known that sleep difficulties are common in many mental health diagnoses including depression and anxiety. A useful tip is that insomnia typically *precedes* a depressive episode and more commonly *follows* an episode of anxiety. Depressive relapses are often predicted by an insomnia prodrome.[15]

Principles of treating sleep disorders

How much sleep is normal? The old adage that everyone needs 8 hours of sleep is commonly believed, but is not true for many people. A range of 6.5–9 hours of sleep is common, and sleep within these parameters does not generally indicate sleep pathology or psychopathology. More or less sleep than this on a regular basis can be indicative of a sleep disorder.

It is crucial to have a diagnosis for the type of sleep disorder being treated or at least to have performed a thorough evaluation to attempt diagnosis, even if a firm diagnosis cannot be made. To prescribe sleeping pills routinely after a minimal or negligible assessment of what kind of sleep problem the patient is having will often mean that underlying medical or psychiatric causes of a sleep disturbance are missed, and will likely result in over-prescription of sleeping medication.

If there is an underlying medical condition (e.g., hypertension, pulmonary problems, cardiovascular disease with cardiac insufficiency, thyroid disease), this must be appropriately evaluated and treated to have reasonable success with improving a patient's sleep. Likewise, if a patient is suffering from depression, bipolar disorder, an anxiety disorder or psychosis, these too must be appropriately evaluated and treated in order for the sleep to improve. If there is any evidence of a primary sleep disorder, including restless leg syndrome/periodic limb movement disorder, sleep apnea or narcolepsy, these must be adequately evaluated rather than simply prescribing sleeping medications that may actually worsen the condition.

Before sleeping medication can be prescribed, the patient's personal history of alcohol and drug use should be assessed and any family history of alcohol or drug abuse noted. Persons with a family history of substance abuse are at more risk for abusing sleep medications than those without. If sleeping medication is prescribed for a patient with a personal or family history of substance abuse, extra vigilance should be maintained for misuse of medication (see Chapter 22).

Treatment of sleep problems

When sleeping medications are prescribed, the least amount of medication that permits restorative sleep should be used for the shortest period of time until the patient's normal sleep pattern re-emerges.

For the responsible patient who is having transient or short-term sleep problems secondary to a clear personal stressor and who does not have a substance abuse problem, or underlying medical or psychiatric illness, sleeping medications can generally be prescribed safely. In these patients there is minimal risk and the clinician can generally feel comfortable prescribing sleeping medications for several days to several weeks.

It is also important to warn patients about possible side effects such as:

• dizziness or lightheadedness, which may lead to falls
• headaches
• gastrointestinal problems, such as diarrhea and nausea
• prolonged drowsiness, more so with drugs that help you stay asleep
• sleep-related behaviors, such as driving or eating when not fully awake
• daytime memory and performance problems.

It is also warranted to mention potential interactions with other sedative medications and increased sensitivity to alcohol's intoxicating effects. The clinician can reassure the patient about the lack of habituation if the medication is taken in the dose prescribed for a several-week period. Over this timeframe, there is also minimal risk of rebound insomnia.

If a short-term trial of medications is insufficient to resolve the patient's problem, or if the patient has had a history of sleep difficulties for longer than 3 weeks, a more in-depth evaluation is necessary. This intensity of the sleep problem is often a sign of a more serious underlying medical illness, psychiatric disorder or primary sleep disorder. Asking the patient to record bedtimes, hours of sleep and times of arising in a sleep diary for 2 weeks may also elicit further useful information. It is essential, in patients with long-term sleep problems, to get historical information from the patient's sleep partner.

Non-pharmacological treatment

The following suggestions should be made to patients routinely, whether or not sleeping medication is ultimately prescribed. These issues are especially crucial in dealing with patients who experience chronic insomnia:

- Advise a regular schedule with approximately the same bedtime and morning arising time each day. Counsel against "sleeping in" on weekend days, and marked variations in bedtime.
- Avoid naps during the day.
- Although a light snack may be useful at bedtime (particularly for geriatric patients with insomnia), heavy meals should be avoided prior to sleep.
- Suggest regular exercise three to four times per week, although it is best not done after dinner since adrenaline stimulation may exacerbate sleep difficulties. Inform the patient that any exercise regime that aids sleep will take up to 6 weeks to have a beneficial sleep effect.
- Control the bedroom temperature and surroundings. Patients generally do not sleep well in rooms that are excessively hot or cold, noisy or brightly lit. If necessary, advise the use of earplugs, sleep masks, white-noise machines or fans to maintain comfortable, consistent bedroom conditions.
- Encourage relaxing activities and a "ritual wind down" in the hour or two prior to going to bed. This can involve reading, television, relaxation exercises or yoga. At times, progressive relaxation training is useful.
    - With the proliferation of cell phones, computers and the Internet in general, there are now multiple applications at low or no cost, which will track a person's sleep as well as provide sounds or conversation to assist a person in falling to sleep.
    - Some of these include:
    - Headspace
    - Noisli
    - Pzizz
    - Slumber
    - Calm
    - Sleep Cycle.
- Avoid stimulating or emotionally charged issues (e.g., preparing taxes, reading an excessively arousing book or discussing emotionally loaded issues) before going to bed.

- Avoid caffeine-containing substances after the noontime meal.
- Avoid alcohol after dinner.
- Advise that the bed be used only for sleeping or sexual activity, and not as a place for watching television, eating or other activities.
- If the patient has not fallen asleep within 30 minutes of going to bed, advise him/her to get up and do a pleasant, relaxing activity, such as reading, listening to music or watching television, until drowsy. Only then return to bed. Advise against staying in bed, tossing, turning and looking at the clock.
- Similarly, if the patient awakens in the middle of the night and has not fallen back to sleep within 30 minutes, advise him or her to get up, do a relaxing pleasant activity until drowsy then return to bed. Avoid simply staying in bed and repetitively looking at the clock (which often prolongs the insomnia).

In patients with a phase-shift sleep problem, a sufficient number of sleep hours are experienced but patients sleep and awaken at inconvenient or unusual times. They may fall asleep very early in the evening and wake up very early in the morning (advanced-phase sleep, which is common in seniors), or stay up until the middle of the night and then sleep until noon (delayed-phase sleep, which is common in younger people). These patients may benefit from the use of high-intensity artificial light therapy, which can gradually readjust the timing of their abnormal phase. For advanced-phase sleep (e.g., 7 p.m. to 3 a.m.), use 10,000 Lux of light in the early evening beginning with a 30-minute exposure and gradually increasing to 90 minutes. For delayed-phase sleep (e.g., 4 a.m. to noon), instruct the patient to arise 30 minutes earlier every 3 days and begin using a 10,000 Lux light for 30 minutes each day at that time. *Medication is seldom a satisfactory treatment for phase-shifted sleep patterns.*

Pharmacological treatment

Once it has been determined that medication would be beneficial and is indicated for a patient's sleep problems, the clinician can choose from one of the following categories:

- over-the-counter/herbal sleep aids
- sedative hypnotics (benzodiazepines, non-benzodiazepines)
- psychotropic medications that may be used for sedation in addition to their mental health effect
- non-psychotropic prescription medications used for their sedative properties.

For a patient who does not have a primary psychiatric disorder, and for whom a "pure" sleeping medication is desired, over-the-counter alternatives may first be considered for mild sleep disorders. These can include antihistamines (such as diphenhydramine and hydroxyzine), melatonin or valerian root. L-tryptophan, which was temporarily banned in the United States because of contamination in the production process, has again been made legal since 2005 and is a useful option.

If the patient fails a trial with an OTC preparation or experiences severe sleep problems, a prescription medication is needed.

If a patient has a primary psychiatric disorder with a sleep problem as one of its symptoms, consider "killing two birds with one stone" by using a sedative medicine that has activity in treating the primary psychiatric illness as well. For example, for depression, an antidepressant with sedative properties (such as mirtazapine or trazodone) may, for some patients, help the sleep disorder when given as a once-daily dosage at bedtime.

Other medications used off-label for sleep, even though this is not their primary indication, are other sedative antidepressants (particularly doxepin, amitriptyline or trimipramine) and clonidine (an antihypertensive). With appropriate monitoring, these medications may be used effectively as sleep aids. When used in this context, these medicines are used solely for their sedative and non-habituating properties. Although using these medications as sedatives is an off-label usage, it can be a safe and rational prescription for some patients with intermittent sleep problems, even if no other medical or psychiatric diagnosis is present. Sedative antipsychotic medications such as quetiapine, asenapine and lurasidone can be chosen for their sleep-inducing properties when treating a psychotic or bipolar patient. In general, however, off-label use of antipsychotics solely as a sleep aid is not recommended for non-psychotic patients.

Medications specifically designed for sleep are generally divided into benzodiazepine compounds and non-benzodiazepine compounds. Benzodiazepines are discussed in Chapter 10, pp. 140–144.

Non-benzodiazepine hypnotics are listed in Table 15.2, and are currently limited to six compounds: eszoplicone (Lunesta), zolpidem (Ambien and Ambien CR), zaleplon (Sonata), zolpiclone (Zimovane and generic, available in the UK only), ramelteon (Rozerem) and suvorexant (Belsomra). The first four of these medications are presumed to exert their mechanism of action at the benzodiazepine receptor site in the brain, but have some advantages over benzodiazepines themselves. Compared to benzodiazepines, the habit-forming potential is less and is relatively low, although some measure of physical dependence has been reported with long-term use of very high doses. Disruption of normal sleep architecture, medication interactions and rebound insomnia are minimal compared to benzodiazepines.[16–21] Their primary downside is cost, as they are considerably more expensive than generic benzodiazepines. Zaleplon's very short half-life makes medication hangover very unlikely. This same property may render it predominantly excreted by the middle of the night, when it might be needed for patients with middle-of-the-night sleep continuity disturbance. It can, however, be taken as a repeat dose in the middle of the night. Although the incidence of side effects and dependence is less than with benzodiazepines, these medications may cause confusion or memory impairment when used in large doses or in sensitive individuals (e.g., seniors or brain-injured individuals.) None of these non-benzodiazepine agents has shown the muscle relaxation and anxiolytic effects typical of benzodiazepines.

Ramelteon, marketed as Rozerem, is in a new class of sleep agents that selectively binds to the MT_1 and MT_2 receptors in the suprachiasmatic nucleus (SCN), instead of binding to GABA-A ("benzodiazepine") receptors. It has been shown to be effective for

Table 15.2 Non-benzodiazepine sedative hypnotics

- Eszoplicone (Lunesta)
- Zolpidem (Ambien, Ambien CR, Edluar, Intermezzo, Zolpimist)
- Zaleplon (Sonata)
- Zolpiclone (Zimovane, Imovane)
- Suvorexant (Belsomra)

insomnia, particularly delayed sleep onset. Ramelteon has not been shown to produce dependence and has shown no potential for abuse, withdrawal or rebound insomnia. Some clinicians also use ramelteon for the treatment of delayed sleep phase syndrome.

Suvorexant (Belsomra) is the newest sleep medication which has been in use since 2014. It works by a different mechanism of action than previous medications. It is the only orexin receptor antagonist for the treatment of insomnia. It selectively blocks orexin receptors, which is thought to inhibit wake drive, thereby inducing sleep. Controlled trials of this medication have shown that compared to non-medication patients, suvorexant-treated individuals patients fell asleep 6 minutes faster and slept 16 minutes longer. Its primary side effect is daytime sleepiness and it is non-habit-forming.

Old-line sleep medications, particularly phenobarbital or other barbiturates, are poor choices of sleep medication due to their high risk of habituation and the availability of multiple alternative safer medications.

Recent research which has uncovered an intracellular signaling mechanism that regulates the sleep–wake cycle opens the possibility for a new generation of target-specific medications for insomnia.

Necessity of follow up

Follow-up assessment of response and/or side effects is important whenever a sleep medication is prescribed. The patient must be evaluated for daytime sleepiness, lack of attention or coordination, or other side effects of overdosage/drug accumulation. Also, a patient should virtually never be prescribed chronic sleep medications without several trials off medication at varying intervals to assess continued need. Unfortunately, patients in institutional care settings or nursing homes have often been prescribed sleep medication with minimal follow up, and can remain on such medication for months, years or indefinitely without appropriate follow up and attempts to discontinue the medication. When a trial off medication is attempted, it should continue for a long enough period of time to allow any rebound insomnia to resolve, since this is temporary and should not be confused with ongoing therapeutic necessity.

Although every effort should be made to stop sleeping medication, for some responsible patients (particularly those with documented psychiatric and/or medical co-morbidity that exacerbates their sleep problems) long-term, chronic prescription of sleep medication may not be poor medication practice.[22] This is especially true when trials off the medication have consistently resulted in clinical deterioration.

Sleep problems in special populations

Patients with substance abuse

Those patients who have a history of substance abuse or have otherwise abused medications are, in general, poor candidates for benzodiazepine and other sedative hypnotics. When these individuals are sleep disordered and non-pharmacological methods have been unsuccessful, some appropriate medication considerations would be:

- ramelteon
- over-the-counter preparations such as antihistamines, melatonin, l-tryptophan or valerian root

- suvorexant
- trazodone, doxepin, trimikpramine or quetiapine.

Patients undergoing withdrawal from alcohol can expect to have disrupted sleep for several days to several weeks. In general, it is not helpful routinely to prescribe sedative hypnotics to such patients except as part of a detoxification profile. If a patient has elevated vital signs, including rapid pulse and raised blood pressure, benzodiazepines are often used to manage withdrawal (see Chapter 16). When used this way, these medications may simultaneously have a beneficial effect on sleep.

There is a select small number of patients who have had a history of substance abuse, but have been substance-free for extended periods of time, and who are dependable and reliable. If the above measures have been tried and are unsuccessful, these patients could be carefully tried on sedative hypnotics, including benzodiazepines. When this is the case, it should only be done with careful assessment, follow up and patient education about the potential risk of habituation. Patients with a history of substance abuse should be encouraged to use sleeping medications intermittently rather than on a regular basis, even if they do not sleep well on the nights when they do not take medication. The clinician should be acutely aware of any signs of medication misuse, "lost" prescriptions or requests for increasing dosage of sleeping medications in this patient group (see Chapter 22).

Liver-impaired patients

Patients who have significant liver impairment from hepatic disease have limited medication options for sleep, as most of these medications are hepatically metabolized. Gabapentin is one good choice for such patients, since the majority of its excretion is through the kidneys. A hepatically impaired patient with bipolar disorder might be tried on lithium or lamotrigine as a mood stabilizer, which might also assist with sleep. Other hepatically metabolized medications, such as atypical antipsychotics, are not totally contraindicated for liver-impaired patients, but should be prescribed in small doses with frequent follow-up evaluation when other measures have failed (see Chapter 5).

Older patients

As seen in Chapter 14, geriatric patients are at increased risk for insomnia and are often at greater risk for side effects from medications.[23-24] In choosing sleeping medications for elderly patients, shorter-acting medications and intermittent dosing are always preferable to longer-acting preparations and nightly dosing, which may lead to drug accumulation. Shorter-acting preparations such as zaleplon or triazolam in small doses may be helpful.

In addition to medication, clinicians should consider the following non-pharmacological issues with elderly patients:

- Increase the patient's exercise, decreasing a sedentary lifestyle.
- Evaluate the patient's daily routine. Particularly if the patient lives alone, he or she may have developed an excessively unusual routine that contributes to sleep difficulty (e.g., staying up very late, performing routine activities in the middle of the night, eating at unusual times).

- Advise the patient to avoid daytime naps.
- Suggest removing a clock from the patient's room so he or she is not constantly looking at the clock and worrying about sleep.
- Suggest a light snack before bed, but avoid a heavy meal.
- Control patient's pain and medical illnesses, such as cardiovascular disease.
- Eliminate any unnecessary medications that may be complicating sleep.
- Avoid late-day diuretics, which increase the need for night-time urination.
- Evaluate for substance abuse that can disrupt sleep (most clinicians do not wish to believe that anyone their grandmother's age abuses alcohol or drugs, even though the prevalence in this age group is significant!).
- Evaluate closely for medication-induced drug hangover, poor balance or coordination, which can lead to falls.
- Re-evaluate the patient frequently to attempt discontinuation of any sleep medication started.

Notes and references

1   Centers for Disease Control and Protection (2017) Short sleep duration among US adults, available at: www.cdc.gov/sleep/data_statistics.html
2   Chattu VK (2019) The global problem of insufficient sleep and its serious public health implications. *Healthcare* 7(1): 1. doi: 10.3390/healthcare7010001
3   Radecki SE and Brunton SA (1993) Management of insomnia in office-based practice: national prevalence and therapeutic patterns. *Archives of Family Medicine* 2: 1129–1134.
4   Gillin JC (1992) Relief from situational insomnia: pharmacologic and other options. *Postgraduate Medicine* 92: 157–160.
5   Lippman S *et al.* (2001) Insomnia: therapeutic approach. *Southern Medical Journal* 94(9): 870–872.
6   Clark MM (2001) Restless leg syndrome. *Journal of the American Board of Family Practioners* 14(5): 368–374.
7   Yoshihawa N *et al.* (1998) A case of insufficient sleep syndrome. *Psychiatry and Clinical Neurosciences* 52(2): 200–201.
8   Ibid.
9   Meyer TJ (1998) Evaluation and management of insomnia. *Hospital Practice* 33(12): 75–86.
10 Hartmann PM (1995) Drug treatment of insomnia: indications and newer agents. *American Family Physician* 51: 191–194.
11 Becker PM *et al.* (1993) Insomnia: use of a "decision tree" to assess and treat. *Postgraduate Medicine* 93: 66–85.
12 Ancoli-Israel S (1996) *All I Want Is a Good Night's Sleep*, Mosby Year Book Inc., p. 116; Salzman C (1998) Benefits versus risks of benzodiazepine. *Psychiatric Annals* 28: 139.
13 Brunton SA (1992) When your patient can't sleep. *Family Practice Recertification* 14: 149–170; Salzman C (1998) Benefits versus risks of benzodiazepine. *Psychiatric Annals* 28: 139.
14 Ohayon MM and Roth T (2003) Place of chronic insomnia in the course of depressive and anxiety disorders. *Journal of Psychiatric Research* 37(1): 9–15; Salzman C (1998) Benefits versus risks of benzodiazepine. *Psychiatric Annals* 28: 139.
15 McGee M and Pres R (2002) Benzodiazepines in primary practice: risks and benefits. *Resident Staff Physician* 48(4): 42–49; Roth T and Roehrs T (2003) Insomnia: epidemiology, characteristics, and consequences. *Clinical Cornerstone* 5 (3): 5–15.
16 Gillin JC (1992) Relief from situational insomnia: pharmacologic and other options. *Postgraduate Medicine* 92: 157–160.

17 Stimmed GL (1999) Future directions in drug treatment of insomnia. *Psychiatric Times* (Suppl.): 1–8.

18 Darcourt G (1999) Safety and tolerability of zolpidem: an update. *Journal of Psychopharmacology* 13(1): 81–93.

19 Bowes M (1999) Sedative hypnotic medications for insomnia. *Psychiatric Times* (Suppl.): 9–16.

20 Doghranji K (1999) Treatment of insomnia in aging patients. *Sleep Disorders* (July): 5–6.

21 Richardson GS *et al.* (2002) Management of insomnia: the role of Zaleplon. *General Medicine* 4(1), available at: www.medscape.com /viewarticle/429607_4

22 Schenck C and Mahowald MW (1996) Long-term benzodiazepine treatment of injurious parasomnias and other disorders of disrupted nocturnal sleep in 170 adults. *American Journal of Medicine* 100: 333.

23 Mosier WA *et al.* (1998) Wanted: a good night's sleep. *Advance for Nurse Practitioners* 6: 30–35.

24 Nakra BRS *et al.* (1991) Insomnia in the elderly. *American Family Physician* 43: 477–483.

16 Alcohol, tobacco, recreational drugs and psychotropic medication

• Ingesting chemicals – a human activity	233
• Alcohol use	234
• Routine warnings regarding alcohol use and psychotropics in the non-substance abusing patient	238
• Early detection of substance abuse	239
• The CAGE assessment tool	241
• Polysubstance abuse	241
• Evaluation of the intoxicated and withdrawing patient	242
• Psychotropic medications and dual diagnosis patients	242
• Psychotropics used in the treatment of substance use disorders	245
• Psychotropics in the treatment of alcohol withdrawal	249
• Other interventions for the prescriber with a substance abusing patient	249
• Smoking, tobacco and nicotine	250
• Routine warnings for other recreational drugs	252
• References	255

This chapter focuses on the complex and dangerous situation of combining prescribed medication with non-prescribed substances. Polypharmacy, the intentional use of multiple medications to treat mental health problems has been discussed in various sections of this book. In these instances, it is the expressed intent of the prescriber to enhance the therapeutic benefit to the person by using multiple substances together. This can be accomplished in a controlled and safe way with oversight and instruction from the prescriber. *Combining medications with non-prescribed substances, some of which have the potential for habituation, is a totally different situation.* Recognizing, assessing and, when necessary, remedying this common clinical situation can present a complicated and difficult challenge for the prescriber.

Ingesting chemicals – a human activity

The intake of both naturally occurring and synthetic substances for the purpose of altering one's mental and physical state has been occurring since the dawn of time. Throughout recorded history, virtually every tribe of people has used one or more drugs to elicit desired mental and emotional outcomes. At times, substances have been used in an intentional fashion for ceremonies, often of a religious or spiritual nature. Far more common, however, has been the use of these substances in an uncontrolled manner either by individuals and groups. Some of the substances are utilized intermittently for "recreation," or as we would say today, to feel good or "get high." Even with intermittent and isolated use, ingestion of some of these compounds can cause significant intoxication and dangerous behavior. Because of the physiological and psychological habit-forming nature of some of these recreational drugs, additionally, their use can intensify and accelerate to the point where they are used frequently and repeatedly. With these substances, frequent use and repeat ingestion may become necessary to prevent physiological withdrawal and/or ever-increasing amounts of the substance must be used to obtain the desired mental effect. The clinical terms used to describe these situations, including the terms *substance abuse, tolerance* and *substance dependence* are defined and discussed in depth in Chapter 22 on the misuse of medication

A partial list of substances which are commonly used (and abused) by people worldwide is listed in Table 16.1. By necessity, this is only a partial list as new "recreational" substances are being discovered and synthesized frequently. This table also lists examples of commercial and street names of the various substances, how the drug is administered, its acute effects and health risks. In this text, the terms "recreational drugs" and "drugs of abuse" will be used interchangeably. Other terms used similarly to identify the same group of chemicals include "street drugs," "habit-forming drugs" or "drugs to get high."

Alcohol use

Alcohol abuse and alcohol dependence are extraordinarily common. According to the World Health Organization,[1] the world population drank the equivalent of 6.4 liters of pure alcohol per person in 2016, with some of the former Soviet states imbibing as much as 10–18 liters per person. Not only purchased in commercial establishments, home-brewed liquor or "moonshine" accounts for almost 30 percent of the world's drinking. The WHO estimates that alcohol results in 2.8 million deaths a year, more than AIDS or tuberculosis. Depending on the study and the definitions used, the prevalence of alcohol abuse and dependence ranges from 10 to 16 percent of the American population (28 percent in men and 8 percent in women).There is also a strong overlap of persons with an alcohol use disorder and a co-morbid mental disorder, being as high as 53 percent in one study.[2–3] In the UK in 2007, 73 percent of men and 57 percent of women reported drinking an alcoholic drink on at least one day in the week; 13 percent of men and 7 percent of women reported drinking every day; 41 percent of men drank more than four units on at least one day of the week. In the United States, deaths from alcohol-related causes increased from 12.0 to 17.6 per 10,000 during the period 2011–2017.[4] Although clearly a "drug of abuse" and a "recreational drug," at times in this text alcohol will be separated out from other drugs of abuse because of its almost universal usage and unique properties.

Many times, alcohol and recreational drugs are used indiscriminately without the knowledge or consent of the prescriber and in amounts which may present a hazard. In order to assist the clinician to effectively and safely deal with this problem, the various elements which constitute interactions between recreational drugs and prescribed psychotropic medications must be detailed separately.

Table 16.1 Common drugs of abuse

Category and name	Examples of commercial and street names	How administered
Alcohol		
• Alcohol (ethyl alcohol)	Found in liquor, beer and wine	Swallowed
	Acute effects – in low doses, euphoria, mild stimulation, relaxation, lowered inhibitions; in higher doses, drowsiness, slurred speech, nausea, emotional volatility, loss of coordination, visual distortions, impaired memory, sexual dysfunction, loss of consciousness	
	Health risks – increased risk of injuries, violence, fetal damage (in pregnant women); depression; neurological deficits; hypertension; liver and heart disease; addiction; fatal overdose	
Cannabinoids		
• Marijuana	Blunt, dope, ganja, grass, herb, joint, bud, Mary Jane, pot, reefer, green, trees, smoke, sinsemilla, skunk, weed	Smoked, swallowed
• Hashish	Boom, gangster, hash, hash oil, hemp	Smoked, swallowed
	Acute effects – euphoria; relaxation; slowed reaction time; distorted sensory perception; impaired balance and coordination; increased heart rate and appetite; impaired learning, memory; anxiety; panic attacks; psychosis	
	Health risks – cough, frequent respiratory infections; possible mental health decline; addiction	
Opioids		
• Heroin	*Diacetylmorphine*: smack, horse, brown sugar, dope, H, junk, skag, skunk, white horse, China white; cheese (with OTC cold medicine and antihistamine)	Injected, smoked, snorted
• Opium	*Laudanum, paregoric*: Big O, black stuff, block, gum, hop	Swallowed, smoked
	Acute effects – euphoria; drowsiness; impaired coordination; dizziness; confusion; nausea; sedation; feeling of heaviness in the body; slowed or arrested breathing	
	Health risks – constipation; endocarditis; hepatitis; HIV; addiction; fatal overdose	
Stimulants		
• Cocaine	*Cocaine hydrochloride*: blow, bump, C, candy, Charlie, coke, crack, flake, rock, snow, toot	Snorted, smoked, injected

(*continued*)

Table 16.1 Cont.

Category and name	Examples of commercial and street names	How administered
• Amphetamine	*Biphetamine, Dexedrine*: bennies, black beauties, crosses, hearts, LA turnaround, speed, truck drivers, uppers	Swallowed, snorted, smoked, injected
• Methamphetamine	*Desoxyn*: meth, ice, crank, chalk, crystal, fire, glass, speed	Swallowed, snorted, smoked, injected
	Acute effects – increased heart rate, blood pressure, body temperature and metabolism; feelings of exhilaration; increased energy, mental alertness; tremors; reduced appetite; irritability anxiety; panic; paranoia; violent behavior; psychosis; severe dental problems	
	Health risks – weight loss; insomnia; cardiac or cardiovascular complications; stroke; seizures; addiction; nasal damage from snorting	
Club drugs		
• MDMA (methylenedioxy-methamphetamine)	Ecstasy, Adam, clarity, Eve, lover's speed, peace, uppers	Swallowed, snorted, injected
	Acute effects – mild hallucinogenic effects; increased tactile sensitivity; empathic feelings; lowered inhibition; anxiety; chills; sweating; teeth clenching; muscle cramping	
	Health risks – sleep disturbances; depression; impaired memory; hyperthermia; addiction	
• Flunitrazepam	*Rohypnol*: forget-me pill, Mexican Valium, R2, roach, Roche, roofies. Roofinol, rope	Swallowed, snorted
	Acute effects – sedation; muscle relaxation; confusion; memory loss; dizziness; impaired coordination	
	Health risks – addiction	
• GHB	*Gamma-hydroxybutyrate*: G, Georgia home boy, grievous bodily harm, liquid ecstasy, soap, scoop, goop, liquid X	Swallowed
	Acute effects – drowsiness; nausea; headache; disorientation; loss of coordination; memory loss	
	Health risks – unconsciousness; seizures; coma	
Dissociative drugs		
• Ketamine	*Ketalar SV*: cat Valium, K, Special K, vitamin K	Injected, snorted, smoked
	Acute effects – analgesia; impaired memory; delirium	
	Health risks – respiratory depression and arrest; death	

Table 16.1 Cont.

Category and name	Examples of commercial and street names	How administered
• PCP and analogs	*Phencyclidine*: angel dust, boat, hog, love boat, peace pill *Acute effects* – analgesia; psychosis; aggression; violence; slurred speech; loss of coordination; hallucinations	Swallowed, smoked, injected
• Salvia divinorum	Salvia, Shepherdess's Herb, Maria Pastora, magic mint, Sally-d	Chewed, swallowed, smoked
• Dextromethorphan (DXM)	Found in some cough and cold medications: Robotripping, Robo, Triple C *Acute effects* – euphoria; slurred speech; confusion; dizziness; distorted visual perceptions	Swallowed
All dissociative drugs	*Acute effects* – feelings of being separate from one's body and environment; impaired motor function *Health risks* – anxiety; tremors; numbness; memory loss; nausea	

Hallucinogens

• LSD	*Lysergic acid diethylamide*: acid, blotter, cubes, microdot, yellow sunshine, blue heaven *Health risks* – flashbacks; Hallucinogen Persisting Perception Disorder	Swallowed, absorbed through mouth tissues
• Mescaline	Buttons, cactus, mesc, peyote	Swallowed, smoked
• Psilocybin	Magic mushrooms, purple passion, shrooms, little smoke *Acute effects* – nervousness; paranoia; panic	Swallowed
All hallucinogens	*Acute effects* – altered states of perception and feeling; hallucinations; nausea; increased body temperature, heart rate, blood pressure; loss of appetite; sweating; sleeplessness; numbness, dizziness, weakness, tremors; impulsive behavior; rapid shifts in emotion	

Other compounds

• Anabolic steroids	*Anadrol, Oxandrin, Durabolin, Depo-Testosterone, Equipoise*: 'roids, juice, gym candy, pumpers *Acute effects* – no intoxication effects *Health risks* – hypertension; blood clotting and cholesterol changes; liver cysts; hostility and aggression; acne; in adolescents – premature stoppage of growth; in males – prostate cancer, reduced sperm production, shrunken testicles, breast enlargement; in females – menstrual irregularities, development of beard and other masculine characteristics	Injected, swallowed, applied to skin

(continued)

Table 16.1 Cont.

Category and name	Examples of commercial and street names	How administered
• Inhalants	*Solvents (paint thinners, gasoline, glues); gases (butane, propane, aerosol propellants, nitrous oxide); nitrites (isoamyl, isobutyl, cyclohexyl):* laughing gas, poppers, snappers, whippets *Acute effects* – (varies by chemical) stimulation; loss of inhibition; headache; nausea or vomiting; slurred speech; loss of motor coordination; wheezing *Health risks* – cramps; muscle weakness; depression; memory impairment; damage to cardiovascular and nervous systems; unconsciousness; sudden death	Inhaled through nose or mouth

Source: Adapted from the American National Institutes of Health, the National Institute on Drug Abuse, available at: www.drugabuse.gov/drugs-abuse/commonly-abused-drugs/commonly-abused-drugs-chart; The Centers for Disease Control and Prevention, available at: www.cdc.gov/nchs/fastats/alcohol.htm

Note: Prescription drugs are in italics.

Routine warnings regarding alcohol use and psychotropics in the non-substance abusing patient

Alcohol

Fortunately, the majority of patients seen for psychotropic medications, who do not have an abuse history, will use alcohol responsibly. Some will not use it at all at the time of the initial prescription, but may do so at a later date. Even if the patient does not expect that substance use will be a problem, any patient who begins psychotropic medication should receive information on the possible safe concomitant use of alcohol with their prescription.

In general, *patients should be advised to refrain from alcohol for the first several weeks of medication prescription while they accommodate to the medication and its effect is being evaluated.* Once stable on the medication, the general rule of thumb for non-substance abusing patients is that they may have *no more than one drink in an evening and no more than four drinks in a week* without seriously compromising the effect of their mental health medication or creating a serious health hazard for themselves. This is discussed in the following dialogue. Specifically, note that the clinician must define the term "moderation" or "moderate drinking." If the clinician uses undefined terms such as "you can drink a little," "only drink in moderation," "don't drink too much" or "don't have more than a few," the patient will utilize their own standard for what these terms mean. The patient may have a significantly different definition of "moderation" from the clinician!

Box 16.1 Talking to patients

"For the first several weeks, while you are adjusting to the medication, I would prefer that you do not drink any alcohol. If and when you do choose to drink alcohol, I would recommend that it be in moderation. I am defining

moderation as no more than one drink in an evening and no more than four in a week. If you stay within this framework while you are taking medication, you are unlikely to have problems from use of alcohol. Do be aware that approximately 20 percent of patients notice increased intoxication if they drink while taking medication.

If you are in that 20 percent, your ability to drive or perform coordinated activities could be affected when you drink. The majority of patients, however, will experience no significant increased intoxication. Remember that the medication I am prescribing is still in your system and may be affected by alcohol regardless of when you took your dose." (The latter fact is important, since some patients think that if medication is taken in the morning, it is no longer in their system at night, and they can therefore drink freely.)

"*There are two significant effects of heavier alcohol intake that you need to be aware of when taking medications.*

First, heavy drinking may work against the effect of the medication. More than just feeling hung-over, you may feel the medication is 'not working' for several days after heavy alcohol intake. It is similar to trying to drive a car with one foot on the gas and one foot on the brake.

Second, if you drink heavily, you may unpredictably experience an alcoholic blackout in which memory is lost for activities surrounding the drinking episode. You can wake up the next morning and not realize how you got home or what you did. You may not have 'passed out,' and may have continued to do potentially dangerous activities such as drinking and driving.

If your intake of alcohol remains moderate, as I have defined, you are not likely to have either of these two problems."

The above guidelines are appropriate for the patient who does not have a past history of significant alcohol use. As part of the initial evaluation, the clinician will have asked for a history of prior substance abuse. *If this has been present, the clinician should advise against any concomitant use of alcohol and medication, and observe the patient carefully during follow up for the emergence of signs of alcohol use or abuse.*

Early detection of substance abuse

When prescribing psychotropic medications, the clinician should always be alert to possible signs or symptoms of substance abuse in their patients. The index of suspicion should be higher in patients who have a past personal history of substance abuse or have a family history of substance abuse. Table 16.1 includes the physiological signs of drug use which might be detected by the prescribing clinician. Because of its extensive frequency throughout the world's population, alcohol overuse and abuse deserve special and more detailed description.

Signs of alcohol abuse

When prescribing psychotropics, it is important that the clinician be vigilant for indications of excessive alcohol use. People's drinking behavior does not always match what they describe in the office. Patients may drink more heavily on weekends or vacations such that overt signs and symptoms are not present when the patient is seen in the office. The clinician should be attuned to the quality of the patient's speech in any phone conversations as well as, when necessary, obtaining input from family members about the patient's alcohol use. Patients' alcohol intake may also change over time with their emotional state. Many signs of alcohol overutilization are well known and easy to discern in a clinical setting.[5–7] These can include:

1   alcohol on the patient's breath
2   staggering gait
3   slurred speech
4   reddened eyes
5   signs of mild to moderate alcohol withdrawal, including:
    • hand and body tremors
    • sweating
    • rapid pulse
    • elevated blood pressure
    • dilated pupils
    • elevated temperature
    • behavioral restlessness or overactivity
    • clouding of consciousness.

Some more subtle signs that may alert the clinician to possible covert alcohol abuse can include the following:

1   *Abnormal laboratory findings* – an abnormal laboratory test may be the first sign to an otherwise unsuspecting clinician that a patient is overutilizing alcohol. Laboratory screening for elevated liver functions can easily be included in the other laboratory work which the clinician requires. While normal liver function tests do not rule out the presence of alcohol abuse, the presence of abnormal values requires further evaluation. Laboratory tests which may indicate abuse of alcohol include:
    • Elevated serum gammaglutamyl transferase (GGT), which is raised in 80 percent of those who overutilize alcohol. If the GGT is greater than 30 units, 70 percent of these individuals will have been involved in persistent heavy drinking (more than eight drinks per day).
    • Carbohydrate-deficient transferase (CDT) greater than 20 units also indicates persistent heavy drinking. Both of these two tests revert to normal within several days to 1 week of cessation of heavy alcohol intake.
    • High-normal or elevated erythrocyte mean corpuscular volume (MCV). Elevated MCV is a direct toxic effect of alcohol on the formation of red blood cells.
    • A broad range of increased liver function tests will gradually occur with long-term and persistent alcohol usage.
    • Increased triglyceride and lipoprotein levels may also be present.
2   The clinician should also be alert to evidence *of cross-tolerance with other addictive medications*. Patients who show an elevated need for narcotic pain medications, sedative/hypnotics and benzodiazepine anti-anxiety medications may also have developed a measure of cross-tolerance because of abuse of alcohol. When this

elevated need for other medications is documented by the prescribing clinician or another healthcare provider, further investigation by the prescriber may be required.

3   *Lack of intoxication when it would be expected* can also signal high regular usage. If a person has a blood alcohol level of greater than 100 milligrams of ethanol per deciliter and does not show some sign of intoxication, this indicates a degree of alcohol tolerance. At a blood alcohol of greater than 200 milligrams per deciliter, most non-tolerant individuals will be severely intoxicated. While blood alcohol levels are not regularly drawn in an outpatient practice, a clinician may get reports from an emergency room or hospital that document a blood alcohol level and lack of signs of intoxication, which can alert the clinician to the possibility of alcohol abuse.

While not all of these signs or symptoms are pathognomonic or automatically valid indicators of alcohol abuse in isolation, several of the signs present together should alert the clinician to the suspicion that alcohol abuse is occurring.

The CAGE assessment tool

A useful brief assessment tool for evaluating the potential problem drinkers is the use of the CAGE questionnaire developed by JA Ewing[8] and shown in Table 16.2. This exceptionally simple set of screening questions was introduced in 1970 and has been in common usage since. As a screening tool, a score of 2 to 3 indicates a high index of suspicion for problem drinking and a score of 4 is virtually diagnostic for alcoholism.

Polysubstance abuse

An increasingly common problem confronting clinicians today is the patient who abuses multiple recreational substances simultaneously – polysubstance abuse. From the list of substances in Table 16.1 alone, the various permutations and combinations of substances which may be ingested simultaneously is almost limitless. It is beyond the aim of this text to fully document all possible signs and symptoms of mixed substance abuse. Each patient in each situation must be evaluated individually. While intentional polysubstance use is common, at times, a drug user will not know the precise chemicals that they ingest and/or take multiple substances unknowingly.

As part of a polysubstance abuse assessment, the prescriber should utilize the patient's self-report even though this may be unreliable or incomplete. The clinician should also utilize:

*   urine and serum drug screens
*   liver function tests and other baseline laboratory measures
*   a thorough, recent physical examination by a clinician familiar with drug abuse.

Table 16.2 The CAGE questionnaire to detect alcohol use disorders

Cut down	"Have you ever felt you ought to cut down on your drinking?"
Annoyed	"Have people annoyed you by criticizing your drinking?"
Guilt	"Have you ever felt bad or guilty about your drinking?"
Eye-opener	"Have you ever had a drink first thing in the morning to steady your nerves or get rid of a hangover?"

Evaluation of the intoxicated and withdrawing patient

Of special note in this section on evaluation is the clinical problem of attempting to do a mental health evaluation in a patient who is alcohol/drug intoxicated or is in the throes of withdrawal. The presence of acute alcohol or drug intoxication or withdrawal will confound the diagnostic acumen of even the best clinicians. The physiological state of intoxication and withdrawal generally lasts no more than several hours to several days. During these times, however, competent assessment for psychotropic medications is difficult, if not impossible. Given the short length of time it takes for these states to resolve, evaluation for psychotropic medication should almost always be delayed until the patient is sober and free from the acute signs and symptoms of withdrawal.

There has been an ongoing belief by some clinicians, which continues to persist, that persons with substance abuse problems must be totally substance-free for an *extended* period of time in order to assess them accurately and potentially treat their emotional problems with psychotropic medication. While this opinion is not totally without merit, the wisest course of action depends on the clinical situation. The willingness of practitioners today to medicate with psychotropics patients who are abusing alcohol will vary markedly from practitioner to practitioner. There are practitioners who insist on patients being completely substance-free for weeks or months before they will medicate at all. Once acute intoxication or withdrawal symptoms have passed, other practitioners (including the author) are willing to prescribe for clearly diagnosed mental health conditions despite the presence of mild to moderate alcohol usage. The hope in this latter situation is that when the patients are appropriately medicated, they will be better able to decrease or eliminate their alcohol usage.

The premise of reduced substance usage once psychotropics are prescribed requires constant re-evaluation, and is certainly not true for all patients. For those patients who, despite an adequate medication regimen, continue to abuse alcohol, ongoing medication prescription may not be in their best interest and may indeed present some medical hazard.

Months or years of sobriety are not necessary, however, prior to a mental health evaluation and the possible prescription of targeted psychotropic medications. While some risk of blurred diagnosis or interaction between alcohol and medication may occur, these risks are relatively small compared to the much larger risk of untreated emotional illness (including suicidal and homicidal behavior, lost jobs and disrupted families). It is reasonable to undertake an evaluation for medication within several days of an episode of acute intoxication, and within a week after a period of significant alcohol withdrawal.

To expect that patients who have been using alcohol for a long time, particularly as "self-medication" (see below), will cease their habit for a lengthy period prior to being medicated is, in most cases, unlikely and unreasonable. Often such a prerequisite with an alcohol-dependent person, if strictly enforced, will drive a patient from treatment before medication can offer improvement. If, however, the clinician has obtained a past history suggesting that this person has abused the combination of medication and alcohol before, it is reasonable to insist that he or she be detoxified before medication is prescribed.

Psychotropic medications and dual diagnosis patients

Once the above-mentioned evaluation techniques are completed, or in some cases after treatment has begun, it may become clear to the clinician that the patient has both at least one diagnosable mental health condition *and* a diagnosable substance use disorder. Often, but not exclusively, the substance abused is alcohol. Individuals with both diagnoses are referred to as "dual diagnosis" patients, and create significant practical issues for the prescriber. As many as 53 percent of individuals with an alcohol use disorder have a co-morbid mental disorder.[9–10] Individuals with alcohol abuse suffer from mood disorders at significantly higher rates than in the general population.

Dual diagnosis – the co-morbidity of mental health and substance abuse diagnoses – can overlap in several ways:

- A person with a psychiatric disease can use alcohol as "self-medication" for emotional symptoms which occur. The alcohol use may be episodic or continuous.
- A psychiatric disorder co-exists with a separate alcohol abuse disorder (which can occur sporadically or continuously) regardless of the presence of mental health symptoms.
- A continuous alcohol use disorder co-exists with ongoing episodic psychiatric symptomatology.

In the past, clinicians have attempted to sort out which illness came first – the substance abuse or the mental illness. This differentiation is less important than ensuring that both conditions are adequately treated. What is unequivocally clear is that the presence of dual diagnoses has a negative impact on a variety of measures including:

- medication adherence
- time to recovery, which is lengthened
- increased rate of relapse for both conditions
- increased (20-fold) utilization of inpatient hospitalization and emergency services
- increased rates for homelessness.

Conversely, adequate treatment of one problem improves the outcome of the other.

Biases of philosophy, training and experience have unfortunately complicated the principles of treatment for dual diagnosis patients. There is a common tendency of purely mental health clinicians to miss the seriousness of and necessity of treatment for alcohol abuse. Primary substance abuse clinicians often inadequately assess and undertreat emotional illnesses, focusing solely on the abuse. These biases have led to two opposite and equally *untrue* conclusions:

1 Mental health medications will treat alcoholism.
2 Appropriate alcohol treatment will solve most mental health symptoms.

Since there is significant overlap between many emotional illnesses and substance abuse, there is much "self-medication" with alcohol. Certain mental health patients, once they begin feeling better as a result of psychotropic medication treatment, no longer feel the need for increased alcohol use. *It is not reasonable, however, to assume that all persons with substance abuse problems will necessarily decrease their substance abuse when they are appropriately medicated for their emotional illness.* Some may continue to abuse alcohol despite their mental health improvement. These individuals will need independent substance abuse treatment. Similarly, patients engaged actively in substance abuse treatment (whether within the 12-step Alcoholics Anonymous model or some other treatment program) will not *automatically* resolve any underlying mental illness by stopping their substance use. In fact, some patients become even more acutely aware of their mental health symptoms when they are clean and sober.

One of the most common clinical situations involving a mental health diagnosis and substance abuse is the overlap of depressive symptoms in a substance abusing patient.[10] The use of antidepressants in the substance abusing population has been studied extensively. Results of these studies suggest that antidepressants do decrease depressive symptoms in a substance abusing population, but once these effects are factored out, there is no evidence showing that depression treatment decreased substance use. Subgroups within this dually diagnosed population show that those with depression and alcohol use benefited somewhat more than those with depression and cocaine or opioid abuse. In general, it was found that as depressive symptoms improved, substance or alcohol use declined, but it rarely declined to the point of clinical remission. There is also some evidence that patients who received tricyclic antidepressants, SNRIs and bupropion showed a more robust clinical improvement of dual diagnosis symptoms than those who received treatment with an SSRI alone.[11–12]

Although this text focuses on the use of psychotropic medications and teaches the principles of prescription, prescribers who routinely treat substance abusing patients should avoid being drawn into the mindset that medications (prescription or OTC) are necessary for treating a negative affect. As noted above, antidepressants do provide some increased benefits to the substance-using depressed patient, but abstinence in conjunction with a structured clinical milieu and psychotherapy using a wide variety of formal treatment methodologies are also significantly associated with improvement in affective symptoms, independent of pharmacological antidepressant treatment.[13] Some time-efficient brief interventions for a prescriber to use with the substance abusing patient are described at the end of the chapter.

After medicating substance abusing patients who also have a primary psychiatric diagnosis, it is reasonable to allow several weeks to several months for adequate symptom control to occur before determining that separate substance abuse treatment is necessary.[14–15] If ongoing substance usage is occurring at that time, specific substance abuse treatment should be recommended and undertaken. Even with considerable symptom relief from emotional symptoms, some patients' substance abuse will take on a life of its own and persist indefinitely without treatment. Substance abuse is a chronic recurring illness with frequent relapses and remissions. Therefore, waiting many months or years for the psychotropic medications to "do their job" while expecting substance use to stop is not reasonable.

Additional evaluation issues in dual diagnosis patients

During an initial evaluation, the prescriber will perform a thorough evaluation of mental health symptoms as well as alcohol and other substance abuse. In addition, the clinician should be alert to the high prevalence of other medical illnesses in patients who abuse substances. These include:

- HIV
- tuberculosis
- hepatitis
- sexually transmitted diseases.

Falls, motor vehicle accidents, homicides and suicides are also more common in patients with substance abuse disorders.

Another issue of relevance to medication prescription for a substance abusing patient is the presence of family history of mood or psychiatric disorder. A positive family history should alert the clinician to the possibility of a genetic predisposition toward an underlying psychiatric disorder, and thus the clinician should be even more vigilant than usual regarding a possible underlying anxiety or mood disorder that could be treated with medication.

Some clinicians with a strong background in substance abuse treatment, particularly the 12-step model, believe that using medications in patients with a history of substance abuse is simply "trading one chemical dependency for another." This is not generally true. If mental health symptoms persist and if a diagnosis can be made, particularly in light of a positive family history of emotional disorder, the clinician should not hesitate to utilize appropriate psychotropics in the treatment of the dual diagnosis patient. Antidepressants, mood stabilizers and antipsychotics are, in general, not abused and may be of significant benefit to an appropriately diagnosed patient.

Habituating medicines, particularly benzodiazepines and stimulants, should *not* be used liberally with dual diagnosis patients.[16] Non-pharmacological means and non-habituating medicines should be tried first. If these fail, however, and the patient is firmly engaged in treatment and shown to be responsible in the use of medication, it may be reasonable to judiciously use small amounts of compounds from these medication groups with close monitoring.

Some patients, when given psychotropics, will correlate side effects from the medication with uncomfortable feelings they have experienced with intoxication or withdrawal from their substance usage. Sedation can mimic a hangover, and nervousness can mimic withdrawal. To minimize this problem in dual diagnosis patients, start with low doses of medications and titrate very gradually with an aim toward a modest final therapeutic dosage and minimal side effects.

Psychotropics used in the treatment of substance use disorders

The above sections have focused on the interaction between alcohol and psychotropic medications, issues of co-morbidity, and the place of medications in the treatment of co-morbid conditions. The latter part of this chapter will discuss the direct usage of psychotropics in the treatment of various syndromes associated with substance use, abuse and withdrawal. Each of the medications used in these disorders – disulfiram, naltrexone, acamprosate, methadone and buprenorphine – are used clinically in different ways from the majority of psychotropics otherwise discussed in this book.

Disulfiram

Disulfiram (Antabuse) is unique in psychopharmacology in that its purpose is to discourage a particular behavior (alcohol intake) by causing intense negative physiological symptoms when alcohol is ingested. Disulfiram has neither a direct effect on psychiatric symptoms, nor a direct effect on the patient's craving for alcohol. Its sole purpose is as a negative deterrent to drinking alcohol, such that the patient knows that drinking while taking disulfiram will lead to severely unpleasant sensations. Disulfiram is usually dosed between 250 mg and 500 mg a day on a daily basis, or three to four times a week for some patients sensitive to its effect.[17]

Disulfiram disrupts alcohol metabolism and inhibits the action of aldehyde dehydrogenase, thus blocking the conversion of acetaldehyde to acetate. Alcohol, when ingested by a person who is taking disulfiram, will bring about an accumulation of acetaldehyde, leading to distinct unpleasant physical sensations, including:

- sweating
- flushing
- difficulty breathing
- nausea and vomiting
- throbbing headache
- weakness and hypotension.

After alcohol ingestion, several of the above symptoms will occur rapidly within 15 to 60 minutes, and persist for 30 minutes to 2 hours.

An important part of the prescription of disulfiram is educating the patient about "hidden" sources of alcohol that, in particularly sensitive individuals, can cause an alcohol–Antabuse reaction. Common but unexpected sources of alcohol include tonics, liquid potions, aftershave lotion, mouthwash, colognes and perfumes. The patient must also be advised to be assertive regarding food preparation, particularly when foods are being prepared by another source (at a restaurant or at another person's home). Such inquiry is necessary to ensure that alcohol is not included in the food ingredients, which could precipitate a reaction (e.g., coq au vin, bratwurst in beer, or liquor-based sauces).

Naltrexone

In substance abuse treatment, naltrexone (Revia, Depade and Vivitrol) is utilized to reduce craving and prevent relapse in both alcohol abusing and narcotic abusing patients. Naltrexone is an opiate antagonist, and binds to the opioid receptors, but rather than activating them, blocks them. In narcotic abuse, it prevents opioid receptors from being activated by agonist compounds, such as heroin or narcotic analgesics.

On the theory that the endogenous opioid system may have been involved in the development of alcohol dependence, naltrexone has also been tested in alcoholics. Although its mechanism of effect in alcohol treatment is poorly understood, several large-scale studies have shown naltrexone to be useful in decreasing alcohol craving, lowering the number of drinking days and reducing the rate of full-blown relapse.[18]

It is available in oral form (Revia, Depade) and monthly injectable extended-release form (Vivitrol). As opposed to other medications used for opioid dependence (methadone and buprenorphine), naltrexone can be prescribed in America by any individual who is licensed to prescribe medicine (e.g., physician, doctor of osteopathic medicine, physician assistant and nurse practitioner).

Acamprosate

Taken as an oral medication three times a day, acamprosate calcium is FDA approved for the maintenance of abstinence from alcohol. It has only been shown to be effective in patients who are currently abstinent from alcohol; that is, they have completed detoxification. Acamprosate reduces the physical and emotional discomfort (e.g., sweating, anxiety, sleep disturbances) many people feel in the weeks and months after they've stopped drinking which makes it easier for them not to drink after the immediate withdrawal period.[19–21] It does not, however, prevent the symptoms of acute alcohol withdrawal (as benzodiazepines do), or cause the unpleasant reaction when alcohol is ingested, similar to disulfiram.

Alcoholics who have stopped alcohol consumption show hyper excitability in the glutamate system. Structurally resembling the naturally occurring amino acid mediator aminobutryic acid (GABA), acamprosate restores normal receptor tone in the glutamate system. Numerous studies involving over 4500 patients have shown acamprosate to decrease alcohol craving, prolong abstinence and reduce the rate of relapse.

Methadone

Methadone is a strong pain reliever and is also used in the treatment of opiate addiction. As a synthetic opioid that blocks the effects of heroin and other narcotic prescription drugs containing opiates, methadone has been shown to eliminate withdrawal symptoms and relieve drug cravings from heroin and prescription opiate medications.

Having cross-tolerance with other opioids but a longer duration of action, methadone has been used successfully for more than 40 years in the treatment of *opioid dependence*. At higher doses it can also block the euphoric effects of heroin, morphine and similar drugs.

Methadone Maintenance Treatment (MMT) is a form of *opiate replacement therapy* where methadone is given to replace an illicit opiate.[22–24] Ideally, once substituted, methadone is gradually tapered to the point where the patient becomes drug free. Methadone tapering works best when done as a slow and gradual reduction in dose, dropping 5 mg every 3–14 days. Once the dose is lowered to 20 mg, the tapering may be slowed down to an even more gradual reduction, to reduce or eliminate any symptoms. Typical reduction rates vary and are adjusted based on patient response. Many methadone providers allow a patient to choose the rate at which the dose is reduced, and adjustments are monitored on a daily basis.

Many MMT patients never become drug free, but are stabilized on a chronic dose of methadone. Methadone maintenance reduces and/or eliminates the use of heroin, reduces the death rates and criminality associated with heroin use, and allows patients to improve their health and social productivity. In addition, enrollment in methadone maintenance has the potential to reduce the transmission of infectious diseases associated with heroin injection, such as hepatitis and HIV. A majority of patients require 80–120 mg/d of methadone, or more, to achieve these effects, and require treatment for an indefinite period of time. According to Harvard Medical School,[25] approximately 25 percent of persons admitted to a methadone maintenance program will, over time, become abstinent from methadone if they choose to have themselves weaned off it. Another 25 percent will continue using methadone while the remainder will stop using methadone and resume its use when they enter another substance abuse treatment program.

Practitioners wishing to administer and dispense approved Schedule II controlled substances such as methadone for maintenance and detoxification treatment must obtain a separate DEA registration as a Narcotic Treatment Program from the Drug Enforcement Administration (DEA). The practitioner must also receive approval from the Center for Substance Abuse Treatment (CSAT) within the Substance Abuse and Mental Health Services Administration (SAMHSA), as well as the applicable state methadone authority.

Buprenorphine

Buprenorphine is a semi-synthetic opioid that was initially developed to control acute pain. Chemically, buprenorphine is an opioid partial agonist and therefore occupies the opioid receptor site, but produces less effect than full agonists such as heroin and methadone. It therefore carries a lower risk of abuse, addiction and side effects when compared to full agonists. At low doses, buprenorphine produces sufficient agonist effect to enable opioid-addicted individuals to discontinue the misuse of opioids without experiencing withdrawal symptoms. The agonist effects of buprenorphine increase linearly with increasing doses of the drug until at moderate doses it reaches a plateau and no longer continues to increase with further increases in dose – the so-called "ceiling effect." These maximal effects of buprenorphine appear to occur in the 16–32 mg dose range for sublingual tablets. Higher doses are unlikely to produce greater effects. Because of its ceiling effect and poor bioavailability, buprenorphine is safer in overdose than opioid full agonists. Buprenorphine has been licensed for detoxification and long-term replacement therapy in opioid dependency since 2002. Some clinicians feel that buprenorphine prescription is preferable to methadone treatment in opiate-addicted individuals.

Buprenorphine is available in a variety of formulations: Subutex, Suboxone (typically used for opioid addiction), Temgesic, Buprenex (solutions for injection often used for acute pain in primary care settings), Norspan and Butrans (transdermal preparations used for chronic pain). Buprenorphine has poor oral bioavailability due to very high first-pass metabolism and therefore is not prescribed orally.

Buprenorphine sublingual tablets (Suboxone and Subutex) have a long duration of action, which may allow for dosing every 2 or 3 days compared with the daily dosing required to prevent withdrawal with methadone. In the United States, following initial management, a patient is typically prescribed up to a 1-month supply for self-administration.

Analogous to MMT, buprenorphine treatment can last from several days (for detoxification purposes) to an indefinite period of time (opiate substitution for life-long maintenance). Although somewhat less prone to abuse, also similar to methadone, buprenorphine itself can be abused.

If a practitioner wishes to prescribe, administer or dispense Schedule III, IV or V controlled substances approved for addiction treatment such as buprenorphine, the practitioner must request a waiver (Form SMA-167) and fulfill the requirements of the CSAT. The DEA will review each request and if approved, the practitioner will receive a Unique Identification Number. If a practitioner then chooses to dispense controlled substances, the practitioner must utilize this number on all buprenorphine prescriptions. He/she must also maintain, separate from all other records, for a period of at least 2 years, all required records of receipt, storage and distribution of buprenorphine.

Psychotropics in the treatment of alcohol withdrawal

Acute alcohol withdrawal syndrome is a serious medical condition. In its milder forms it is characterized by sweating, tremors, elevated blood pressure, tachycardia, insomnia, elevated body temperature and irritability. In its more severe form, it can be accompanied by delirium tremens, hallucinations, grand mal seizures progressing to status epilepticus and, rarely, death. Various psychotropics have been used to modulate the progress of alcohol withdrawal. For much of the past four decades, benzodiazepines have been the mainstay of treatment for alcohol withdrawal (alcohol detoxification or "Detox") especially in North America. In Europe, the anticonvulsants carbamazepine (Tegretol), valproic acid (Depakene and others) and phenytoin (Dilantin) have also been used successfully to treat alcohol withdrawal[26] and are effective in reducing the severity of withdrawal symptoms and emotional distress related to withdrawal.[27] In the past, other psychotropics (e.g., barbiturates) had been used to manage withdrawal; however, use of these agents has fallen out of favor.

Various institutions and academic bodies have developed many benzodiazepine protocols using diazepam, lorazepam and chlordiazepoxide to treat withdrawal.[26–27] Some of the protocols have fixed decreasing doses of the benzodiazepine as the patient's withdrawal symptoms improve. Others have flexible dose regimens depending on the presence or absence of certain measurable criteria, such as elevated pulse, elevated blood pressure and elevated body temperature (see Table 16.3).

Because of nutritional deficiencies and possible deficiency-related disease, thiamine, folic acid and vitamin B12 are given during the detoxification process. Other agents such as beta blockers (atenolol, propranolol) and alpha-agonists such as clonidine are often used adjunctively to improve vital signs, reduce alcohol craving and further decrease the severity of withdrawal symptoms.

Other interventions for the prescriber with a substance abusing patient

Most interventions to identify and treat problem drinkers have been aimed at the primary care arena because primary care practitioners are often the only medical professionals that problem drinkers encounter. Several strategies and interventions have been found helpful in the primary care setting although they can be easily adapted for a mental health practitioner.

Evaluation and counseling for substance abuse should be based on a style of "motivational interviewing."[20,28] In this technique providers use therapeutic empathy, deal actively with resistance, ambivalence and risk, assess motivation to change, emphasize patient responsibility and provide a menu of specific strategies to reduce alcohol use.

Clinicians do not, in general, advise abstinence, but recommend reducing intake for problem drinkers. When reduced intake is not successful, the clinician can recommend more specific alcohol treatment and provide a referral for further therapy. Compared with matched controls, problem drinkers who receive a brief intervention are twice as likely to moderate their drinking within a 6–12-month period. Likewise, brief interventions significantly decrease the fraction of individuals whose alcohol intake exceeds recommended levels.[29] They also decrease the incidence of suicide attempts, domestic violence, child abuse, assaults and motor vehicle accidents associated with the alcohol use.[19,30]

Table 16.3 Examples of diazepam and lorazepam protocols

Mild withdrawal	Moderate withdrawal	Severe withdrawal
Diazepam	*Diazepam*	*Diazepam*
5–10 mg p.o.	*Day 1*: 15–20 mg p.o. q.i.d. *Day 2*: 10–20 mg p.o. q.i.d. *Day 3*: 5–15 mg p.o. q.i.d. *Day 4*: 10 mg p.o. q.i.d. *Day 5*: 5 mg p.o. q.i.d.	10–25 mg p.o. every hour while awake PRN
Lorazepam	*Lorazepam*	*Lorazepam*
1–2 mg p.o. every 4–6 hours PRN for 1–3 days	*Days 1 and 2*: 2–4 mg p.o. q.i.d *Days 3 and 4*: 2 mg p.o. q.i.d. *Day 5*: 1 mg p.o. b.i.d. (may need to adjust, based on signs and symptoms of alcohol withdrawal)	1–2 mg i.v. every hour while awake PRN for 3–5 days (to sedate)
Systolic blood pressure	Systolic blood pressure	Systolic blood pressure
>150 mmHg	150–200 mmHg	200 mmHg
diastolic blood pressure	diastolic blood pressure	diastolic blood pressure
>90 mmHg	100–140 mmHg	>140 mmHg
Pulse >100 bpm	Pulse 110–140 bpm	Pulse >140 bpm
Temperature >100 °F	Temperature 100–101 °F	Temperature >101 °F
Tremulousness	Tremulousness	Tremulousness
Insomnia	Insomnia	Insomnia
Agitation	Agitation	Agitation

Source: Miller NS (1997) Pharmacological detoxification from alcohol and other drugs. *Essent Psychopharmacology* 1(3): 273–290.

Note: Monitoring in intensive care is recommended for cardiac and respiratory function, fluid and nutrition replacement, vital signs and mental status. Restraints are indicated in the confused and agitated state to protect the patient from self and others. (Delirium tremens can be a terrifying and life-threatening state.)

The overall approach to dealing with problem drinkers is summarized by Whitlock et al.[21] as "The 5 As" shown in Table 16.4.

Smoking, tobacco and nicotine

Although smoking rates are declining, 14.4 percent of adults in the United States still smoke cigarettes.[31] Given this figure as well as the prevalence of the use of psychotropic medications, one would expect multiple overlaps of these two situations in many patients. The situation is complex, however, since cigarette smoking has been implicated in the causation and progression of a number of mental health disorders.

Cigarette smoking is estimated to be two to five times higher in patients with schizophrenia, mood disorders, anxiety disorders, ADHD, binge eating disorder, bulimia dementia and substance use disorders. Although the statistical evidence is clear, the

Table 16.4 The 5 As of brief interventions for alcohol use

Ask: screen for use
- "Do you sometimes drink beer, wine, or alcohol?"
- "In the past year, how many times have you had 5 or more drinks in a day?"

Advise: provide strong direct advice to change
- Empathic, non-confrontational feedback on the consequences of continued drinking with the current pattern
- Relate the consequences to patient's current health, family, social and legal issues
- Clinician states a concern for current condition and recommends change

Assess: determine the willingness to change
- Discuss what the patient likes and dislikes about drinking
- Discuss patient's life goals
- Determine how willing the patient is to change and *what* he or she is willing to change
- Agree on a mutually acceptable goal

Assist: help the patient make a change if he or she is ready
- Set mutually agreed-upon specific goals (how many days, how many drinks)
- Encourage a risk reduction agreement. Write it down – the "prescription for change"
- Identify high-risk situations
- Identify supports and supporters (family, friends)

Arrange: reinforce change effort with follow up
- Make a follow-up appointment
- Provide supportive telephone consultations
- Refer patients to a specialty treatment if necessary

Source: Adapted from Whitlock EP *et al.* (2004) Behavioral counseling interventions in primary care to reduce risky/harmful alcohol use by adults: a summary of the evidence for the U.S. Preventive Services Task Force. *Annals of Internal Medicine* 140(7): 557–568.

exact mechanism by which cigarette smoking may cause deterioration in many psychiatric disorders is as yet not known with precision. At a minimum, studies have shown alteration in the function of neural circuitry involved in inhibitory control, attentional system and risky decision-making compared with non-smoking controls. Therefore, brain structure and neural circuitry in brain regions clearly implicated in many psychiatric disorders are affected by cigarette smoking. It is now well known that smoking is a potential confounding issue with medication dosing. Drug interactions are caused by components of tobacco smoke itself, rather than nicotine.[32] This means that nicotine replacement therapy (NRT) can be used without concern regarding drug interactions and medication changes.

It makes clinical sense that since cigarette smoking causes worsening of psychiatric conditions that the prescriber and/or the primary care provider should work to attempt smoking cessation in the patient if at all possible. While a lessening of the amount of smoking is desirable, this is not always a simple procedure to undertake successfully. There are multiple factors that need to be considered when working with the patient regarding his/her smoking – including the psychiatric clinical stability of the patient, willingness on the part of the patient as well as the support of family or friends for the process.

Tobacco smoke induces many CYP-450 enzymes in the liver, which play an important role in medication absorption, distribution, metabolism and elimination. Perhaps the most significant of these enzymes is CYP1A2; these enzymes are induced by smoking (therefore increasing the activity of this enzyme, resulting in lower blood levels for a specific dose than if a person is a non-smoker). (See Chapter 20 on "Danger Zones" for a more detailed discussion of Cytochrome P-450 interactions.)

Psychiatric medications such as antipsychotics, antidepressants, hypnotics and anxiolytics are widely affected by cigarette smoking. For these classes, the drug concentration in the blood can be decreased with smoking, and reduction in efficacy may lead to the need for upward dosing to obtain therapeutic effect. Common psychotropic medications metabolized by CYP1A2 include duloxetine, clozapine, diazepam, haloperidol, mirtazapine, nortriptyline and olanzapine.

Beyond the metabolic changes induced by cigarette smoking, the physical risks of smoking include lung cancer, chronic obstructive pulmonary disease (COPD), stroke, and coronary heart disease, to name a few. It may fall to the psychotropic medication prescriber and/or the primary care provider to discuss and perhaps initiate smoking cessation

Routine warnings for other recreational drugs

Regardless of the patient's personal or family history of recreational drug use, the prescriber must also make a brief statement about the risks of using recreational drugs while taking psychotropic medications. The advice is simple and direct – "DO NOT USE RECREATIONAL DRUGS WHILE TAKING THIS MEDICATION" (regardless of what medication is being prescribed and which recreational drug is used). Even without a personal past history of drug use, no knowledgeable clinician will expect that this prohibition will prevent some patients from experimenting with, or at times, regularly using recreational drugs while taking a psychotropic. The possible interactions between the wide variety of prescribed medications and the multitude of possible recreational substances are many. Since the potential number of these combinations and possible reactions are myriad and often unknown, it is beyond the substance of this text to attempt to describe them. In addition, any interactional effects are dependent on the amount of a recreational drug that is ingested and the purity/impurity of the preparation (many street drugs contain a mixture of chemicals which may not be known to the user). In many situations, there is virtually no research or evidence to cite documenting particular combinations of prescription medication and recreational drugs.

It is best to say that *"you cannot predict the outcome of mixing recreational drugs and prescription medications* (which you cannot), *but that almost all the outcomes are negative and potentially dangerous."*

Some particularly knowledgeable patients may counter this statement by saying *"Aren't some street drugs being used for positive purposes in the treatment of mental health conditions?"* While such research on psilocybin, LSD and ecstasy has been started, it remains purely investigational and until significant results are obtained and replicated, you do not recommend use of any of these chemicals as treatments.

Some of the most commonly used and abused recreational drugs include marijuana, K2/spice and Kratom. Therefore, some mention of these recreational drugs and possible interactions with psychotropics is warranted.

Specific recreational drugs

Ketamine – a special case

Ketamine got its start as an anesthesia medicine in the 1960s. It was used on the battlefields of the Vietnam War since, at lower doses, it can help ease pain. Since the

1970s, ketamine has been marketed in the United States as an injectable, short-acting anesthetic for use in humans and animals

Ketamine also produces hallucinations. It distorts perceptions of sight and sound and makes the user feel disconnected and not in control for a relatively short time, lasting approximately 30–60 minutes. Because of these properties, the substance became one of a number of "club drugs" which were used and abused at raves or dance parties. Therefore, for a long time, it was seen as a recreational drug and a drug of abuse, known alternatively as Special K, Cat Valium, Kit Kat, K, Super Acid, Super K, Purple, Special La Coke, Jet and Vitamin K on the street.

Searching for treatments for "treatment-resistant depression" (TRD), researchers began investigating its use because it had a different mechanism of action than other antidepressant substances. It was found to have rapid antidepressant effects in TRD patients, confirming the active role of glutamate in the pathophysiology of the complex condition of depression. In addition to its antidepressant properties, ketamine was also found to be effective in reducing suicidality in TRD samples.

Ketamine is a DEA controlled drug and a DEA Schedule III controlled substance which during the last 10 years has only been available as an intravenous medication which needed to be delivered under a physician's care in specialized clinics. Nonetheless, it became useful for patients who had not responded to other treatments.

In 2019, the Food and Drug Administration approved a new formulation which could be given as a nasal spray. By the parameters of its approval, the patient must administer the spray under medical supervision in the doctor's office once or twice a week, and it cannot be used at home.

Side effects include dizziness, nausea, sedation, vertigo, anxiety, lethargy, increased blood pressure, vomiting and feeling drunk.

Marijuana

Marijuana with its active ingredient (tetrahydrocannabinol) and its derivative cannabidiol (CBD) have been used for various medical therapeutic and recreational uses for centuries. Marijuana used "to get high" (Weed, Mary Jane, grass, reefer, pot, and many other names) is the most widely used psychoactive recreational substance in the world. It is also the third most commonly abused drug[33] in the United States after alcohol and tobacco. Although marijuana contains over 100 separate chemical compounds called cannabinoids, THC or tetrahydrocannabinol is the compound which creates the "high" associated with its use. It has been an object of intense focus in many U.S. states because of progressive legalization of both medical and recreational use.

Driven in part by the push for legalization of marijuana in Western countries, the efficacy and safety of cannabis-based medicines have been investigated for treatment or alleviation of mental conditions such as a variety of anxiety disorders – PTSD, psychosis/schizophrenia, anorexia nervosa and ADHD. Used as an oil and ingested orally as well as mucosally through a nasal spray, CBD shows promising results even though double-blind placebo-controlled studies documenting its uses are often isolated and utilize a small sample size.

Perhaps the best studied therapeutic mental health effect has been on several anxiety disorders including generalized anxiety disorder, social phobia, PTSD and panic disorder. Zuardi *et al.* have reviewed the controlled studies[34] and opine:

Taken together, most studies clearly suggest an anxiolytic-like effect of CBD, both in animal models and in healthy volunteers. In addition, this cannabinoid was shown to decrease anxiety in patients with social phobia. Novel clinical trials involving patients with other anxiety disorders, such as panic, obsessive-compulsive, social anxiety, and posttraumatic stress disorders are now necessary. Studies documenting the optimal therapeutic window of CBD and the mechanisms involved in its anxiolytic action remain to be determined.

These studies as with most studies on naturally occurring compounds have the difficulty of varying concentrations of active ingredient in the samples tested.

While the medical uses (for help with the spasticity of multiple sclerosis, the nausea and vomiting of chemotherapy, neuropathic pain and seizures) are relatively well documented and have led to the movement of legalizing medical marijuana, many people believe that medical marijuana legalization is simply the first step on the path to legalization of social and recreational use. Although technically the possession, distribution and use of marijuana are illegal under U.S. federal law, at the time of this edition, 33 states have legal medical marijuana and 11 have legal recreational marijuana. This number is likely to increase over the next 3 to 5 years.

A major factor in assessing marijuana's effect on mental health (either positively or negatively) is the dramatic increase in the potency of marijuana which is now ingested, compared to the potency in the past century. In addition to the recent cultivation of stronger strains of marijuana, the proliferation of hashish and THC concentrates (often called "dabbing") have increased the amount of THC which a person may ingest quickly and simply. The use of these stronger preparations has intensified the frequency and extent of mental health consequences, including paranoia, anxiety, panic attacks and hallucinations. Even when psychotropic medications aimed at potentially counteracting these symptoms are also taken, it is very difficult to predict how often such symptoms will break through.

There is substantial evidence of a statistical association[35] between cannabis use and the development of schizophrenia or other psychoses, with the highest risk among the most frequent users. These data, although moderately substantial, are confounded by the question that has yet to be answered; namely, does this heavy use of cannabis *cause* schizophrenia or are there other genetic or environmental factors which would have resulted in schizophrenia whether or not the drug use existed. Significant research evidence also substantiates[36–37] that regular use of high-potency marijuana products can also lead to increased symptoms of bipolar disorder and social anxiety. The question of mere association versus causality exists with this body of evidence as well.

Spice or K2

Although looking similar to marijuana and packaged in fancy ways, K2 (also known as spice or "fake weed") usually does not include any true THC. Fundamentally, it consists of dried plant materials which are sprayed with mind-altering chemicals which are cannabinoids but not THC. These chemicals bind to the same brain receptors as THC, but do so in a much stronger fashion with potentially deadly outcomes. Although consumers may assume that "fake" marijuana is safer than real marijuana, it is in fact much more dangerous. The user has no idea how many or which chemical cocktails may have been sprayed on the plant materials. Although in some cases a user may experience relaxation, euphoria and increased awareness of his or her environment, spice can lead to severe bleeding, agitation, psychosis, hypertension, seizures, nausea and vomiting. Several U.S. states have banned this product. Even in those states where it is legal, the packages will state "Not for human consumption." This, however, does not stop its use. The vast majority of emergency department visits because of "marijuana" are, in fact, due to the use of spice. Since every sample of K2 contains a different mixture of cocktails, it is virtually impossible to ascertain how this substance interacts with psychotropic medications. Most of the serious side effects are usually due to the various sprayed-on chemicals and not due to any interaction of the plant base with appropriately prescribed medicines.

References

1 World Health Organization (2018) *Global Status Report on Alcohol and Health*, available at: https://apps.who.int/iris/bitstream/handle/10665/274603/9789241565639-eng.pdf
2 Pettinati HM *et al.* (2013) Current status of co-occurring mood and substance use disorders: a new therapeutic target. *American Journal of Psychiatry* 170(1): 23–30.
3 Substance Abuse and Mental Health Services Administration (SAMHSA) (2014) Mental and substance use disorders, available at: www.samhsa.gov/disorders (accessed February 21, 2018).
4 Centers for Disease Control and Prevention (2019) *QuickStats*: Rate of alcohol-induced deaths among persons aged ≥ 25 years, by age group – National Vital Statistics System, 1999–2017. *Morbidity and Mortality Weekly Report* 68(33), available at: www.cdc.gov/mmwr/volumes/68/wr/mm6833a5.htm
5 Arndt T (2001) Carbohydrate-deficient transferrin as a marker of chronic alcohol abuse: a critical review of preanalysis, analysis and interpretation. *Clinical Chemistry* 47: 13–27.
6 Kessler RC *et al.* (1997) Lifetime co-occurrence of DSM-III-R alcohol abuse and dependence with other psychiatric disorders in the National Comorbidity Survey. *Archives of General Psychiatry* 54(4): 313–321.
7 Stratowski SM *et al.* (1998) Twelve-month outcome after a first hospitalization for affective psychosis. *Archives of General Psychiatry* 55(1): 49–55.
8 Steinweg DL and Worth H (1993) Alcoholism: the keys to the CAGE. *American Journal of Medicine* 94: 520–523.
9 Tohen M *et al.* (1998) The effect of comorbid substance use disorders on the course of bipolar disorder: a review. *Harvard Review of Psychiatry* 6(3): 133–141.
10 Nunes EV *et al.* (2004) Treatment of depression in patients with alcohol or other drug dependence: a meta-analysis. *Journal of the American Medical Association* 291: 1887–1896.
11 Helstrom AW *et al.* (2016) Reductions in alcohol craving following naltrexone treatment for heavy drinking. *Alcohol and Alcoholism* 51(5): 562–566.
12 Anton RF (2008) Naltrexone for the management of alcohol dependence. *New England Journal of Medicine* 359(7): 715–721. doi: 10.1056/NEJMct0801733
13 Boothby LA and Doering PL (2005) Acamprosate for the treatment of alcohol dependence. *Clinical Therapeutics* 27(6): 695–714.
14 Torrens M *et al.* (2005) Efficacy of antidepressants in substance use disorders with and without comorbid depression. *Drug Alcohol Dependency* 78(1): 1–22.
15 Albanese MJ (2001) Assessing and treating comorbid mood and substance use disorders. *Psychiatric Times* 18(4): 55–58.
16 Pelc I *et al.* (1997) Efficacy and safety of acamprosate in the treatment of detoxified alcohol: a 90-day placebo-controlled dose-finding study. *British Journal of Psychiatry* 171: 73–77.
17 Skinner MD *et al.* (2014) Disulfiram efficacy in the treatment of alcohol dependence: a meta-analysis. *PLoS One* 9(2): e87366. doi: 10.1371/journal.pone.0087366

18   Volpicelli JR *et al.* (1992) Naltrexone in the treatment of alcohol dependence. *Archives of General Psychiatry* 49(11): 876–880.

19   Willenbring ML *et al.* (2009) Helping patients who drink too much: an evidence-based guide for primary care clinicians. *American Family Physician* 80(1): 44–50.

20   Carroll KM *et al.* (2006) Motivational interviewing to improve treatment engagement and outcome in individuals seeking treatment for substance abuse: a multisite effectiveness study. *Drug and Alcohol Dependence* 81(3): 301–312.

21   Whitlock EP *et al.* (2004) Behavioral counseling interventions in primary care to reduce risky/harmful alcohol use by adults: a summary of the evidence for the U.S. Preventive Services Task Force. *Annals of Internal Medicine* 140(7): 557–568.

22   Joseph H *et al.* (2000) Methadone maintenance treatment (MMT): a review of historical and clinical issues. *Mount Sinai Journal of Medicine* 67(5–6): 347–364.

23   NSW Methadone Clinic Accreditation Standards, available at: www.health.nsw.gov.au/aod/resources/Publications/methadone-cas.pdf

24   Harvard Health Publishing (2019) Treating opiate addiction, part 1: detoxification and maintenance, available at: www.health.harvard.edu/mind-and-mood/treating-opiate-addiction-part-i-detoxification-and-maintenance

25   Harvard Health Publishing (2014) In brief: opiate maintenance alternatives: two studies, available at: www.health.harvard.edu/newsletter_article/In_brief_Opiate_maintenance_alternatives_Two_studies

26   Sachdeva A *et al.* (2015) Alcohol withdrawal syndrome: benzodiazepines and beyond. *Journal of Clinical and Diagnostic Research* 9(9): VE01–VE07. doi: 10.7860/JCDR/2015/13407.6538

27   Benzodiazepines for alcohol withdrawal, available at: www.addictioncenter.com/alcohol/benzodiazepines-alcohol-withdrawal/

28   Medslund G *et al.* (2011) Motivational interviewing for substance abuse. *Cochrane Database Systematic Reviews* 11(5): CD008063.

29   Fleming MF *et al.* (2010) Brief physician advice for heavy drinking college students: a randomized controlled trial in college health clinics. *Journal of Studies on Alcohol and Drugs* 71(1): 23–31.

30   U.S. Department of Health and Human Services (2005) Helping patients who drink too much: a clinician's guide, available at: https://pubs.niaaa.nih.gov/publications/practitioner/cliniciansguide2005/guide.pdf

31   Centers for Disease Control and Prevention (2020) Current cigarette smoking among adults in the United States, available at: www.cdc.gov/tobacco/data_statistics/fact_sheets/adult_data/cig_smoking/index.htm

32   Zevin S and Benowitz NL (1999) Drug interactions with tobacco smoking: an update. *Clinical Pharmacokinetics* 36(6): 425–438. doi: 10.2165/00003088-199936060-00004

33   Discover Recovery (2021) The most commonly used recreational drugs in America, available at: https://discoverrecovery.com/the-most-commonly-used-recreational-drugs-in-america/

34   Zuardi AW *et al.* (1982) Action of cannabidiol on the anxiety and other effects produced by Delta 9 THC in normal subjects. *Psychopharmacology* 76: 245–250.

35   Patel S *et al.* (2020) The association between cannabis use and schizophrenia: causative or curative? A systematic review. *Cureus* 12(7): e9309. doi: 10.7759/cureus.9309

36   Sewell R *et al.* (2009) Cannabinoids and psychosis. *International Review of Psychiatry* 21(2): 152–162.

37   Johns A (2001) Psychiatric effects of cannabis. *British Journal of Psychiatry* 179: 270–271.

17 The confused and cognitively impaired patient – medication pitfalls

• General principles of dealing with the confused patient	258
• Cognitive disorders – delirium and dementia	259
• Management of delirium and dementia	262
• Medication use in delirium and dementia	263
• Dementia of the Alzheimer's type	265
• Current medications for Alzheimer's dementia	267
• Mild cognitive impairment	268
• Psychiatric diseases that may present with confusion	270
• References	270

While not a specific diagnosis, mental confusion may be caused by any of a variety of conditions, both medical and psychiatric. Either self-referred or brought by their families, patients with mental confusion, poor memory and cognitive disorganization will frequently present to clinicians for mental health evaluation, in the hope that medication will help their cognitive difficulties. At other times, patients present for an evaluation of physical or mental health symptoms and the clinician perceives a confused state during the evaluation process. When aware of their deficiencies, patients may use phrases such as "I'm spacey," "I just can't focus," "My memory is going" or "I'm losing my mind." Other profoundly confused and forgetful patients are almost oblivious to their mental state, despite ample evidence to those around them. Behavioral historical information from family or caregivers may alert the clinician to possible cognitive problems. The family may identify that the patient is having difficulty with finances, transportation, taking medication, grooming, organization, planning or performing tasks of daily living.

Clinical tip-offs that may alert the clinician to the presence of mental confusion that is not a primary complaint are listed in Table 17.1.

Primary care and non-mental health providers, when confronted with a patient who is disorganized, forgetful, confused or inattentive, can often quickly jump to the diagnostic assumption that this is a "psych" case with need of a treatment referral to a mental health specialist. If consultation is unavailable, reaching for the prescription pad to treat the symptoms can also be a common, but unhelpful, solution.

Table 17.1 Signs and symptoms that can alert the clinician to patient confusion

---

- Perplexed, confused facial appearance
- Disorganized thinking
- Disorientation to person, place or time
- Poor memory for details
- Rambling, disjointed speech
- Seeming inability to understand or respond appropriately to questions
- Easy distractibility
- Easy startle response

Table 17.2 Causes of confusion

---

1 Cognitive disorders
  - Delirium
  - Dementia
2 Substance use
  - Alcohol intoxication or withdrawal
  - Intoxication or withdrawal from other drugs of abuse
3 Psychiatric causes
  - Psychosis
  - Mania
  - Depression
4 Anxiety
5 Attention deficit disorder

The role of medications in the treatment of disorders of cognitive impairment is quite variable and, in general, different from the target symptom approach described in most of the other portions of this text. Although psychotropic medications may help for specific diagnoses and indirectly decrease confusion, in general, psychotropic medications are at best neutral, and may actually cloud the initial assessment process of the confused patient. As will be seen, medication prescription is often *not* one of the appropriate first steps in dealing with a confused patient unless that person is acutely, behaviorally out of control.

This chapter will discuss the stepwise assessment of confusion, and recognition of the limited number of situations when medication may be appropriate.

General principles of dealing with the confused patient

Mental confusion has many causes (see Table 17.2). While some are traditionally thought of as "psychiatric," many confused people have a medical problem that results in delirium, which has mental confusion as one of its symptoms.
Assessment and evaluation to discover the cause of the mental confusion is essential to appropriate management.

Recent onset confusion, particularly when severe, is cause for an urgent medical evaluation. This is especially true in an adult without a past history of a definitive psychiatric disorder. *Unless urgent behavioral control is necessary for the patient, evaluation of the cause of confusion is the primary task and the use of psychotropic medications should be minimized.*

Cognitive disorders – delirium and dementia

Cognitive disorders (disorders that affect thinking, learning and memory) are one of the most common causes of mental confusion, forgetfulness and inattention. Cognitive disorders are broadly divided into *delirium* and *dementia*, which are described here.

Delirium and dementia are symptom complexes of an underlying medical condition, and are not illnesses in and of themselves. There is a vast array of systemic medical conditions, as well as direct illnesses of brain tissue, that affect normal brain functioning and cause delirium or dementia. In the past, cognitive disorders have often been referred to as "organic" brain disorders or "organic brain syndromes." This classification is not particularly helpful, since it implies that these conditions are due to "organic" causes and that other "functional" conditions (such as psychosis, bipolar disorder and depression) are a separate, clearly differentiated group without medical cause. As our understanding of these latter so-called "functional" illnesses has progressed, it has become clear that they too have clear biological underpinnings, and therefore are also "organic."

Box 17.1 Primary care

In the mentally confused patient, especially when there is no history of previous psychiatric illness (and at times, even if there is), think of delirium and dementia first and psychiatric disease second.

During an evaluation, when a clinician detects that a patient being evaluated has mild or moderate confusion, a formal assessment of mental status should be promptly performed (see Chapter 3 and Appendix 1) to document the level of confusion and disorganization. If the patient is significantly confused, further history taking from the patient will be at best inaccurate, and may be an inefficient use of the clinician's time. Rather than gathering information from a significantly confused patient, initial history should be obtained from other sources, including patient records, family members, friends, caretakers and other individuals familiar with the patient's day-to-day life. If the confused patient shows signs of intoxication, regardless of the source, it is usually of little use to attempt to elicit extensive historical information. Beyond simple basics such as medications taken, recent ingestions, substance use and medical illnesses, detailed history taking should be postponed to a later time when the patient is not intoxicated.

Because psychotropic medications take an entirely different role with delirium and dementia as opposed to other conditions, further detail about the evaluation of delirium and dementia is necessary at this time. In almost all situations discussed in this text, medications are used to treat specific symptoms or a diagnosis in a positive, symptom-specific way. However, when treating problematic behavior associated with delirium and dementia, most psychotropic medications do not treat the diagnosis or the underlying cause. Any excess medication may complicate the assessment process and potentially worsen the patient's clinical state. The sole exceptions to this are the cholinesterase inhibitors that target one possible underlying mechanism of Alzheimer's dementia (see below).

After a clinical description, the appropriate evaluation process and treatment for delirium will be outlined.

Delirium

Delirium is defined as an acute mental syndrome primarily involving changes in cognition, disturbance of consciousness and impaired attention. It is divided into two groups, depending on the cause:

1   delirium secondary to a medical condition
2   delirium secondary to drug intoxication or withdrawal.

Delirium is considered a sign of acute dysfunction of the brain and should be considered a medical emergency requiring urgent diagnostic evaluation and treatment. Delirium is quite common in emergency room settings, intensive care units and on medical/surgical wards. The common symptoms of delirium are listed in Table 17.3.

In general, a delirium develops quickly and progresses rapidly. It may be highly reversible once the medical cause is discovered and corrected. Although there are intracranial causes of delirium, as can be seen in Table 17.4, *the majority of causes of delirium exist outside the central nervous system.*

Delirium may precede the symptoms of its medical cause. If the cause is not immediately identified in a first round of diagnostic tests, but delirium continues to be present, it is incumbent on the clinician periodically to re-evaluate the patient's medical condition to attempt specifically to identify the cause.

Dementia

Dementia is a cognitive disorder that involves global impairment of many aspects of memory, judgment and cognition. As it progresses, higher cortical functions (such as abstract reasoning, language and ability to follow directions) deteriorate. In contrast

Table 17.3 Symptoms of delirium

- Rapid onset
- Usually lasts for several days to several weeks
- Clouding of consciousness, which often fluctuates
- Patient may act bewildered or confused
- Activity level varies; the patient may be restless and hyperactive, psychomotorically slowed or show changing activity level
- Prominent deficits in attention, distractible in thought
- Frequent perceptual disturbances, visual hallucinations or illusions
- Alteration in sleep/wake cycle, may be drowsy
- Often disoriented to time, but may also be disoriented to place or person; orientation may fluctuate over time
- Marked impairment in memory, particularly for recent events
- Speech may be incoherent, confused, unintelligible or unclear
- Changes of setting (including overstimulation or understimulation) can worsen the condition
- The patient may be acutely aware of his or her disorganization, but not always
- Can present at any age

Sources: Adapted from Andreason NC and Black DW (2010) *Introductory Textbook of Psychiatry*, 5th edn., American Psychiatric Association Press; Gilder M (ed.) (2012) *New Oxford Textbook of Psychiatry*, Oxford University Press; Hales RI (ed.) (2008) *American Psychiatric Association Textbook of Psychiatry*, 5th edn., American Psychiatric Association Press; Sadock BJ and Sadock VA (2009) *Kaplan and Sadock's Comprehensive Book of Psychiatry*, 9th edn., Lippincott, Williams & Wilkins; Keltner NL and Folks DG (2005) *Psychotrophic Drugs*, 4th edn., Mosby.

Table 17.4 Causes of delirium

Causes within the brain
- Direct brain trauma
- Infections, including meningitis and encephalitis
- Brain tumors
- Vascular disorders
- Epilepsy and postictal states

Causes outside the brain
- Drug ingestion (prescribed and street/recreational drugs)
- Drug withdrawal
- Drug side effects
- Endocrine dysfunction, including:
  - Hyper- and hypo-pituitarism
  - Hyper- and hypo-adrenalism
  - Hyper- and hypo-thyroidism
  - Hyper- and hypo-parathyroidism
- Liver disease (hepatic encephalopathy)
- Kidney disease (uremic encephalopathy)
- Hypoxia
- Congestive heart failure, arrhythmia and hypotension
- Vitamin deficiencies, including folic acid, B12 and thiamine
- Hypoglycemia
- Systemic infections with fever and sepsis
- Electrolyte imbalance from any cause including dehydration
- Post-operative states

Sources: Adapted from Andreason NC and Black DW (2010) *Introductory Textbook of Psychiatry*, 5th edn., American Psychiatric Association Press; Gilder M (ed.) (2012) *New Oxford Textbook of Psychiatry*, Oxford University Press; Hales RI (ed.) (2008) *American Psychiatric Association Textbook of Psychiatry*, 5th edn., American Psychiatric Association Press; Sadock BJ and Sadock VA (2009) *Kaplan and Sadock's Comprehensive Book of Psychiatry*, 9th edn., Lippincott, Williams & Wilkins; Keltner NL and Folks DG (2005) *Psychotrophic Drugs*, 4th edn., Mosby.

to the rapid onset of delirium, dementia has a slow, chronic, insidious onset. Often the level of consciousness is unimpaired until late in the course. Patients typically have a normal level of arousal. Both recent and remote memory are impaired. The speed of psychomotor actions is generally normal. There is less disruption of the sleep/wake cycle than in delirium.

Dementia is an acquired condition, and its incidence increases with age:[1-4]

- 1–6 percent of those 65 to 75 years of age have dementia.
- 7–8 percent of those 75 to 85 years of age have dementia.
- 18–32 percent of those over 85 years of age have dementia.

Clinicians treating the elderly population should therefore be especially attuned to signs, symptoms (see Table 17.5) and evaluation of dementia.

Most dementias are chronic. Sixty-five percent of dementias are progressive, and because of their gradual onset, dementia is often overlooked by patients and families. Some families would prefer not to identify that "grandpa is confused," and show considerable denial. The intellectual deterioration is often attributed to normal aging, particularly early in the course. The patient is often unaware of the loss of cognitive functions, or

Table 17.5 Symptoms of dementia

Initial symptoms
• Subtle personality change – "He/she is just not him/herself"
• Impaired social skills
• Decreased range of interests, loss of interest in hobbies
• Emotional lability and shallow affect
• Somatic complaints
• Gradual loss of intellectual functions
• Depression, which may occur prior to other symptoms

Late symptoms
• Increasing memory loss (recent memory is lost before remote memory)
• Confabulation (the making up of tales, or responding to questions without regard to fact)
• Increasing mood and personality change with exaggeration of previous personality traits
• Loss of orientation to person and place, in addition to loss of orientation to time
• Sleep problems
• Wandering – patient gets lost
• Impulsiveness and compromised judgment with little foresight and planning
• Psychotic symptoms, including hallucinations, illusions, delusions and ideas of reference
• Language impairment, thought blocking, occasionally mute

Sources: Adapted from Andreason NC and Black DW (2010) *Introductory Textbook of Psychiatry*, 5th edn., American Psychiatric Association Press; Gilder M (ed.) (2012) *New Oxford Textbook of Psychiatry*, Oxford University Press; Hales RI (ed.) (2008) *American Psychiatric Association Textbook of Psychiatry*, 5th edn., American Psychiatric Association Press; Sadock BJ and Sadock VA (2009) *Kaplan and Sadock's Comprehensive Book of Psychiatry*, 9th edn., Lippincott, Williams & Wilkins; Keltner NL and Folks DG (2005) *Psychotrophic Drugs*, 4th edn., Mosby.

denies that changes are occurring. Knowledgeable families will sometimes bring a relative in for an evaluation saying, "I think he/she is depressed," because they know that many depressions are treatable. They often do not emphasize symptoms of confusion because they also may know that many causes of dementia are not treatable.

As with delirium, *dementia indicates a serious underlying medical problem affecting the functioning of the brain*. Even though most are not treatable, searching for the underlying cause is the most important issue for the clinician (see Table 17.6). Dementia patients are poor historians, and it is always essential to interview significant others and family to obtain valid historical information.

As the condition progresses, the person has few complaints of cognitive loss, and often appears unconcerned about his or her own condition. The patient may show wandering, pacing, repetitive or stereotypic behaviors, temper outbursts and complaining. More aggressive actions, such as pushing, biting, scratching or kicking, may also occur.

Management of delirium and dementia

Unless a patient is acutely disruptive, uncontrollable or unsafe, medication should take fifth place in the treatment of delirium and dementia behind the following four considerations:

1   *Ensure the safety of the patient*. If the patient remains out of the hospital, discuss safety issues with the family or caregivers. Include assessment of the risks in the residence, such as accessibility of medications/toxins/poisons, access to cooking appliances (stove/oven) and other dangerous items such as weapons or tools. Assess

Table 17.6 Causes of dementia

- Brain tumors (both primary and metastatic)
- Brain trauma
- Chronic brain infection, including syphilis and AIDS
- Jacob-Creutzfeld disease
- Cardiovascular causes, including single or multiple infarctions ("multi-infarct dementia")
- Congenital or hereditary diseases, including Huntington's disease
- Epilepsy
- Normal pressure hydrocephalus
- Vitamin deficiencies
- Chronic metabolic disturbances
- Chronic anoxia
- Degenerative dementias, including
  - Alzheimer's disease
  - Parkinson's disease
  - Pick's disease
  - Wilson's disease
  - Progressive supranuclear palsy
- Demyelinating diseases, such as multiple sclerosis
- Intoxication and poisoning from various elements including alcohol, carbon monoxide, heavy metals, medications or irradiation

Sources: Adapted from Andreason NC and Black DW (2010) *Introductory Textbook of Psychiatry*, 5th edn., American Psychiatric Association Press; Gilder M (ed.) (2012) *New Oxford Textbook of Psychiatry*, Oxford University Press; Hales RI (ed.) (2008) *American Psychiatric Association Textbook of Psychiatry*, 5th edn., American Psychiatric Association Press; Sadock BJ and Sadock VA (2009) *Kaplan and Sadock's Comprehensive Book of Psychiatry*, 9th edn., Lippincott, Williams & Wilkins; Keltner NL and Folks DG (2005) *Psychotrophic Drugs*, 4th edn., Mosby.

and discuss the patient's risk of wandering or getting lost, including at night. In the hospital, keep the patient near the nursing station. Have frequent orientation by consistent staff members, or have family members stay with the patient. If the behavior is more disruptive, the patient may need a sitter or be secluded/restrained.

2   *Perform a thorough medical evaluation* as described in Table 17.7, with appropriate neurological consultation. Serial mental status examinations will help to document the progression and course of the illness (see Appendix 1).

3   *If the dementia is due to drug intoxication or side effects, stop the offending agent.* If it is due to drug withdrawal, manage the withdrawal.

4   *Correct whatever medical problem is occurring* to whatever extent it is correctable.

Medication use in delirium and dementia

As emphasized earlier in this chapter, medication is not usually the first or second intervention for confused patients. Ensuring safety, a thorough medical evaluation, removing any intoxicating substances and treating any underlying medical causative factors are initially more important. Psychotropic medication *is* used for a confused and disorganized patient, however, in two circumstances:

- medication for non-specific behavioral control (acute or chronic)
- medication aimed at mediating one of the possible causes of the Alzheimer's type dementia.

Table 17.7 Medical work-up for delirium and dementia

- Complete medical history, usually provided or supplemented by information from family or caregivers
- Thorough physical and neurological examinations
- Detailed standardized mental status examination (see Appendix 1)
- Laboratory studies, including complete blood count, serum electrolytes, serum glucose, calcium, albumin, magnesium, blood urea nitrogen, creatinine, liver function tests
- Screening for syphilis and HIV, thyroid function tests, vitamin B12 and folate levels, EKG and chest X-ray
- Urinalysis and urine drug screen
- Arterial blood gases
- Baseline psychological testing may be helpful
- If the clinical condition warrants it, lumbar puncture, CT scan or MRI, EEG, blood cultures, lupus prep or antinuclear antibody levels

---

Source: Adapted from Trzepacz P (chair) (2002) Practice guidelines for the treatment of patients with delirium, in *American Psychiatric Association Practice Guidelines for the Treatment of Psychiatric Disorders: Compendium 2002*, American Psychiatric Association, pp. 29–60.

Many, but not all, patients with delirium or dementia will show agitation and problematic disruptive behaviors. Agitation is a general term, akin to the terms fever or pain, and is not a diagnosis in itself. While the behaviors of some agitated patients may be signs of an underlying psychiatric disorder (for example, psychosis or depression), these behaviors may be a result of social disinhibition or ignoring social norms and cues. These behaviors, while disturbing to caregivers, may not be reflective of specific underlying diagnoses. Such agitated behaviors may be purposeful but performed in an uncoordinated or erratic way, or appear purposeless to the observer. However, some behaviors may have a stereotypical, repetitive quality, and others are random. If the behaviors are not clearly acutely dangerous, it may be most beneficial initially to observe the patient medication-free while undertaking the diagnostic evaluation. Some behaviors can be violent and harmful, however, and can be acute, persistent, self-directed or directed at other persons or property. Specific medications have been used to attempt to control or manage these agitated behaviors, and are discussed by class. Anxiolytics, antipsychotics, antidepressants and anticonvulsants have all been used to some degree beneficially in the agitated patient.

Whenever medication is used, the patient must be carefully monitored for signs of clouding of consciousness, worsening of disorientation, excess sedation and fall risk. (See Chapter 14 for further discussion of medication treatment as behavioral control for the elderly agitated patient.)

Anxiolytics

Benzodiazepines alone seldom control delirium and dementia. Acutely anxious patients may benefit from a short-acting benzodiazepine, however, particularly when used in combination with a traditional or atypical antipsychotic (see Chapters 5, 6). Longer-acting benzodiazepines should generally be avoided with cognitively impaired persons. Chronic or repeated administration of benzodiazepines can lead to further clouding of consciousness and worsening of attention problems. Benzodiazepines may, however, be the medication of choice for a delirium associated with seizures, or precipitated by withdrawal from alcohol or sedatives. Although some practitioners may recommend buspirone as an alternative to benzodiazepines, it is at best modestly useful and generally considered a poor choice for acute control of agitation.[5]

Antipsychotics

Antipsychotic medications have long been the mainstay of treating agitated patients, particularly in the elderly. Although the use of atypical antipsychotics is rapidly replacing conventional antipsychotics, the combination of 2–5 mg of haloperidol plus 1–2 mg of lorazepam remains a standard treatment in many institutional care facilities for agitation. Unfortunately, typical antipsychotics have been used rather indiscriminately for sedation and behavioral control, rather than being targeted to diagnosed *psychotic* patients. This has created significant problems when conventional antipsychotics are used long term, because of their propensity to cause movement disorders and tardive dyskinesia. There is now ample evidence for the positive benefit of using atypical antipsychotics in agitated behavioral disturbances and confused patients. These agents (especially olanzapine, quetiapine and risperidone) have beneficial side-effect profiles compared with typical or first-generation antipsychotics. The use of these agents in demented patients has been complicated by the Food and Drug Administration "black box warning" on increased risk of sudden death when used in these patients (see Chapter 19 for a full discussion).

Clozapine, because of its risk of agranulocytosis, hypotension, excess sedation and anticholinergic side effects, is generally not a first-line choice for the agitated, demented elderly.

Antidepressants

Some antidepressants, such as mirtazapine and trazodone, have been found to be useful in treating depression in the elderly as well as, to some extent, for sedation and behavioral control.[6]

Anticonvulsants

Valproic acid and carbamazepine, in smaller doses, have been useful for sedation and behavioral control. There are limited controlled data on the use of any other anticonvulsants.

Dementia of the Alzheimer's type

Dementia of the Alzheimer's type is the most common form of dementia, affecting more than 5.5 million persons in the United States and 24 million worldwide with a prevalence that has been estimated as high as 10 percent for individuals over 65 years of age.[7] A total of 12.8 percent of the population in the UK suffers from Alzheimer's and it was the cause of death in every 1 in 8 persons in 2019.[8] The exact cause of this devastating illness is still being elucidated, although a combination of genetic, lifestyle and environmental factors is suspected.

The large size and extreme polarization of neurons is crucial to their ability to communicate at long distances and to form the complex cellular networks of the nervous system. Brain cells depend on an internal support and transport system to carry nutrients and other essential materials throughout their cell bodies. One of the major systems of intracellular transport is the microtubule-based transport system. Intracellular transport requires the normal structure and functioning of the so-called "Tau" protein which binds to *microtubules* and assists with their formation and stabilization. In addition to this transport within the neuron, there must be extensive communication between individual cells for normal neurological functioning.

In Alzheimer's dementia, two neuroanatomical features are prominent – *plaques* and *neurofibrillary tangles*. *Plaques* are clumps of a beta-amyloid protein which may damage and destroy brain cells in several ways, including specifically interfering with cell-to-cell communication. Intracellularly when Tau protein is hyperphosphorylated, it is unable to bind. The cell's microtubules become unstable and begin disintegrating. In Alzheimer's disease, threads of Tau protein twist into abnormal *neurofibrillary tangles*. Some researchers believe that when the Tau proteins are thus hyperphosphorylated, it leads to failure of the transport system and is implicated in the decline and death of brain cells. Others note that persons whose brains display tangles can survive for decades and that tangles can appear in healthy individuals. Therefore, it is felt that tangles may not play a causative role in the disease process, but rather are actually protective in nature.[9]

New guidelines and recommendations regarding Alzheimer's dementia have been introduced by the National Institute on Aging and the Alzheimer's Association (NIA-AA).[10] The guidelines state that genetic risk and biomarkers, including chemical and neuroimaging markers, be used in research settings. Many clinicians, however, will not have access to such biomarkers as yet in clinical practice. Even when available, the guidelines emphasize that no single finding or combination of findings define the disease state. In this rapidly advancing field of investigation, some combination of genetic testing and biomarkers may in the future be useful as a surrogate for neuropathologic changes or functional decline.

Other important conclusions from these national guidelines:

- There is a preclinical stage of Alzheimer's dementia which shows amyloid accumulation, neurofibrillary change and neuritic plaques.
- For individuals without cognitive impairment at the time tissue was obtained, it is possible that neuropathologic changes of Alzheimer's dementia may predate onset of symptoms by years.
- For individuals with cognitive impairment at the time tissue was obtained, an "intermediate" or "high" level of AD neuropathologic change should be considered to be an adequate explanation of cognitive impairment or dementia.
- When a "low" level of AD neuropathologic change is observed in the setting of cognitive impairment, it is likely that other diseases are present. Co-morbidities are common and include Lewy body disease (LBD), vascular brain injury (VBI) and hippocampal sclerosis (HS).

Although there is still controversy about the precise cause of the disease, there is ample evidence to suggest that there is degeneration in the cholinergic neurons, more rapidly and more consistently than in other neurotransmitter systems.[11] There is a prominent loss of cholinergic markers in the cortex and hippocampus, which are involved in cognition and memory. It is thought that the decrease of neurotransmission in these acetylcholine-dependent neurons leads to many of the functional deficits of Alzheimer's disease, including memory impairment, aphasia, apraxia, agnosia and disturbance in executive functions (planning, organization, sequencing and abstracting).[12]

There is no doubt that as the mechanisms underlying the pathogenesis of Alzheimer's dementia are more fully known, novel treatments and medications will be developed with actions quite different from those currently available. One of many initiatives seeks to diminish the levels of the amyloid beta peptide (sometimes referred to as A-beta peptide). A-beta peptide results from the formation of amyloid plaques and has protofibrils that are neurotoxic. A-beta's presence (or at least the ratio of the various subtypes of this peptide) is highly correlated with Alzheimer's dementia[13] and believed to be a major cause of the neurodegeneration that occurs. Medications are being developed to inhibit two enzymes essential to the formation of this peptide, BACE-1 and BACE-2. Such inhibition could lead to minimized neurotoxicity and clinical improvement.[14–15]

Current medications for Alzheimer's dementia

Cholinesterase inhibitors

Because of the seeming increased loss of cholinergic neurons, medication development has focused on different methods of increasing levels of acetylcholine. Early efforts to increase the production of acetylcholine by providing precursors to acetylcholine formation were unsuccessful. More recent efforts have been directed at blocking acetylcholinesterase, the enzyme that breaks down acetylcholine, thereby leading to a functional increase in acetylcholine levels. Tacrine, the first drug developed for this problem, was effective, but was hampered by severe liver toxicity and the necessity of giving four separate daily doses. Because of these disadvantages, it has largely fallen out of favor.

There are currently four medications in common usage for treating dementia of the Alzheimer's type: donepezil (Aricept), rivastigmine (Exelon), galantamine (Razadyne) and memantine (Namenda). Donepezil and galantamine inhibit acetylcholinesterase, while rivastigmine inhibits both acetylcholinesterase and butyrylcholinesterase, which may provide a more broad-spectrum activity and increased efficacy. Rivastigmine is available as a transdermal patch in addition to oral forms. Memantine has a much more complex pharmacological profile than originally described. It does work by a similar mechanism to the other three drugs in affecting acetylcholine-related signaling. In addition, it has weak actions on glutamate which may or may not confer added effectiveness. Each of these agents has shown benefits for Alzheimer's patients in improving overall assessments of behavior functioning, anxiety, aggression, agitation and wandering. When the patient's memory, cognition and ability to maintain activities of daily living improve, confusion and agitated behaviors decrease.

Within the three cholinesterase inhibitors, effectiveness is statistically approximately equal, although medication B may provide more benefit than medication A in any given individual. The combination of memantine plus a cholinesterase inhibitor together may confer added beneficial effect.[16] Dosage is started small and gradually increased based on clinical effect and tolerability as side effects (nausea, vomiting, diarrhea and/or weight loss) can increase with larger doses (see Table 17.8).[17] The extent of therapeutic benefit from each of these medications/combinations in particular patients can vary significantly – from minimal to moderate effectiveness.[18–20]

These medications slow the progression of acetylcholine-dependent neurotransmission loss, thus delaying the intensification of Alzheimer's symptoms. There is evidence

Table 17.8 Dosing schedules of medication in medications used to treat dementia of the Alzheimer's type

Medication	Dosing schedule
Galantamine	Tablet: initial dose of 8 mg/day (4 mg twice a day); may increase dose to 16 mg/day (8 mg twice a day) and 24 mg/day (12 mg twice a day) at minimum 4-week intervals if well tolerated
	Oral solution: same dosage as tablet
	Extended-release capsule: same dosage as tablet but taken once a day
Rivastigmine	Capsule: initial dose of 3 mg/day (1.5 mg twice a day); may increase dose to 6 mg/day (3 mg twice a day), 9 mg/day (4.5 mg twice a day) and 12 mg/day (6 mg twice a day) at minimum 2-week intervals if well tolerated
	Patch: initial dose of 4.6 mg once a day; may increase to 9.5 mg once a day after minimum of 4 weeks if well tolerated
	Oral solution: same dosage as capsule
Donepezil	Tablet: initial dose of 5 mg once a day; may increase dose to 10 mg/day after 4–6 weeks if well tolerated, then to 23 mg/day after at least 3 months
	Orally disintegrating tablet: same dosage as above
Memantine	Tablet: initial dose of 5 mg once a day; may increase dose to 10 mg/day (5 mg twice a day), 15 mg/day (5 mg and 10 mg as separate doses) and 20 mg/day (10 mg twice a day) at minimum 1-week intervals if well tolerated
	Oral solution: same dosage as above
	Extended-release tablet: initial dose of 7 mg once a day; may increase dose to 14 mg/day, 21 mg/day and 28 mg/day at minimum 1-week intervals if well tolerated

that in some limited number of patients there is an actual reversal of symptoms, although this effect is modest. There is no pharmacological cure for Alzheimer's disease. Since the cause of the disease remains unclear, no treatment is as yet positively aimed directly at an underlying mechanism.

Mild cognitive impairment

Because of the dramatic rise in the diagnosis and public awareness of Alzheimer's dementia, patients have become sensitive to identifying small mild changes in cognition, both in themselves and their loved ones. Patients with mild cognitive impairment (MCI) often present with vague and subjective symptoms of declining cognitive performance, which may be difficult to distinguish from the age-related decline in performance affecting healthy older individuals. Appropriate assessment of these complaints becomes important for the prescriber since patients will often seek a medication remedy for their perceived symptoms.

The following advice from the Mayo Clinic[21] can be helpful to the clinician in assessment and possible treatment:

> Mild degrees of cognitive impairment, particularly when self-reported by patients, pose a substantial challenge to the clinician. The physician may be dealing with a patient with a mild or transient condition, a drug-induced adverse effect, or a

depressive disorder; the patient may be in the early stages of a condition that will eventually lead to a dementia; or the complaint may be due to a psychological condition rather than an organic brain disorder. Because a variety of conditions may result in a complaint of cognitive impairment, an individualized workup for such conditions and a consensus on a therapeutic approach should be sought.

To demonstrate that cognitive function is worse than that expected for one's age, neuropsychological testing is necessary so that a patient's performance can be compared with that of an age-matched (and ideally education-matched) control group. Important facts about MCI and dementia include the following:

- A practice parameter recommendation by the American Academy of Neurology states that patients with MCI should be identified and monitored because of their increased risk for Alzheimer's disease and, to a lesser extent, other dementing conditions.
- MCI represents a stage of cognitive decline that exceeds the normal expected age-related changes, but where functional activities are largely preserved. MCI itself, therefore, does not meet the criteria for dementia, but in some individuals it may be an intermediate step in an ultimate progression to dementia.
- Different subtypes of MCI are recognized. One common classification distinguishes between amnestic and non-amnestic forms of MCI. The amnestic form, where memory impairment predominates, is often a precursor for clinical Alzheimer's disease. A variety of cognitive impairments may occur in the non-amnestic forms of MCI, with the most common deficit being impaired executive function. This form of non-amnestic MCI may be associated with cerebrovascular disease or may be a precursor for some front temporal dementias.
- A substantial number of patients initially assessed to have MCI may be judged to have normal cognition on a repeat visit. A follow-up examination with the clinician is, therefore, indicated before further extensive diagnostic and/or therapeutic measures are undertaken.

There is no medication that has been FDA-approved for MCI. Even with modest symptoms of MCI, patients may urge the clinician to try existing treatments in hopes of improving cognitive functioning and/or delaying what they fear – the onset of full-blown dementia. In similar fashion to the modest improvements in symptoms shown in Alzheimer's disease, utilization of cholinesterase inhibitors in patients with MCI may show some clinical improvement. Since these medications are not without side effects, patients with MCI are not, however, routinely prescribed cholinesterase inhibitors. The potential side effect–benefit ratio must be evaluated individually for each patient. Also, follow-up assessment of clinical improvement, if any, must be documented, so as to prevent unnecessary chronic prescription if benefit is not seen. Unfortunately, the use of cholinesterase inhibitors in patients with MCI has not been found to delay the onset of Alzheimer's disease or other dementias.[22–24] The presence of depression with MCI is thought to be predictive of progression from amnestic mild cognitive impairment (AMCI) to Alzheimer's disease. In one study, treatment with donepezil did delay progression to Alzheimer's disease among depressed subjects with AMCI, without affecting their symptoms of depression.[25]

Psychiatric diseases that may present with confusion

While it is not the intent of this text to detail a full psychiatric differential diagnosis, or medication recommendations for the spectrum of psychiatric disease, some patients with major psychiatric disorders present with confusion or inattention as one of the symptoms. If delirium/dementia have been ruled out, and a psychiatric cause for the patient's disorganization is considered, some of the following additional symptomatic cues may be useful in assessing the cause of mental confusion, making a tentative diagnosis and, when appropriate, prescribing psychotropic medication.

With *psychosis*, the patient often has the presence of hallucinations. Auditory hallucinations are common, but they may be visual, olfactory or tactile. There may be delusions (fixed false beliefs that do not change despite factual information to the contrary). The patient's affect is often flattened. There may be a history of previous psychotic episodes.

In *mania*, in addition to mental disorganization and confusion there can be rapid, pressured speech, excess energy or physical motion, and a lack of need for sleep. The patient may be grandiose in ideation or plans. At other times there is little grandiosity and the patient is primarily angry or pressured, with intense irritability out of proportion to the circumstances.

Confusion and cognitive impairments associated with *depression* have the specific label of "depressive pseudodementia." The differentiation of pseudodementia from true dementia is often difficult. However, a depressed patient will often have sad, dysphoric or depressed affect. In addition, these patients have psychomotor slowing and, at times, suicidal thoughts or actions.

The intensely *anxious patient* who is also somewhat confused and distractible will often have other physical signs of anxiety, including pacing, sweating, tremor or shaking. There may be a history of overt panic attacks.

In *Attention Deficit Hyperactivity Disorder* (ADHD), acute confusion is not prominent, although a patient with ADHD may have chronic difficulty with attending to details or memory. This topic will be discussed in more detail in Chapter 18.

More detailed discussion of the diagnosis of psychiatric conditions can be found in any of the widely used, authoritative textbooks on psychiatry such as:

Kaplan and Sadock's Comprehensive Textbook of Psychiatry (2017), 10th edn., Lippincott, Williams & Wilkins.
The American Psychiatric Association Textbook of Psychiatry (2019), 7th edn., edited by Hales *et al.*, American Psychiatric Publishing.

References

1 Breteler MMB *et al.* (1992) Epidemiology of Alzheimer's disease. *Epidemiology Review* 14: 59–82.
2 Aronson MK *et al.* (1991) Dementia: age-dependent incidence, prevalence, and mortality in the old. *Archives of Internal Medicine* 151: 989–992.
3 Canadian Study of Health and Aging Working Group (1994) Canadian study of health and aging: study methods and prevalence of dementia. *Canadian Medical Association Journal* 150: 899–913.
4 Bachman DL *et al.* (1992) Prevalence of dementia and probable senile dementia of the Alzheimer type in the Framingham Study. *Neurology* 2: 115–119.

5 Semla T *et al.* (2000) *Geriatric Dosage Handbook, Including Monitoring, Clinical Recommendations and OBRA Guidelines*, 5th edn., Lexi-Comp.

6 Rawling JN and Verma S (2001) Behavioral disturbances in older patients: guidelines for management. *Psychiatric Times* (October): 72–74.

7 Kaschkow J (2002) Cognitive enhancers for dementia: do they work? *Current Psychiatry* 1(3).

8 Office for National Statistics (2020) Dementia and Alzheimer's disease deaths including comorbidities, England and Wales: 2019 registrations, available at: www.ons.gov.uk/releases/dementiaandalzheimersdiseasedeathsincludingcomorbiditiesenglandandwales2019registrations

9 Lee HG *et al.* (2005) Tau phosphorylation in Alzheimer's disease: pathogen or protector? *Trends in Molecular Medicine* 11(4): 164–169.

10 Diagnostic Criteria & Guidelines, available at: www.alz.org/research/diagnostic_criteria/

11 Katzman R (1986) Alzheimer's disease. *New England Journal of Medicine* 314: 964–973.

12 Kar S *et al.* (2004) Interactions between β-amyloid and central cholinergic neurons: implications for Alzheimer's disease *Journal of Psychiatry and Neuroscience* 29(6): 427–441.

13 Koyama A *et al.* (2012) Plasma amyloid-β as a predictor of dementia and cognitive decline: a systematic review and meta-analysis. *Archives of Neurology.* doi:10.1001/archneurol.2011.1841

14 Evin G and Kenche VB (2007) BACE inhibitors as potential therapeutics for Alzheimer's disease. *Recent Patents on CNS Drug Discovery* 2(3): 188–199.

15 Vassar R (2001) The beta-secretase, BACE: a prime drug target for Alzheimer's disease. *Journal of Molecular Neuroscience* 17(2): 157–170.

16 Alzheimer's: drugs help manage symptoms, available at: www.mayoclinic.org/diseases-conditions/alzheimers-disease/in-depth/alzheimers/art-20048103

17 How is Alzheimer's disease treated?, available at: www.nia.nih.gov/health/how-alzheimers-disease-treated

18 Zurad EG (2001) New treatments for Alzheimer's disease: a review. *Drug Benefit Trends* 13(7): 27–40.

19 Borson S (2002) New strategies for management of behavioral disturbances and psychosis in older patients. Presented at the American Association for Geriatrics Society 15th Annual Meeting, Orlando, Florida, February.

20 Brandt MJ (2001) Pharmacotherapy for dementias. Presented at the American Pharmaceutical Association 148th Annual Meeting, San Francisco, California, March.

21 Mild cognitive impairment, available at: www.mayoclinic.org/diseases-conditions/mild-cognitive-impairment/symptoms-causes/syc-20354578

22 Raschetti R *et al.* (2007) Cholinesterase inhibitors in mild cognitive impairment: a systematic review of randomised trials. *PLoS Medicine* 4(11): e338. doi:10.1371/journal.pmed.0040338

23 Parminder R *et al.* (2008) Effectiveness of cholinesterase inhibitors and memantine for treating dementia: evidence review for a clinical practice guideline. *Annals of Internal Medicine* 148(5): 379–397.

24 Farlow MR (2009) Treatment of mild cognitive impairment (MCI). *Current Alzheimer Research* 6(4): 362–367.

25 Panza F *et al.* (2010) Effect of donepezil on the continuum of depressive symptoms, mild cognitive impairment, and progression to dementia. *Journal of the American Geriatrics Society* 58(2): 389–390.

18 Inattention and hyperactivity – ADHD and stimulants

- ADHD – a diagnosis which is increasing rapidly 272
- What are the syndromes of ADHD and why is it confusing? 274
- What are the causes of ADHD? 274
- How is ADHD diagnosed in children? 276
- ADHD in adults 277
- Stimulant medication and its appropriate uses 279
- Other medications used in ADHD 280
- Additional treatments for ADHD beyond medication 281
- Other alternative/home remedies for ADHD 282
- Abuse of stimulants 284
- Notes and references 284

Perhaps nowhere in the realm of twenty-first-century mental health prescribing is there more controversy than in the area of diagnosing and treating Attention Deficit Hyperactivity Disorder (ADHD) and the prescription of stimulants. The pharmacology of stimulants itself is not difficult. As will be seen in this chapter, the controversy and complexity have to do with the process of diagnosing the disorder prior to prescription. With a class of medication such as stimulants, a prescriber is unlikely to rely solely on another clinician's diagnostic assessment. To be a competent prescriber, the clinician must be knowledgeable about the elements of the diagnostic process. While this text is not intended to be a comprehensive psychiatric diagnostic manual, before delving into the psychopharmacology and medication prescription for ADHD we must first discuss the issues, nuances and confounding elements in the diagnosis of inattention and overactivity. This will be followed by recommendations for the competent prescription of stimulants and its pitfalls.

ADHD – a diagnosis which is increasing rapidly

Although overactivity and periods of poor concentration have been part of the human condition throughout recorded history, diagnosing these behaviors and attempting to treat them in a coherent manner is a relatively new phenomenon. This cluster of symptoms has carried many names including "minimal brain damage," "minimal brain dysfunction," "learning/behavioral disability" and "hyperactivity." The term "Attention Deficit Disorder (ADD) with or without hyperactivity" first appears in DSM-III published in 1980. In 1987, the revised edition, DSM-III-R changed the term to

Table 18.1 Signs of inattention

The person:
- Often fails to give close attention to details or makes careless mistakes in schoolwork, at work or with other activities
- Often has difficulty holding attention in tasks or play activities
- Often does not seem to listen when spoken to directly
- Often does not follow through on instructions and fails to finish schoolwork, chores or duties in the workplace
- Often has trouble organizing tasks and activities
- Often avoids, dislikes or is reluctant to do tasks that require mental effort over a long period of time (such as schoolwork or homework)
- Often loses things necessary for tasks and activities (e.g., school materials, pencils, books, tools, wallets, keys, paperwork, eyeglasses, mobile telephones)
- Is often easily distracted
- Is often forgetful in daily activities

Source: American Psychiatric Association (2013) Attention-deficit/hyperactivity disorder diagnostic criteria. In *Diagnostic and Statistical Manual of Mental Disorders DSM-V*, 5th edn., American Psychiatric Association.

Table 18.2 Signs of hyperactivity and impulsivity

The person:
- Often fidgets with hands or feet or squirms in seat
- Often leaves seat in classroom or other situations in which remaining seated is expected
- Often runs about or climbs excessively in situations where it is inappropriate
- Often has trouble playing or engaging quietly in leisure activities
- Is often "on the go" or often acts as if "driven by a motor"
- Often talks excessively
- Often blurts out answers before questions have been completed
- Often has difficulty awaiting their turn
- Often interrupts or intrudes on others (e.g., butts into conversations or games)

Source: American Psychiatric Association (2013) Attention-deficit/hyperactivity disorder diagnostic criteria. In *Diagnostic and Statistical Manual of Mental Disorders DSM-V*, 5th edn., American Psychiatric Association.

"Attention Deficit Hyperactivity Disorder" (ADHD), which has remained in common usage since that time. Three subtypes of ADHD – predominately impulsive type, predominately inattentive type and combined type – have been described. As can be seen in Tables 18.1 and 18.2, each diagnosis is made through patient observation and self-reported symptoms. Each of the following conditions must be met:

- Six (or more) of the following symptoms have persisted for at least 6 months to a degree that is inconsistent with his or her developmental level and that negatively impact directly on social and academic/occupational activities.
- The symptoms are not solely a manifestation of oppositional behavior, defiance, hostility, or failure to understand tasks or instructions.
- For older adolescents and adults (age 17 and older), at least five symptoms are required:
  - Several inattentive or hyperactive-impulsive symptoms were present before the age of 12.

- Several symptoms are present in two or more settings (such as at home, school or work; with friends or relatives; in other activities).
- There is clear evidence that the symptoms interfere with, or reduce the quality of, social, school or work functioning.
- The symptoms are not better explained by another mental disorder (such as a mood disorder, anxiety disorder, dissociative disorder or a personality disorder). The symptoms do not happen only during the course of schizophrenia or another psychotic disorder.

Estimates vary, but globally a mean worldwide prevalence of ADHD of 6.1 percent overall (range: 0.1–8.1 percent in children and adolescents [aged <18 years]) is reported. The mean prevalence of ADHD in adults (aged 18–44 years) from a range of countries in Asia, Europe, the Americas and the Middle East was reported as 4.4 percent overall (range: 0.6–7.3 percent).[1]

What are the syndromes of ADHD and why is it confusing?

ADHD is a chronic neurobehavioral condition that begins in childhood and often persists into adulthood.[2]
    The subtypes are categorized as follows:

- predominantly inattentive type ADHD – a child that has at least six signs and symptoms from Table 18.1.
- predominantly hyperactive-impulsive type ADHD – a child that has at least six signs and symptoms from Tables 18.2 and 18.3.
- Combined type ADHD – a child that has six or more signs and symptoms from each of the two above criteria.

While the above behaviors are potentially observable and able to be documented, the diagnostic confusion exists in part because almost all children at one time or another display some of these behaviors for short or intermittent periods during their development. Periods of poor attention, overactivity and impulsive behavior are totally normal behaviors for children when they occur sporadically and for a short time. The diagnosis, therefore, should not be made based on any one or two behaviors, nor on any symptoms that do not continue chronically and with regularity. To make the diagnosis, symptoms must present themselves early in life (before the age of 7), and persist. This is particularly important as a prescriber begins to evaluate adolescents or adults with possible ADHD.

What are the causes of ADHD?

For a decade the rate of diagnosis increased rapidly, showing approximately a 3 percent increase every year from 1997 to 2006. In the same interval, parent-reported incidence of symptomatic children between 4 and 17 years of age went from 7.8 to 9.5 percent.[3] Because of this exceptional increase and an initial lack of tangible laboratory proof, many in the mental health field were skeptical about the validity of the diagnosis and questioned whether the condition was being overdiagnosed.

With the advent of more sophisticated gene analysis and MRI specificity, it has been shown that genetic abnormalities are at least a partial likely cause for this condition; and gradually we are identifying these genetic errors.[4] A plethora of magnetic resonance imaging studies have shown that ADHD is characterized by multiple functional and structural neural network abnormalities.[5] Now, not only can ADHD be identified on MRI, but the various subtypes can be differentiated.[6] Nonetheless, it is not yet possible for clinicians to use a single MRI test to make the diagnosis. In the future, researchers expect to see deep learning models improve through artificial intelligence as they are exposed to larger neuroimaging datasets. When and if this occurs with sufficient precision, neural imaging may become the backbone of diagnostic information.

Although usually thought to be at least in part a genetically mediated disease, the behaviors associated with ADHD can also arise from environmental factors that disrupt normal brain growth before, during and after birth, such as fetal alcohol syndrome, maternal smoking, maternal alcohol and drug use, and severe childhood deprivation. Approximately 25 percent of children with exposure to environmental toxins, particularly lead, develop ADHD.[7–8] Parents who meet the formal diagnostic criteria for ADHD have approximately a 50 percent chance of siring a child with ADHD.[9–10] Twin studies have placed the heritability of ADHD in the range of 80 percent.[11] *A child or adolescent who has had extended periods of normal, non-hyperactive and non-inattentive behavior in his/her early life does not develop ADHD as an acquired condition in adolescence or adulthood.*

It is suspected that the children with ADHD also show a delay in the development of the frontal cortex accompanied by rapid maturation of the motor cortex.[12] This combination of a brain which is slow to develop in the areas of impulse control and focal thinking, but overdeveloped in areas of motor activity could account for ADHD's symptom complex of impulsive decision-making with motor restlessness and hyperactivity. Other brain abnormalities found in these children include deficits in dopamine release in the caudate and limbic regions,[13–14] changes in neuron connectivity particularly in the temporal lobe,[15] reduced blood circulation and low neural activity in the striatum,[16] differential EEG tracings[17] and lowered glucose metabolism.[18] It is yet to be determined as to which of these features are core biological changes for the disorder. Most clinicians and researchers now believe that abnormal genetics play a crucial role in as many as 75 percent of all identified cases.[19] As with most mental health disorders, it is unlikely that one unitary genetic cause will be found.

Following a paper published in the UK in 2007,[20] consideration has been given to a possible causative link between certain food additives such as artificial colors or preservatives and ADHD. Further research is necessary to learn if, and in what manner, these food additives may be a potential cause. Based on this information, some governments have restricted the use of artificial food colorings (AFCs), although this practice has not been consistently adopted worldwide. Even the most recent summary data from collated studies about the role of artificial food colorings lead to mixed results. The author of the best fairly recent study[21] suggests at least the following two conclusions:

- "AFCs are not a main cause of ADHD, but they may contribute significantly to some cases, and in some cases may additively push a youngster over the diagnostic threshold."
- The current status of evidence is inconclusive "but too substantial to dismiss."

Other studies have suggested that environmental exposure to organophosphate pesticides between pregnancy and grade school may play a factor. Although there are several suggestive studies,[22-23] this link, too, remains unproven.

Brain injuries are thought by some theoreticians to be involved in the development of ADHD. A portion of children who have experienced such injuries may show behaviors similar to those with ADHD. In males, children with moderate and severe ADHD had increased odds of having had a TBI (traumatic brain injury). No associations between severity and TBI were found in girls.[24]

Perhaps the most controversial, but widely purported causative environmental issue involves the use of refined sugar in children's diets. Although there is widespread popular belief that refined sugar causes or worsens ADHD, much more research discounts this theory than supports it.[25-26]

Another controversial yet at times widely publicized possible cause for ADHD is as a side effect of childhood vaccinations. Sometimes grouped together with other childhood diseases whose incidence is increasing such as autism, allergies and asthma, ADHD has been suggested to be primarily caused by vaccinations or the combined effect of vaccinations and genetic predisposition. While this connection has been proposed by a few writers and seen on various Internet websites, there is virtually no scholarly research to support this conclusion.[27-28] Based on current evidence, there is no reason to avoid routine vaccinations against childhood diseases because of the potential for ADHD.

How is ADHD diagnosed in children?

With school-age children, a multifactorial approach to diagnosis is necessary. The clinician must obtain a full history of symptoms, including their onset, and course over time. If at all possible, the clinician should observe the child directly in structured and unstructured activities to evaluate the child's attention, concentration and overall activity level. In addition, separate interviews with the parents or caregivers are useful to discuss the child's behavior in a variety of circumstances. Such information should also include whether there have been any significant recent events in the child's life such as the death of a family member, a divorce or parental job loss which could lead to emotional and/or behavioral disruption. Written or verbal reports from the child's teachers describing school-related activities and behaviors are also crucial.

Box 18.1 Primary care

The necessity of extensive data collection and comprehensive evaluative procedures when diagnosing ADHD is often not feasible for busy family/general practitioners. Clinicians who see large numbers of children and adolescents would benefit from the establishment of a consistent relationship with one or more mental health providers who can assist with, or provide, the necessary evaluation. These clinicians can then also participate in a team-oriented approach to treatment. Large practices might find it useful and cost-effective to contract with a mental health clinician on an ongoing basis.

Beyond this historical information, a thorough medical examination of the child must be performed to rule out other causes unrelated to ADHD for the child's behavior. These can include:

- undetected seizures
- middle-ear infections causing hearing problems
- learning disabilities
- undetected vision problems
- anxiety, depression or other independent mental health diagnoses.

Because of concern about possible cardiac effects of stimulants, some clinicians have considered an electrocardiogram (EKG) as a necessary component of the prescriptive evaluation process. The latest recommendation which carries the backing of the American Academy of Child and Adolescent Psychiatry is that routine EKGs are not necessary unless a cardiac history and/or a physical examination suggest cardiac risk.[29]

Rating charts and evaluation forms for the child and/or parents and teachers are often used by many clinicians. These include:

- ADHD Rating Scale-IV (ADHD-IV)[30]
- Vanderbilt ADHD Diagnostic Parent Rating Scale[31]
- SNAP-IV Rating Scale-Revised (SNAP-IV-R).[32]

When assessing many mental health diagnoses, the use of the DSM-V criteria or the use of ICD-10 criteria (*International Classification of Diseases*, 10th revision, which is used in the UK and the rest of Europe) makes little difference. With ADHD, this is not the case. The ICD-10 uses different terminology for these syndromes, listing them as "Hyperkinetic Disorders." Although there is significant overlap between the two classifications, statistically the use of DSM-V criteria (listed in Tables 18.1 and 18.2) makes the diagnosis three to four times more likely than if the ICD-10 parameters are used.[33] The ICD-10 wording can be seen in Table 18.3.

ADHD in adults

Depending on the study used, 30–60 percent of children diagnosed with ADHD are thought to show continued symptoms as adults.[34-35] For a significant period of time, however, this purported incidence was not uniformly accepted by clinicians. Since the diagnosis of "Adult ADHD" did not appear until the late 1980s and because of the rapid and somewhat sensationalistic presentation through print and video media, some professionals felt that this diagnosis did not represent individuals with a true mental illness. Their perspective was that Adult ADHD represented a "medicalization" of poor performance and lack of personal responsibility.[36] This skepticism notwithstanding, the advent of functional and structural neuro-radiological evidence of changes in the brains of these individuals, as well as genome-wide association studies, twin, family and adoption studies have led to common acceptance of the diagnosis. Professional bodies such as the American National Institutes of Mental Health and the World Health Organization, now endorse the validity of Adult ADHD as a recognizable and treatable mental disorder.[37-39] Symptoms might look different at older ages. For example, in adults, hyperactivity may appear as extreme restlessness or wearing others out with

Table 18.3 ICD-10 wording of criteria for hyperkinetic disorders

This group of disorders is characterized by:

Early onset; a combination of overactive, poorly modulated behaviour with marked inattention and lack of persistent task involvement; and pervasiveness over situations and persistence over time of these behavioural characteristics.

Hyperkinetic disorders always arise early in development (usually in the first 5 years of life). Their chief characteristics are lack of persistence in activities that require cognitive involvement, and a tendency to move from one activity to another without completing any one activity, together with disorganized, ill-regulated, and excessive activity. These problems usually persist through school years and even into adult life, but many affected individuals show a gradual improvement in activity and attention.

Several other abnormalities may be associated with these disorders. Hyperkinetic children are often reckless and impulsive, prone to accidents, and find themselves in disciplinary trouble because of unthinking (rather than deliberately defiant) breaches of rules. Their relationships with adults are often socially disinhibited, with a lack of normal caution and reserve. They are unpopular with other children and may become isolated. Cognitive impairment is common, and specific delays in motor and language development are disproportionately frequent.

Source: available at: www.who.int/classifications/icd/en/ (Neurological Diseases section).

their activity. The overall prevalence of current adult ADHD is 4.4 percent with the prevalence higher for males (5.4 percent) versus females (3.2 percent).[40]

Co-morbidities with ADHD are common and include social anxiety disorder, bipolar disorder, major depressive disorder and alcohol dependence.[41] A confounding factor in ADHD diagnosis in adults is that there have been no formally drafted diagnostic criteria for adults. The DSM criteria were developed for children only, although many clinicians have presumed that they apply equally to adults.

ADHD symptoms in adults can be subtle and the assessment process can be subjective from one clinician to another. Evaluation of adults with symptoms of ADHD requires integration of a range of data, including patient history, patient self-report of current symptoms and mental status testing (see Chapter 3 and Appendix 1). A thorough history should include an emphasis on past school performance and conduct, previous and current psychiatric therapies, and reports of specific symptoms of inattention, distractibility and disorganization. Adult patients should be asked to provide any available school records and to gather information from parents and other adults who knew them as children. A family history of possible ADHD symptoms should also be obtained as siblings, parents or children frequently have similar behaviors. Because adults with ADHD may not fully recognize their symptoms, the patient's spouse or partner should ideally be included in the evaluative interview. Even though patients with ADHD may have difficulty accurately recalling relevant history, *an extended, consistent pattern of ADHD symptoms dating to early childhood is essential in making the diagnosis. A recent onset of symptoms without significant past history of symptoms, or sporadic episodes of symptoms, should raise concern about the appropriateness of an ADHD diagnosis.*

The medical evaluation should include a neurologic examination. There are suggestions that patients with ADHD exhibit a greater incidence of "soft neurologic signs" including problems with right–left discrimination, motor overflow movements and sequencing difficulties. Laboratory tests may include a serum lead level and thyroid function tests.[42]

Table 18.4 Rating evaluation forms for ADHD in adults

- The Wender Utah Rating Scale[1]
- The Copeland Symptom Checklist[2]
- The Brown Adult ADD Scale[3]
- The Connors Adult ADHD Rating Scales (CAARS – one for patients and a second for observers)[4]
- The Barkley Adult ADHD Rating Scale[5-6]

Sources:
1 Gentile JA and Gillig PM (2006) Adult ADHD: diagnosis, differential diagnosis, and medication management. *Psychiatry* 3(8): 25–30.
2 Kessler RC *et al.* (2006) The prevalence and correlates of adult ADHD in the United States: results from the National Comorbidity Survey Replication. *American Journal of Psychiatry* 163: 716–723.
3 Brown TE (1996) *ADD Scales.* Psychological Corp., pp. 5–6.
4 Available at: www.wpspublish.com/caars-conners-adult-adhd-rating-scales
5 Available at: www.guilford.com/books/Barkley-Adult-ADHD-Rating-Scale-IV-BAARS-IV/Russell-Barkley/9781609182038
6 Available at: www.russellbarkley.org/

There are numerous questionnaires developed for clinician use in diagnosing ADHD in adults (see Table 18.4). Corroborative information on organization, attention to detail and capacity for accuracy can be obtained from the manner and thoroughness with which a patient completes one of these questionnaires. The report of a spouse or significant other may also help the prescriber. A patient may subjectively report that they have difficulty at work or in school, but there is often no objective work or school performance information available to the clinician. *Therefore, at this time, the diagnosis of Adult ADHD is solely a clinical assessment and formulation.*

Stimulant medication and its appropriate uses

While the diagnosis of ADHD can be somewhat complicated and challenging, the medication prescription decisions for this disorder are relatively simple. While not the only treatment, medication is a central feature of ADHD treatment for many patients. At least two-thirds of children with current ADHD are taking medication for the disorder and the percentage is increasing. Stimulant medications (sometimes referred to as "psychostimulants") are generally thought to be the medication treatment of choice by most clinicians.[43-44] See also Chapter 10 for more information on stimulants.

The general term "stimulant" refers to properties of certain drugs or medications which "stimulate" or enhance a particular body system, such as cardiac stimulants or respiratory stimulants. In mental health, however, the term is used specifically to identify a group of medications which have a variety of neurological and physical effects and are postulated to act by affecting brain catecholamine neurotransmitters, especially norepinephrine and dopamine. Benzedrine was first used with behaviorally disturbed children in 1937. Eleven years later, dexedrine was introduced, with the advantage of having equal efficacy at half the dose. Methylphenidate (marketed as Ritalin) was introduced in 1954 with the hope that it would have fewer side effects and less abuse potential.

Currently, there are a staggering array of branded stimulants. The underlying chemicals contained in these brands, however, are closely related and/or stereoisomers of the parent compounds – amphetamine, dextroamphetamine, lisdexamphetamine, methylphenidate and dexmethylphenidate. Other than the speed with which the medication enters the system (immediately or time release) and the modality of preparation (pills, capsules, liquid or patch) these medications have generally similar effects, uses, side effects and prescriptive patterns. Although, as with all psychotropics, there is individual variability of response to any particular drug in this medication class, there is little statistical therapeutic advantage to one medication over another. It is often useful for the beginning clinician initially to learn one or two preparations/medications well and be less concerned with the remainder of the list. With experience, other preparations can be learned.

Other uses of stimulant medication

This chapter focuses on Attention Deficit Hyperactivity Disorder and treatment with stimulants. However, because of stimulants' wide effects in the central and peripheral nervous systems (such as increased alertness, wakefulness and arousal; enhanced endurance, productivity and motivation; increased motor activity, heart rate and blood pressure) they have been used in mental health practice in a variety of additional clinical situations. These include:

- to counteract lethargy and fatigue
- to reduce sleepiness and increase wakefulness
- to decrease appetite and promote weight loss
- to treat narcolepsy
- off-label as a third- or fourth-line treatment for clinical depression
- as a remedy for the side effect of dizziness due to lowered blood pressure.

The "me too" concept of medication development, explaining why there are so many stimulants on the market, and information on the dosing of stimulants and their side effects can be found in Chapter 10.

Other medications used in ADHD

While stimulants are the mainstay of ADHD prescription, several other medications are used to treat this condition. The most prominent of these is atomoxetine (Strattera). Atomoxetine, a non-stimulant norepinephrine reuptake inhibitor, has been available since 2005. It has shown effectiveness in ADHD treatment for children above the age of 6, as well as adolescents and adults. It is not a controlled substance and has minimal abuse potential. Unlike stimulants whose effects are seen quickly (often with a single dose), atomoxetine takes a minimum of 7 days to build up in the system and generally should be continued for 6–8 weeks to assess effectiveness. It is often used in patients who have not responded to stimulants, are at high risk for abuse, are averse to taking stimulants or have side effects from taking them. The starting atomoxetine dosage for adults, as well as children or teens weighing more than 154 pounds, is 40 mg once daily or 20 mg twice daily. Children and teenagers weighing less than 154 pounds typically start with 0.25 mg of atomoxetine per pound of body weight, rounded to the nearest available strength. Side effects to the medication include dry mouth, nausea, decreased appetite, constipation, dizziness, sweating, decreased libido, urinary hesitancy, palpitations, increased heart rate and blood pressure.[45]

Certain antihypertensive medications including guanfacine (Intuniv and Tenex) and clonidine (Catapres) have shown efficacy in treating ADHD. Although guanfacine, an alpha-2 agonist, has been used off-label for several years to treat ADHD, it has now received American FDA approval in an extended-release formulation. It has shown effectiveness primarily in younger children with the hyperactive form of the condition, beingless effective with the inattentive form. Clonidine has been used to decrease impulsivity and aggression, primarily in children. These medications have also been prescribed to reduce tics or insomnia caused by other ADHD medications.

Last, antidepressants have shown some treatment effectiveness. Although the evidence is limited, there is support for utilizing tricyclic antidepressants and bupropion in ADHD.

Additional treatments for ADHD beyond medication

As with virtually all mental health conditions, medication alone is less effective without additional treatment modalities. ADHD is no exception. Beyond the benefits that medication can provide, specific behavioral suggestions and interventions can be helpful to both the child and adult patient. Depending on who prescribes the medication, a second mental health clinician with appropriate training and experience may be primarily involved in providing non-medication treatment. In other situations, the prescriber may also provide the patient with elements of non-medication treatment. Types of non-medication interventions for ADHD are listed in Table 18.5.

Table 18.5 Non-medication interventions for ADHD patients

- Behavior therapy – teachers and parents follow specific behavior-changing strategies to deal with problematic behavior. Such strategies can include reward/penalty systems to reinforce desired behaviors.
- Individual psychotherapy – adult and child patients can benefit from exploring and sharing upsetting behaviors and situations. They can explore negative behavioral patterns and ways to deal with their symptoms. Patients learn to monitor themselves and their own behavior while giving themselves positive rewards when appropriate.
- Practical skills training – individuals benefit from help in organizing tasks to complete schoolwork and/or occupational work while sustaining themselves through emotionally difficult events.
- Social skills training – children need to learn how to wait their turn, share their toys/belongings, ask for help and respond to teasing. Many ADHD patients have not learned to appropriately read facial expressions and voice tone from others and hence do not respond appropriately. These are, however, teachable and learnable skills.
- Parenting skills training – many parents, particularly young parents or those with emotional problems themselves, have not learned the most effective ways to understand and guide their child's behaviors. Training parents often focuses on:
  - giving children immediate positive or negative feedback on specific behaviors
  - the use of "timeouts"
  - avoiding overstimulation of a child
  - showing the child considerable affection in spite of frustrating behavior
  - practicing patience and keeping events in perspective
  - keeping a regular schedule for meals, naps and bedtimes to ensure that the child gets adequate rest
  - planning ahead to anticipate difficult or problematic situations for the child

(continued)

Table 18.5 Cont.

- finding ways to improve their child's self-esteem
- being simple and straightforward with directions and discipline
- learning stress management techniques for themselves.
- Family therapy – in addition to the above modalities, bringing the entire family constellation together, including parents, the identified patient and siblings, can often further treatment goals most efficiently and effectively.
- Support groups – most metropolitan areas have ADHD support groups for patients and families.

Source: Brown CS (1991) Treatment of attention deficit hyperactivity disorder: a critical review. *DICP* 25(11): 1207–1213.

Table 18.6 ADHD therapy references

Print books
- *CBT Toolbox for Depressed, Anxious & Suicidal Children and Adolescents: Over 220 Worksheets and Therapist Tips to Manage Moods, Build Positive Coping Skills & Develop Resiliency* (D Pratt [2019] PESI Publishing & Media)
- *Flipping ADHD on Its Head: How to Turn Your Child's Disability into Their Greatest Strength* by (J Poole [2020] Greenleaf Book Group Press)
- *ADHD, Executive Function & Behavioral Challenges in the Classroom: Managing the mpact on Learning, Motivation and Stress* (C Goldrich and C Goldrich [2019] PESI Publishing & Media)
- *Parenting Children with ADHD: 10 Lessons that Medicine Cannot Teach* (APA Lifetools) (VJ Monastra [2014] American Psychological Association)
- *The ADD & ADHD Answer Book: Professional Answers to 275 of the Top Questions Parents Ask* (S Ashley [2005] Sourcebooks Inc.)
- *Learning to Slow Down & Pay Attention: A Book for Kids About ADHD* (KG Nadeau *et al.* [2004; 3rd edn.] Magination Press)
- *More Attention, Less Deficit: Success Strategies for Adults with ADHD* (A Tuckman [2009] Specialty Press)
- *Taking Charge of ADHD: The Complete, Authoritative Guide for Parents* (RA Barkley [2000; Revised edn.] Guilford Press)
- *The Disorganized Mind: Coaching Your ADHD Brain to Take Control of Your Time, Tasks, and Talents* (NA Ratey [2008] St. Martin's Griffin)
- *ADD-Friendly Ways to Organize Your Life* (J Kolberg and K Nadeau [2002] Routledge)

Internet website
- Children and Adults with ADHD (www.chadd.org/)

There are many books, authoritative pamphlets and articles which provide helpful strategies for patients and parents. A selection of them is listed in Table 18.6; however, a further Internet or bookstore search will reveal many more.

Other alternative/home remedies for ADHD

Other therapies that may benefit ADHD include those discussed in Table 18.7. Even though advocated by various sources (including some of those in the previously cited list of references), treatments listed in Table 18.8 have *not* conclusively been shown to be effective in ADHD. For any given treatment modality, there may be case reports,

Table 18.7 ADHD therapies that have some evidence-based support

---

- *Fish oil (essential fatty acids)* – as has been stated elsewhere in this text, the use of omega-3 fatty acids has shown a limited but useful role in minimizing symptoms of mood disorders. As precursors of neuronal development, there is limited evidence that omega-3 fatty acids may have a beneficial effect in ADHD, but at the time of this writing, the issue remains unclear and further research is necessary.[1–3]

- *EEG biofeedback/neurofeedback training* – this modality involves connecting the patient to an electroencephalograph while performing designated tasks. The patient "learns" to train his/her brain by monitoring changes in EEG wave patterns as certain behaviors are performed. Although still early in its development and utilization, there is evidence-based support that this treatment may be helpful for ADHD. Further larger-scale studies and refinement of the technique are necessary.[4–6]

Sources:

1 Richardson AJ *et al.* (2002) The Oxford-Durham study: a randomized, controlled trial of dietary supplementation in children with specific learning difficulties. *Progress in Neuro-Psychopharmacology and Biological Psychiatry* 26(2): 233–239.
2 Sinn N and Bryant J (2007) Effect of supplementation with polyunsaturated fatty acids and micronutrients on learning and behavior problems associated with child ADHD. *Journal of Developmental & Behavioral Pediatrics* 28(2): 82–91.
3 Richardson AJ and Montgomery P (2005) Children with developmental coordination disorder. *Pediatrics* 115(5): 1360–1366.
4 Monastra VJ (2008) *Unlocking the Potential of Patients with ADHD: A Model for Clinical Practice*, American Psychological Association.
5 Monastra VJ *et al.* (2006) Electroencephalographic biofeedback in the treatment of attention-deficit/hyperactivity disorder, investigations in neuromodulation, neurofeedback and applied neuroscience. *Journal of Neurotherapy* 9(4): 5–34.
6 Lubar JF *et al.* (1995) Evaluation of the effectiveness of EEG neurofeedback training for ADHD in a clinical setting as measured by changes in T.O.V.A. scores, behavioral ratings, and WISC-R performance. *Applied Biofeedback and Psychophysiology* 20(1): 83–99.

Table 18.8 Purported ADHD therapies that in general are *not* adequately evidence based

---

- *Yoga and meditation* – while intuitively it might seem that activities such as yoga and meditation with their calming properties would reduce ADHD symptoms, there is no conclusive evidence that this is so.

- *Vitamin, mineral or herbal supplements* – vitamins and mineral supplementation may be important for overall good health particularly in those children who have extremely poor diets. There is no evidence, however, that supplemental vitamins and minerals, including so-called "megadoses" of vitamins, are helpful for ADHD. "Megadoses" may actually be harmful. St. John's Wort has specifically been shown not to be helpful.

- *ADHD special diets* – a wide variety of dietary regimens have been suggested as treatment for ADHD, including those that limit caffeine, sugar, artificial food colorings and common allergens such as wheat, milk and eggs. Although there are sporadic research studies for any given special diet, consistent and replicable evidence has not been shown for any one dietary plan being helpful. Specifically, limiting refined sugar in the diet does *not* help ADHD children.

Sources: Sawni A (2008) Attention-deficit/hyperactivity disorder and complementary/alternative medicine. *Adolescent Medicine: State of the Art Reviews* 19(2): 313–326, xi; Brue AW and Oakland TD (2002) Alternative treatments for attention-deficit/hyperactivity disorder: does evidence support their use? *Alternative Therapies in Health and Medicine* 8(1): 68–70, 72–74; www.mayoclinic.com/health/adult-adhd/DS01161/DSECTION=treatments-and-drugs

Table 18.9 Warning signs of possible stimulant misuse

• Frequent or continuous requests for increased dosage levels
• Missed appointments and inconsistent attendance at follow-up appointments
• Repeated lost prescriptions or requests for an early refill
• Calls for an emergency supply of medication
• Symptoms of psychosis (especially hallucinations which can occur at high doses of stimulants)
• Syncope, shortness of breath and palpitations (all of which can occur at elevated stimulant doses)
• Insistent demands for immediate-release stimulants as opposed to time-release preparations
• Other behavioral signs of substance abuse (see Chapter 22)

Source: Narconon (2021) Signs and symptoms of amphetamine abuse, available at: www.narconon.org/drug-abuse/amphetamine-signs-symptoms.html

anecdotal evidence or small studies. To date though, none of these modalities has sufficient conclusive, replicable research to warrant recommendation for ADHD patients.

Abuse of stimulants

As outlined above, the process for prescribing stimulant medications is generally straightforward and not difficult. There is, however, one significant area relevant to stimulant prescription that can potentially create significant problems – medication misuse, abuse and diversion. This topic has been discussed in Chapter 10. The warning signs and behaviors of potential misuse are listed in Table 18.9.

When reading Table 18.9, further information on stimulant misuse and abuse, screening for these disorders and the use of clinician "Contracts" and "Advisories" when prescribing stimulants can be found in Chapter 10.

Notes and references

1 National Institute of Mental Health (2017) Attention-Deficit/Hyperactivity Disorder, available at: www.nimh.nih.gov/health/statistics/attention-deficit-hyperactivity-disorder-adhd.shtml

2 Centers for Disease Control (2008) Diagnosed attention deficit hyperactivity disorder and learning disability: United States, 2004–2006. *Vital and Health Statistics* 10(237): 1–14.

3 Bruchmüller K *et al.* (2012) Is ADHD diagnosed in accord with diagnostic criteria? Overdiagnosis and influence of client gender on diagnosis. *Journal of Consulting and Clinical Psychology*, 80(1): 128–138; Brain & Behavior Research Foundation (2019) The first robust genetic markers for ADHD are reported, available at: www.bbrfoundation.org/content/first-robust-genetic-markers-adhd-are-reported

4 Brain & Behavior Research Foundation (2019) The first robust genetic markers for ADHD are reported, available at: www.bbrfoundation.org/content/first-robust-genetic-markers-adhd-are-reported

5 Rubia K *et al.* (2014) Imaging the ADHD brain: disorder-specificity, medication effects and clinical translation. *Expert Review of Neurotherapeutics* 14(5): 519–538.

6 Joszt L (2017) Brain MRIs can identify ADHD and distinguish among subtypes, available at: www.ajmc.com/newsroom/brain-mris-can-identify-adhd-and-distinguish-among-subtypes

7 Biederman ME *et al.* (2002) Case-control study of attention-deficit hyperactivity disorder and maternal smoking, alcohol use, and drug use during pregnancy. *Journal of the American Academy of Child and Adolescent Psychiatry* 41(4): 378–385.

8   Braun J *et al.* (2006) Exposures to environmental toxicants and attention-deficit/hyperactivity disorder in U.S. children. *Environmental Health Perspectives* 114(12): 1904–1909.

9   Ibid.

10 Voeller KKS (2004) Attention-Deficit Hyperactivity Disorder, available at: www.medscape.com/viewarticle/495640_3

11 Ibid.

12 Arnsten AFT *et al.* (2009) The emerging neurobiology of attention deficit hyperactivity disorder: the key role of the prefrontal association cortex. *Journal of Pediatrics* 154(5): I–S43. doi: 10.1016/j.jpeds.2009.01.018

13 Volkow ND *et al.* (2009) Evaluating dopamine reward pathway in ADHD: clinical implications. *Journal of the American Medical Association* 302: 1084–1091.

14 Ibid.

15 Konrad K and Eickhoff S (2010) Is the ADHD brain wired differently? A review on structural and functional connectivity in attention deficit hyperactivity disorder. *Human Brain Mapping* 31: 904–916.

16 Ibid.

17 Clarke AL *et al.* (2003) Hyperkinetic disorder in the ICD-10: EEG evidence for a definitional widening? *European Child & Adolescent Psychiatry* 12(2): 92–99.

18 Ibid.

19 Khan SA and Farone SV (2006) The genetics of attention-deficit disorder: a literature review of 2005. *Current Psychiatry Reports* 8: 393–397.

20 McCann D *et al.* (2007) Food additives and hyperactive behaviour in 3-year-old and 8/9-year-old children in the community: a randomized, double-blinded, placebo-controlled trial. *Lancet* 370(9598): 1560–1567.

21 Arnold LE *et al.* (2012) Artificial food colors and Attention-Deficit/Hyperactivity symptoms: conclusions to dye for. *Neurotherapeutics* 9(3): 599–609.

22 Kanarek RB (2011) Artificial food dyes and attention deficit hyperactivity disorder. *Nutrition Reviews* 69: 385.

23 Krull KR (2019) Attention deficit hyperactivity disorder in children and adolescents: epidemiology and pathogenesis, available at: www.uptodate.com/contents/attention-deficit-hyperactivity-disorder-in-children-and-adolescents-epidemiology-and-pathogenesis

24 Karic S *et al.* (2019) The association between attention deficit hyperactivity disorder severity and risk of mild traumatic brain injury in children with attention deficit hyperactivity disorder in the United States of America: a cross-sectional study of data from the National Survey of Children with Special Health Care Needs. *Child: Care, Health and Development* 45(5): 688–693. doi: 10.1111/cch.12684

25 Busting the sugar–hyperactivity myth, available at: www.webmd.com/parenting/features/busting-sugar-hyperactivity-myth#

26 Kim Y and Chang H (2011) Correlation between attention deficit hyperactivity disorder and sugar consumption, quality of diet, and dietary behavior in school children. *Nutrition Research and Practice* 5(3): 236–245. doi: 10.4162/nrp.2011.5.3.236

27 CHADD (2018) Vaccines have no role in ADD, available at: https://chadd.org/adhd-weekly/vaccines-have-no-role-in-adhd/

28 Brennan D (2020) Do vaccines cause autism?, available at: www.webmd.com/brain/autism/do-vaccines-cause-autism

29 Perrin JM *et al.* (2008) Cardiovascular monitoring and stimulant drugs for attention-deficit/hyperactivity disorder. *Pediatrics* 122(2): 451–453.

30 Available at: www.addwarehouse.com/shopsite_sc/store/html/product52.html

31 Available at: https://dss.mo.gov/mhd/cs/psych/pdf/adhd_scoring_parent.pdf

32 Available at: www.adhdclinicjeeva.com/diagnosis/snap-iv-C-6160C-80tems.pdf

33 Schneider H and Eisenberg D (2006) Who receives a diagnosis of attention-deficit/hyperactivity disorder in the United States elementary school population? *Pediatrics* 117(4): e601–e609.

34 Barbaresi WJ *et al.* (2013) Mortality, ADHD, and psychosocial adversity in adults with childhood ADHD: a prospective study. *Pediatrics* 131(4): 637–644. doi: 10.1542/peds.2012-2354

35 Agnew-Blais JC *et al.* (2016) Persistence, remission and emergence of ADHD in young adulthood: results from a longitudinal, prospective population-based cohort. *JAMA Psychiatry* 73(7): 713–720. doi: 10.1001/jamapsychiatry.2016.0465

36 Conrad P and Potter D (2000) Hyperactive children to ADHD Adults, 2000. *Social Problems* 4(4): 559–582.

37 Tom CM (2005) Recognizing and treating ADHD in adolescents and adults. *US Pharmacist* 30(1): 67–76.

38 Gentile JA and Gillig PM (2006) Adult ADHD: diagnosis, differential diagnosis, and medication management. *Psychiatry* 3(8): 25–30.

39 Kessler RC *et al.* (2006) The prevalence and correlates of adult ADHD in the United States: results from the National Comorbidity Survey Replication. *American Journal of Psychiatry* 163: 716–723.

40 National Institute of Mental Health (2017) Attention-Deficit/Hyperactivity Disorder, available at: https://www.nimh.nih.gov/health/statistics/attention-deficit-hyperactivity-disorder-adhd.shtml

41 Ibid.

42 Searight HA *et al.* (2000) Adult ADHD: evaluation and treatment in family medicine. *American Family Physician* 62(9): 2077–2086.

43 Cleveland Clinic (2016) Attention Deficit Hyperactivity Disorder (ADHD): stimulant therapy, available at: https://my.clevelandclinic.org/health/treatments/11766-attention-deficit-hyperactivity-disorder-adhd-stimulant-therapy

44 Bhandari S (2021) Stimulant medications for ADHD, available at: https://www.webmd.com/add-adhd/adhd-stimulant-therapy#1

45 Simpson D and Plosker GL (2004) Spotlight on atomoxetine in adults with attention-deficit hyperactivity disorder. *CNS Drugs* 18(6): 397–401.

Part IV

Medication dilemmas and their clinical management

19 Side effects of psychotropic medications and their treatment

- During the initial evaluation   290
- Useful advice to patients   292
- Side-effect assessment in follow-up visits   293
- How much of a problem is it?   293
- Other issues to consider in evaluating side effects   294
- Changing medication due to side effects   295
- Severity of side effects   295
- Side effects and clinical response   296
- The novice clinician and side effects   296
- Side effects seen most frequently   297
- Sedation   298
- Overactivation/anxiety   299
- Nausea and gastrointestinal problems   304
- Sexual interference   306
- Weight gain   311
- Headaches   318
- Asthenia/weakness   318
- Dry mouth   319
- Hair loss   319
- Skin reactions   321
- Prolactin elevation   322
- Hypotension   324
- Falls   324
- Elevation of blood sugar and lipids   325
- Hyponatremia   326
- Suicidality   328
- Side effects and medication combinations   329
- References   329

Any healthcare practitioner who is legally authorized to prescribe medication can write a prescription for a psychotropic medication. One of the distinguishing characteristics of the knowledgeable practitioner, who will maintain greater success with mental health patients, is the practitioner who can successfully manage the side effects of a medication. The manner in which a practitioner discusses side effects can have a major impact on whether the person takes the medication, or becomes a frightened, non-compliant patient. Some practitioners will ignore or fail to assess side effects because they don't know how to offer solutions if the patient admits to having them. This chapter will discuss the common and potentially uncomfortable side effects that occur with psychotropic medications, and how the astute clinician can manage them. Less common, but potentially more serious, adverse reactions are discussed in Chapter 20.

During the initial evaluation

For many patients, the risk of side effects is *a* major, or in some cases, *the* major issue in taking psychotropic medications. The popular press now describes many mental health medications in detail, including possible side effects. With the vast amount of information available on the Internet, patients often come to the office armed with a series of questions about what potential unwanted effects may be associated with a prescribed medication. If a patient brings up the issue of side effects early in the initial interview, it is wise to suggest that the evaluation first be completed to determine *if* medication is needed and *which* medication might be most helpful. The clinician should reassure the patient that side-effect issues will be covered before treatment decisions are made.

Discussing the side effects of a medication

For the typical physically healthy individual, serious side effects with psychotropics are remarkably rare and the clinician can be genuinely optimistic that medications prescribed are unlikely to cause significant harm. For physically compromised patients, or for patients taking a complicated medical regimen, there may be some risk of adding a psychotropic. When present, these risk issues need to be individualized and discussed with each patient as their situation dictates. Table 19.1 lists some facts regarding psychotropics and side effects.

When the time comes to introduce the issue of side effects, toward the end of the initial evaluative session for a routine patient without special risk factors, the concept can be introduced as suggested here.

 Box 19.1 Talking to patients

"Most people take this medication without side effects, and that is what I expect for you. As with any medication, however, there can be some unwanted effects. Fortunately, if these unwanted effects occur, they are usually of the annoying, short-term variety, and are not serious or life-threatening. If anything is not mild or is not going away, I want you to call me, so together we can decide how to proceed."

Table 19.1 Facts regarding psychotropics and side effects

- Most side effects of psychotropics are more annoying than serious
- Life-threatening or irreversible side effects are rare
- Many side effects are remediable or pass with time

If patients have read about or heard of specific side effects, or are especially fearful of a particular adverse reaction, these possibilities must be addressed specifically. Many times, the patient's concerns can be alleviated with simple reassurance and, in fact, the side effect of concern may be of minimal likelihood with the medication to be prescribed. If the side effect the patient is concerned about *is* a possibility with the particular medication chosen, acknowledge this with:

Box 19.2 Talking to patients

"Yes, that has been reported with some, but not most, patients. [Include any data or statistics to approximate the frequency, if known.] *I know you are concerned about this and we will be watching for this possibility carefully. If it emerges as a problem, we will deal with it at that time. However, I do not believe the small possibility of the problem should stop you from beginning the medication. How do you feel about this plan?"*

Usually this is sufficient to have the patient begin treatment. If the patient does remain resistant or highly skeptical, the clinician should outline what, if any, other medication alternatives might be tried and the reasons the initial recommendation has been made. Often, having heard the clinician's thinking and rationale, the patient can proceed with a trial of the first-choice medication. On occasion, a patient may insist on a second-line choice, even when its therapeutic potential is less, because it avoids or minimizes a particular side effect. As long as the clinician feels the choice has some reasonable chance of success, it is a good idea to form a contract to use a second choice of medication initially if it means the patient can be adherent. If, because of side effect fears, a patient is requesting a clinically inappropriate medication, of course the clinician needs to discuss why he or she will not agree to this prescription. The death of singer Michael Jackson, when he was inappropriately prescribed proprofol for sleep, shows the potentially serious problems which can result when a clinician agrees to prescribe an inappropriate medication at a patient's request.

Even if the patient brings no information about side effects, it is important to cover a few common side effects that might occur with any medication prescribed. The key to success is striking a balance between identifying some possible side effects while refraining from frightening the patient with a litany of possible, but unlikely, adverse consequences.

Box 19.3 Talking to patients

For example, when prescribing an SSRI antidepressant, you might say: *"Most people take these medicines without problem. If there are going to be any side effects, the most common ones tend to be upset stomach, diarrhea, headaches, sleepiness, agitation or some interference with sexual arousal. If you get any of these problems and they are mild, bear with them because they will often pass within several days to a week. If the side effects are not mild or are not passing, be sure to let me know so that we can decide how to fix the problem."*

For a discussion of a side effect that is serious and carries significant risk for this patient, the representative presentations shown here can serve as models.

Box 19.4 Talking to patients

To an elderly schizophrenic patient in the hospital who might be at risk for a fall: *"Mrs. Fisher, I am going to prescribe* [name of medication] *to help decrease the voices in your head that you have told me about. This medicine is a good choice for you. However, the medicine has the possibility of making you somewhat sleepy or lightheaded.*

Therefore, we will start with a small dose and evaluate how you tolerate it. I do not want you to fall or lose your balance. Please get up slowly when you have been lying down or sitting, or ask for assistance from the nursing staff. Also, tell them if you feel light-headed or dizzy."

When prescribing carbamazepine (which could lower the estrogen levels via P-450 enzyme induction – see Chapter 20) to a patient on birth control pills: *"In prescribing carbamazepine, there is a possibility that this medication may cause your body to break down estrogen more quickly and could lower the birth control protection from your low-dose estrogen pills. We have tried several other mood stabilizers without success, and your symptoms remain significant. I believe carbamazepine is now the best choice to help you feel more stable. I want you to contact your Ob/Gyn practitioner to change your birth control pill to one with a higher strength of estrogen before we begin this medication. If you like, I will call him/her to explain why I am suggesting this."*

Useful advice to patients

While some side effects will occur despite the best efforts of the prescriber and the patient, two useful recommendations should be made to all patients. These can prevent inadvertent side effects or, in rare cases, serious Danger Zones as discussed in Chapter 20:

> *"Before you leave the pharmacy (or when you receive the medication in the mail), be sure your name is on each container's label. Also be sure the right drug name and dose is on the label."*
>
> *"If the pills look different or unfamiliar, or if you have any questions or concerns, speak with the pharmacist or call the mail-order pharmacy service before taking any dose."*

Some practitioners hand out a small sheet with these precautions to patients when they are given prescriptions. Others have ancillary staff make these reminders or large-lettered signs are posted where they can be seen as the patients exit the office.

Side-effect assessment in follow-up visits

If a clinician does not ask about side effects and intervene when necessary, the patient will stop the medication or drop out of treatment!

Asking the patient if he or she is experiencing any unwanted effects from the medicine is mandatory for each of the first several follow-up appointments, at least until such time as the patient is stabilized and is clearly tolerating the medicine without problem. *Do not assume that the patient will spontaneously volunteer side-effect information.*

When the practitioner learns of any side effects, the following questions will help to identify a course of action and/or remedy:

- What changes, sensations or symptoms are you experiencing? (Have the patient first describe facts, not their own assessment, beliefs or assumptions about the cause.)
- How often do you feel this?
- Is there any pattern to when this occurs?
- When, in relation to taking the medication, does the problem occur?
- Is the problem diminishing or intensifying with time?
- Does anything make the problem better or worse?
- How troublesome is this for you? (Use a 1–10 numerical scale.)

For example, if a patient complains of nausea, this fact alone is insufficient information. The clinician needs to know when the nausea occurs. Is it constant? Does it occur at specific times of the day? Does it occur within an hour or two of taking the pill, or at other times as well? Does it interfere with sleep, or occur in the middle of the night? Is it accompanied by vomiting? Have the patient's eating habits been affected by the nausea? Only with these data can the clinician decide to lower or split the dose, prescribe it at bedtime, add an antinauseant, or change the psychotropic medication.

How much of a problem is it?

With any given side effect, it is crucial to find out how severe and troublesome this particular side effect is to this particular patient. Individuals have very different tolerances for adverse effects of medication. For example, some people are remarkably tolerant of gastrointestinal side effects and others are intensely bothered. Likewise, headache, sexual interference and weight gain may be acceptable consequences for some individuals, and be absolutely intolerable, even when mild, to others. As discussed in Chapter 6, quantification of the patient's words is often helpful to the clinician in evaluating side effects as well.

 Box 19.5 Clinical tip

It is useful to have the patient quantify the amount of the particular side effect on a scale of 0–10, with 0 being no side effects at all, 1 being minimal and 10 being maximal. Such clarification can help the clinician decide if a side effect is of a magnitude to require intervention or a change of medications.

Box 19.6 Talking to patients

Ask the patient: *"On a scale of 0 to 10, where zero is 'I am never bothered by this problem' and 10 is 'I am extremely bothered by this problem all the time,' how does this affect you?"* In general, side effects rated by the patient as a 4 or above will almost always require intervention. A patient rating of 1 to 3, particularly if the side effect is beginning to wane, is often tolerable, at least for a short time. Mentally, the clinician may adjust the patient's rating of a side effect up or down the scale depending on the clinician's assessment of the consequences of the side effect. For example, headache, fatigue or sexual interference are bothersome, but usually do not have serious imminent sequelae for healthy patients. The clinician may mentally move the patient's rating down slightly, even though it is bothersome to the patient. The occurrence of a seizure, changes in blood cell counts, severely decreased or increased blood pressure, repetitive vomiting, marked changes of liver function or the onset of tardive dyskinesia have potential serious outcomes and sequelae. The clinician may mentally move the rating of this type of side effect higher, even if the patient's rating is not particularly high (patients do not always appreciate the gravity of some side effects).

Other issues to consider in evaluating side effects

Just because a patient complains of a side effect that he or she believes is a direct effect of the medication, this may or may not be the case. Further detailed inquiry is essential. The clinician should first look for other causes besides the prescription that may account for the unwanted effect. Inquire about any recent medications prescribed by other practitioners, herbal or over-the-counter medications, food intolerances or changes in sleep and/or activity schedules that correlate in time with the onset of the complaint.

The clinician should next consider possible indirect effects relative to the medication prescribed. For example, P-450 interactions may change the blood levels of other medications the patient is taking, and these blood level changes can result in the patient experiencing adverse effects without them actually being a direct side effect of the medication prescribed (see Chapter 20).

Third, the practitioner should assess the frequency of the particular side effect described: Is it continuous or intermittent? Does it occur most or all days, or relatively infrequently?

Fact: Most psychotropic medication side effects are typically continuous or very frequent. Side effects that occur once a week or several times a month are often, at least in part, related to other causes, and are not solely due to the psychotropic. Side effects that occur for several days and then are totally absent for weeks or months are again much less likely to be related directly to the psychotropic.

Occasionally a psychotropic can predispose an individual to a side effect that can then be precipitated by a second independent cause. If this is the case, modifying the second external cause may allow the patient to continue taking the psychotropic without a need to change medication. For example, a psychotropic may cause loose bowel movements. While this may be tolerable in general to the patient, significant diarrhea occurs only when certain foods are eaten. Rather than discontinuing the psychotropic, the simple solution is to identify and temporarily avoid the offending food while the medication is being prescribed.

Fourth, the timing of the side effect in relation to ingestion should be assessed. Side effects that occur within 30 minutes to an hour after taking the pills are often related to a rapid rise in blood concentration to a high peak level and/or irritation of the stomach lining by the medication. Symptoms such as an upset stomach, headache, nausea or nervousness that only occur shortly after taking the pill may be minimized if the medication is taken at bedtime. As long as the side effect is not severe enough to awaken the patient, the problem may have diminished enough to be tolerable upon waking. Side effects from high peak blood levels can also be improved by lowering the total daily dose, or dividing the dose into two or more smaller quantities taken at different times of the day.

Changing medication due to side effects

A frequent dilemma facing a clinician is whether or not to change medications because of side effects. In addition to the severity of the side effect, the clinician should take into account:

- the patient's therapeutic response to the medication so far
- the presence or absence of suitable alternatives
- the length of time that the patient has been on the medication
- the patient's individual concerns and wishes.

Severity of side effects

Side effects can be classified as mild, moderate, significant or serious. The clinician's response will vary depending upon the classification. For *mild* side effects (1 to 2 on the scale previously mentioned), education and labeling the symptom as a side effect, along with reassurance, is all that is usually necessary. Sometimes a watch-and-wait approach will allow the symptom to disappear, but, in any case, the course of the side effect should be re-evaluated at follow-up visits.

For *moderately intrusive* side effects (3 to 5 on the scale), there may be ways to remedy the problem without actually changing medications. These may include splitting the dosage, taking the medication at a different time of day, changing to a long-acting formulation of the medication or recommending changes in diet and/or exercise.

For more *significant* side effects, either because of the patient's discomfort or the clinician's assessment of possible risk (6 to 8 on the scale), it is absolutely essential that the side effects be addressed specifically and promptly. If not, the patient may drop out of treatment or, at the very least, stop the medication, sometimes without telling the clinician.

For *serious* side effects, again either because of the patient's discomfort or the clinician's assessment of risk (9 or 10 on the scale), it is imperative that the clinician responds quickly and decisively. For example, with the onset of a seizure or a fainting episode leading to unconsciousness, it is essential to address the issue, discontinue the medication or significantly reduce the dosage. Specialty consultation with a neurologist or internist may be necessary to evaluate other causes for such symptoms. Other examples requiring prompt action would be serious abnormalities of laboratory testing, such as drops in white blood count (to less than 1500 absolute neutrophil count),[1] platelet count (below 100,000 per cubic millimeter) or a marked increase in liver function tests (above two or three times normal). The clinician needs to communicate the need for a prompt evaluation to the patient and, if appropriate, to the patient's family. These more serious risk issues will be covered in more detail in Chapter 20. Even if the medical risk of the side effect is small, when a patient rates a side effect at 4 or above on the basis of discomfort and/or frequency, the clinician should act promptly if adherence is to be maintained.

When serious side effects occur, the clinician's written records are crucial and provide documentation of his or her assessment, thinking and interventions. In the event of medico-legal action because of serious adverse consequences from medication, the written medical record provides the best defense. Such documentation should reflect:

- the onset of the symptoms/side effects; i.e., when did they start?
- when the clinician was made aware of these complaints
- exactly what recommendations were made regarding remediation
- any dosage changes instituted
- when, and if, the medication was recommended to be stopped
- any specific behavioral precautions that were advised.

Side effects and clinical response

When the patient is receiving a strong positive therapeutic response to a medication and/or there are few or poor alternatives available, a mild to moderate side effect should generally be managed by watching and waiting, adding a non-prescription remedy or adding a prescription remedy. Ultimately, if these interventions are unsuccessful, changing medications may be the only option, even if the alternatives are less desirable.

If, on the other hand, the patient is having a mediocre response and/or there are good alternatives for change, the clinician will likely change medications sooner. It is always possible to return to medication A, if medication B is tried unsuccessfully. If the patient is only having a mediocre or poor therapeutic response, changing medications may provide two benefits – engendering a more positive treatment response, as well as minimizing side effects. Therefore, with a mediocre response, changing medications should be tried before trying non-prescription or prescription remedies for the side effect itself. These alternatives were summarized in Table 6.1.

The novice clinician and side effects

If a patient complains of side effects, it is appropriate to empathize with the patient's discomfort without denial or defensiveness. The novice clinician may feel uncomfortable at having caused seeming harm or discomfort to the patient. Side effects are possible with the prescription of any medication, and the presence of side effects does not necessarily indicate bad practice or poor decision-making.

When beginning the practice of psychotropic prescription, the volume and variation of multiple side effects for the spectrum of mental health medications may seem overwhelming to the novice clinician. To recognize and manage side effects effectively, novice clinicians and non-mental health practitioners initially do well to become knowledgeable about one or two medications in each class of psychotropic. Understanding the medication side-effect profiles for several medications will form an effective knowledge base that can be broadened once the clinician has more experience. If, alternatively, at the outset of a career, the novice clinician attempts to learn and prescribe, for example, eight different mood stabilizers, it will be difficult and confusing to remember the side-effect profile of each.

Box 19.7 Primary care

If you do not prescribe psychotropics commonly, it is better to know one or two medications from each class well, rather than attempting to be superficially familiar with the universe of psychotropics.

Is it a side effect or not?

The use of print, media and Internet resources, as well as personal consultation from colleagues, are important ways to learn about side effects. The *Physician's Desk Reference* (*PDR*), the USP formulary and package-insert prescribing information can be helpful in sorting out what may or may not be a side effect of a particular drug. Additionally, all pharmaceutical companies maintain telephone support lines for medication prescribers that can be useful sources of data about potential side effects of their products. These telephone numbers are listed by company at the beginning of the *PDR*. Ultimately, even with appropriate input, a clinician may not know whether a side effect or complaint is actually related to a medication. *At times, the only way to assess whether a side effect is related to a particular medication is to stop the medication and observe.*

When appropriate, the practitioner should not hesitate to admit lack of certainty about a particular drug fact or possible side effect. It is better for the practitioner to investigate the question and get back to the patient rather than attempt to appear assured when he or she is not, and guess.

Almost all side effects referable to psychotropic medications pass quickly and should be totally eliminated within 7–14 days of stopping the medication. If a patient continues to complain of side effects weeks or months after discontinuation of the medication, it is highly unlikely that such a side effect was related to the psychotropic, and other etiologies should be evaluated.

Side effects seen most frequently

The most common side effects of psychotropic medications are listed in Table 19.2. Assessment and remedies are discussed in the following text.

The first two sections focus on opposite side effects; namely, sedation and overactivation. Both are common, but each presents different challenges to the prescriber. Sedation is usually a relatively simple and straightforward side effect.

Overactivation is more complicated, and may have widely differing root causes with markedly differing remedies.

Table 19.2 Common side effects of psychotropic medications

- Sedation
- Overactivation
- Nausea and other gastrointestinal problems
- Sexual dysfunction
- Weight gain
- Headaches
- Asthenia (weakness)
- Dry mouth
- Hair loss
- Skin reactions
- Prolactin elevation
- Hypotension
- Falls
- Elevation of blood sugar and lipids
- Hyponatremia
- Suicidality

Sedation

When taking psychotropic medication, sedation (often perceived as sleepiness or grogginess) is one of the single most commonly reported side effects. Sedation that occurs when starting medication may or may not be related directly to the medication itself. When patients have been deprived of sleep from their illness, sleeping longer than normal for up to a week may represent them "catching up" on lost rest. During the first week, if it is not incapacitating, a wait-and-watch approach is appropriate, as their normal sleep pattern may emerge.

Sedation, when present, is not always undesirable. In an agitated or anxious patient, some daytime sleepiness may contribute to calmness during the initial period of symptom resolution. This then becomes a specific application of the general principle mentioned above, which states that side-effect tolerance is very individualized for each patient. In this case, what may be intolerable for one patient may be tolerable and even desirable for another.

There are, however, patients with no history of sleep deprivation who become sleepy with psychotropics that cause daytime sleepiness at the outset or with dosage increase. If the sedation is medication related and mild, allowing 7–14 days for accommodation is prudent and may allow patients to adjust satisfactorily.

Historically, patients were dosed with psychotropics throughout the day in the belief that this was necessary in order to achieve optimal therapeutic response. Current practice is that antidepressant, antipsychotic or mood-stabilizing response can usually be obtained with once-daily dosing.

Box 19.8 Clinical tip

The vast majority of psychotropic medications do not need to be given multiple times a day to be effective.

If medication doses taken during waking hours cause daytime sleepiness, a simple remedy may be to move all the medication to bedtime dosing. In this way, the sedative side effect may provide a useful sleep aid. For patients who require daytime dosing of potentially sedative medications, consider giving a smaller daytime dose and a larger bedtime amount. For example, a patient may tolerate 10–25 percent of their full dose in the morning and receive 75–90 percent at bedtime without daytime sleepiness. This plan can, however, present problems for the patient who complains of grogginess in the morning after taking the larger dose of medicine at bedtime. Moving the evening medication dose to earlier in the evening, particularly if the sedative effect of the medication takes several hours to emerge, may minimize morning hangover. Taking the medication at 8 p.m. or at dinner often significantly decreases morning grogginess. As a last resort, for a medication that is very effective and for which there are not available alternatives, divide the total dose into three or four small doses throughout the day, and have the patient tolerate a consistent mild to moderate amount of daytime sedation.

If a medication causes marked intolerable sleepiness, or several weeks of attempts at accommodation have not met with success, a change in medication should be undertaken. Fortunately, within each of the major classes of medications there are generally alternatives that will be less sedative to individual patients. It may take several trials to find a medication that is minimally sedative to each particular patient. Within the *antidepressants*, there are several choices that for most patients will be less sedative. These include bupropion, desipramine, fluoxetine and venlafaxine. Within the *atypical antipsychotics*, ziprasidone may be a less sedating choice. Within the *traditional antipsychotic* class, molindone or loxapine may be less sedating. Within the *mood-stabilizer* category, each medication in general comes from a different chemical class and their tendency to promote sedation may vary greatly. Therefore, individual tolerances for the sedative effect of mood stabilizers may also vary, and it may be necessary to try several different medications to find a non-sedative option for a particular patient. Benzodiazepine *anti-anxiety medications*, as a class, offer no options that are "non-sedative." Here, patient tolerance becomes the crucial variable. Shorter half-life drugs such as lorazepam or alprazolam may sedate for less time than their longer-acting cousins – diazepam, clorazepate or chlordiazepoxide.

It should be noted that, *although these generalizations are made, individual sensitivity to the sedative effect of any particular medication can vary greatly.* Some patients may experience significant sleepiness on any of the medications listed above, even if that medication is less sedative in general.

Overactivation/anxiety

An overactivated response to psychotropic medication may show itself in a variety of forms, and may be signaled by different symptoms, including:

- feelings of mental nervousness or agitation
- internal restlessness
- difficulty in falling or staying asleep
- shakiness/tremor
- feeling emotionally "out of control"
- feeling mentally speeded/pressured or "unable to slow down."

Table 19.3 Potential causes of overactivation as a side effect

---

- Nervousness
- Akathisia
- Hypomania
- Sleeplessness
- Tremor alone

Before automatically assuming that the cause of a complaint of overactivation is the medication, the patient should be evaluated for other causes that are not directly related to the medication, such as:

- excessive caffeine intake
- ingestion of non-prescribed stimulants, including appetite suppressants, diet pills and "energizing" herbs
- use of recreational drugs, including cocaine and amphetamines
- excessive work pressure, family or life stressors.

If all these causes have been ruled out or are minimal, medication side effect should be suspected and the various possibilities considered separately.

The five potential causes of overactivation are shown in Table 19.3. Each is a separate entity, and has a markedly different solution. In order to remedy overactivation satisfactorily, accurate assessment is essential to decide which cause is present.

Nervousness

A patient who is prescribed a psychotropic may complain of mental anxiety, of feeling agitated or being restless. The nervousness can be solely internal without external signs, or may additionally show tremor and/or sweating externally.

Such nervousness is most commonly associated with non-sedating antidepressants (see above), but can also occasionally occur with mood stabilizers and antipsychotics. In general, if nervousness alone is present (without any of the other symptoms of overactivation, discussed in the following subsections) and is mild, the patient should be reassured that this most likely will pass. If the symptom persists, decreasing the dose of the medication may, for some patients, make the regimen tolerable. As a last resort, the addition of a small dose of a benzodiazepine (lorazepam 0.25–1 mg/day or clonazepam 0.25–1 mg/day) to the regimen for a several-week period of time may allow accommodation to the anxiety-causing medication.

For example, a patient on fluoxetine for depression may feel agitated and nervous. Using a small dose of a benzodiazepine for several weeks can allow the patient to accommodate to this nervousness, which will often pass with time. If the nervousness persists beyond the first several weeks when the benzodiazepine is withdrawn, switching antidepressants is the next alternative. On some occasions when switching is not desirable or possible, it may be necessary to continue taking the benzodiazepine for the entire period the patient is taking the offending primary psychotropic. While this is less desirable, if it allows a patient to take an antidepressant that is otherwise working well for depression it may be a satisfactory trade-off.

Anxiety and nervousness, as a side effect from medication, may not be mild and can present as frank panic attacks – either singly or in groups. This development may occur as a flare-up of previously quiescent panic attacks or occur *de novo* in a patient who has never previously experienced panic attacks. Panic attacks are acutely distressing and uncomfortable for the patient, and require a prompt response from the clinician. A PRN dose of a benzodiazepine (e.g., alprazolam, clonazepam or lorazepam 0.5–1 mg) will usually quell the immediate symptoms, but the medicine causing this side effect should be decreased in dose or discontinued entirely.

While this reaction may occur in patients who have never experienced an anxiety attack, it is more commonly seen in patients previously prone to these attacks. These individuals may be acutely sensitive to SSRIs or other antidepressants. A panic attack may occur with even the first dose. Should this occur, the medication should be decreased to a fraction of the usual starting dose and very gradually increased as tolerated by the patient. The patient usually accommodates to the slowly increasing dose with minimal discomfort.

There are rare patients who are exquisitely sensitive to antidepressants, and may react with excessive anxiety/panic to even a small amount. Such patients may be *very* slowly titrated on the medication using a liquid preparation, beginning with only a drop or two to start. Although it may take several months to reach a traditional therapeutic dose, the use of liquid medication does allow such depressed patients to be treated with an antidepressant. Patients who have previously experienced panic attacks with antidepressant medication therapy are understandably afraid of starting any antidepressant for fear it will again precipitate the attacks. Such patients benefit from being given wide latitude in when, and by how much, their antidepressant dosage is increased. With this sense of control, these patients develop confidence and proceed to a higher dose only when they are ready. Carrying a PRN "emergency" dose of benzodiazepine also provides extra assurance to these patients.

Akathisia

Akathisia, a sense of internal restlessness, is a common side effect with traditional antipsychotics, and may be perceived as overactivation. It is less typical with second-generation antipsychotics, but may still occur. Some antidepressants, particularly fluoxetine, bupropion and some tricyclics, may also cause akathisia. Patients with akathisia often have difficulty in describing their condition clearly. They will feel uncomfortable, at times intensely so, but have trouble articulating the source of their discomfort. They have difficulty sitting still, may pace and will become more agitated if they are not permitted to do so. They may describe the sense that their intestines are agitated or moving, even though no frank gastrointestinal symptoms are present. Such patients often present as fidgety in the office, and may have difficulty sitting in a chair throughout an interview. Persons with akathisia can be uncomfortable to the point of attempting drastic solutions to rid themselves of the feeling. Serious akathisia has been linked to attempted or completed suicide. It is critical for the clinician to have a high index of suspicion for akathisia with traditional antipsychotics. Immediate intervention is vital, since failing to diagnose this symptom can lead to fatal consequences.

Once akathisia is diagnosed, a reduction in dosage of the offending drug may help. Unfortunately, this side effect may continue, even at a lower dose, and a change to another class of antipsychotic is indicated. Akathisia with a traditional antipsychotic may abate with a change to an atypical antipsychotic.[2-4] If the patient has a particularly positive response to a medication *and* the clinician is hesitant to alter positive results, the addition of a beta blocker (for example, propranolol 20–60 mg), an anticholinergic (benztropine 1–2 mg) or a benzodiazepine (alprazolam 0.25–0.5 mg) may be a useful countermeasure to the akathisia.[5] In all cases, the patient should be closely monitored over time.

Hypomania

Antidepressants, atypical second-generation antipsychotics and even medications thought to be mood stabilizers can induce mania or hypomania (partial, mild manic symptoms). Hypomania can present with symptoms similar to other causes of overactivation discussed above, such as anxiety, panic attacks, internal restlessness, fidgeting and pacing. Hypomania, however, is also accompanied by other symptoms, including rapid speech, increased speed of thought, inability to sleep, a lack of need to sleep, impulsive behavior, displays of unusual energy or feelings of exceptional well-being.

The onset of such signs shortly after beginning an antidepressant points to a diagnosis of hypomania, although such mania may present at any time during the treatment with an antidepressant. Other classes of medications with antidepressant properties, including some mood stabilizers (for example, lamotrigine and topiramate) or atypical antipsychotics (ziprasidone, risperidone, olanzapine and quetiapine), may also cause hypomania as a side effect. This is paradoxical, since the intent of these medications is to stabilize mood and reduce mania.

Once new or unexpected manic/hypomanic symptoms present, a reconsideration of the diagnosis may be required. Patients who may have been previously assessed as having unipolar depression or dysthymia should often now be given a bipolar or cyclothymic diagnosis. Although some clinicians consider mania that solely occurs in the presence of an antidepressant as a separate subcategory of bipolar disorder, most clinicians will respond to antidepressant-induced mania in the same way as they would treat other subtypes of bipolar disorder.

Beyond re-diagnosing the patient, the clinician can remedy the hypomanic response by:

*   decreasing the dosage of the antidepressant
*   discontinuing the antidepressant
*   adding a mood stabilizer to the current dose of antidepressant.

It should be noted that most (if not all) patients with an antidepressant response leading to hypomania will revert to depression when the antidepressant is withdrawn.

Sleeplessness as a side effect

Another common overactivation side effect to antidepressants, but which may occur with some mood stabilizers as well, is sleeplessness. Patients may complain of difficulty falling asleep, sleep continuity disturbance or a worsening of a pre-existing sleep disturbance. If there are no other symptoms of akathisia or hypomania, sleeplessness alone may be treated in several ways. Moving the antidepressant dose away from bedtime to an earlier time in the day may minimize the sleep-disturbing effect. More often, however, some other remedy must be instituted. A sedative antidepressant, such as trazodone, mirtazapine, doxepin, nefazodone or trimipramine, can be added at bedtime to promote sleep. Other sedatives/hypnotics, such as a benzodiazepine, zolpidem or zaleplon, may be added briefly. A third option is to add valproic acid or an atypical antipsychotic (e.g., quetiapine) in small doses for the purposes of sleep alone. Particularly activating antidepressants may require some form of sleep medication frequently in the early stages of their use. Some depressed patients who are particularly sensitive to the sleep disruption may require sleep medication on a more chronic basis while they are treated.

Attention to sleep patterns is important, since adequate sleep is not just a comfort in patients with serious anxiety or depressive disorders; it is also healing and restorative. When an antidepressant is working well otherwise, it is reasonable to continue sleep medication on a longer-term basis if it is needed and if the alternative is sleep deprivation. (See Chapter 15 for further information about medication and sleep difficulties.)

Tremor

Some patients may interpret the presence of a tremor as suggestive of anxious overactivity, since it has been common in Western culture to assume that someone who shakes is anxious. While this may be true for some people, there are many patients with tremor who are minimally anxious or not anxious at all. Conversely, many anxious people will never experience tremor. Unaddressed, pronounced tremors may interfere with fine motor activities such as writing, eating, grasping objects or serving food, and be of significant embarrassment to patients. Psychotropics that have been associated with tremors are listed in Table 19.4.

If a patient develops a tremor while taking psychotropic medication, his or her caffeine intake should be assessed. Many patients may develop tremors or have existing tremors worsened for several hours by the ingestion of caffeine.

If caffeine is not the culprit and a tremor is deemed to be medication induced, small amounts of a beta blocker (e.g., propranolol 10–60 mg) or small amounts of a benzodiazepine (e.g., lorazepam or alprazolam 0.5 mg) can be considered. Since the anti-tremor effect of these remedies will only last for 3–6 hours, it may be necessary to repeat the dose several times to achieve control throughout the day.

Table 19.4 Medications used in mental health that can cause tremor

---

- Lithium
- SSRIs and other new-generation antidepressants
- Stimulants
- TCAs
- Thyroxine
- Traditional and atypical antipsychotics
- Valproic acid
- Verapamil

Source: Adapted from Conner GS (2001) Essential tremor: mechanisms and management, *Proceedings of a Symposium of Southern California Neurological Society*, ILab Publications, p. 30.

Several other antidotes with "effective" or "probably effective" ratings for essential tremor are identified by the American Academy of Neurology.[6] By extrapolation, although without hard evidence, they would probably be useful for medication-induced tremor. These include primidone, atenolol, gabapentin and topiramate. This latter list has not generally been used solely for medication-induced tremor, although if medications from these classes were being used for treatment of ancillary non-mental health diagnoses, it might be helpful to choose a specific medication on this list which might "kill two birds with one stone."

Patients with tremor may not need to have the tremor controlled throughout a 24-hour period. Many patients, for example, are only concerned about tremor during working hours, at times when their behaviors are observed or on occasions when they feel self-conscious. A beta blocker or benzodiazepine for tremor may be needed only at certain times during the day, or on certain days of the week, in order to make the situation bearable for the patient. Some patients may only use anti-tremor medication during the work week and omit the medication on weekends. Still others may use the anti-tremor medication only sporadically and intermittently, when they feel the tremor would be a particular hindrance. Responsible patients can be given significant latitude as to when, and how often, to use anti-tremor medication. Once-daily use of long-acting beta-blocker preparations (e.g., Inderal-LA 60 mg) may give satisfactory tremor control through most or all of the day without repeating the dose.

Careful questioning may reveal the patient to have had an "essential" or familial tremor that has worsened with the use of psychotropic medication. Such "essential" tremors may not respond to the above remedies, and a separate neurological evaluation is indicated to rule out potentially more significant neurological illness.

Nausea and gastrointestinal problems

Gastrointestinal (GI) side effects from gastric and bowel reactions to medications are common. They may present as upper gastrointestinal problems, such as:

- nausea or upset stomach
- dyspepsia
- gastric pain
- increased gas
- vomiting

Or as:

- lower GI distress and cramps
- diarrhea
- constipation.

Except for vomiting, recurrent diarrhea and severe constipation, these symptoms are not in general dangerous; however, they are often quite uncomfortable for the patient. GI side effects may also result in changes in appetite, eating habits and weight. Patients who, by history, tend to be concerned about bowel function may react strongly to even mild changes in bowel-movement frequency or consistency.

Nausea

As noted earlier, when patients complain of nausea with medication it is important to assess *when* the nausea occurs in relation to taking the dose, *how long* it lasts and when, if ever, it remits. Nausea that occurs shortly (30–90 minutes) after taking a dose of medication may result from an irritated stomach lining. In this situation, several remedies are useful:

- take the medication with food
- take the medication at bedtime; as long as the nausea does not disrupt sleep, it can disappear or be minimal by morning
- split one larger dose of medication into several smaller doses
- take over-the-counter antacids at the time of dosing.

If the nausea is severe, occurs throughout most of the day or does not remit with the above treatments, the psychotropic medication should be changed.

Constipation

For patients who experience constipation with psychotropic medications, the clinician must evaluate the medication in the context of the patient's lifestyle, including diet, activity level and other medications/foods that could be contributing to the problem. Although not limited to older adults, constipation is common in this population, particularly when multiple constipating medications are taken simultaneously. A geriatric lifestyle may be sedentary, and dietary preferences for dairy products and cheese may add to hardened stools and decreased bowel motility. When constipation occurs with the initiation of a psychotropic, remedies include:

- increased physical activity
- increased fluid intake
- increased dietary intake of fruits and vegetables
- psyllium husk (Metamucil) or other generic bulk-promoting preparations
- stool softeners such as bisacodyl
- preparations of senna, 20–60 mg per day
- a cholinesterase inhibitor (donepezil 5–10 mg) which often has diarrhea as a side effect.

If constipation is severe or is unresponsive to the above remedies, a change of medication is necessary.

Diarrhea

Mild diarrhea (or looser-than-normal stools) is not uncommon after beginning many psychotropic medications. If this is mild and infrequent, it is prudent to wait for up to a week to determine if bowel habits normalize. A slightly altered bowel habit, including more frequent or looser bowel movements, is not physiologically a serious problem, and reassurance to such individuals may be sufficient. If diarrhea persists beyond a few days, wakes the patient in the middle of the night or creates urgency resulting in fecal accidents, the patient's situation must be addressed promptly. Bulk preparations, while useful in constipation, may also be of some use in mild diarrhea. Over-the-counter antidiarrheal preparations such as loperamide hydrochloride (Imodium and others) may also be somewhat helpful for mild loose stools. A prescription medication such as diphenoxylate with atropine (Lomotil) is useful as a short-term treatment for diarrhea. Such preparations, however, are not appropriate long-term remedies. If diarrhea persists despite these remedies, or if the diarrhea recurs anytime the remedy is withdrawn, a change of medications is usually necessary.

Rarely, a medication may cause intense diarrhea or multiple episodes of diarrhea in a single day. Especially in children or individuals who might be affected by excessive fluid loss, the amount of diarrhea should be monitored carefully. Such intense diarrhea should not be allowed to continue for more than several days and it usually requires a change of medication

Sexual interference

As psychotropic medications have been used more commonly, their ability to interfere with sexual arousal, desire and performance has been well publicized. While previously, sexuality may have been an unspoken issue between prescriber and patient, it is now clearly within the purview of prescribing clinicians to address sexual issues, and it is a necessary area to be discussed when prescribing psychotropics.

Selective serotonin specific reuptake inhibitor (SSRI) antidepressants, as well as other antidepressants, mood stabilizers (particularly lithium and carbamazepine) and traditional and atypical antipsychotic medications are well known for sexual interference.[7] Decrease in desire for sex, decrease in physical arousability (male erection, female vaginal lubrication), increased time to ejaculation/orgasm and impaired ability to orgasm are common possible side effects of various psychotropics. Ideally, a patient's sexual functioning should be evaluated and documented prior to starting any medication. Since a decrease in sexual functioning or arousability is common in depressed, anxious and psychotic patients,[8-9] it is useful to ask about the level of sexual activity at the time of initial evaluation. Often because of time constraints, however, and particularly if the patient did not complain of sexual problems, the details of the patient's sexual behavior may not have been assessed or recorded. If a patient complains of a change in sexual behavior after a medication is started, it is important to assess the patient's level of sexual functioning prior to the medication as well as currently.

Even when the change in sexual behavior coincides with beginning medication, the clinician should inquire about other qualitative changes in the patient's sexual relationships, since not all changes in sexual activity are directly related to the medication. As patients begin to experience the benefit of psychotropic medications, they may also change partners, change the frequency of sexual activity or otherwise change their sexual behavior in a way that affects their arousability.

When evaluating potential sexual interference from medication, *the clinician must ask detailed, pointed questions about the frequency and quality of sexual activity, elucidating facts and behaviors rather than accepting broad statements.* Patients can often state: "This pill knocked the heck out of my sex life" or "I'm just not into sex anymore," or "I can't do it with my partner anymore." The clinician's questions must then be specific and direct about what changes have occurred in the patient's mental interest or physical arousal, to determine the etiology and possible remedies for the problem. Such questions include the following

1 *For both males and females*:
   • Are you mentally not interested in engaging in sexual activity as much as before?
   • Are you mentally interested, but have difficulty achieving essential physical elements of arousal?
   • Is there any evidence to suggest that a new or recent onset medical condition may be affecting sexual functioning? (Common medical and surgical conditions that can cause sexual dysfunction are listed in Table 19.5.)
   • Has there been a recent introduction of a non-psychotropic medication that could be affecting sexual function (such as those listed in Table 19.6)?

Table 19.5 Medical and surgical causes of sexual dysfunction

Medical illnesses associated with sexual dysfunction:
1 Cardiovascular
   • Atherosclerotic diseases
   • Hypertension
   • Myocardial infarction
   • Cardiac failure and angina
2 Renal
   • Chronic renal failure
3 Genitourinary
   • Pelvic-genital infection
   • Atrophic vaginitis
   • Endometriosis
   • Peyronie's disease
   • Testicular disease
   • Genital trauma
4 Endocrine
   • Diabetes mellitus
   • Hypogonadal states
   • Hyperprolactinemia
   • Pituitary dysfunction
   • Thyroid dysfunction
   • Adrenal disease
5 Neurological
   • Multiple sclerosis
   • Peripheral neuropathy
   • Central nervous system tumors
   • Stroke
   • Spinal cord disease
   • Substance use disorder
Surgical procedures associated with sexual dysfunction:
   • Prostatectomy
   • Mastectomy
   • Vaginal surgeries
   • Episiotomy
   • Lumbar sympathectomy

Source: Adapted from Keltner NL and Folks DG (2001) *Psychotropic Drugs*, 3rd edn., Mosby, p. 349.

Table 19.6 Classes of medication that may affect sexual response

Drug	Sexual response
Antihypertensives	Libido, erectile, ejaculation problems
Diuretics	Libido, erectile, ejaculation problems
Timolol (ocular)	Libido, erectile, low ejaculate problems
Central-acting adrenergic inhibitors	Libido, erectile, ejaculation problems
Peripheral-acting adrenergic inhibitors	Libido, erectile, ejaculation problems
Alpha-adrenergic blockers	Low incidence of sexual dysfunction
Combined alpha- and beta-adrenergic blockers	Erection, ejaculation, delayed detumescence problems
Angiotensin-converting enzyme (ACE) inhibitors	Worsening of sexual dysfunction
Hormones	
Androgens	Libido decreased, impotence, testicular atrophy
Anabolic steroids	Azoospermia
Estrogens	Decreased vaginal atrophy, decreased libido in males
Cancer agents	
Alkylating chemotherapy agents	Gonadal dysfunction in males and females
Other chemotherapeutic agents	Gonadal dysfunction in males and females with procarbazine and vinblastine; suppressed testicular and adrenal androgen synthesis with ketoconazole
Carbonic anhydrase inhibitors	Libido, erectile problems
Antiepileptic drugs	
Carbamazepine, phenytoin	Decreased libido or erectile problems

Source: Adapted from Buffum J (2001) Prescription drugs and sexual function, *Psychiatric Medicine* 10: 181.

2   *For males*:
   • Can you gain and maintain an erection long enough for sexual intercourse? How long can you maintain an erection? Are you unable to ejaculate? How long does it take to ejaculate? If it takes more time to ejaculate than before, how much longer? Have you noticed a change in the quality of the ejaculatory sensation? (The word "ejaculation" may or may not be understood by the patient. If not, the clinician might use "come," "orgasm" or "climax" to be understood.)
3   *For females*:
   • Have you noticed a change in ability to obtain vaginal lubrication? Are you able to reach orgasm? What percentage of the time do you reach orgasm? How long does it take to reach orgasm? Is this different from before medication? Has the quality of orgasm changed?

If, after gaining the above information, it appears that there is no other obvious cause for the change in sexual drive or behavior, and if the timing is consistent with starting psychotropic medications, it is probable that the medications are having a direct effect on the patient's sexual functioning. When this occurs, it is often soon after starting the medication, but it may also occur at some later interval – particularly after a dosage increase.

If it is the clinician's assessment that the medication is interfering with sexual functioning, it is crucial to determine how important the interference is to *this* patient at *this* time. The clinician can never assume that his or her own level of concern about sexual interference is the same as the patient's. Particularly when patients are feeling better emotionally, it may not be a problem for some individuals temporarily to undergo a limited amount of diminished capacity for sexual arousal. Other patients may simply not put a high priority on sexual activity, and for them this side effect is of minimal importance at this point in life.

The reverse is also true. There are many patients who cannot tolerate even small changes in sexual functioning. For them, sexual activity and prowess may be an extraordinarily important part of their day-to-day life, and any diminishment in functioning may have significant ramifications to their self-esteem and their relationship with their partner. Such individuals, if not dealt with sensitively, will discontinue medication very quickly, at even the earliest sign of sexual interference. A significant number of patients who prematurely terminate medication do so because of sexual side effects that are not evaluated by the clinician.

If the clinician decides that sexual interference is likely caused by medication, the elements of Phase I interventions should be instituted as in Table 19.7.

If the Phase I strategies are unsuccessful, or the patient is unwilling to comply, the clinician can go to Phase II, as shown in Table 19.8.

Table 19.7 Phase I: first responses to medication-induced sexual interference

---

The clinician should:

1 Clearly state that he or she believes the patient's sexual interference *is* likely connected to the medication. This information should also be given to the patient's partner by the patient or, with consent, by the clinician. This is quite important since, without this information, the partner may ascribe the sexual dysfunction to causes which are not true such as lack of their own attractiveness, extramarital sexual activity or excessive masturbation.

2 Tell the patient that initial medication-induced sexual interference may diminish and pass with time. When such accommodation occurs, it usually does so within several weeks to several months.

3 Clearly state that, even if the interference is due to the medication, there will be no permanent change in sexual functioning. When the medication is discontinued, the person's baseline level of sexuality will return.

4 Assess the patient's response to this information. If acceptable, agree on a timeframe for further observation after which, if the situation has not resolved, other action will be considered.

5 Consider "drug holidays," particularly for shorter-acting medications. If the sexually offending drug is a short to medium half-life antidepressant (sertraline, venlafaxine and possibly citalopram, paroxetine), a "drug holiday" may solve the problem. This is accomplished by having the patient omit the medication dosage on the morning before planned sexual contact, which permits the blood level of medication to drop over the ensuing 12–18 hours. The amount of medication in the body may be sufficiently low by evening to avoid significant interference in sexual functioning. The patient then takes the regular dose of medication the following morning. It is unnecessary to take the missed dose. Surprisingly, many patients can satisfactorily accomplish this without any serotonergic withdrawal syndrome, and without loss of antidepressant activity. While a drug holiday requires planning as to the time of sexual activity and minimizes sexual spontaneity, this remedy can be an effective and simple tool for some patients.

Table 19.8 Phase II: remedies for medication-induced sexual interference

---
- Lower the dose of the offending psychotropic
- Change to another psychotropic
- Stop all psychotropics, if clinically possible
- Add a pharmacological antidote

Sexual interference that persists despite waiting and education may respond to dosage change or a change of medication. Lowering the dose of the psychotropic may help some patients, but is seldom totally effective. If the medication causing the problem is an antidepressant, a change to mirtazepine or bupropion may be effective in lessening sexual problems.[7] Since the sexual interfering effects of antipsychotics or mood stabilizers are quite variable from patient to patient, any change of medication or category may, in some individuals, reverse medication-related sexual dysfunction. There are some data to suggest that medications that increase prolactin (notably traditional antipsychotics and risperidone) may cause a higher rate of sexual dysfunction than others. Beyond that, there are very limited data as to which specific antipsychotic and mood-stabilizing medications are consistently less sexually interfering. Therefore, there is no one recommended change, and any change may or may not be useful.

When changing medications, the other important consideration is maintaining the desired antidepressant, mood-stabilizing or antipsychotic effect. When the medication is changed because of persistent sexual interference, any changes should, in general, be done gradually and with a graduated crossover method (as discussed in Chapter 6) to give the patient the highest likelihood of maintaining symptom remission.

When the previous remedies are inadequate and medication change is contraindicated (or has been tried and failed), use of pharmacological antidotes is the next step. Pharmacological remedies that have shown some usefulness in modulating or reversing psychotropic-induced (especially antidepressant-induced) sexual interference are shown in Table 19.9. Unfortunately, with the exception of the phosphodiesterase-5 inhibitors for erectile dysfunction, none of these pharmacological remedies is consistently or significantly effective

The four phosphodiesterase-5 inhibitors (sildenafil – Viagra, tadalafil – Cialis, vardenafil – Levitra and avanafil – Stendra) for erectile problems are effective in reversing antidepressant-induced erectile dysfunction by 75–90 percent.[10] Bupropion is 50–70 percent effective in improving orgasmic function in women.[11–12] Unfortunately, each of the remaining antidotes, individually and collectively, is only effective for a limited number of patients. When use of the phosphodiesterase-5 inhibitors or bupropion is ineffective, switching the offending psychotropic medication may be a more successful strategy than trying repeated add-on pharmacological antidotes.

With an aggressive pharmacological approach, patients can often obtain both adequate anxiety/mood effect and satisfactory sexual functioning. There are, however, some patients who, despite all attempts and strategies, will have to make a choice between emotional health and full sexual response. While not desirable, emotional stability may have to take preference over sexual satisfaction for some severely ill patients. This is a marginally tolerable situation for some patients, and is totally intolerable for others.

Table 19.9 Drugs used to treat antidepressant-induced sexual dysfunction

Drug	Symptom/indicator	Dosage
Bethanecol	Erectile dysfunction	10–40 mg PRN
Amantadine	Anorgasmia	100 mg PRN 1 h before sexual activity
	Erectile dysfunction	100 mg bid
	Hypoactive desire	100 mg bid
Avanafil	Erectile dysfunction	50–200 mg before sexual activity
Bupropion	Anorgasmia	75–150 mg PRN 1–2 h before sexual activity
	Hypoactive desire	75–150 mg bid
	Arousal	75–150 mg bid
Buspirone	Anorgasmia	20–60 mg/day
	Hypoactive desire	20–60 mg/day
	Erectile dysfunction	20–60 mg/day
Cyproheptadine	Anorgasmia	4–16 mg PRN 1 h before sexual activity
	Hypoactive desire	4–16 mg/day
Dextroamphetamine	Anorgasmia	5–20 mg PRN
	Hypoactive desire	2.5–5 mg bid
Granisetron	Anorgasmia	1 mg PRN 1 h before sexual activity
Gingko biloba	Hypoactive desire	60 mg bid–qid
Methylphenidate	Anorgasmia	5–20 mg PRN
	Hypoactive desire	5–20 mg/day
	Arousal	5–20 mg/day
Pemoline	Anorgasmia	18.75 mg PRN
	Hypoactive desire	18.75–75 mg/day
	Arousal	18.75–75 mg/day
Sildenafil	Erectile dysfunction	50–100 mg before sexual activity
Tadalafil	Erectile dysfunction	5–20 mg before sexual activity or 2.5–5 mg daily
Vardenafil	Erectile dysfunction	2.5–20 mg before sexual activity
Yohimbine	Anorgasmia	5.4–10.8 mg PRN
	Hypoactive desire	5.4 mg/day to 5.4 mg tid
Avanifil	Erectile dysfunction	5.4 mg/day to 5.4 mg tid
Alprostadil	Erectile dysfunction	50–100 mg
Testosterone replacement	Erectile dysfunction	Injected or via cream
Flibanserin (for women)	Hypoactive desire	Per practitioner's instruction
Bremelanotide (for women)	Hypoactive desire	Per practitioner's instruction
		Per practitioner's instruction

Source: Keltner NL and Folks DG (2001) *Psychotropic Drugs*, 3rd edn., Mosby, p. 349.

Weight gain

Maintenance of reasonable body weight is a medical health and safety issue. Additionally, body image is both a health issue and an important matter of self-esteem for both men and women. From a cultural standpoint, staying slim is a virtual obsession for many people in Western society. From a medical perspective, obesity can lead to a worsening incidence of hypertension, cardiovascular disease, diabetes and stroke. The issue of how a psychotropic medication may affect weight, particularly if it may cause weight gain, is a major concern for many patients.

Obesity is generally defined via the Body Mass Index (BMI), which is a person's weight in kilograms divided by his or her height in meters squared. A BMI of 30 or greater is a commonly accepted definition of obesity. A person is overweight when the BMI is between 25 and 29.9.[13]

Some patients will ask about possible weight gain even before a medicine is prescribed. Other patients will only raise the issue when, and if, they begin to gain weight on the medication. A smaller group of patients will be almost oblivious to a possible connection between the medication and weight changes. Therefore, it will be important for the clinician to discuss the issue of weight maintenance prior to prescribing any medication likely to cause weight gain.

Chronically mentally ill patients are already two to three times more likely to be obese than the general population.[14] Depression, schizophrenia and bipolar disorder carry their own burden of increased obesity.[15-20] Therefore, the management of weight when prescribing antidepressant, antipsychotic and mood-stabilizing medications becomes even more crucial.

For psychotropic medications with an "average" incidence of weight gain, the majority of patients either do not gain weight or lose it, or gain small amounts. Most psychotropics have an "average" incidence of weight gain, with the exceptions noted in Table 19.10.

Table 19.10 Psychotropics and weight gain

Antidepressants causing a higher than average amount of weight gain:
- Paroxetine
- Mirtazepine[1]
- TCAs
- MAOIs[2]

Antidepressants causing less than average weight gain:
- Bupropion
- Reboxetine (UK only)

Mood stabilizers causing a higher than average weight gain:
- Valproic acid[2]
- Lithium carbonate[2]

Mood stabilizers causing less than average weight gain and/or weight loss:
- Topiramate

Antipsychotic medications causing higher than average weight gain:
- Clozapine
- Olanzapine[4]
- Low potency traditional antipsychotics, such as thioridazine[4]
- Risperidone[3,5]
- Quetiapine[3]
- Iloperidone

Antipsychotics causing less than average weight gain:
- Ziprasidone[4]
- Molindone[3]
- Lurasidone
- Asenapine
- Aripiprazole[6]
- Amisulprid[6]

Sources:

1 Sussman N and Ginsberg D (1998) Weight gain associated with SSRIs. *Primary Psychiatry* 1: 28–37.
2 *The Maudsley Prescribing Guidelines* (2001), 6th edn., Informa Healthcare, p. 195.
3 Malhotra S and McElroy S (2002) Medical management of obesity associated with mental disorders. *Journal of Clinical Psychiatry* 63 (Suppl. 4): 26.
4 Allison DB *et al.* (1999) Antipsychotic induced weight gain: a comprehensive research synthesis. *American Journal of Psychiatry* 156: 1686–1696.
5 Ratzone G *et al.* (2002) Weight gain associated with olanzapine and risperidone in adolescent patients: a comparative prospective study. *Journal of the American Academy of Child and Adolescent Psychiatry* 41: 337–343.
6 *The Maudsley Prescribing Guidelines* (2009), 10th edn., Martin Dunitz, p. 96.

Weight gain or loss with psychotropic medication is usually reported as the average or mean collected from a group of patients. When dealing with patients and psychotropics clinically, there can be considerable variability among individuals. Many patients will not gain weight on drugs that have "higher than average" statistical weight gain; conversely, some individuals may gain weight on medications with "low or moderate" statistical averages.

When patients do gain weight from medications, leaner patients (with a lower BMI) statistically gain more weight than obese persons (with a high BMI).[21]

Therefore, patients who are obese should not automatically be excluded from using medications with a "higher than average" risk of weight gain if the medication is otherwise indicated.

The mechanism of psychotropic weight gain is unclear.[22] It may be related to increased appetite, a direct influence on calorie metabolism or, at least in part, from the development of insulin resistance, altered blood glucose levels or blood leptin levels.

Box 19.9 Talking to patients

If a patient raises the possibility of weight gain when using medications of "average" weight gain, the clinician can discuss the issue in the following way: *"Most people on [name of medication] do not gain weight. I do not expect that to be a significant issue for you. There is, however, almost no mental health medication that has not been alleged for some people, at some time, to cause weight gain. I, too, am interested in making sure that you maintain a reasonable body weight. There are good reasons why we are prescribing this medicine at this time, and I believe that those reasons are more important than the slight risk of possible weight gain. We will, however, be monitoring this together. Please notify me if there is any significant change in your weight, and we will discuss our options at that time."*

Box 19.10 Talking to patients

When selecting a medication that does have a risk of higher than average weight gain, early attention and prevention are crucial. Therefore, the discussion can proceed as follows: *"I am prescribing [name of medication] for you. I believe this is a good choice for you and that it can make a significant improvement in your symptoms. We know that one possible side effect of [name of medication] is an increase in appetite* [see discussion below]. *It is important that, if possible, we avoid making future decisions about your medication based solely on this factor. Therefore, I want both of us to keep track of your eating habits, exercise and weight. Be sure to maintain a nutritious, low calorie diet and minimize significant intake of fruit juices and full-calorie soda. Let's discuss the amount of physical activity that you now do."* Then map a plan for physical exercise. Use a dietitian, if necessary, to discuss which foods are low and high calorie if the patient is not knowledgeable in these areas.

Even though weight gain may be the concern in the clinician's mind, notice that the clinician warns of increased *appetite*, not specifically increased *weight*. This presentation is often much more palatable to patients (who can then feel some control over the process) than specifically identifying that they will gain weight (over which they are likely to feel they have little control).

At the time of initial evaluation, the patient's baseline weight and BMI should be noted so that any changes in weight can be accurately correlated to their premedication weight.

"It must be the medication…"

Once a medication is prescribed, and if a weight increase is noticed, it is common for the patient quickly to suspect that the medication is the cause of the problem. However, although weight gain from medication is possible, patients often find medication an easy and convenient target to blame for possible weight gain when there may be other causes to consider. Rather than immediately accepting the patient's assumption that any weight gain is caused by medication, the clinician should ask and document responses to the following questions:

- What is your previous weight history over time?
- How has your weight fluctuated with your emotional state in the past?
- What exercise, if any, do you do? How often? For how long?
- Has your level of exercise changed since you began the medication?

In the interval until the next visit, the clinician should ask the patient to:

1   Weigh him- or herself twice a week until the next visit. Describe the most accurate method for obtaining weight, which is to weigh oneself first thing in the morning, after using the bathroom and before having anything to eat or drink.
2   Maintain a written, detailed history of food intake (a "food diary") that lists everything put into the mouth for a 10-day period, including all snacks and beverages. Have the patient bring the diary and record of weight measurements to the next visit.

With this information, there may be clear indications of possible factors contributing to weight gain:

- There may have been a marked increase in food intake once the patient began feeling better.
- The overall diet may be high in fatty or caloric items.
- The amount of exercise may be minimal or non-existent.
- An anxious or manic patient may have slowed the amount of physical activity to "normal." This may have led the patient's weight to increase from a subnormal level to a more normal level now that the anxiety or mania is improving and physical overactivity is waning.
- Some depressed patients who lost appetite and have eaten poorly for weeks or months may have been below baseline weight. After medication, patients become less depressed, and a weight gain to baseline is not only normal, but also a sign of return to health.

Some patients who lose weight because of their illness enjoy the weight loss that may have returned them to a more personally desirable level, reminiscent of weight when they were an adolescent or young adult. An increase in weight as they recover on the medication, however, moves them away from this idealized earlier weight. They should be counseled that this goal may not be realistically achievable as an adult.

Intervention helps

If, on evaluation of the above data, no other primary cause is apparent and the patient's weight is increasing, the medication may be playing a role. A crucial clinical fact is that advice, intervention and monitoring of the patient's diet and activity level by the clinician can make a difference. Several studies[23-25] now conclude that if the clinician takes an active role in helping patients to manage their weight, results are significant. These interventions can occur as the patient starts a possible weight-gaining medication (and thus minimizing or preventing the gain), or after the weight gain has started. They include:

- a thorough discussion of weight management and the possible effect of medication
- nutrition counseling – directly or through referral to a dietitian
- monitoring and reporting weekly weight
- a gradual increase in vigorous physical exercise.

Approaches to medication-induced weight gain

When it is suspected that weight gain is due to the medication, the following remedies should be considered:

- If the weight gain is minimal (1–5 lb; 0.5–2.5 kg), a wait-and-see approach combined with appropriate diet and/or exercise may be sufficient.
- If the patient's diet is not healthy and/or the patient's exercise is minimal, a frank discussion about the connection between calorie intake, physical activity and body weight is necessary. If the patient is doing well on a medication and the clinician feels it should be continued, it can be useful to consider forming a contract with the patient for appropriate lifestyle changes to allow for ongoing medication. For some patients, the course of medication is time-limited and a minor weight gain can be tolerated, or even reversed, with appropriate diet and exercise during that time.
- Lowering the dose of medication to the smallest possible amount that satisfactorily treats the mental health symptoms may decrease any appetite enhancement and/or weight gain. (This may not be an effective strategy for weight gain associated with antipsychotics.)[21]
- For new or significant weight gain which starts only after the patient has been taking medication for a substantial period of time, the clinician should consider whether it is time to discontinue the medication, even if it is earlier than initially planned. If the patient can safely taper off the medication, medication-induced weight gain may no longer be an issue.
- If lowering of dose, appropriate diet and increase in exercise cannot stem weight gain, and it would be premature to discontinue the medication, a change of

medications and/or class of medications is indicated, considering the options presented in Table 19.10.

- Group support programs for weight loss may also be beneficial. Commonly used weight loss support programs include: Weight Watchers (www.weightwatchers. com); Richard Simmons (www.richardsimmons.com); Overeaters Anonymous (Telephone: 505-891-2664; https://oa.org/); TOPS Club, Inc. (www.tops.org).
- Use of eating manuals/plans, diet and nutrition books. Although new books and weight-loss plans are published every year, many effective principles are time-honored and remain valid. A book's recent publication date does not ensure a more successful result. Some useful self-help books on diet and nutrition include:[26]
  - *The Blue Zones Kitchen: 100 Recipes to Live to 100*, by D Buettner (2019)
  - *Mini Habits for Weight Loss: Stop Dieting. Form New Habits. Change Your Lifestyle Without Suffering*, by S Guise (2016)
  - *The Pescatarian Cookbook*, by C Harbstreet (2018)
  - *The South Beach Diet*, by A Agatston (2005, St. Martin's Griffin)
  - *Eat More, Weigh Less*, by D Ornish and JS Brown (2001, HarperCollins)
  - *Dr Shapiro's Picture Perfect Weight Loss*, by HM Shapiro (2000, St. Martin's Press)
  - *Eating Well for Optimum Health*, by A Weil (2000, Alfred A Knopf).

Even when medications are changed, continued watchful diligence is required by both the clinician and patient. Monitoring is necessary, and weight should be regularly recorded.

Pharmacotherapy of weight gain

Appetite suppressants can be utilized in select patients on a time-limited basis. These include:

- Phentermine (30 mg before breakfast)
- Desoxyn (5 mg before each meal).
- Contrave 8 mg/90 mg tablets twice daily
- Qsymia (phentermine and topiramate) 11.25 mg/69 mg daily
- Belviq 10 mg twice a day.

Many weight loss/appetite suppressant medications are sympathomimetic stimulants or have stimulant properties. They are FDA scheduled drugs that can have the same habit-forming potential of other stimulants. Because of abuse potential, desoxyn, especially, is closely regulated. In addition to their ability to decrease appetite, they can cause physical side effects such as agitation, insomnia, tremor or anxiety. In some individuals, they can have antidepressant effects, cause hypomania or aggravate psychosis, and they are contraindicated for use with MAOIs. They are not generally used long term.

Other weight loss medications include Xenical (orlistat), which is a weight loss medication that acts by an entirely different mechanism from stimulants, and does not include central nervous system activity. The medication is a reversible inhibitor of gastric and pancreatic lipases, which convert dietary fat into absorbable free fatty acids in the gut. When not transformed in this way, triglycerides are not digestible into the systemic circulation and pass out through the feces, so calorie reduction results. The dose is 120 mg three times a day.

Topirimate, an anti-epileptic medication used for partial seizures, has mood-stabilizing properties. Because of its weight-reduction property, it may be useful in a regimen of bipolar or antipsychotic medications.[27-29] If there is clinical necessity for the use of multiple mood stabilizers, the weight-reduction effect can be maintained when topirimate is used as an add-on to other drugs The dose is 50–100 mg per day. Another new anticonvulsant with some anti-manic properties, Zonisamide, may also be helpful as an agent in the treatment of weight gain in mood disorder patients, although the results are still preliminary.[30]

A relatively "new" medication for weight loss (marketed in America as Qysmia) received FDA approval in 2012. It is a timed-release capsule combination product of two existing products mentioned above – phentermine and topiramate. In initial studies, the combination showed significant weight loss – up to 10 percent of total body weight in the first year of use – when compared to placebo. Side effects of the combination were dry mouth, tingling, abnormal taste sensation, insomnia, increased heart rate and palpitations. Of concern was a two- to fivefold increased incidence of cleft lip in babies born to pregnant women who were taking the drug. The FDA has recommended a strict policy of pregnancy testing before and during use. Given that it combines two medications that are individually effective, it would be expected to be useful in appetite suppression and weight loss. It remains to be seen if the time-release brand-name combination is sufficiently superior and cost-effective when compared to prescribing the two existing generic products together. Also approved in America in 2012 was lorcaserin (marketed as Belviq). It has been approved for persons with a BMI of 27 or greater who also have one weight-related condition such as Type-2 diabetes, hypertension or high cholesterol. In testing, 10 mg two times a day was twice as effective as placebo in providing a loss of up to 5 percent of body weight; it should be used in conjunction with a weight-reduction diet and exercise. Lorcaserin's purported mechanism of action is to reduce appetite and food consumption by activation of brain Serotonin 2C receptors. As a serotonergic drug, lorcaserin could theoretically be associated with Serotonin Syndrome when co-administered with other serotonergic or anti-dopaminergic agents, such as serotonergic antidepressants, antipsychotics or MAOIs (see Chapter 20). The most common adverse reactions associated with its use (greater than 5 percent) are headaches, dizziness, fatigue, nausea, dry mouth, constipation, back pain, cough and fatigue. Hypoglycemia is also reported in diabetic patients.

There are several small studies showing that amantadine (100–300 mg daily)[31-32] and H_2 antagonist nizatidine (300 mg twice daily)[33] may possibly be useful in reducing weight in patients taking antipsychotic medications.

Several studies of the use of the oral hypoglycemic agent metformin (glucophage), 500 mg two to three times daily, showed significant weight reductions in children taking olanzapine, risperidone, quetiapine and valproic acid[34] and adult women with first-episode schizophrenia taking antipsychotics.[35] Of additional positive note is that in the latter study, there was also restoration of menstruation and improvement in insulin resistance, which have not heretofore been demonstrated with other treatments.

Hoodia, a succulent plant from the Kalahari Desert, has had significant marketing and sales on the Internet as an appetite suppressant. Although there are some small studies supporting effectiveness, it is marketed as a dietary supplement rather than a prescription appetite suppressant and therefore does not require formal FDA approval and/or scrutiny. Allegedly, the underlying chemical deceives the brain into feeling that fullness has been achieved and therefore further food intake is not necessary. Although the compound appears to have few side effects, there is little replicable scientific evidence of its effectiveness at this time.[36]

Old sayings are still true

Whether or not weight changes are due to medication, two adages apply to weight loss remedies: *"There is no such thing as a free lunch"* and *"If it sounds too good to be true, it probably is."* Inexpensive, over-the-counter weight loss preparations often do not work, or contain potentially harmful ingredients. Products that promise significant "amazing" weight loss "without dieting or exercise" are likely, at best, to have little solid research to support their efficacy. At worst they may contain ephedra (or *Ma Huang*, an herbal form of ephedrine), which can interact problematically with prescription antidepressants, stimulants and other herbal products, such as St. John's Wort. Ephedra has been linked to hypertension, stroke, myocardial infarction, nephrotoxicity and sudden death.[37–38] "Fad" or "crash" diets are seldom helpful, and may be metabolically dangerous. Even if a patient manages to lose a significant amount of weight in a short timeframe, the weight loss is seldom maintained and the patient will often regain weight rapidly when a crash diet is stopped.

Headaches

Headaches have been reported with many psychotropic medications. Sometimes the headaches are migrainous in type, with all the consequent sequelae of migraines, but at other times they may have non-migrainous qualities and patterns. Some patients who start psychotropics will notice a worsening of pre-existing headaches/migraines, while other patients will start headaches anew. Not all patients with pre-existing headaches will have them worsen, and some patients' headaches may improve with the addition of an SSRI antidepressant or lithium.[39]

When headaches do occur and they are mild, taking the medication at bedtime may allow the headache to occur during sleep, such that it is minimal during the day when the patient is awake. Headaches that emerge within an hour or two of taking the medication may benefit from splitting the dosage into two or three smaller amounts that are dosed throughout the day. Such smaller dosages may eliminate the headache altogether, or allow the patient to live with very mild pain. Over-the-counter pain relievers such as aspirin, ibuprofen or acetaminophen may be sufficient to treat milder headaches. If none of these remedies is effective, a change of medication is often necessary.

Patients with pre-existing migraine headaches that worsen with mental health medication can require close cooperation between the mental health prescriber and a neurologist, since many of the most useful psychiatric drugs can alter the frequency or intensity of headaches. Likewise, many medications used to treat headache can have significant mood effects or create psychiatric mood instability in the psychiatric patient.

Asthenia/weakness

Asthenia, or weakness, may occur, particularly with strongly serotonergic antidepressants. Patients with normal mood can also develop a "frontal lobe-like" syndrome characterized by apathy, lack of motivation, intermittent fatigue and mental dulling. Generally, this is thought to result from excess serotonergic stimulation. Decreasing the dosage of the SSRI may limit and improve the apathy and dulling. Adding a stimulant or bupropion, both of which increase norepinephrine and dopamine activity, may also increase motivation and minimize fatigue. If these remedies fail, changing the medication is often necessary.

Dry mouth

With strongly anticholinergic medications such as TCAs and traditional antipsychotics, dry mouth can be a considerable problem. In its mildest form, it is an annoyance. When more severe and persistent, however, dry mouth is quite uncomfortable, may make speech and swallowing difficult, and lead to increased dental caries.

The clinician should, whenever possible, decrease the anticholinergic load by choosing medications that may be less anticholinergic. Switching from a TCA to an SSRI or other new-generation antidepressant, or switching from a traditional antipsychotic to an atypical antipsychotic, may help in this regard. Other remedies for this problem include asking the patient to use chewing gum or sugar-free candy, or to drink increased amounts of water. Last, a cholinergic agent such as bethanechol hydrochloride (10–20 mg per day) or a cholinesterase inhibitor (e.g., donepezil 5–10 mg per day) may modulate the dryness.

Hair loss

While statistically uncommon, hair loss (alopecia) has been reported with a wide variety of psychotropic medications. When it does occur, it can be markedly distressing to the patient, and the clinician will be queried. The patient will complain of noticing increased amounts of hair on a hairbrush, or seeing hair in the drain when taking a shower or bath.

Surprisingly little research has been done on this side effect, and much of our information on the subject is anecdotal or is based on isolated case reports. It is helpful to explain to the patient important facts that we do know about hair, hair growth and hair loss:

- Of the roughly 100,000 hairs on the scalp, loss of up to 150 strands per day is normal.[40–41]
- Before it becomes clinically evident, 25 to 50 percent of a person's hair must be lost.[40, 42]
- Patients unfortunately associate any discussion of psychotropic medication-related hair loss with cancer chemotherapy hair loss, which is not a valid comparison. Hair loss due to cancer chemotherapy is generally much more severe than that which occurs with psychotropic medications, and is a result of a different mechanism.[40–43]
- Mental health patients will report idiopathic hair loss even when they are not on any psychotropic medication.
- Drug-induced hair loss is actually hair breakage, or shedding at the scalp line. The patient's hair follicles remain intact, and new hair will grow back to replace that which breaks off.[40, 44]

Table 19.11 Psychotropic medications causing hair loss with significant frequency

---

- Lithium carbonate
- Valproic acid
- Fluoxetine

Source: Adapted from Gautem M (1999) Alopecia due to psychotropic medication. *Annals of Pharmacotherapy* 33: 631–636.

Table 19.12 Psychotropic medications with at least one case of possible medication-related hair loss

---

• Amitriptyline	• Loxapine
• Bupropion	• Methylphenidate
• Carbamazepine	• Maprotiline
• Citalopram	• Mirtazepine
• Clonazepam	• Nefazodone
• Silbutramine	• Olanzapine
• Desipramine	• Oxcarbazine
• Donepezil	• Paroxetine
• Fluvoxamine	• Propranolol
• Gabapentin	• Risperidone
• Haloperidol	• Sertraline
• Iloperidone	• Topirimate
• Imipramine	• Tranylcypromine
• Lamotrigine	• Venlafaxine

Source: Adapted from *Physician's Desk Reference* (2002), Medical Economics Company.

- Most medication-induced hair loss is generally time-limited, and will resolve spontaneously within several weeks or months.[40, 43, 45–46]
- Hair lost due to psychotropic medications will grow back within 2–5 months after the offending medication is stopped.[40]
- The hair that grows back has been reported for some patients to be a different texture when the offending agent is lithium or valproic acid. This has not been reported with other medications.[47]

The strongest psychotropic medication offenders in causing hair loss are shown in Table 19.11.

Many other medications have had a low incidence of case reports of hair loss associated with their use. The medications are shown in Table 19.12.

On evaluation of hair loss, other causes must be considered besides medication-induced alopecia. Since hypothyroidism is a known cause of hair loss, a thyroid function panel and thyroid stimulating hormone (TSH) level should be obtained on any patient who makes this complaint. Trichotillomania (compulsive hair pulling) is another possible cause.

Unfortunately, there is no definitively curative treatment for alopecia caused by medication. Since the hair loss is usually transient and self-limited, if the medication is significantly beneficial to the patient for mental health symptoms, encourage the patient to continue taking the medication if possible. In mild cases, the patient may be willing to do this, and the condition will resolve spontaneously. Other remedies that have been recommended include taking oral selenium (100 μg/day) and zinc (15 mg/day). Application of a selenium-containing shampoo (for example, brand name Selsun Blue) directly to the scalp can also be tried. Finasteride and minoxidil have been used to treat hair loss, but the results are quite variable. With more significant hair loss, patients are often more reluctant to continue the medication, and the clinician should decrease the dose or change medicines.

Skin reactions

Many psychotropics have reported a modest incidence of skin rashes or skin reactions as potential side effects. These may be described as maculopapular rashes, dermatitis, skin itching or exacerbation of acne. In general, the majority of these skin problems are annoying but minor, and the incidence is no greater than 1–2 percent for any given medication. It is difficult to interpret the literature to know how many of these skin rashes are associated with actual drug allergy, since a skin rash is such a prominent part of allergic drug reactions. Even though some of these rashes might be more accurately described as a side effect and not represent a true drug allergy, the appearance of a rap-idly spreading rash in a patient on medication should be treated as an allergy, and the principles outlined in Chapter 20 followed. Some compounds, however, have a higher incidence of non-allergic skin problems, and these are listed in Table 19.13.

In contrast to the benign rashes at a fairly low incidence that occur with many psychotropics, there are three mental health medications that have significant, frequent and potentially serious skin complications – lamotrigine, carbamazepine and lithium.

Lamotrigine has a documented incidence of severe rash (classified as Stevens-Johnson syndrome, or toxic epidermal necrolysis) in a small number of patients. In addition, up to 10 percent of patients taking lamotrigine may have a benign rash, which often does not progress or relate to the more serious forms. Because the clinician may have diffi-culty in distinguishing the more benign rash from the more serious variety, any patient who develops a rash on lamotrigine should have the medicine discontinued unless there is a strong clinical indication for continuing. This is unfortunate, since upwards of 95 percent of these rashes will turn out to be benign, will eventually disappear and do

Table 19.13 Psychotropic medications with an incidence of skin rash greater than 3 percent

Generic name (brand name)
- Alprazolam (Xanax)
- Bupropion (Wellbutrin)
- Silbutramine (Meridia)
- Fluoxetine (Prozac)
- Lamotrigine (Lamictal)
- Naltrexone (Revia)
- Pimozide (Orap)
- Iloperidone (Fanapt)
- Quetiapine (Seroquel)
- Sertraline (Zoloft)
- Tacrine (Cognex)
- Topirimate (Topamax)
- Valproic acid (Depakote)
- Venlafaxine (Effexor)
- Ziprasidone (Geodon)

not progress to Stevens-Johnson syndrome. Several clinical facts have evolved regarding the incidence of rash with lamotrigine that have led to clinical guidelines. The incidence of serious rash is significantly higher in the pediatric population than in adults (1 percent in patients under 16 years old, and 0.3 percent in adults older than 16 years). High initial dosage or rapid dosage escalation are also associated with increased risk of serious rash. Therefore, the following recommendations are used with lamotrigine:

- Lamotrigine should not be used in patients under 16 years of age.
- Lamotrigine should not be started at more than 50 mg per day and dosages should be increased by modest amounts every week or two (see lamotrigine product information for further description of a normal dosing schedule).
- The presence of valproic acid will increase the blood level of lamotrigine, whenever the two are prescribed simultaneously. Therefore, a patient who is already taking valproic acid should have lamotrigine started at 25 mg every other day and the dosage increased gradually from there.
- Most lamotrigine-precipitated serious rashes occur in the first 2–8 weeks of administration; however, a few have occurred after 6 months of continuous use.

Carbamazepine also has a small, but well-known, incidence of severe dermatological reactions, including toxic epidermal necrolysis or Stevens-Johnson syndrome. Rarely, these syndromes have led to death, but most of these fatal reactions occurred in the past, during the first years of usage of this compound. Other skin reactions occurring with carbamazepine include pruritic and erythematous rashes, urticaria, photosensitivity reactions, exfoliative dermatitis, erythema multiforme and erythema nodosum. Unlike lamotrigine, no other obvious precipitating factors leading to an increased incidence of rash have, to date, been uncovered. These serious skin rashes appear to be an idiosyncratic response in certain individuals.

Lithium has long been known to be a medication that can cause skin irritation, skin rash or other skin problems. In addition to a rash per se, lithium may cause dryness of the skin, pruritus, exacerbation of acne and a worsening of psoriasis. Because of this propensity, lithium should be a third- or fourth-line choice of mood stabilizer for patients with existing psoriasis. In rare cases, psoriasis has been precipitated *de novo* by taking lithium on a regular basis.

Despite the known incidence of these serious skin conditions with these three compounds, it must be reiterated that their frequency is small – certainly less than 1 percent, and in many cases less than 0.1 percent. Therefore, it is not necessary for clinicians to avoid the usage of these otherwise valuable mood stabilizers.

Prolactin elevation

Prolactin, a hormone secreted from the anterior pituitary gland, is, as its name suggests, responsible for breast milk production, and also stimulates breast epithelial cell proliferation. It does have a number of other functions as well, related to menstruation, sexual functioning and fertility. Several antipsychotic medications, specifically all traditional antipsychotics, lurasidone and risperidone, have been known to increase prolactin secretion, presumably through a mechanism of dopamine receptor blockade and dopamine D_2 receptor occupancy. Except for risperidone and lurasidone, the other seven atypical antipsychotics – olanzapine, clozapine, quetiapine, aripiprazole, iloperidone, asenapine and ziprasidone – have no detectable prolactin elevation, or a minimal transient elevation lasting no more than a few hours.[48]

Studies suggest that when typical antipsychotics and risperidone are given to a patient there is an immediate and pronounced increase in prolactin level within 15–30 minutes, and in general, women have a greater elevation than men.[49–52]

When the offending medication is stopped, prolactin levels show a rapid decline, reaching normal levels within 3 days of stopping.

The amount of prolactin secretion caused by the administration of these antipsychotics is significantly less than the amount of prolactin released through primary hyperprolactinemia or prolactin-secreting tumors. In general, the side effects due to the elevated prolactin levels from antipsychotics are also much less intense and less severe than in these medical conditions. In primary hyperprolactinemia there are more severe manifestations of hypogonadism, leading to decreased serum testosterone levels and estrogen deficiency in women. These symptoms and the sequelae of these lowered gonadal functions have only been shown in other causes of elevated prolactin level, and have not been shown in medication-induced hyperprolactinemia.

The clinical side effects listed in Table 19.14 are presumably caused by elevated prolactin levels, although the exact chemical connection has not been proven by research.

When any of the side effects mentioned in Table 19.14 present in a patient taking a traditional antipsychotic, lurasidone or risperidone, elevated prolactin should be considered a possible cause. The patient should be screened with a random, non-fasting serum prolactin level test, and the following measures of treatment considered:

1   If it is time to stop the antipsychotic medication and clinically indicated, do so.
2   Reduce the dose of the offending medication to the lowest possible effective dose.
3   Switch the patient to a non-offending psychotropic including clozapine, olanzapine, quetiapine, aripiprazole or ziprasidone.
4   If the offending medication cannot be stopped or switching medication has failed:[53]
    •   If the prolactin level is high-normal or mildly elevated (<50 mg/ml), watch and wait. Recheck the prolactin level in 3 months and periodically thereafter, as long as the offending medication is continued.
    •   If the prolactin level is greater than 0.50 mg/ml, consider an endocrinologic consultation and/or CT or MRI of the head (cone-down sella turcica).
5   If symptoms in Table 19.14 persist and treatment is necessary, treat with bromocriptine 5–12.5 mg/day.

Table 19.14 Clinical effects of elevated prolactin

• Menstrual irregularity, infrequent or lack of menstrual periods
• Sexual side effects, including decreased libido, impaired arousal and erectile function, and possible ejaculatory and orgasmic dysfunction
• Infertility
• Gynecomastia (breast enlargement)
• Galactorrhea (leaking of breast milk and breast tenderness)
• Weight gain

Source: Adapted from Compton MT and Miller AH (2002) Antipsychotic-induced hyper prolactinemia and sexual dysfunction. *Psychopharmacological Bulletin* 36(1): 15.

Whenever a switch of medications is made or treatment for the hyperprolactinemia is instituted, women patients should be educated about the possible increase in fertility potential. Patients who have been infertile and perhaps have become lax in using contraception while on the offending medication may find themselves more fertile, and pregnancy becomes an increased possibility when the medication is stopped.

Hypotension

Patients taking MAO inhibitors, TCAs, traditional and some atypical antipsychotics may show lowered systolic and diastolic blood pressure with consequent dizziness and lightheadedness. If the amount of lowering is not dramatic, and does not lead to near-fainting or passing out, several remedies may be helpful to allow the patient to live with the mild symptoms. Postural hypotension (lightheadedness that only occurs when getting up quickly from a seated or lying position) occurs because of blood pooling in the distensible veins of the legs. Before getting up, have the patient clench the calf and thigh muscles to compress leg veins and then arise slowly. If the dizziness is non-positional and occurs when walking or standing, the patient can also be instructed to wear support hosiery to compress leg veins continuously. In more severe cases, and when the offending drug cannot be changed, the patient can be instructed to use a stimulant. A small dose of methylphenidate or other stimulant (2.5–10 mg) several times a day will often boost blood pressure sufficiently so that lightheadedness is a minimal problem.

Falls

Falls in patients who take mental health medications are often assumed to be due primarily to hypotension. While this is one cause, there are others – sedation, psycho-motor impairment, dizziness, impaired or blurred vision. All of these alone or in combination can increase the fall risk for medicated patients, particularly the elderly and individuals compromised by other medical illnesses. When medications are used in combinations, the risk of falls is known to increase, even in young or middle-aged patients.[54-55] Other, non-psychotropic medications such as antihypertensives, anti-Parkinsonian medication, diuretics, anti-arrhythmics and anti-angina medications are also well known to create increased fall risk. Patients who take these medications in addition to psychotropics should be monitored vigilantly.

With psychotropic prescription, *the clinician should always give consideration to the fall risk in this particular patient with this particular medication*. It is usually unreasonable to withhold appropriate psychotropic medication solely because of concern for falling, even in vulnerable patients. However, it may be necessary to consider a second-line medication choice with lower risk, give specific warnings to the patient/caregiver about falls and/or initiation of a medication in smaller than normal doses. In situations where a psychotropic is essential to good mental health but the fall risk is great in a vulnerable patient, other interventions must be considered including the use of a helmet, a multi-prong cane, a walker, a wheelchair or advising caregivers not to allow patients to walk unassisted.

Virtually all psychotropic medication categories increase the risk of falls. These include:

- antipsychotics, both first and second generation
- all classes of antidepressants

- benzodiazepines and other sedative hypnotics
- anticonvulsants used as mood stabilizers.

In patients deemed to be at greater than average risk for falls, the prescriber's evaluation should include:

- a thorough understanding of all medications taken, prescription and non-prescription
- a history of alcohol use
- the patient's history of falls
- a comprehensive physical evaluation, including:
  - a gait and balance assessment
  - a vision examination
  - a measurement of postural blood pressure
  - a targeted neurologic, musculoskeletal and cardiovascular examination.

Elevation of blood sugar and lipids

Psychiatric patients have long been known to have multiple risk factors for obesity, cardiovascular disease and poor blood sugar regulation. These include:

- sedentary lifestyle with lack of exercise
- smoking
- poor dietary habits
- hypertension
- impaired motivation for change.

Patients with schizophrenia and other psychotic illnesses are statistically two to three times as likely to be overweight even without psychotropic medication.[56] While these facts have been evident, the issue of metabolic concerns in the mental health patient has only come to the forefront in the last three decades with the advent of second-generation antipsychotic agents.[57] These second-generation "atypical" antipsychotics have both therapeutic benefits on so-called "negative" symptoms of schizophrenia and safety improvements related to lessened movement disorders and tardive dyskinesia. The Achilles' heel of these medications, however, is that to varying degrees, they all cause metabolic effects which can lead to obesity, Type-2 diabetes and hyperlipidemia with all their subsequent health consequences.

Psychotropic-induced weight gain is associated with increased fat deposition in the visceral adipose tissue. Excess visceral fat leads to dyslipidemia, hypertension, increased risk for Type-2 diabetes. It is, therefore, a key factor in the development of cardiovascular disease and associated morbidity and mortality, although the exact mechanism behind visceral fat increasing cardiovascular risk and impairing glucose metabolism is still unclear.[58]

It is no longer competent clinical mental health practice to prescribe these medications without assessing baseline lipid and blood sugar levels with additional monitoring over time.

Each medication within this class has a differing risk of causing metabolic interference, as noted in Table 19.15.[59]

Table 19.15 Metabolic effects of atypical antipsychotics

Medication	Weight gain	Risk for diabetes	Dyslipidemia
Clozapine	+++	+	+
Olanzapine	+++	+	+
Risperidone	++	IR	IR
Quetiapine	++	IR	IR
Aripiprazole	+/–	–	–
Ziprasidone	+/–	–	–
Amisulpride (UK only)	–	–	–

Note: + increasing effect; – no effect; IR inconclusive results.

Table 19.16 Monitoring protocol for patients on second-generation antipsychotics

	Baseline	4 weeks	8 weeks	12 weeks	Quarterly	Annually	Every 5 years
Personal/family history	X					X	
Weight (BMI)	X	X	X	X	X		
Waist circumference	X					X	
Blood pressure	X			X		X	
Fasting plasma glucose	X			X		X	
Fasting lipid profile	X			X			X

Source: American Diabetes Association, American Psychiatric Association, American Association of Clinical Endocrinologists *et al.* (2004) Consensus development conference on antipsychotic drugs and obesity and diabetes. *Diabetes Care* 27: 596–601.

Note: More frequent assessments may be warranted based on clinical status.

Newer atypicals, including asenapine, iloperidone and lurasidone, all have promising, shorter-term data suggesting that their metabolic profiles are good to excellent with minimal effect on weight, blood sugar and lipid levels. While this is reassuring and likely to put them in a more favorable group which already includes aripiprazole, ziprasidone and amisulpride, as always, real-world longer-term experience is necessary to bear out this assessment.

A protocol for assessment and monitoring of blood sugar and lipid levels from the American Diabetic Association is shown in Table 19.16.

Hyponatremia

Hyponatremia, a low level of serum sodium, is a moderately common side effect of psychotropic prescription in certain vulnerable populations. This condition most commonly occurs with the use of highly serotonergic antidepressants (especially SSRIs and venlafaxine), but has also been reported with carbamazepine, various traditional and second-generation antipsychotics and clozapine.[60]

When prescribing psychotropics, there are many risk factors for hyponatremia. Some of the most important include:

- concomitant use of thiazide diuretics
- female gender
- older age, especially age >80
- low BMI
- psychotropic polypharmacy
- CYP 3A4 interactions
- low basal levels of sodium
- decreased renal function
- hyperkalemia.

Most importantly from this list, concomitant use of SSRIs and thiazides may pose a 13-fold increase in hyponatremia risk

Normal serum sodium is between 136 and 145 mmol/L. Mild hyponatremia (serum sodium of 125–135 mmol/L) can be asymptomatic or show the following symptoms:

- weakness, lethargy
- confusion
- headache
- anorexia.

More severe symptoms occur when the sodium level drops rapidly (within 48 hours) and/or falls below 125 mmol/L. In this situation, delirium, seizures, coma and death can occur.

Medication-induced hyponatremia generally appears during the first 2 weeks of treatment and may progress gradually or rapidly. Some of the initial symptoms of hyponatremia can be mistaken for worsening of depressive symptoms. The clinician who fails to recognize SSRI-induced hyponatremia might increase the antidepressant dose instead of reducing it, leading to a more severe form of hyponatremia.[61]

In most patients without additional risk factors, routine measurement of sodium is not necessary when beginning a psychotropic medication. The most important consideration for the prescriber is to maintain vigilance for the possibility of hyponatremia in those individuals with one or more risk factors. In these patients, if minimal or no symptoms are present, a baseline sodium level, a repeat test in 2–3 weeks, then quarterly rechecks are appropriate.

The sudden emergence of symptoms warrants more urgent action, and care is often best referred to a specialist colleague. Once significantly lowered levels of sodium are detected, the suspected drug must be stopped and restriction of fluid intake to 1.5 liters per day may correct mild hyponatremia.[62–64]

Re-challenge with an offending antidepressant may or may not cause a recurrence of hyponatremia. Prescription of an antidepressant with stronger noradrenergic action (reboxetine, desipramine, lofepramine or an MAO inhibitor) or use of ECT is recommended.

Suicidality

All of the other side effects mentioned in this chapter are physical in nature and it may seem unusual to consider the mental issue of suicidality as a "side effect" of medication therapy. Because of the seriousness of this issue as well as the residue of controversy about it, further discussion is warranted beyond the initial discussion in Chapter 2.

Despite numerous data analyses and scholarly articles on the subject of quantifying suicidal behavior in relation to the use of psychotropic medications (and particularly antidepressants), confusion continues to persist. Much of this controversy relates to articles published in 2003 and 2006 by Hammad *et al.*[65-66] which suggested that there was an increase in suicidality in children and adolescents who had begun antidepressant medication therapy. At the time, this created considerable attention in the popular press and obvious concern among mental health practitioners. In the original paper, the incidence of "suicidality" was approximately doubled from 2 percent in placebo-treated patients to 4 percent in those taking antidepressant medications.

Several studies surveying large populations have subsequently challenged the conclusion of this study and have called into question whether, in fact, there is any increase in suicidality with antidepressant medication. A further methodological problem with the 2006 study was that it included the concept of "suicidality" without clarification as to whether this reflected suicidal ideation, suicidal attempts or completed suicides. It is well known to clinicians that suicidal ideation is very common in mental health patients, particularly those who are depressed. The presence of suicidal ideation may have little statistical relationship to suicidal behavior and/or completion. The most recent large-scale study by Gibbons and Mann in 2011[67] concluded that there was little evidence of psychotropic drugs increasing the risk of suicide and related behavior. The study went on to state that "numerous lines of evidence in adults clearly demonstrate that *the inadequate treatment of depression* (pharmacotherapy and/or psychotherapy) is associated with increased risk of suicidal behavior." A further publication by the same group states:[68]

> Fluoxetine and venlafaxine decreased suicidal thoughts and behavior for adult and geriatric patients. This protective effect is mediated by decreases in depressive symptoms with treatment. For youths, no significant effects of treatment on suicidal thoughts and behavior were found, although depression responded to treatment. No evidence of increased suicide risk was observed in youths receiving active medication.

The "black box warning" issued in America by the Food and Drug Administration for all antidepressants in 2004 is active and prominently displayed in American psychopharmacology textbooks. Many clinicians now believe that this warning was based on minimal solid evidence, and further evidence shows markedly differing results. While a prescriber cannot be cavalier with regard to this possibility, virtually all would agree that the incidence of increased suicidal ideation or behavior in patients treated with antidepressants remains a rare event. It is as likely, and perhaps more likely, that suicidal ideas or behavior in a newly medicated patient may reflect poor adherence to the medication or choice of a non-effective medication rather than a true "side effect" of the medication. Based on the evidence to date, the wise clinician will continue to prescribe antidepressants in appropriately diagnosed depressed patients. He/she should not avoid these medications solely because of a purported small increase in suicidal risk. This is true even when the patient may have suicidal ideation as a presenting symptom of their mental health problem. There is ample evidence to suggest that the competent prescription of antidepressants, in combination with psychotherapy and other non-medication treatments, benefits such patients and diminishes suicidal thoughts and behavior in the vast majority of situations.

Nonetheless, the clinician will need to inform the patient that there have been reports of a small increase in suicidal thoughts in some patients, and if that were to happen, to report any such occurrence promptly to the prescriber. Close monitoring of a depressed patient's condition for all symptoms, including suicidal thoughts, during the first several weeks of treatment is, of course, recommended and is the standard of care.

Assuming that a medicated patient improves with the use of an antidepressant, there is no evidence that medication-related suicidal action or ideation occurs later in a course of medication. Any flare-up of suicidal ideation or behavior after a substantial period of improvement is due to other factors and is not a medication side effect.

Side effects and medication combinations

Prescribing several medications simultaneously for a patient is the rule rather than the exception in modern mental health. It is not at all uncommon for patients to be taking several medications simultaneously. Intuitively, most clinicians have assumed that if a single medication caused one or more side effects, the number and intensity of side effects would increase if multiple medications were prescribed. The most recent study to assess this, however, in treatment-resistant depression revealed a surprising result. In this study,[69] 1300 patients who had not responded to citalopram alone were divided into two groups. The first group was switched to another antidepressant and the second group had citalopram augmented by bupropion or buspirone. Unexpectedly, there was no significant difference in the number or strength of side effects between the two groups. While this conclusion cannot be applied to other diagnoses or other medication combinations, it does give some reassurance to the prescribing clinician. As the authors state (p. 16), "For treatment resistant depression, the decision to augment or switch medications should be based on [an] individual patient's clinical status, as well as the possible benefits and risks of each treatment." Although there is no specific research to support or undermine the recommendation, in general, prescribers should not be dissuaded from using medication combinations by the *theoretical* possibility that more side effects may occur. Increased side effects may or may not occur and each specific situation should be evaluated individually. (See Chapter 5 for further discussion of medication combinations.)

References

1 Silverstein FS *et al.* (1983) Hematological monitoring during therapy with car-bamazepine in children [letter]. *Annals of Neurology* 13: 685–686.
2 Miller CH *et al.* (1996) The prevalence and severity of acute extrapyramidal side effects in patients treated with clozapine, risperidone or conventional antipsychotics. In American Psychiatric Association (ed.) *New Research Program and Abstracts of the 149th Annual Meeting of the American Psychiatric Association, May 8 1996, New York* (Abstract NR542: pp. 217–218), APA.

3   Rosebrush PI and Mazurek MF (1999) Neurologic side effects in neuroleptic-naïve patients treated with haloperidol or risperidone. *Neurology* 52: 782–785.

4   Kapur S *et al.* (1999) Clinical and theoretical implications of 5-HT2 and D2 receptor occupancy of clozapine, risperidone and olanzapine in schizophrenia. *American Journal of Psychiatry* 156: 286–293.

5   Fleuschacher WW *et al.* (1990) The pharmacologic treatment of neuroleptic induced akathisia. *Journal of Clinical Psychopharmacology* 10: 12–21.

6   Available at: www.neurologyreviews.com/Article.aspx?ArticleId=1t3blPEVOLI=& Full Text=1

7   Seagraves R (1998) Antidepressant-induced sexual dysfunction. *Journal of Clinical Psychiatry* 59 (Suppl. 4): 48–54.

8   Bartlik B *et al.* (1999) Sexual dysfunction secondary to depressive disorders. *Journal of Gender-Specific Medicine* 2(2): 52–60.

9   MacLean F and Lee A (1999) Drug induced sexual dysfunction and infertility. *Pharmaceutical Journal* 262 (7047): 780–784.

10   Nurnberg HG *et al.* (2001) Sildenafil citrate in extension of a double-blind placebo-controlled study for serotonergic reuptake inhibitor-induced sexual dysfunction: open-label results. Presented at the American Psychiatric Association Conference.

11   Ashton AK and Rosen RC (1998) Bupropion as an antidote for serotonin reuptake inhibitor-induced sexual dysfunction. *Journal of Clinical Psychiatry* 59: 112–115.

12   Labbate LA *et al.* (1997) Bupropion treatment of serotonin reuptake antidepressant-associated sexual dysfunction. *Annals of Clinical Psychiatry* 9: 241–245.

13   Aquila R (2002) Management of weight gain in patients with schizophrenia. *Journal of Clinical Psychiatry* 63 (Suppl. 4): 33–36.

14   Coodin S (2001) Body mass index in persons with schizophrenia. *Canadian Journal of Psychiatry* 46: 549–555.

15   McElroy S *et al.* (2002) Correlates of overweight and obesity in 644 patients with bipolar disorder. *Journal of Clinical Psychiatry* 63(3): 207–213.

16   Weissenburger J *et al.* (1986) Weight changes in depression. *Psychiatry Research* 17: 275–283.

17   Pine DS *et al.* (2001) The association between childhood depression and adulthood body mass index. *Pediatrics* 107: 1049–1056.

18   Elmslie JL *et al.* (2000) Prevalence of overweight and obesity in bipolar patients. *Journal of Clinical Psychiatry* 61: 179–184.

19   Elmslie JL *et al.* (2001) Determinants of overweight and obesity in patients with bipolar disorder. *Journal of Clinical Psychiatry* 62: 486–491.

20   Allison DB *et al.* (1999) The distribution of body mass index among individuals with and without schizophrenia. *Journal of Clinical Psychiatry* 60: 215–220.

21   Kinon BJ *et al.* (2001) Long term olanzapine treatment: weight changes and weight-related health factors in schizophrenia. *Journal of Clinical Psychiatry* 69: 92–100.

22   Casey DE and Zorn SH (2001) The pharmacology of weight gain with antipsychotics. *Journal of Clinical Psychiatry* 65 (Suppl. 7): 4–10.

23   Litrell KH *et al.* (2002) *Educational Interventions for the Management of Antipsychotic-Related Weight Gain*, The Promedica Research Center.

24   O'Keefe C *et al.* (2001) Reversal of weight gain associated with antipsychotic treatment. Presented at the American Psychiatric Association Annual Meeting, New Orleans, May.

25   Ball PM *et al.* (2001) A program for treating olanzapine-related weight gain. *Psychiatric Services* 52: 967–969.

26   Maren M (2001) Evaluating weight loss programs. Presented at National Conference of Nurse Practitioners, Baltimore, MD, November.

27   Dursun SM and Devarajan S (2000) Clozapine weight gain plus topirimate weight loss [letter]. *Canadian Journal of Psychiatry* 40: 198.

28 Privitera MD (1997) Topirimate: a new antiepileptic drug. *Annals of Pharmacotherapy* 31: 1164–1173.

29 Hussain MA *et al.* (2000) Topirimate as an anti-obesity agent. In American Psychiatric Association (ed.), New Research Abstracts of the 153rd Annual Meeting of the American Psychiatric Association, May 18 2000, Chicago (Abstract NR709: 249), APA.

30 Gadde KM *et al.* (2002) Zonisamide in obesity: a 16-week randomized trial. Presented at the American Psychiatric Association Meeting, Philadelphia, May.

31 Correa N *et al.* (1987) Amantadine in the treatment of neuroendocrine side effects of neuroleptics. *Journal of Clinical Psychopharmacology* 7: 91–95.

32 Floris M *et al.* (2001) Effect of amantadine on weight gain during olanzapine treatment. *European Neuropsychopharmacology* 11: 181–182.

33 Breier A *et al.* (2001) Nizatidine for the prevention of weight gain during olanzapine treatment in schizophrenia and related disorders: a randomized controlled double-blind study. Presented at the Meeting of the Colleges of Psychiatric and Neurologic Pharmacists, San Antonio, March, 23–26.

34 Morrison JA *et al.* (2002) Metformin for weight loss in pediatric patients taking psychotropic drugs. *American Journal of Psychiatry* 159(4): 655–657.

35 Wu RR *et al.* (2012) Metformin for treatment of antipsychotic-induced weight gain in women with first episode schizophrenia: a double-blind, randomized, placebo-controlled study. *American Journal of Psychiatry* 169: 813–821.

36 Hoodia: lots of hoopla, little science, available at: www.webmd.com/diet/guide/hoodia-lots-of-hoopla-little-science

37 Centers for Disease Control and Prevention (1996) Adverse effects with ephedra containing products: December 1993–September 1995. *Morbidity and Mortal Weekly Report* 45: 689–692.

38 Sussman N and Ginsberg D (1998) Weight gain associated with SSRIs. *Primary Psychiatry* 1: 28–37.

39 Saper JR *et al.* (1993) *The Handbook of Headache Management*, Williams and Wilkins, pp. 104–109.

40 Warnock JK (1991) Psychotropic medications and drug-related alopecia. *Psychosomatics* 32: 149–152.

41 Azrin N *et al.* (1978) Drug causes of hair loss. *Drug and Therapeutics Bulletin* 16: 77–79.

42 Blankenship ML (1983) Drugs and alopecia. *Australian Journal of Dermatology* 24: 100–104.

43 Maguire HC (1979) Drug-induced alopecia. *American Family Physician* 19: 178–179.

44 Gautam M (1999) Alopecia due to psychotropic medication. *Annals of Pharmacotherapy* 33: 631–636.

45 Brodin M (1987) Drug related alopecia. *Dermatology Clinics* 5: 571–579.

46 Barth J and Dawber R (1989) Drug induced hair loss [letter]. *British Medical Journal* 298: 675.

47 Potter WZ and Ketter TA (1993) Pharmacological issues in the treatment of bipolar disorder: focus on mood stabilizing compounds. *Canadian Journal of Psychiatry* 38 (Suppl. 2): S51–S56.

48 Compton MT and Miller AH (2002) Antipsychotic-induced hyper prolactinemia and sexual dysfunction. *Psychopharmacological Bulletin* 36(1): 143–164.

49 Meltzer HY and Fang VS (1976) The effect of neuroleptics on serum prolactin in schizophrenic patients. *Archives of General Psychiatry* 33: 279–286.

50 Yasui N *et al.* (1998) Prolactin response to bromperidol treatment in schizophrenic patients. *Pharmacology and Toxicology* 82: 153–156.

51 Kuruvilla A *et al.* (1992) A study of serum prolactin levels in schizophrenia: comparison of males and females. *Clinical and Experimental Pharmacology and Physiology* 19: 603–606.

52 Grunder G *et al.* (1999) Neuroendocrine response in antipsychotics: effects of drug type and gender. *Biological Psychiatry* 45: 89–97.

53 *Family Practice Notebook*, available at: www.fpnotebook.com

54 Rubenstein LZ *et al.* (2001) Quality indicators for the management and prevention of falls and mobility problems in vulnerable elders. *Annals of Internal Medicine* 135: 686–693.

55 Leipzig RM *et al.* (1999) Drugs and falls in older people: a systematic review and meta-analysis, Part I and II. Psychotropic drugs. *Journal of the American Geriatric Society* 47: 30–50.

56 Coodin S (2001) Body mass index in persons with schizophrenia. *Canadian Journal of Psychiatry* 46: 549–555.

57 Dayabandara M *et al.* (2017) Antipsychotic-associated weight gain: management strategies and impact on treatment adherence. *Neuropsychiatric Disease and Treatment* 13: 2231–2241. doi: 10.2147/NDT.S113099

58 Tschoner A *et al.* (2007) Metabolic side effects of antipsychotic medication. *International Journal of Clinical Practice* 61(8): 1356–1370.

59 American Diabetes Association, American Psychiatric Association, American Association of Clinical Endocrinologists *et al.* (2004) Consensus development conference on anti-psychotic drugs and obesity and diabetes. *Diabetes Care* 27: 596–601.

60 Appiani F (2011) Hyponatremia. *Psychiatry Weekly* 6(14).

61 Appiani F (2009) *Efectos adversos y seguridad en psicofármacos*, Akadia.

62 Alanen HM *et al.* (2011) Hyponatremia due to psychoactive drugs is common in the elderly. *Duodecim laaketieteellinen aikakauskirja* 127(4): 406–413.

63 Vucicevic Z *et al.* (2007) Fatal hyponatremia and other metabolic disturbances associated with psychotropic drug polypharmacy. *International Journal of Clinical Pharmacology and Therapeutics* 45(5): 289–292.

64 *The Maudsley Prescribing Guidelines* (2009), 10th edn., Informa Healthcare, pp. 119–120, 193–194.

65 Hammad TA *et al.* (2003) Incidence of suicides in randomized controlled trials of patients with major depressive disorder. *Pharmacoepidemiology and Drug Safety* 12 (Suppl. 1): S156.

66 Hammad TA *et al.* (2006) Suicidality in pediatric patients treated with antidepressant drugs. *Archives of General Psychiatry* 63: 332–339.

67 Gibbons RD and Mann JJ (2011) Strategies for quantifying the relationship between medications and suicidal behavior: what has been learned? *Drug Safety* 34(5): 375–395.

68 Gibbons RD *et al.* (2012) Suicidal thoughts and behavior with antidepressant treatment reanalysis of the randomized placebo-controlled studies of fluoxetine and venlafaxine. *Archives of General Psychiatry* 69(6): 580–587.

69 Hansen RA *et al.* (2011) Risk of adverse events in treatment-resistant depression: propensity-score-matched comparison of antidepressant augment and switch strategies. *General Hospital Psychiatry* (November): 11–14.

20 Danger zones – areas of risk with psychotropics

• P-450 issues made easy	333
• Serotonin syndrome	340
• Anticholinergic intoxication	343
• Lithium toxicity	346
• QTc interval issues	349
• Sudden death and antipsychotics	354
• Extrapyramidal symptoms, neuroleptic malignant syndrome and tardive dyskinesia	355
• Extrapyramidal symptoms	356
• Neuroleptic malignant syndrome	359
• Tardive dyskinesia	361
• Monoamine oxidase inhibitor reactions	364
• Other potentially dangerous side effects	368
• Notes and references	373

Statistically, and in day-to-day clinical practice, most psychotropic medication side effects can be uncomfortable and bothersome but do not present areas of serious risk to health and safety. As with all medications, however, there are some psychotropic medication interactions and certain clinical situations that present serious risk of morbidity or, rarely, mortality. This chapter will focus on these areas of more significant risk, their symptoms, prevention and treatment.

Other than issues of P-450 interactions which are better understood in a different format, each condition will be further divided to address:

- the syndrome and its cause
- signs and symptoms
- clinical situations of increased risk
- prognosis
- prevention
- treatment.

P-450 issues made easy

Virtually unknown to most mental health practitioners several decades ago, P-450 enzyme interaction issues are now well known and are a potentially important clinical consideration when clinicians prescribe psychotropics, particularly antidepressants.

Although P-450 interactions are not limited to antidepressants, the majority of such interactions that concern mental health prescribers involve this group of medications. Broadly, *P-450 interactions are those interactions that affect a drug's pharmacokinetics – that is, a drug's metabolism or elimination.*

The P-450 enzyme system is a cytochrome enzyme system located primarily in the liver, but also present in the small intestine, lungs and kidneys. The system got its name – cytochrome P-450 (CYP-450) – because this enzyme makes a "peak" at 450 nm when analyzed by spectrophotometry. The names used to identify each individual enzyme within the system include several numbers and letters. Some books will preface the numbers and letters with the abbreviation CYP, meaning "cytochrome P-450 system." The first number indicates the family of the enzyme, the letter indicates the subfamily within that family, and the second number indicates the specific enzyme within that family. Therefore, CYP1A2 indicates the cytochrome P-450 enzyme of the first family, the A subfamily and the second enzyme in the A subfamily.

The P-450 enzyme system is involved in the breakdown and metabolism (through hydroxylation) of medications. At present over 34 such enzymes have been identified, although only a small number of them are important to the mental health prescribing clinician. Metabolism of many psychotropics occurs by hydroxylation, which becomes the "rate limiting step" of medication breakdown; that is, when speed of hydroxylation is affected, the entire process of breakdown and excretion may either be accelerated or slowed. When the effectiveness of a P-450 enzyme is either inhibited or induced (see below), it affects the speed of metabolism of any medication broken down by that enzyme. This can lead to significant changes in the serum blood concentration of that specific medication in the body.

It is suggested that the most effective way to learn about and clinically manage P-450 enzyme interactions is to understand certain key definitions, understand the principles of enzyme interaction, and be familiar with some of the more common interactions in mental health prescription. Beyond this basic understanding, it is best to use a chart that documents known P-450 interactions, since memorizing the list is very difficult.

Important definitions

A *substrate* is the site where an enzyme works; i.e., a medication that will be acted upon or broken down by an enzyme.

An enzyme is *inhibited* if its activity is blocked or slowed, resulting in a *raised* blood level of any substrate medication that is metabolized by that enzyme. Enzyme *inhibition* occurs when two or more drugs compete for the same enzyme. It can be reversible or irreversible. Usually, it begins after the first dose of the inhibitor; its maximum effect is reached at steady state (usually within four to seven half-lives).

An enzyme is *induced* if more of the enzyme is produced or its activity is increased, which results in a *lowered* blood level of any substrate medication that is metabolized by this enzyme. Enzyme *induction* usually occurs because of increased synthesis of an enzyme when exposed to particular drugs or substances. This usually begins within 2 days, but takes more than a week to reach its maximum effect.

The conveyor belt analogy

A useful analogy to the understanding of the pharmacokinetic interactions associated with the P-450 enzyme is that of a conveyor belt used by workers to remove boxes of product from a factory. In this analogy, the boxes of product are medications to be metabolized and excreted from the body (moved outside the factory). P-450 enzymes are the workers that package the product into boxes and place the boxes on the conveyor belt for exit from the factory. Once outside the factory, the boxes (medications) have been excreted. On a normal workday (when the patient is taking a steady dose of a psychotropic medication), there is a regular inventory of boxes put on the assembly line by the workers (enzymes) at a predictable rate that leads to a steady removal (metabolism and excretion). The workers (enzymes) work at a fixed speed, leading to excretion at a predictable rate. When a worker is inhibited (for example, if a ball and chain is put on his leg), he is unable to do his job as rapidly. Less product is packaged and placed on the conveyor belt and, therefore, the inventory of boxes inside the factory grows and may become abnormally high. At times this excess inventory may become so large as to cause problems inside the factory (drug accumulation side effects or toxicity).

When a worker (enzyme) is induced (for example, by offering him higher pay), he works faster and more efficiently. More product is packaged and placed on the conveyor belt for exit (excretion). Inventory of product in the factory becomes low (substrate medication levels drop). Because of this low inventory in the factory (low blood levels of medication), the medication may become clinically less effective or stop working.

Common P-450 facts and principles

The following statements are some of the more prominent issues relevant to psychiatric prescription, taken from a long list of possible P-450 issues and interactions.

- Two enzymes, 3A3/4 and 2D6, account for 50 percent and 30 percent respectively of all P-450 phase 1 metabolism. All other enzymes combined account for the remaining 20 percent. Of the remaining 30+ enzymes, only 1A2, 2C9 and 2C19 have clinically relevant interactions for the mental health prescriber.
- The most common significant inhibitors of P-450 enzymes are antidepressants – fluoxetine, paroxetine and bupropion (which inhibit 2D6), and nefazodone and fluvoxamine (both of which inhibit 1A2 and 3A3/3A4). Several antidepressants have minimal or no documented P-450 interactions. These include mirtazapine and venlafaxine.
- Grapefruit juice blocks enzyme 1A2. No medication should be taken with grapefruit juice. This includes all forms of grapefruit and grapefruit juice – fresh, canned or frozen. All other juices are safe and do not result in significant P-450 interactions.
- Of the human population, 10–20 percent have no 2D6 enzyme (7–10 percent of Caucasians and up to 15 percent of Asians). Because they have no 2D6, these persons may have an initial serum blood concentration of any medication metabolized by 2D6 (including all SSRIs and tricyclics) that is significantly higher than usual on a small oral dose. This is one of the explanations for a person who gets exaggerated side effects and/or clinical effects to what is otherwise a small dose of medication. A test for the presence or absence of 2D6 as well as the presence of various alleles is available through the Mayo Clinic laboratories.
- Several minor inhibitors of a particular enzyme may result in a clinically significant reaction when taken simultaneously, even if anyone inhibitor does not significantly block metabolism.
- The most common psychotropics to cause enzyme (induction) are carbamazepine and lamotrigine.

- The metabolism of estrogen and oral contraceptives is accomplished primarily via 3A4. Potent inducers of 3A4 (such as carbamazepine and lamotrigine) may accelerate the metabolism of estrogen and diminish the effectiveness of hormone replacement therapy and/or oral contraceptives.
- Cigarette smoking and eating charbroiled meats induce enzyme 1A2, and may therefore decrease blood levels of all psychotropics metabolized by 1A2 (such as clozapine, fluvoxamine, haloperidol, imipramine, olanzapine and theophylline).
- Medication with a narrow therapeutic index (a small difference between therapeutic serum levels and toxic serum levels) may result in clinically significant problems from P-450 interactions. Common drugs with a narrow therapeutic index include tricyclic antidepressants, cardiac anti-arrhythmics and prescription pain medications.

Using blood levels to assist with P-450 interactions

If a substrate medication subject to a P-450 interaction is measurable through serum blood level monitoring (for example, TCAs, carbamazepine and clozapine), use of blood levels is helpful in readjusting the dose of these medications. A clinical example will illustrate. If paroxetine (a known inhibitor of 2D6) is added to a stable regimen of imipramine (a TCA metabolized by 2D6), the clinician can expect inhibition of the enzyme and decreased metabolism of the imipramine – leading to higher blood levels of imipramine. To prescribe safely in this situation and avoid toxicity, the clinician should obtain a blood level of imipramine before the paroxetine is started, then add paroxetine and prescribe only half of the current imipramine dose. The imipramine serum level should be rechecked in 4–7 days. Based on the result, the imipramine dose may be increased (or decreased), checking the blood level with each adjustment until a therapeutic imipramine level is achieved.

If the combination is started in reverse order (i.e., the imipramine is added to a stable paroxetine dose), the imipramine should be started at half the usual starting dose, the serum blood level checked (expecting it to be higher than usual for this dose) and the imipramine dosage readjusted to reach a therapeutic level based on the serum blood level results. Several adjustments and serum level rechecks may be necessary.

Use of a chart

In the last *Physician's Desk Reference*, over 1000 prescription drugs are listed. This results in a potential 2.8×1015 combinations of medications. With each new drug approved, another 4.4 trillion possible multiple drug combinations become available.[1] While many of these interactions are clinically insignificant, it is clear that attempting to learn all of them is impossible.

Since it is not possible to memorize all P-450 enzyme interactions, and new interactions are being discovered almost monthly, beyond the common interactions noted in this section, the clinician should utilize a chart that is current and keep a copy of this chart on hand in the office for consultation during medication prescription. A particularly helpful website that is actively updated and contains a number of possible P-450 interactions is maintained by Dr. David Flockhart at the University of Indiana. The website address is http://medicine.iupui.edu/flockhart/. An example of a list of clinically relevant P-450 interactions, available at this website, is shown in Table 20.1.

Table 20.1 Drugs with known P-450 enzyme metabolism

1A2	2B6	2C19	2C9	2D6*	3A
Clozapine	Bupropion	Amitriptyline	Celecoxib	Amitriptyline	Alprazolam
Cyclobenzapine	Cyclophosphamide	Citalopram	Diclofenac	Carvedilol	Buspirone
Fluvoxamine	Ifosfamide	Diazepam	Flurbiprofen	Clomipramine	Calcium channel blockers
Haloperidol		Imipramine	Ibuprofen	Codeine	Carbamazepine
Imipramine		Lansoprazole	Losartan	Desipramine	Cyclosporine
Mexiletine		Nelfinavir	Naproxen	Dextromethorphan	Efavirenz
Olanzapine		Omeprazole	Phenytoin	Fluoxetine	Haloperidol
Tacrine		Phenytoin	Piroxicam	Metoprolol	HIV protease inhibitors
Theophylline		Pantoprozole	Torsemide	Nortriptyline	Statins (not pravastatin)
Zileuton			Tolbutamide	Oudaasetrun	Midazolam
Zolmitriptan			Warfarin	Oxycodone	Nevirapine
				Paroxetine	Tacrolimus
				Propafenone	Triazolam
				Risperidone	Zolpidem
				Timolol	
Inhibitors					
Cimetidine	Thiotepa	Cimetidine	Amiodarone	Amiodarone	Andodarone
Ciprofloxacin		Felbamate	Fluconazole	Chlorpheniramine	Diltiazem and verapamil
Fluvoxamine		Fluoxetine	Fluoxetine	Fluoxetine	Grapefruit juice
Levofloxacin		Fluvoxamine	Fluvostatin	Haloperidol	HIV protease inhibitors
		soniazid	Metronidazole	Indinavir	Itraconazole
		Ketoconazole	Paroxetine	Paroxetine	Ketoconazole
		Lansoprazole	Zafirtukast	Ritonavir	Macrolide antibiotics (not azithromycin)
		Omeprazole		Terbinatine	
		Ticlopidine		Ticlopidine	Nefazodone
Inducers					
Carbamazepine	Phenobarbital	Carbamazepine	Phenobarbital	Carbamazepine	Chargrilled meat
Phenytoin	Rifampin	Rifampin	Efavirenz and nevirapine	Rifampin	Rifampin
Rifabutin and rifampin	Tobacco	Ritonavir	St. John's Wort		

Source: Flockhart DA (2007) Drug interactions: cytochrome P-450 drug interaction table, Indiana University School of Medicine, available at: http://medicine.iupui.edu/flockhart/

*Note: Absent in 15–30% of Asians, absent in 7% of Caucasians.

A more detailed list, including less common interactions, is also available for download at that site.

Further detailed information on P-450 interactions can be seen in review articles.[2-3] As discussed in Chapter 3, commercially available tests of cytochrome P-450 enzyme levels do not currently help the prescriber make clinical decisions about medication metabolism.

Another way to slice the pie

Although P-450 interactions are best learned by understanding the definitions and principles and then using a chart, as outlined above, some clinicians may find it helpful to look at selected P-450 data and important interactions by particular medication class and specific medication. Therefore, the next two sections are organized in that way, and are included to assist those who prefer this style.

Antidepressants

Much of the data on P-450 interactions has been obtained from the usage of antidepressants. The P-450 effects are substantially different from class to class, and within each class.

SSRIs

Fluoxetine is an inhibitor of 2D6. Therefore, all 2D6 substrates may be elevated when fluoxetine is added. TCAs are in this group of substrates. The potential dramatic increase in TCA blood levels (which has led to toxicity and potential death) by the addition of fluoxetine is one of the classic examples of P-450 interactions.

Paroxetine is also a potent inhibitor of 2D6, and would likewise affect blood levels of tricyclics and other 2D6 substrates.

Sertraline is a relatively weak inhibitor of 2D6 and 3A4. In moderate doses its effect on 2D6 substrates is minimal; however, at high doses it may have inhibitory effects and similarly affect blood levels of tricyclics and other 2D6 substrates.

Fluvoxamine is a potent inhibitor of 1A2 and 3A4. Therefore, it will inhibit the metabolism of clozapine, TCAs, theophylline, alprazolam and triazolam. When fluvoxamine is added to a steady regimen of any of these medications, substantial blood level increase of the substrate can be expected.

Citalopram is a relatively weak inhibitor of 2D6, and in general is thought not to affect tricyclic blood levels, although there is one reported case of elevated concentrations of desipramine and clomipramine when citalopram was added. The exact mechanism of this interaction is unclear.

Other, newer antidepressants

Bupropion is a potent inhibitor of 2D6, and will elevate the blood levels of tricyclic antidepressants and other 2D6 substrates.

Nefazodone is a potent inhibitor of 3A4, and will increase the concentration of 3A4 substrates including triazolam, alprazolam and protease inhibitors used in HIV therapy.

Mirtazepine has insignificant interactions with specific cytochrome P-450 enzymes, and is thought not to cause meaningful interactions.

Venlafaxine has minimal interactions with 2D6, 3A4 or other cytochrome enzymes; however, it has been reported to increase plasma concentrations of haloperidol by up to 70 percent and desipramine up to fourfold by unknown mechanisms.[4]

Monoamine oxidase inhibitors (MAOIs), although they have another set of potential interactions that will be discussed later in this chapter, do not have known P-450 interactions.

Mood stabilizers

Lithium has many medication interactions that are summarized later in the chapter under lithium toxicity, but no specific P-450 interactions are known.

Carbamazepine is both a substrate of CYP 3A4 and an inducer of 3A4. These characteristics lead to the phenomenon of "auto-induction," where the concentration of carbamazepine is gradually diminished over time as the body's ability to metabolize it is increased by induction of more 3A4 enzyme. As a potent inducer of 3A4, carbamazepine can reduce the concentrations of alprazolam, triazolam, clonazepam, cyclosporine, lovastatin, protease inhibitors, verapamil, estrogen and oral contraceptives. Carbamazepine also decreases the concentration of lamotrigine by up to 40 percent by a different mechanism.

Oxcarbazepine, which is structurally similar to carbamazepine, can also induce metabolism of estrogen and oral contraceptives, and decrease lamotrigine levels by other mechanisms.

Valproic acid has multiple potential drug interactions with other anticonvulsants, particularly lamotrigine; however, these are not thought to result from P-450 interactions. The addition of carbamazepine to valproic acid may decrease valproic acid concentrations.

Lamotrigine can have decreased concentration caused by the addition of carbamazepine, and increased concentration by the addition of valproic acid, but neither of these is related to P-450 interactions.

Topirimate has its concentration decreased by carbamazepine, but not by a P-450 interaction.

Stimulants

Methylphenidate has caused increased tricyclic levels suggestive that there may be a P-450 interaction; however, this has not been specifically documented. When stimulants are added to a steady tricyclic regimen, it is prudent to decrease the tricyclic dosage.

Anti-anxiety medication

Benzodiazepines, particularly alprazolam, triazolam and, to some degree, diazepam, can have their metabolism inhibited via the 3A4 system when nefazodone, fluvoxamine or erythromycin is added – each of which is a potent 3A4 inhibitor. This may lead to increased sedation and side effects from these anti-anxiety medicines.

Buspirone may have its concentration increased by 3A4 inhibitors such as nefazodone or fluvoxamine, grapefruit juice or ketoconazole.

Antipsychotics

Haloperidol's metabolism has been studied for many years, but is still somewhat unclear. There is evidence that 2D6, 3A4 and 1A2 may all be involved to various degrees in its metabolism. Nefazodone and fluvoxamine (3A4 inhibitors) may raise the blood level of haloperidol. The addition of haloperidol to tricyclics may show mutual metabolic inhibition, necessitating a reduction in doses of both drugs.

Clozapine has shown interaction with 1A2, 3A4 and, to some degree, 2D6. Addition of 3A4 inhibitors, such as fluvoxamine and nefazodone, increases plasma concentrations of clozapine. 2D6 inhibitors, such as fluoxetine and paroxetine, have also increased concentrations of clozapine. Additionally, erythromycin, a potent 3A4 inhibitor, has raised clozapine doses.

Risperidone, although metabolized primarily via 2D6 and, to some degree, by 3A4, has not shown clinically significant interactions in a number of studies, and may have a relatively benign P-450 profile.

Olanzapine is principally metabolized via 1A2, although clinical interactions via the P-450 system have not currently been shown.

Quetiapine is primarily metabolized via 3A4. In theory, inducers of 3A4 could decrease its plasma concentration, although clinical reports have not been noted.

Ziprasidone, although metabolized primarily via a non-P-450 enzyme (aldehyde oxidase) and to a limited degree by 3A4 and 1A2, has shown little interaction with major P-450 enzymes.

Serotonin syndrome

The syndrome and its cause

Serotonin syndrome is a hyper serotonergic state caused by the addition of two or more medications that increase serotonin (5-hydroxytryptamine) concentrations in the brain. This leads to hyper stimulation at serotonin receptors of the brainstem and spinal cord, particularly the 5HT1A sub-receptor.

Signs and symptoms of serotonin syndrome

Symptoms of serotonin syndrome fall under five symptom clusters:

1   mental status changes
2   motor abnormalities
3   cardiovascular changes
4   gastrointestinal symptoms
5   miscellaneous other symptoms.

Specific symptoms that could occur in the context of the recent addition of a strongly serotonergic medication or a precursor of serotonin synthesis (such as L-tryptophan) are listed in Table 20.2.

Table 20.2 Symptoms associated with serotonin syndrome

1 Mental status changes	• Confusion, restlessness, coma
2 Motor abnormalities	• Myoclonus (recurrent muscle twitching or spasm) • Hyperreflexia • Muscle rigidity • Restlessness • Tremor • Ataxia and incoordination • Shivering
3 Cardiovascular changes	• Sinus tachycardia • Hypertension
4 Gastrointestinal problems	• Nausea
5 Other symptoms	• Diaphoresis • Unreactive pupils • Fever

Medical situations of risk

Although the majority of cases of serious serotonin syndrome have occurred when monoamine oxidase inhibitors are combined with SSRIs, L-tryptophan, lithium or other strongly serotonergic medications, there are a number of psychotropics and other medications that have also been implicated. These are listed in Table 20.3.

Serotonin syndrome and neuroleptic malignant syndrome (NMS – see below) share many symptoms/clinical features, and are thought to exist on a continuum of the same disorder. NMS, however, is an idiosyncratic drug reaction, whereas serotonin syndrome is an effect of drug toxicity. Patients with NMS have higher fevers and pronounced extrapyramidal signs with muscle rigidity. In general, patients with serotonin syndrome have lower fevers, gastrointestinal dysfunction and myoclonus.

Prognosis

Mild to moderate cases of serotonin syndrome usually resolve within 24–72 hours.[5] Most cases can be treated, and are completely resolved within a week, although some patients can become acutely and severely ill. Hospitalization, admission to intensive care and mechanical ventilation may be necessary in such cases. Mortality associated with severe cases of this condition is estimated to be 11 percent.[6]

Prevention

The most important element of preventing serotonin syndrome is knowing which medications are strongly serotonergic, and avoiding combinations of multiple strongly serotonergic medications. If combinations of strongly serotonergic medications are clinically necessary, it is important to start with small doses and make any dosage increases gradually.

Serotonin syndrome can occur even after a patient has stopped a drug if its clinical effect persists, or if a long-lasting metabolite remains in the body. This especially applies to MAOIs and fluoxetine. When stopping MAOIs, a 2-week "wash out" period should be maintained before beginning another strongly serotonergic medication. When

Table 20.3 Drugs that affect serotonin levels and have been implicated in serotonin syndrome

Effect	Drug
Increases serotonin synthesis	L-tryptophan
Decreases serotonin metabolism	Isocarboxazid Phenelzine Selegiline Tranylcypromine
Increases serotonin release	Amphetamines Cocaine Reserpine
Inhibits serotonin uptake	Amitriptyline Amphetamines Clomipramine Cocaine Desipramine Dextromethorphan Doxepin Fluoxetine Fluvoxamine Imipramine Meperidine Nefazodone Nortriptyline Paroxetine Protriptyline Sertraline Trazodone Venlafaxine Vilazodone
Direct serotonin receptor agonists	Buspirone Lysergic acid diethylamide (LSD) Sumatriptan
Non-specific increases in serotonin activity	Lithium
Dopamine agonists	Amantadine Bromocriptine Bupropion Levodopa Pergolide Pramipexole

Sources: Adapted from Mills K (1995) Serotonin syndrome. *American Family Physician* 52: 1475–1482; Sternbach H (1991) The serotonin syndrome. *American Journal of Psychiatry* 148: 705–713.

stopping fluoxetine and beginning an MAOI, a 4–5-week "wash-out" period should be allowed before beginning the MAOI, since a long-lasting metabolite (norfluoxetine) may still be present for that period of time.

Treatment

For most mental health practitioners, the most important elements of treatment are *recognition* of the syndrome and *discontinuation of one or more of the suspected serotonergic agents*, including any over-the-counter medications (e.g., dextromethorphan, pseudoephedrine or phenylpropanolamine). However, if the patient is severely ill, referral for hospitalization is appropriate. While in intensive care, supportive measures including a cold blanket to reduce hyperthermia, antihypertensive medications for elevated blood pressure and mechanical ventilation may be used. Pharmacological countermeasures include short-acting benzodiazepines or dantrolene for myoclonus and resulting hyperthermia, Cyproheptadine, propranolol or methysergide can be used if the symptoms persist.[7-8]

Anticholinergic intoxication

The syndrome and its cause

Anticholinergic intoxication (alternately referred to as anticholinergic psychosis, "toxic delirium," anticholinergic syndrome or "atropine psychosis") is an acute delirium caused by the ingestion of excessive amounts of medications with strong anticholinergic properties. There are over 600 different legal and illegal plants, various chemicals and psychotropic medications that can have anticholinergic properties.[9-11] Ingestion may occur from iatrogenic polypharmacy, when the clinician prescribes multiple medications with highly anticholinergic properties (e.g., a traditional antipsychotic plus an anticholinergic agent for extrapyramidal symptoms and an antihistamine for cold symptoms).

The patient may precipitate anticholinergic intoxication through an intentional or accidental overdose of anticholinergic agents. Anticholinergic drugs have been overused for recreational purposes and to potentiate the effects of other psychoactive substances (most notably heroin). Acute overdose is likely to occur more frequently in populations that abuse anticholinergic medication. The syndrome can also result from chronic over usage of anticholinergic medications for purposes of abuse.[12] Some schizophrenic patients have been observed to overutilize anticholinergic drugs in preference to an antipsychotic because of what they perceive as the stimulant or euphorigenic properties of anticholinergics, using them orally, intravenously or by smoking the drug.

Signs and symptoms

After ingestion of moderate amounts of medications or substances with strong anticholinergic properties, a patient will, within 20 minutes to 3 hours, develop the following signs:[13-16]

1   agitation or euphoria
2   mental confusion or obtundation
3   paresthesia of fingers and toes
4   motor incoordination
5   mild drowsiness.

In cases of more severe intoxication, the patient will show:

•   hot dry skin or hyperthermia
•   urinary retention
•   aggressive, paranoid or delirious behavior
•   visual and/or auditory hallucinations

- muscle spasms
- progressive central nervous system depression
- tachycardia
- blurred vision
- dried mucosal services.

Gastrointestinal disturbances, including abdominal pain, nausea, vomiting and constipation, occur occasionally and may vary in severity, but at times may be acute. Elderly
patients with cerebrovascular disease are particularly prone to develop anticholinergic
confusional states, even when taking therapeutic doses of medications with anticholinergic properties.

The signs and symptoms of anticholinergic intoxication have been incorporated into
a mnemonic that has many variations when taught in different geographic locales. One
of the more common versions describes the patient with anticholinergic intoxication
as "Mad as a Hatter, blind as a bat, red as a beet, hot as a pistol and plugged with a
cork" – meaning mental status changes, blurred vision, hyperthermia, hot dry skin and
urinary retention.

Clinical situations of risk

Situations particularly likely to lead to anticholinergic intoxication include:

1   Simultaneous prescription of strongly anticholinergic medications from various
    classes. This can include any of the medications shown in Table 20.4.
2   Schizophrenic patients who abuse anticholinergic medications on a short-term or
    long-term basis.
3   Persons who ingest significant amounts of plants with anticholinergic activity*
    such as: *Datura* (Jimson weed, angel's trumpet), *Atropa belladonna* (deadly night-
    shade), *Hyoscyamus niger* (henbane) and *Mandrogana officiarum* (mandrake).

A useful chart, reproduced as Table 20.5, shows the approximate anticholinergic equivalent of various medications to trihexyphenidyl. For example, 75 mg of imipramine has
the same anticholinergic effect as 10 mg of amitriptyline and 1 mg of Cogentin, 50 mg
of Benadryl and 2.5 mg of trihexyphenidyl. Using the chart can give the clinician an
approximation of the "anticholinergic load" occurring with the prescription of various
medications.

Table 20.4 Medications that have strong anticholinergic properties

- TCAs
- Traditional antipsychotics
- Antihistamines
- Cycloplegics (medications that temporarily paralyze the ciliary muscle of the eye for dilation)
- Antispasmodics
- Antiparkinsonian medications
- Belladonna alkaloids*
- Some H_2 blockers (for example, cimetidine or ranitidine) have also produced a syndrome
  indistinguishable from anticholinergic intoxication, particularly in high doses

Table 20.5 Anticholinergic effect of commonly prescribed psychotropic drugs compared with trihexyphenidyl

Drug	Equivalent (in mg)	Typical use
Atropine	0.5	Given before surgery
Benztropine (Cogentin)	1.0	Antiparkinsonism
Trihexyphenidyl (Artane)	2.5	Antiparkinsonism
Biperiden (Akineton)	1.0	Antiparkinsonism
Amitriptyline (Elavil)	10	Antidepressant
Doxepin (Sinequan)	30	Antidepressant
Nortriptyline (Pamelor)	60	Antidepressant
Imipramine (Tofranil)	75	Antidepressant
Desipramine (Norpramin)	150	Antidepressant
Amoxapine (Asendin)	600	Antidepressant
Clozapine (Clozaril)	15	Antipsychotic
Thioridazine (Mellaril)	50	Antipsychotic
Chlorpromazine (Thorazine)	370	Antipsychotic
Diphenhydramine (Benadryl)	50	Antihistamine

Source: Keltner NL and Folks DG (2001) *Psychotropic Drugs*, 3rd edn., Mosby, p. 436.

Prevention

Prevention of anticholinergic intoxication involves knowledge of which medications are strongly anticholinergic and, whenever possible, avoiding their combination. Clinicians treating patients in a geriatric setting must be particularly alert to the sensitivity of this group to anticholinergic side effects. Likewise, clinicians who treat chronically psychotic and schizophrenic individuals need to be aware of anticholinergic intoxication when using multiple neuroleptics and/or anticholinergic medications for side effects. This patient group is also at high risk for abuse of anticholinergics. In vulnerable populations, consider using atypical antipsychotics that have less anticholinergic activity. When using anticholinergics or antihistamines for side effects, discontinue them whenever possible to observe whether they are still necessary. If an antidepressant is needed in someone already on a strong mix of anticholinergic medications, consider an SSRI or other new-generation antidepressant rather than a TCA.

Prognosis

Mild anticholinergic intoxication can usually be managed by stopping the offending agents. In most cases, the condition will resolve on its own without pharmacological management. Even if the patient has developed significant sensory changes or psychosis, these conditions will usually clear within 36–48 hours of stopping the causative agents.

Treatment

The first and most important element of treatment is to *recognize the source of anticholinergic load* (medications or plants) *and stop the offending agents*. Patients experiencing an acute psychotic episode or other strong symptomatology after a significant overdose of anticholinergic drugs may require constant supervision in hospital for several days to prevent accidental injury or aspiration of vomitus, and to control hyperthermia (particularly in children).

Physostigmine, a cholinesterase inhibitor, has both central and peripheral *cholinergic* actions, and can be used specifically to counteract the *anticholinergic* symptoms.[15–17] Generally, the patient is given a slow 2 mg test dose intravenously over 2 minutes. Because physostigmine has a short duration of action, the patient's symptoms may recur and repeated doses may be necessary every 30–60 minutes.

If the cause of intoxication is overdose, management also includes the usual modes of treatment, such as gastric lavage, cathartics and activated charcoal. When medication is necessary for control of agitation or delirium because of the overdose, traditional phenothiazine antipsychotics should be avoided as they increase anticholinergic load. A benzodiazepine, orally or by injection, may be helpful for behavioral control, and is less cholinergic.

Lithium toxicity

The syndrome and its causes

Lithium is commonly used for a variety of psychiatric and medical conditions, including:[18]

- acute and prophylactic treatment of bipolar affective disorder
- as an augmentation agent with antidepressants for depression
- to treat rage reactions
- as a prophylactic agent for chronic cluster headache
- as a therapeutic agent to treat thyrotoxicosis.

Lithium toxicity (also referred to as lithium intoxication or lithium poisoning) is one of the more common of the potentially serious psychotropic side effects. Lithium toxicity occurs with some frequency because lithium has a narrow therapeutic index (a small difference between safe levels and toxic levels) and has a number of common interactions that cause increased blood levels of lithium.

Lithium is 95 percent excreted in the urine, 4 percent in the sweat and 1 percent in feces. Eighty percent of the lithium filtered in the kidney is reabsorbed in the proximal tubules and is not reabsorbed in the distal tubules. By antagonizing the effects of antidiuretic hormone, the patient's urine output may increase, leading to dehydration. To compensate for this, proximal tubular reabsorption of water increases, along with increased reabsorption of lithium and consequent further toxicity.[18] Therefore, once initiated, lithium intoxication may start a vicious cycle of increasing toxicity.

Signs and symptoms

Early signs of lithium toxicity include:[19]

1 vomiting
2 diarrhea
3 coarse tremor
4 sluggishness or sleepiness
5 vertigo

6   poor coordination
7   dysarthria with slurred and indistinct speech.

If untreated or ignored, further elevation of lithium levels leads to:

- muscle twitching and hypertonia
- confused sensorium or coma
- asymmetrical deep tendon reflexes
- seizures
- a grayish hue to the skin.

Medical situations of risk

A variety of medical situations/causes may lead to lithium toxicity, including:

1   a single large overdose of lithium with suicidal intent
2   an accidental overdose (often by a manic patient with a wish to "improve quickly")
3   a decrease in renal lithium clearance without a corresponding reduction in dose, which may occur in the presence of:
   - kidney disease
   - sodium deficiency
   - water deprivation
   - medication interactions leading to elevated lithium levels.

Common clinical circumstances that lead to the above problems for a patient on lithium include:

- the initiation of a low-salt/no-salt diet
- a weight-reduction diet (without the addition of extra salt) and reduced fluid intake
- use of diuretics
- fever and excessive sweating
- vomiting and diarrhea from gastrointestinal illnesses
- prescription of inappropriately high oral doses of lithium
- failure to regularly monitor serum blood levels of lithium
- use of concomitant non-steroidal anti-inflammatory agents (20 percent of patients using non-steroidals when on lithium will have increased lithium levels; 80 percent will have no change in levels).

Most lithium toxicity occurs at serum levels of 2.0 meq per liter; however, it is possible that patients will have some symptoms of toxicity at lower levels. Some patients will have symptoms of mild lithium intoxication even at technically "therapeutic" levels (below 1.5 meq per liter). It has been estimated that serious toxicity occurs at levels between 2.5 and 3.5 meq per liter, and that life-threatening toxicity occurs at serum levels over 3.5 meq per liter. This latter level can result from an acute overdose of as few as 20 300-mg pills.[20]

Prognosis

Patients with mild lithium toxicity will generally completely recover without after-effects.[20] Patients with moderately severe or life-threatening lithium toxicity, however, can have residual neurological signs, including ataxia, broad-based gait, lack of coordination, tremors and nystagmus. Also reported with extensive lithium toxicity are cognitive damage, poor short-term memory and dementia. If the signs continue for 6 months or longer, they are generally permanent.[21] In general, the seriousness of the syndrome as well as the likelihood of residual symptoms occurs in proportion to the elevation of blood level and the length of time the patient is exposed to the toxic dose.[22]

In the past, mortality rates in acute lithium overdosage have been estimated to be between 25 and 33 percent.[22-23] With better recognition and treatment, including the use of dialysis, this figure has been dramatically lowered to 16 percent.[24-25]

Prevention

Keys to preventing lithium toxicity include patient education, clinician vigilance to potential situations of risk and regular monitoring of serum blood levels.

All patients started on lithium should be thoroughly educated about the early signs and symptoms of lithium toxicity and possible medication interactions that could raise their serum lithium level. The signs of mild lithium intoxication can be often conceptualized for patients by telling them that the signs are *similar to those that a person may experience from drinking too much alcohol and waking up hung over*. These include:

- nausea and vomiting
- tremor
- slurred speech or "thick tongue"
- difficulty with walking or gait.

If patients notice any of these signs or symptoms, they must be instructed to withhold further lithium doses and contact the clinician at once. The clinician will order a serum lithium level and adjust the dosage downward.

The other elements of education include the identification of common medications or conditions that may increase lithium level, with particular focus on the concomitant use of diuretics or non-steroidal anti-inflammatory agents, gastrointestinal illnesses leading to diarrhea or vomiting, and the initiation of a low-salt diet.

Regular lithium levels should be followed in all patients, but particularly in patients at risk, including geriatric patients, medically fragile patients or patients with a complicated medication regimen. For long-term patients on a stable lithium regimen and who have had consistent lithium levels, these levels can be monitored every 3–6 months. Levels should be monitored more frequently in patients at higher risk for toxicity, such as those who have a fluctuating salt and fluid balance, those who are prone to be non-adherent with medication, geriatric patients, patients with neurological or cognitive illness and patients prone to dehydration. If any of the early warning signs of lithium toxicity occur, the patient's lithium level should be checked immediately and, if elevated, the dosage lowered.

Treatment

Treatment should be individualized depending on the extent of toxicity. Regardless of the level of intoxication, when signs of toxicity are seen or suspected, *all lithium treatment should be temporarily stopped* until a blood level result is reported and the clinical signs are beginning to wane.

In the event of acute overdosage, gastric lavage or induced emesis should be used to remove unabsorbed lithium. Repeated lithium levels should be followed to ensure that the serum level is diminishing. In severe overdose, hemodialysis is the treatment of choice.[25] It is highly effective in removing lithium from the body with the goal of reducing the level to 1.0 meq per liter 6–8 hours after dialysis.[26]

In general, when the acute symptoms are minimal and the clinical situation dictates continued lithium therapy, the patient is gradually restarted on the lithium, leading to a target therapeutic dose within 24–72 hours. Usually, the target dose is less than that which caused the toxicity, unless there were extenuating circumstances (e.g., GI illness or dietary change) that will not reoccur.

QTc interval issues

Another example of a potential serious side effect that was virtually unknown to most practicing mental health practitioners 20 years ago, but is now of significant importance, is the QTc interval and its effect on heart rhythm. With current understanding of the nature of this problem, we may now be able to explain some of the instances of sudden unexplained death from the use of psychotropics, particularly antipsychotic medications, in the past. Because of documented concerns regarding cardiac safety, certain psychiatric and non-psychiatric medications have been appropriately withdrawn from the market because of concerns about their ability to severely alter the QTc interval. It has also become a pharmaceutical company marketing message to identify a medication's propensity to lengthen the QTc interval, as a reason for or against prescribing a particular medication.

The syndrome and its causes

As shown in Figure 20.1, cardiac rhythm begins with depolarization of the heart ventricle (the Q-wave) and ends with completion of repolarization (the T-wave). The time interval between the Q-wave and T-wave is the *QT interval*, measured in milliseconds. The QT interval varies with heart rate, and therefore has been "corrected" for changes in heart rate, thus leading to the term "QT interval corrected" or, more commonly, "QTc interval." Normal QTc intervals run from 400 to 450 milliseconds.

A lengthened QTc interval can lead to an increased risk of ventricular arrhythmias, most notably *torsades de pointes* (literally meaning twisting of the points, from the appearance of the electrocardiogram [EKG] of individuals with this serious and potentially fatally arrhythmia). *All known cases of* torsades de pointes *have been associated with QTc intervals of over 500 milliseconds*. QTc intervals of over 450 msec are considered to be of some concern since they are approaching the 500 msec barrier, but QTc intervals between 450 and 500 msecs have no documented direct incidence of arrhythmias or *torsades de pointes*.

There are several factors that can cause changes in QTc intervals, thereby increasing the risk of a cardiac arrhythmia. These include:

• genetic predisposition (so-called "long QT syndrome")
• electrolyte imbalance
• cardiac disease (see medical situations of risk, below)
• drug-induced lengthening.

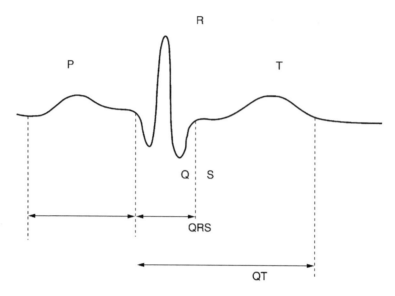

Figure 20.1 QT interval.

QTc interval concerns may involve a psychotropic medication itself or a non-psychiatric medication that has accumulated in the body because a psychotropic is also taken – usually due to P-450 enzyme interactions. In this latter case, the QTc lengthening occurs from the excessive dose of the non-psychotropic drug, although the psychotropic may be the precipitating factor. This situation has led to the withdrawal from the U.S. market of several non-psychotropic medications, including terfenadine (Seldane), astemizole (Hismanal), grepafloxacin (Raxar) and cisapride (Propulsid). One antipsychotic, sertindol (Serlect), was also denied marketing in the United States because of its intrinsic propensity to lengthen the QTc interval. Two other antipsychotics, thioridazine (Mellaril) and mezoridazine (Serentil), received a "black box warning" for their ability significantly to lengthen the QTc interval. Ziprasidone (Geodon in the United States and Zeldox outside the United States) also modestly increases the QTc interval, necessitating a warning in its product information. To be clear about the proportionate risk, the average amount of QTc lengthening should be noted for each of these antipsychotics. Thioridazine and mezoridazine lengthen the QTc interval by approximately 30 msec, Sertindol (which was not marketed) by an average of 22 msec and ziprasidone by 9 msec.

Within our current scope of knowledge, a long QTc interval does not directly cause or lead to *torsades de pointes*. The longer interval is only a statistical marker that *torsades* is more likely. Interestingly, therefore, there are several non-psychotropic medications that cause a lengthened QTc interval but have not been shown to give an increased incidence of *torsades*.

Signs and symptoms

The lengthening of the QTc interval can be seen on an EKG performed before or after a medication is started. Generally, a cut-off of 500 msec is used by most cardiologists, above which there is increased risk of arrhythmia and *torsades de pointes*.[27] No significant increased arrhythmia frequency has occurred in the range between 450 and 500 msec. It is important to note that a QTc interval of between 450 and 500 msec is not, in and of itself, a direct concern, but is a potential warning sign that the 500 msec cut-off could be reached by the addition of an offending medication.

Clinical signs that could alert the patient or clinician that an arrhythmia may be occurring include dizziness, lightheadedness, unexplained syncope or seizure.

Medical situations of risk

In addition to the genetically inherited causes of long QTc interval and the acquired risk with ingesting certain medications, there are other risk factors for a lengthened QTc interval.[28] These include:

- low blood levels of potassium or magnesium
- female gender
- increased age
- alcohol and illicit drug usage that may lead to electrolyte abnormalities
- history of recent myocardial infarction or uncompensated heart failure.

In general, patients with any of these risk factors should have serum magnesium and potassium levels drawn and a baseline EKG performed prior to starting a medication that lengthens the QTc interval. Since 85 percent of congenital long QTc interval is familial, anyone with a family history of this condition or sudden unexplained fainting spells should also have a baseline EKG.

Table 20.6 lists medications that have been potentially associated with prolongation of the QTc interval and a tendency to induce *torsades de pointes*.

Table 20.6 Drugs that prolong the QTc interval and/or induce *torsades de pointes* (TdP)

Drug (brand name®)	Drug class (clinical usage)	↑QT TdP comments
Amiodarone (Corarone, Pacerone)	Anti-arrhythmic (abnormal heart rhythm)	↑QT TdP F > M
Arsenic trioxide (Trisenox)	Anti-cancer (leukemia)	↑QT TdP Cases in Lit
Asenapine	Antipsychotic	↑QT
Bepridil (Vascor)	Anti-anginal (heart pain)	↑QT TdP F > M
Chlorpromazine (Thorazine)	Antipsychotic/anti-emetic (schizophrenia/nausea)	
Cisapride (Propulsid)	GI stimulant (heartburn)	↑QT TdP F > M
Clarithromycin (Biaxin)	Antibiotic (bacterial infection)	Cases in Lit
Disopyramide (Norpace)	Anti-arrhythmic (abnormal heart rhythm)	↑QT TdP F > M
Dofetilide (Tikosyn)	Anti-arrhythmic (abnormal heart rhythm)	↑QT TdP F > M

(continued)

Table 20.6 Cont.

Drug (brand name®)	Drug class (clinical usage)	↑QT TdP comments
Dolasetron (Anzemet)	Anti-nausea (nausea, vomiting)	↑QT
Droperidol (Inapsine)	Sedative/anti-nausea (anesthesia adjunct, nausea)	↑QT TdP Cases in Lit
Erythromycin (EES, Erythrocin)	Antibiotic/GI stimulant (bacterial infection; increase GI motility)	↑QT TdP F > M
Felbamate (Felbatrol)	Anticonvulsant (seizure)	TdP
Flecainide (Tambocor)	Anti-arrhythmic (abnormal heart rhythm)	↑QT TdP Association not clear
Fluoxetine (Prozac, Serafem)	Antidepressant (depression)	↑QT TdP Association not clear
Foscarnet (Foscavir)	Antiviral (HIV infections)	↑QT
Fosphenytoin (Cerebyx)	Anticonvulsant (seizure)	↑QT
Gatifloxacin (Tequin)	Antibiotic (bacterial infection)	
Halofantrine (Halfan)	Antimalarial (malaria infection)	↑QT TdP F > M
Haloperidol (Haldol)	Antipsychotic (schizophrenia, agitation)	↑QT TdP
Ibutilde (Corvert)	Anti-arrhythmic (abnormal heart rhythm)	↑QT TdP F > M
Iloperidone	Antipsychotic	↑QT
Indapamide (Lozol)	Diuretic (stimulate urine and salt loss)	↑QT Cases in Lit
Isradipine	Antihypertensive	↑QT (Dynacirc) (high blood pressure)
Levofloxacin (Levaquin)	Antibiotic (bacterial infection)	TdP Association not clear
Levomethadyl	Opiate agonist (pain control)	↑QT (Orlaam) narcotic dependence
Mesoridazine (Serentil)	Antipsychotic (schizophrenia)	↑QT
TdP Moexipril/hCTZ (Uniretic)	Antihypertensive (high blood pressure)	↑QT
Moxifloxacin (Avelox)	Antibiotic (bacterial infection)	↑QT
Naratriptan (Amerge)	Serotonin receptor antagonist (migraine treatment)	↑QT
Nicardipine (Cardene)	Antihypertensive (high blood pressure)	↑QT
Octreotide (Sandostatin)	Endocrine (acromegaly, carcinoid diarrhea)	↑QT

Table 20.6 Cont.

Drug (brand name®)	Drug class (clinical usage)	↑QT TdP comments
Paroxetine (Paxil)	Antidepressant (depression)	TdP
Pentamidine (NebuPent Pentam)	Anti-infective (pneumocystis pneumonia)	↑QT TdP F > M
Pimozide (Orap)	Antipsychotic (Tourette's tics)	↑QT F > M Cases in Lit
Procainamide TdP (Procan, Pronestyl)	Anti-arrhythmic (abnormal heart rhythm)	↑QT
Quetiapine (Seroquel)	Antipsychotic (schizophrenia)	↑QT
Quinidine (Cardioquin, Quiniglute)	Anti-arrhythmic (abnormal heart rhythm)	↑QT TdP F > M
Risperidone (Risperdal)	Antipsychotic (schizophrenia)	↑QT
Salmeterol (Serevent)	Sympathomimetic (asthmas, COPD)	↑QT
Sertraline (Zoloft)	Antidepressant (depression)	↑QT TdP Association not clear
Sotalol (Betapace)	Anti-arrhythmic (abnormal heart rhythm)	↑QT TdP F > M
Sparfloxacin (Zagam)	Antibiotic (bacterial infection)	↑QT TdP
Sumatriptan (Imitrex)	Serotonin receptor agonist (migraine treatment)	↑QT
Tacrolimus (Prograf)	Immunosuppressant (immune suppression)	Cases in Lit
Tamoxifen (Nolvadex)	Anti-cancer (breast cancer)	↑QT
Thioridazine (Mellaril)	Antipsychotic (schizophrenia)	↑QT TdP
Tizanidine (Zanaflex)	Muscle relaxant	↑QT
Venlafaxine (Effexor)	Antidepressant (depression)	↑QT
Ziprasidone (Geodon)	Antipsychotic (schizophrenia)	↑QT
Zolmitriptan (Zomig)	Migraine treatment	↑QT

Source: Woosley RL *et al*. (2021) QTdrugs list, available at: https://crediblemeds.org/ (accessed April 14, 2021), AZCERT, Inc. 1822 Innovation Park Dr., Oro Valley, AZ 85755.

Notes:
↑QT: prolongation is mentioned in the FDA-approved labeling as a known action of the drug.
TdP: the FDA-approved labeling includes mention of cases or a risk of TdP.
Cases in Lit: there are case reports of TdP in the medical literature.
F > M (Females > Males): substantial evidence indicates a greater risk (usually >twofold) of TdP in women.

Prognosis

Patients may have a mildly prolonged QTc interval (in the 450–480 msec range) without any incidence of clinically significant or serious arrhythmias. When *torsades de pointes* occurs, *it is potentially fatal* (so far only documented in persons with QTc > 500 msec).

Prevention

Prevention of lengthened QTc interval and *torsades de pointes* involves clinician vigilance and knowledge about the causes of elongation. When risk factors are present, baseline blood electrolyte levels and EKGs are useful, as well as follow-up EKGs to measure any changes in QTc interval after medication is added.

Treatment

Even though a direct causative connection cannot be proven between increased QTc interval and arrhythmia, current wisdom suggests that if a patient's QTc intervals exceed 500 msec, the medication regimen should be changed. This usually involves switching to another medication that does not lengthen QTc interval or, in cases where the medication had been particularly useful and no other alternatives are available, to a lower dose. (The incidence of arrhythmias and *torsades de pointes* is dose-related for almost all drugs.)[29] Patients with baseline QTc intervals over 450 msec should not be placed on medications that may further lengthen the QTc interval, unless there is clear clinical necessity. For clinical reasons, when a decision is made to utilize a drug that has the possibility of prolonging the QTc interval in a patient who is already at risk, written informed consent should be obtained and the possible risks explained.

Sudden death and antipsychotics

In 2007, the American Food and Drug Administration issued a class-wide "black box warning" for sudden death with the use of antipsychotic medicines in dementia-related psychosis. While varied, most of the deaths appeared to be precipitated by cardiovascular causes (e.g., heart failure or sudden death) or infectious causes (e.g., pneumonia). It is possible that some of the deaths were related to the QTc issues and arrhythmias discussed in the previous section of this chapter. Since not all of the deaths were cardiovascular, though, there are likely other mechanisms.

Several large-scale studies, largely involving second-generation antipsychotics, revealed an incidence of unexplained death in dementia-related psychosis patients of 1.6 to 1.7 times that seen in placebo-treated patients.[30] Follow-up studies suggest that traditional, first-generation antipsychotics had a similar propensity.[31–32]

Given the data, it seems certain that these individuals, when treated with antipsychotics, do have an increased incidence of death. This creates a quandary for the practitioner since these agents are commonly used and effective off-label for behavioral control in dementia-related psychotic individuals.[33]

While not limiting the risk, recent research has revealed important data which provide some clinical guidance to the prescriber. A large retrospective cohort study was conducted on 33,000 individuals over the age of 65 who were begun on a variety of antipsychotics and followed for 180 days.[34] The mortality risks were then measured and considerable differences occurred. Death rates were as follows:

- haloperidol – 20 percent
- olanzapine – 12.6 percent
- risperidone – 12.5 percent
- valproic acid (as a non-antipsychotic comparison) – 9.8 percent
- quetiapine – 8.8 percent.

Other important conclusions from the study were:

- Mortality rate was highest in the first 30 days for haloperidol, then sharply and significantly declined thereafter.
- For all other agents, the differences in mortality risk were most significant in the first 120 days and then decreased during the remaining 60 days.

It was not clear why quetiapine had a significantly lower mortality rate than the other antipsychotics. Purely from a safety standpoint, quetiapine would appear to have an advantage. Some authors suggested, however,[34-35] that the efficacy evidence for quetiapine in this population is questionable for decreasing behavioral symptoms. Kales *et al.* state that three previous studies have shown a modest but significant improvement in decreasing both aggression and psychosis with the use of risperidone and olanzapine. In the opinion of these authors, risperidone and olanzapine emerge as the best evidence-based options when an antipsychotic is deemed necessary.

Based on its similarly low rate of mortality, valproic acid would seem a logical choice as an alternative to the use of antipsychotics in dementia patients. This is true; however, it should be remembered that valproic acid and its derivatives carry additional associated risks such as sedation, fracture and thrombocytopenia.

Additional clinical recommendations include:

- prescribing the lowest dose possible and avoiding polypharmacy and metabolic interactions
- using informed consent and thorough documentation – if the patient's decision-making ability is impaired, it is recommended that consent for treatment with antipsychotic therapy is obtained from the patient's designated proxy
- *The Maudsley Prescribing Guidelines* suggest that with hospitalized patients, an EKG be performed on admission, before discharge and at a yearly checkup.[36]

Extrapyramidal symptoms, neuroleptic malignant syndrome and tardive

dyskinesia

The following three syndromes – extrapyramidal symptoms, neuroleptic malignant syndrome and tardive dyskinesia – are constellations of symptoms almost totally associated with traditional antipsychotic neuroleptics. Since the use of traditional antipsychotics is gradually decreasing, the incidence of these syndromes will also likely decrease and eventually, in large measure, fade from the clinical landscape entirely. However, since traditional antipsychotics are still in common use in various parts of the world or are required in clinical situations where the patient is intolerant of (or non-responsive to) atypical antipsychotics, clinicians must still be knowledgeable about these conditions. They represent areas of significant risk, discomfort and, rarely, mortality to patients. These three syndromes are divided into early-onset syndromes (extrapyramidal symptoms and neuroleptic malignant syndrome) and a late-onset syndrome (tardive dyskinesia).

Extrapyramidal symptoms

The syndrome and its causes

The term "extrapyramidal symptoms" (EPS) covers three separate conditions – dystonia, akathisia and parkinsonism (also called pseudo parkinsonism). Each is a discrete syndrome involving movement and motor activity associated with initiation of traditional antipsychotics. Dystonia and parkinsonism, as they occur in mental health prescribing, will be discussed in this chapter. Akathisia has already been covered as one possible cause of "overactivation" in Chapter 18.

The pyramidal system in the brain mediates voluntary movements such as walking or sitting. The *extra*pyramidal system is responsible for coordination and for fine-tuning the many involuntary muscle activities necessary to performing these tasks, and is modulated by dopaminergic and cholinergic neurons.

Dopaminergic neurons are generally inhibitory and cholinergic neurons generally excitatory to normal motor function. It has been suggested that functional alteration of the extrapyramidal system is caused by a disruption of this normal balance between dopaminergic and cholinergic neurons.[37] When traditional neuroleptics are introduced, they block dopaminergic neurons, leading to a decrease in dopamine and a relative increase in cholinergic activity, disrupting the balance. The disruption of the normal balance between these neurotransmitters then leads to the loss of certain motor functions and their smooth coordination. This explanation most closely accounts for dystonia and pseudo parkinsonism, but does not clearly explain akathisia.

Dystonia

Dystonic movements (dystonias) are the involuntary contractions of striatal muscle groups. Although any muscle group may be involved, the commonly affected muscle groups are those of the face, head, extremities, neck and back. These reactions are not under voluntary control and may appear suddenly (within minutes or hours of initiation of an offending agent), or may come on in a sporadic fashion over several days or weeks. In general, the symptoms, which wax and wane over time, are made worse by emotionally upsetting experiences, and generally disappear during sleep. Dystonias usually end within a short period of time after discontinuation of antipsychotic medication, but in some cases, it may take days or weeks for them to pass. The symptoms are often quite uncomfortable and anxiety-producing for the patient, and distressing to family members. The incidence varies greatly with the presence of risk factors (see below), and can be anywhere from 2–95 percent.[38–39]

Depending on which muscle group is involved, some dystonic EPS symptoms have specific labels such as:

- oculogyric crisis (a rolling back and upward of the eyeballs toward the back of the head)

- trismus (involuntary jaw clenching)
- torticollis (twisting of the neck secondary to involuntary neck muscle contraction)
- carpopedal spasm (involuntary contraction of the hand or foot musculature, leading to dorsiflexion of the toes and inward contraction of the hands, fingers and wrists)
- opisthotonos (contraction of the back and neck muscles leading to a backwards arching of the back, spine and neck).

Parkinsonism

Drug-induced parkinsonism (or pseudo parkinsonism, as it is sometimes called) is another set of primarily motor symptoms that occurs weeks to months after the onset of dopamine blocking agents such as typical antipsychotics. In general, parkinsonian symptoms are bilateral, although on occasion they are more pronounced on only one side of the body. Symptoms include:

- muscle rigidity
- tremor (often in the hands, and referred to as a "pill rolling" tremor since the hands appear to be rolling a pill)
- bradykinesia (slowed motor movements) with difficulty in starting voluntary muscle activities
- akinesia (lack of motor movement in general)
- abnormal, shuffling gait
- dysarthric speech
- dysphagia (difficulty swallowing)
- micrographia (cramped handwriting)
- decreased motor movements in the facial muscles with lessened facial expression (often referred to as "mask-like facies")
- cog-wheel rigidity (a ratchet-like loss of smooth fluid motion of joints), which may be elicited on examination of the elbows, wrists, knees or neck.

Prognosis

Dystonias are often self-limited within 7–10 days of onset. For some patients they may persist indefinitely without treatment if the offending agent is continued. Despite their time-limited nature, they are sufficiently uncomfortable to the patient and distressing to family members that treatment is often initiated relatively quickly after onset.[40-41] When they occur acutely and strongly, as in oculogyric crisis, acute torticollis and opisthotonos, urgent interventions are necessary to relieve painful symptomatology and the resulting grotesque motor postures. Parkinsonism, once established, tends to persist or worsen with time if the offending medication continues to be taken.

Prevention

Prevention consists of minimizing the use of traditional neuroleptics. Whenever antipsychotic medication activity is required, utilization of atypical antipsychotics will dramatically lessen the incidence of EPS, akathisia and parkinsonism. Because of the possibility of these side effects, it is particularly important, when possible, to avoid the use of traditional antipsychotics for non-psychotic symptoms (e.g., as a hypnotic, for affective disorders which are not psychotic, or as treatment for general behavioral control in delirious or demented patients). When it is necessary to use typical antipsychotic medication, the clinician should prescribe the lowest possible dose and be alert to the onset of any extrapyramidal symptoms in the first week of treatment (90 percent of all EPS occurs within the first 4 days after initiation of the antipsychotic).[38]

Known high-risk statistical predictors of EPS include:

- lower age (<35 years)[42]
- male sex[43]
- use of high-potency antipsychotics (haloperidol, fluphenazine)[44–45]
- use of neuroleptics in a patient with an affective disorder
- patients with a previous history of EPS
- during rapid tranquillization or after large dosage increases.

A useful preventative strategy involves the prophylactic use of anticholinergic medications in patients at high risk for EPS.[46] Benztropine 1–2 mg daily can be started simultaneously with the initiation of a traditional neuroleptic in those patients who are at high risk for EPS (e.g., a young male patient in whom a high-potency neuroleptic is being started at a relatively high dose). When prophylaxis is used, the patient's anticholinergic medication should be gradually discontinued after several weeks. In up to 50 percent of clinical situations, the patient will no longer need the anticholinergic and the EPS will not re-emerge. If the symptoms do re-emerge, the anticholinergic medication can be reinstated.

Treatment

When starting traditional antipsychotics, patient education about the benign course and nature of these side effects is essential to prevent excessive fear and overreaction. Patients and their families should be alerted to the possible signs of early EPS so that, if they occur, treatment can be instituted promptly.

When using a traditional antipsychotic and EPS emerge, the prescriber should switch to an atypical neuroleptic or, if the traditional antipsychotic is to be continued, change to a lower potency neuroleptic (e.g., chlorpromazine or thioridazine), or minimize the dose to the lowest possible therapeutic amount.[40–41] Use of the atypical antipsychotic agents olanzapine, ziprasidone, quetiapine and clozapine will show a marked decrease in the incidence of EPS compared to typical antipsychotics.[47–48] Risperidone also has a lower incidence of EPS than traditional neuroleptics, if the total daily dose is kept below 4 mg per day.[49]

Pharmacological treatment of dystonia and parkinsonism involves the use of several medication groups, including:

- anticholinergics, which decrease the availability of acetylcholine and therefore partially restore the dopamine–choline balance (benztropine, trihexyphenidyl and others)
- antihistamines (diphenhydramine and others) that have central anticholinergic effects and fewer peripheral effects than anticholinergics
- benzodiazepines (lorazepam, diazepam, clonazepam and others) are useful, particularly for akinesia or akathisia
- drugs that enhance the release of dopamine and increase its availability at the synapse (e.g., amantadine) will modulate EPS symptoms

- direct stimulators of dopamine receptor activity (e.g., bromocriptine) are used in NMS and parkinsonism, but not typically for routine EPS.

Benztropine 1–2 mg per day will control modest levels of EPS symptomatology.[50] Up to 6 mg per day may be necessary for severe symptoms. Parkinsonism may also be at least partially improved by the use of similar doses of benztropine[51–52] and amantadine.[53] In the inpatient setting, diphenhydramine (50 mg i.m. or i.v.), amantadine (200–400 mg per day)[54] and diazepam (5 mg i.m. or i.v.)[55] can be equally effective in reversing and preventing dystonias. For dystonias, anticholinergic medication may be given orally if the symptoms are mild and gradual in onset. If acute or intense dystonic symptoms occur rapidly, intramuscular and intravenous dosing of the anticholinergic will give more prompt symptom relief. Parenteral administration also avoids the problem of difficulty in swallowing oral medication, which may be part of the dystonic picture.

When using medication to treat EPS, the treating remedy should be gradually withdrawn after 4–6 weeks to see if its continued use is necessary.

Neuroleptic malignant syndrome

The syndrome and its causes

Although the rarest of the serious adverse reactions to typical antipsychotics (with an incidence of 0.2 percent), neuroleptic malignant syndrome (NMS) is significantly important because it is life-threatening if unrecognized and untreated. This syndrome is neither specific to any one psychiatric diagnosis, nor limited to mental health patients. It can be seen in any patient where the brain is exposed to medication that induces dopamine-2 receptor blockade resulting in sudden decrease in brain dopamine levels. Even when dopamine-blocking medications are used for other non-psychiatric purposes (such as prochlorperazine, promethazine and droperidol, which can be used for blocking emesis, promoting peristalsis or as anesthesia/sedative), NMS can occur. Although most of the cases of NMS have been reported with traditional antipsychotics, the actual incidence of NMS with the use of *atypical* antipsychotics remains unclear[56] (there have been six reported cases involving clozapine and two with quetiapine).

The symptom complex includes:[57]

1 muscle rigidity (often referred to as "lead pipe" rigidity) with cog wheeling, myoclonus and coarse tremors
2 mental status changes, including delirium, stupor and coma
3 hyperthermia (>38 °C) with profuse sweating
4 autonomic activation and instability, with changes in blood pressure and tachycardia
5 rapid and labored breathing
6 drooling, incontinence
7 laboratory test abnormalities, including:
   - elevated serum creatinine phosphokinase (CPK), sometimes increased to extraordinary levels, reflecting significant muscle necrosis (rhabdomyolysis)
   - metabolic acidosis, hypoxia, low serum iron and electrolyte abnormalities.

The syndrome can occur within the first 24 hours after beginning neuroleptic treatment, and two-thirds of all cases occur within the first week. Once symptoms develop, progression is quite rapid and symptoms reach peak intensity within 72 hours. NMS does not generally result from an overdose of neuroleptic medication, and usually occurs when the medication dose is within the therapeutic range.[58]

Medical situations of risk

Although many factors have been evaluated as potential risk factors for NMS, the evidence is neither extensive nor convincing for any one risk factor, other than the recent initiation of a dopamine-blocking agent. There is some evidence to support increased risk with high-potency traditional antipsychotics, high ambient temperatures, male gender, genetic predisposition and possibly an association of concomitant usage of lithium with the neuroleptic. The bottom line, however, is that any medication that blocks dopamine in the brain may precipitate NMS. Patients with a previous history of NMS are at increased risk for future episodes.

Prognosis

Once traditional neuroleptic medication is discontinued, NMS is generally self-limiting, with most patients recovering in 7–10 days.[58–59] Nearly all patients recover within 30 days, and most patients who survive make a full recovery. The course of NMS may be prolonged if the precipitating agent is a long-acting depot neuroleptic.[58] The mortality rate is approximately 5 percent, but has much improved in the last three decades.

Prevention

Clinician vigilance and lowered usage of strong dopamine-blocking agents has already lessened the incidence of NMS in recent years. The wider use of atypical antipsychotic agents will likely further decrease its incidence.

Re-challenging a patient with a neuroleptic after a history of NMS has been a matter of some debate. Current estimates are that approximately 30 percent of patients who recover from NMS will have a recurrent episode following traditional neuroleptic re-challenge. The majority of patients can be re-challenged, however, if this is done in very gradual doses, no sooner than 2 weeks following recovery. It is prudent to consider the use of an atypical antipsychotic or a lower potency traditional neuroleptic if a re-challenge is going to be undertaken. When retrying a typical antipsychotic, the patient should be given a small test dose and carefully monitored for signs of NMS.

Treatment

Specific treatments for NMS include:[60]

- cessation of any dopamine-blocking drugs
- supportive medical/nursing care including fluid replacement, fever reduction, use of cooling blanket and support of cardiac, respiratory and renal function
- with moderate symptoms, use of dopamine agonists can reverse the dopamine blockade – the following agents have been shown to be useful: amantadine 100 mg p.o. via NG tube every 8 hours; bromocriptine 2.5–5 mg p.o. via NG tube every 8 hours; or dantrolene 1–2.5 mg/kg i.v.

- high-dose benzodiazepines such as lorazepam 1–2 mg i.m./i.v. every 8 hours can also be helpful
- electroconvulsive therapy (ECT) remains the definitive treatment for those patients with a syndrome severe enough to be admitted to an intensive care unit.[61–62] The average number of ECT treatments is ten, and response is usually seen after four treatments.

Tardive dyskinesia

The syndrome and its causes

Tardive dyskinesia (TD) literally translated means abnormal involuntary movements of late onset. It is one of several late-onset movement disorders associated with dopamine-blocking agents such as traditional antipsychotics. *Tardive akathisia* and *tardive dystonia* can also occur after months or years of neuroleptic usage; however, the incidence of these latter syndromes is significantly less frequent than tardive dyskinesia, on which most of the clinical investigation has been focused. The signs, symptoms and treatment of late-onset tardive dystonia and tardive akathisia are similar to their early-onset counterparts discussed previously.

The essential element of tardive dyskinesia is brain exposure to drugs that results in strong central dopaminergic blockade, particularly at the dopamine-2 receptor.[63] Although most cases of TD have been related to traditional antipsychotics, other non-psychiatric medications such as levodopa, prochlorperazine (Compazine), amphetamine and metoclopramide (Reglan, Maxelon – UK only) have also been associated with TD. The antidepressant agent amoxapine, which itself blocks dopamine, and Triavil, which contains perphenazine (a dopamine-blocking traditional antipsychotic agent), can also lead to significant dopamine blockade and TD.

Essential to the diagnosis is exposure to the dopamine-blocking agent for at least 3 months (1 month if the patient is older than 60 years). Usually, this syndrome emerges gradually over a number of months, but on occasion it will occur relatively quickly when dopamine antagonists are *decreased* in dosage or withdrawn altogether (withdrawal dyskinesia).

Although exposure to dopamine-blocking agents is thought to be essential to tardive dyskinesia, it is clear that many elderly patients have a spontaneous incidence of dyskinesia. *Schizophrenic patients and patients with dementia may have a higher incidence of spontaneous dyskinesia than the general population, even without exposure to dopamine-blocking agents.* Therefore, estimates of the prevalence rate of tardive dyskinesia have been quite variable. It is currently estimated that TD occurs in 15–30 percent of patients exposed to traditional antipsychotics.[64] Risk of TD has been shown to be considerably lower with use of atypical agents compared to traditional antipsychotics.[65] Although there are some abnormal movement problems, clozapine and olanzapine are associated with very low TD rates.[66–70] Risperidone, with a lower rate of EPS than traditional neuroleptics, should also have lower rates of TD,[71] although there are several case reports of the association of risperidone with TD.[72] Although research evidence can be at times contradictory, several factors do emerge as clear risk factors for an increased incidence of TD.[73] These include:

- advancing age
- higher doses of a typical antipsychotic

- longer duration of exposure to the antipsychotic
- female gender
- smoking
- diabetes
- previous history of neuroleptic-induced parkinsonism
- diagnosis of affective disorder or dementia when compared to a diagnosis of schizophrenia.

Signs and symptoms

The symptoms include hyperkinetic, involuntary movements in a variety of body parts including:

1   orofacial dyskinesia with
    - exaggerated movements of the tongue and mouth
    - grimacing and chewing movements
    - bulging or puffing of the cheeks
    - vermiform ("worm-like") movements of the tongue
    - increased blinking and blepharospasm
2   choreoathetoid (slow, writhing) movements of the hands, arms, legs, feet
3   rocking and swaying of the trunk and pelvis.

Because of the involuntary movements, patients may have trouble eating, speaking or using their hands with dexterity. Occasionally, the patient will make grunting sounds or have difficulty breathing. The movements may be worse during periods of emotional stress and when the patient's attention is distracted away from the movements. The movements usually disappear during sleep.

Since orofacial dyskinesia is the most common presentation of TD, it is important not to misidentify TD in a patient who simply has ill-fitting dentures. Be sure to ask about the presence of dentures in the evaluation process for TD. The AIMS (Abnormal Involuntary Movements Scale), developed by the National Institutes of Mental Health Psychopharmacology Research branch, is the standard tool for evaluation of movement disorders (see Appendix 6).

Situations of medical risk

A patient who is treated with any dopamine-blocking agent is at risk for tardive dyskinesia, particularly if the exposure continues for an extended time. Therefore, vigilance on the part of the clinician is always essential when this group of medications is used. Based on the risk factors identified above, any elderly female diabetic who is a smoker is especially at risk for developing TD. Patients with affective disorders are also a high risk, and strong dopamine-blocking agents should be avoided in their care whenever possible.

Prognosis

Although early wisdom suggested that many cases of tardive dyskinesia were irreversible, further evidence suggests that a large percentage of persons with TD will show remission once the offending agent has been removed for a long period of time. This is particularly true if the length of exposure to the medication was short and the patient is young. The exact persistence rate of TD, once it becomes evident, is difficult to estimate. Most recent studies, however, show that if a long-term timeframe (2–5 years) is used to evaluate the patient after discontinuation of the antipsychotic, 50–90 percent show improvement of at least 50 percent on AIMS ratings.[74] Sixty percent of patients see TD symptoms disappear or improve greatly in the course of 2–3 years. Nevertheless, 30–40 percent of patients who develop TD will continue with TD symptoms on a chronic basis. Direct mortality from TD has not been reported; however, the patient's lifestyle, functional behavior and self-care ability may be significantly hampered.

Prevention

Prevention of TD is the most significant area for clinicians to consider, but is somewhat less urgent with the advent of two successful treatments (see below). Prevention involves minimizing exposure to strong dopamine-blocking agents, both in dose and duration. Of particular importance is avoiding the use of traditional neuroleptics for non-psychotic purposes, such as sedation, anxiety or behavioral control in non-psychotic patients. Whenever possible, atypical antipsychotic medication or other medication groups should be used in preference to traditional antipsychotics.[66, 75]

Involvement in precipitating TD through the use of traditional antipsychotics has long been an area of medico-legal risk for mental health prescribers. Even though the use of these agents is decreasing, it continues to be important that a patient placed on a strong dopamine-blocking agent signs an adequate informed consent document. The alternatives available and the possibility of the emergence of TD should be explained to the patient if he or she is competent; if this is not the case, such risk should be explained to the family or legal guardian.

A patient who is placed on a traditional neuroleptic should have the medication regimen re-evaluated periodically for ongoing necessity. When possible, supplementary agents including lithium, valproic acid, carbamazepine, benzodiazepines or atypical antipsychotic agents should be used to augment antipsychotic activity and allow minimization of the dosage of traditional neuroleptic.

Treatment

Once considered almost untreatable when it emerged, TD has now been shown to be significantly responsive to two new medications – valbenzadrine (Ingressa) and deutetrabenazine (Austedo) which both belong to the class VMAT2 inhibitors. TD responds quickly, often within a week.[76–77] These medications do create some problems for patients who take them, including drowsiness or parkinsonism. Also, when patients stop the medication their TD often recurs. Nonetheless, this is a relatively new development providing relief for a significant number of patients who developed TD from first-generation antipsychotics. Other remediation strategies are based primarily on preventing the onset of the condition[75] and include:

- Discontinuing the offending antipsychotic or switching the patient to an atypical antipsychotic.
- When traditional antipsychotics are necessary, lowering the dose to the least amount necessary for clinical response and maintaining the exposure for the shortest period of time.

- Other pharmacological treatments have included trials with amine-depleting agents, dopamine antagonists, cholinergic agents, GABA agonists, anxiolytics, anticholinergics, vitamin E and beta-adrenergic blocking agents.[66, 75] Except for the above-mentioned VMAT2 drugs, none of these treatments has shown significant clinical response.

Raising the dose of the offending dopamine-blocking agent will temporarily mask or alleviate TD symptoms. While this may provide some short-term benefit, it is obviously not a useful long-term strategy, and is not considered part of good treatment.

Unfortunately, the concept of "drug holidays" – stopping the dopamine-blocking agent medication for days or weeks at a time – does not provide significant protection against the emergence of TD. While logical in concept and appealing in that it minimizes neuroleptic exposure, rigorous evaluation has found that it is not of benefit, and may actually aggravate the symptoms of TD.[78–79]

If the patient is being withdrawn from a traditional neuroleptic because of the onset of TD, this should be done in a gradual fashion to avoid a flare-up of TD (withdrawal dyskinesia) and also to prevent a rapid, florid worsening of the psychosis. The only exception to this gradual tapering principle would be the patient with TD who also develops neuroleptic malignant syndrome, which itself is an emergency. In this situation, the neuroleptic should be withdrawn immediately.

Monoamine oxidase inhibitor reactions

Monoamine oxidase inhibitors (MAOIs) have been used since the 1960s, and are useful antidepressants for bipolar depression, treatment-resistant depression and so-called "atypical depressions" (patients with mood reactivity, hypersomnia, leaden paralysis, hyperphagia and rejection sensitivity). In twenty-first century psychopharmacology, MAOIs represent fourth- or fifth-line choices for most patients because of dietary restrictions and problematic medication interactions. Because of the possibility of strong, sudden and serious interactions, these medications engender apprehension on the part of patients and, at times, clinicians. Nevertheless, certain patients respond to MAOIs when all other medication groups have failed. Understanding their possible interactions is necessary to prescribing or monitoring any patient who is taking them. These interactions occur with *irreversible* MAOIs such as phenelzine, tranylcypromine and selegiline – the only three currently available in the United States. A *reversible* MAOI meclobemide (Manerix) is available in a number of European and Latin American countries, as well as in Canada. Because of its improved safety profile and the lack of dietary restriction that is necessary for irreversible MAOIs, meclobemide has had some popularity in these regions, although there has been some question about its efficacy compared to irreversible MAOIs. Currently, a transdermal delivery system of an irreversible MAOI is in testing. Since this system bypasses the enteric–hepatic circulation, it will not require dietary restrictions. If successfully tested, it may trigger a resurgence of MAOI usage.

The syndrome and its causes

Problematic interactions with irreversible MAOIs are twofold:

1   serotonin syndrome
2   hypertensive crisis

Table 20.7 Strongly serotonergic psychotropics prohibited in conjunction with MAOIs

---

- All SSRIs, including fluoxetine, paroxetine, sertraline, citalopram, vilazodone, fluvoxamine
- Venlafaxine
- Nefazodone

Table 20.8 Dietary restrictions for patients taking irreversible MAOIs

---

Foods to avoid completely
- Aged cheese (all cheeses *except* cottage, farmer, ricotta and cream cheese)
- Pickled or aged meats (fermented and dry sausage, pepperoni, salami), aged poultry or fish (herring), caviar
- Spoiled meat, poultry or fish (such as that left in the refrigerator too long)
- Fava (broad) bean pods
- Concentrated yeast extracts (Marmite or brewer's yeast tablets; yeast used in baking is safe)
- Sauerkraut
- Soy sauce and soy-bean condiments
- Tap beer, red wine, sherry, Chianti, liqueurs
- Liver from beef or chicken (fresh beef or chicken meat is safe)
- Banana peel

Foods to avoid in large quantities
- White wine, bottled or canned beer, vodka, gin
- Ripe avocados
- Anchovies
- Chocolate
- Meat tenderizers
- Beverages containing caffeine

Source: Fiedorowicz JG and Swartz KL (2004) The role of monoamine oxidase inhibitors in current psychiatric practice. *Journal of Psychiatric Practice* 10(4): 239–248.

Note: Dietary restrictions should be maintained for 2 weeks after stopping an MAOI.

Serotonin syndrome, which occurs when strongly serotonergic medications are combined with MAOIs, was discussed earlier in the chapter. Those psychotropic medications with strongly serotonergic properties, which are contraindicated in patients taking irreversible MAOIs, are listed in Table 20.7.

The second set of interactions with MAOIs involves markedly elevated blood pressure (*hypertensive crisis*) when MAOIs are combined with certain medications and foods. This occurs because the MAOI blocks monoamine oxidase, the enzyme that breaks down monoamines in the body. When an irreversible MAOI is taken consistently, monoamine oxidase is irreversibly blocked for up to 2 weeks. During this time, if the patient ingests foods that contain pressor monoamines, these cannot be metabolized, and will accumulate in the body and raise blood pressure. The most common such amine implicated in these reactions is tyramine. Therefore, when irreversible MAOIs are used the patient should be cautioned to avoid eating foods or drinking beverages that are potentially high in tyramine. Substances that are likely to be high in tyramine are listed in Table 20.8.

If an MAOI is stopped, dietary restrictions should still be maintained for 2 weeks. This is because the monoamine-blocking effect may last for up to 14 days after discontinuation of an MAOI.

Table 20.9 Drugs contraindicated for patients receiving irreversible MAOIs

---

Over-the-counter cold and cough medications
- Ephedrine
- Pseudoephedrine
- Phenylephedrine
- Dextromethorphan
- Phenylpropanolamine

Stimulants
- Methylphenidate
- Dextroamphetamine

Diet pills
- Prescription
- Over-the-counter

Street/recreational drugs
- Cocaine
- "Speed" (amphetamines)

Narcotics
- Meperidine is most risky
- Morphine is less dangerous
- Codeine is generally safe

Centrally acting antihypertensives
- Reserpine
- Guanethidine
- a-methyldopa

Serotonergic agents/SSRIs
- All SSRIs
- Clomipramine
- Venlafaxine
- Nefazodone
- Fenfluramine
- Dexfenfluramine
- Sumatriptan (Imitrex)

Anesthetics containing pressors

Source: Fiedorowicz JG and Swartz KL (2004) The role of monoamine oxidase inhibitors in current psychiatric practice. *Journal of Psychiatric Practice* 10(4): 239–248.

Elevated blood pressure and hypertensive crisis can also be precipitated by the combination of an MAOI with various medications. These include over-the-counter cough and cold medications, diet pills, certain street drugs, prescription stimulants, narcotics and centrally acting antihypertensives (see Table 20.9).

In the past, the combination of a tricyclic antidepressant and an MAOI was thought to be risky and was contraindicated. It has been shown more recently that this combination can be tolerable for certain patients if the combination is instituted simultaneously and the TCA used is doxepin, amitriptyline or trimipramine.[80–81] It is contraindicated to add a TCA to an ongoing regimen of an MAOI or to use imipramine as the TCA.

Signs and symptoms

Patients who ingest one of the prohibited foods or medications while taking an irreversible MAOI will, within 15–90 minutes, begin experiencing:

1 severe headache, usually occipital and temporal ("like the top of my head is going to come off")
2 sweating
3 elevation of systolic and diastolic blood pressure
4 mydriasis (dilated pupils).

If the headache and other symptoms do not occur within 2 hours after ingestion of a prohibited compound, it is unlikely that they will occur subsequently. Rarely, during a strong reaction, intracerebral hemorrhage and death can occur.

Medical situations of risk

Given proper prescriptive habits and appropriate education about problematic interactions, the most likely situations in which a patient could still experience a hypertensive crisis or serotonin syndrome are:

1 when the patient *accidentally* ingests one of the prohibited foods
2 when *inappropriate medication combinations* are prescribed by a clinician who is unaware that the patient is taking an MAOI.

Ingestion of prohibited foods most often occurs when patients are outside their usual eating routine, or are unaware of the ingredients in what they are eating. At a restaurant or when ingesting food prepared by someone else, they may unknowingly eat a prohibited ingredient.

Dangerous medications could accidentally be simultaneously prescribed when patients come to the emergency room unconscious, and do not have an ID bracelet or other indication that they are taking an MAOI. The unsuspecting clinician may prescribe a hazardous combination of medications inadvertently.

Prognosis

In general, if small amounts of the prohibited substance are ingested, the patient experiences a severe headache, sweating and moderately elevated blood pressure, but recovers within several hours without ongoing sequelae. Serious consequences of a hypertensive crisis, specifically cerebrovascular accident and death, have had markedly reduced incidence over the last 15 years. This is due in part to better education about the possible problematic interactions, and lessened usage of MAOIs.

Treatment

Instruct patients that if they experience any symptoms of hypertensive crisis, particularly a severe headache, they are immediately to seek emergency medical evaluation and care. Although many hypertensive crises will pass without treatment, patients cannot be assured of how much of the prohibited substance they may have ingested, and how high their blood pressure will rise. In the past, patients were instructed to use an "emergency pill" of nifedipine or another blood pressure lowering agent to prevent severe hypertensive reactions while they were en route to the emergency room. However, this practice led to further complications from severely lowered blood pressure, and has been discontinued.[82]

After arrival at the emergency room, when proper medical care is available, a blood pressure lowering agent such as nifedipine can be given, the effect of which lasts 4–6 hours. Usually, by the end of that time, the crisis has passed and blood pressure will normalize without further treatment. If large amounts of a prohibited substance have been ingested, however, repeat doses may be necessary to maintain a safe blood pressure.

Prevention

The most important preventive measure is ongoing education to the patient about prohibited foods and medications. The patient is strongly urged to be diligent about avoiding ingestion of any prohibited substances *without experimentation*. Each patient taking an MAOI should carry documentation of this fact at all times (e.g., an ID card in the wallet or purse, and/or a medical ID bracelet).

Other potentially dangerous side effects

In addition to those mentioned above, several other side effects present serious, hazardous and, rarely, potentially fatal reactions to psychotropics. These include:

- bleeding and blood dyscrasias
- liver toxicity
- seizures.

Bleeding and blood dyscrasias

Although relatively infrequent, changes in blood parameters (blood dyscrasias) and abnormal bleeding are well-known complications associated with the use of various psychotropics. The most serious of these is an extremely low neutrophil count or agranulocytosis (defined as an absolute neutrophil count of 100 per microliter or less). The presence of very low numbers of white blood cells leaves the patient open to frequent severe infections or sepsis.

Although many cases of incipient agranulocytosis are heralded by gradually decreasing neutrophil counts, some are precipitous and sudden. If a patient has a neutrophil count of under 2000, a hematological consult should be obtained and serious consideration given to switching medications. Those psychotropic medications associated with an incidence of agranulocytosis are listed in Table 20.10.

A baseline level of blood parameters drawn via a complete blood count (CBC) should be performed prior to instituting any of these agents. Follow-up monitoring is as follows:

- For carbamazepine, CBCs should be done 4–6 weeks after initiation and then every 3 months for the first year. There is some evidence that a rash with carbamazepine may be a precursor of a blood dyscrasia.[83] A patient who develops a significant rash with ongoing carbamazepine therapy should have close monitoring of blood count for possible drops in neutrophil count.

Table 20.10 Medications with known risk of agranulocytosis

Antipsychotic medications
Chlorpromazine*
Clozapine*
Prochlorperazine
Thioridazine*
Trifluoperazine*
Mood stabilizers
Carbamazepine*
Miscellaneous
Desipramine
Chlordiazepoxide

Source: Adapted from Distenfeld A (n.d) Agranulocytosis, available at: www.emedicine.com/med/topic82.html

Note: *Worst offenders

- For clozapine, the patient's blood count is monitored once weekly for the first 6 months and every other week thereafter.

Clinical symptoms that may indicate a lowered white blood cell count include:

- frequent, recurrent infections, particularly recurrent sore throats and throat ulcers, infections of the oral mucosa, gums, skin and sinuses
- fever
- sepsis.

Thrombocytopenia (low platelet count) may occur with carbamazepine or valproic acid. In general, normal platelet counts are between 150,000 and 450,000 per cubic millimeter. Platelet counts from 100,000 to 150,000 per cubic millimeter, even though technically in the "low" range, are not worrisome unless unusual or abnormal bleeding is occurring. When platelet counts are lowered, the clinician should be particularly alert to complaints of unusual bleeding, bruising or petechiae. If any of these clinical signs emerge, a CBC should be drawn and the patient's clinical condition monitored more carefully. When platelet counts drop below 100,000 per cubic millimeter, a medication change is usually wise. With valproic acid, there are reports of abnormal bleeding that may occur even with normal platelet levels, due to interference with normal platelet function. When using valproic acid, therefore, evidence of abnormal bleeding may raise a concern even in the face of normal platelet levels.

Abnormal bleeding without a drop in platelet count has been associated with the use of SSRI antidepressants. This complication might have been predicted from the mechanism of action of these antidepressants. SSRIs inhibit the serotonin transporter which is responsible for the uptake of serotonin into platelets. This inhibition will deplete platelet serotonin levels, thus leading to a reduced ability to form clots and a subsequent increase in the risk of bleeding. While modest in overall frequency, such bleeding events are serious when they occur. Patients taking SSRIs have been shown to be at increased risk for upper and lower gastrointestinal bleeding, but the risk may not be limited to the system alone.

The bleeding risk is intensified in those patients who are simultaneously taking ibuprofen or other NSAIDs, aspirin, warfarin or other anticoagulants. In these situations, the use of a proton pump inhibitor may be gastro-protective and reduce the risk of bleeding. An alternative consideration is switching from an SSRI to a tricyclic antidepressant.[84]

Liver toxicity

Most psychotropics are metabolized through the liver. A potential side effect of some psychotropics is gradual damage to the liver (hepatotoxicity) causing increasingly abnormal measures of liver functions over time. Other psychotropics may show an acute fulminant hepatitis with rapidly rising liver enzymes and a clinical picture that resembles viral hepatitis. Rarely, this leads to liver failure.

Psychotropics known to have a significant incidence of liver toxicity are listed in Table 20.11.[85–87]

Although there is a low but measurable incidence of hepatotoxicity with virtually all antidepressants, the frequency is relatively small for most SSRIs and other new-generation antidepressants. The known exception is nefazodone, which has been shown to have an increased incidence of hepatitis with hepatocellular injury in a small number of patients. Traditional antipsychotics, clozapine, carbamazepine, valproic acid and MAOIs have long been known to be potentially hepatotoxic, and should be used with caution in persons with liver disease.

The clinical management of most potential hepatic effects from psychotropics initially involves drawing a baseline set of liver functions prior to instituting medications that have a high incidence of hepatotoxicity (as listed in Table 20.11). A follow-up set of liver functions should be drawn 4–6 weeks after beginning the medication, and every 3–6 months thereafter for the first year. In general, small increases in liver function test values (two to three times above normal) are not necessarily an indication that the medication must be stopped, although it would be prudent to monitor liver functions more frequently in such patients. If the values continue to rise, discontinuation may be necessary. When liver function

Table 20.11 Psychotropics associated with liver toxicity

Antipsychotics
- All traditional typical antipsychotics (neuroleptics)
- Clozapine

Antidepressants
- Nefazodone
- Irreversible MAOIs
- Clomipramine

To a lesser degree:
- Mianserin
- Lofepramine (UK only)
- Trazodone
- Fluvoxamine

Mood stabilizers
- Valproic acid
- Carbamazepine
- Lamotrigine

Table 20.12 Clinical symptoms of liver toxicity

- Jaundice
- Fever
- Ascites
- Nausea
- Vomiting
- Lethargy
- Confusion
- A change in blood-clotting ability

Table 20.13 Psychotropics with a low risk of seizure

Antidepressants
- Fluoxetine
- Paroxetine
- Sertraline
- Venlafaxine
- Trazodone
- Phenelzine
- Tranylcypromine

Antipsychotics
- Risperidone
- Haloperidol
- Fluphenazine
- Pimozide

Source: Adapted from Pisani F *et al.* (2002) Effect of psychotropic drugs on seizure threshold. *Drug Safety* 25(2): 91–110.

elevations reach three times the normal rate, changing medication is almost always necessary. In mild hepatocellular injury, there may be minimal or no observable external clinical signs of hepatocellular disease, other than the laboratory test abnormalities.

Although the serious forms of hepatotoxicity are rare, they are idiosyncratic. Unfortunately, laboratory monitoring is a poor indicator of these rare toxic episodes. Serious hepatic toxicity can occur after repeated laboratory monitoring showing normal or only minimally elevated liver enzymes. Such serious toxicity is often heralded by physical signs and symptoms as shown in Table 20.12. When these occur, liver function tests are markedly abnormal.

Seizures

The rate of unprovoked seizures in the general population is 0.07 to 0.09 percent.[88] In large studies, the rate of seizure occurrence during use of therapeutic doses of most commonly used antipsychotics and antidepressants ranges from 0.1 to 1.5 percent. Because of methodological differences in research, however, the data are confusing. The exact range is hard to specify, the variability is large and precise differences between drugs is hard to discern.[88] Although an absolute increase in risk is measurable, the clinical risk of seizure in the non-epileptic, non-head-injured patient when using psychotropics is small. Medications that have a relatively low risk of causing a *de novo* seizure in an otherwise healthy patient are shown in Table 20.13.

Use of anticonvulsant mood stabilizers and benzodiazepines (which can raise seizure threshold and make seizures *less* likely) are even less problematic. Patients who, at baseline, are more at risk for seizures are those with:

- a history of head injury
- a history of seizure or epilepsy
- bulimia
- an overdose of medications
- alcohol/street drug use, abuse and withdrawal
- a strong family history of seizure disorder.

Some of the more common mental health scenarios potentially leading to seizure include:

- A bulimic patient whose vomiting decreases intracellular fluid volume such that the epileptogenic effect of medications may be increased. This is particularly noticeable with bupropion.
- Patients who take large doses of benzodiazepines, either chronically or in overdose, then have a precipitous drop in benzodiazepine blood level due to suddenly stopping the medication. Short half-life benzodiazepines create a greater risk than long half-life compounds for seizure in this situation.
- Precipitous alcohol withdrawal from high chronic usage.
- Accidental or intentional overdose of large doses of medication or mixed overdose.

Except for drug overdose (in which the rate of seizures may be as high as 30 percent), such at-risk patients show only a small absolute risk of a psychotropic causing a new or increased frequency of seizure. Several studies now show that if a psychotropic is introduced at low doses, with slow, gradual increases, the targeted mental health condition improves with minimal change in seizure threshold. In up to one-third of studied patients, the frequency of seizures actually decreases.[88–90]

Other clinical guidelines for psychotropic prescription in patients at risk for seizure include maintaining the minimal effective dose, since the frequency of seizures is dose proportionate. Also, complex polypharmacy should be avoided.

There are some psychotropics associated with a higher-than-average incidence of seizure. These are listed in Table 20.14, and should be considered second-line choices in patients at higher baseline risk for seizures.

For purposes of illustration, it is useful to look at absolute percentages within this table. While the incidence of seizures with bupropion is greater when compared to other

Table 20.14 Psychotropic medications associated with a higher-than-average seizure risk

Antidepressants
- Maprotiline
- Clomipramine
- Bupropion

Antipsychotics
- Clozapine
- Traditional antipsychotics, particularly chlorpromazine

antidepressants, its total incidence of seizures (0.4 percent when the dosage is less than 400 mg per day) is still small compared to the seizure incidence of clozapine, which has a 1–2 percent incidence of seizures at doses less than 300 mg, 3–4 percent at doses between 300 and 600 mg and 5 percent incidence of seizures at doses over 600 mg.[91] Therefore, at typical doses, clozapine is over ten times as likely to induce a seizure than is bupropion.

If a patient has a seizure when taking a psychotropic

If a patient has a first seizure during psychotropic prescription, it is almost never clear without further evaluation whether or not the medication is absolutely implicated. Therefore, in the event of seizure, the patient should be referred for urgent medical evaluation and psychotropic medication doses should be held until such evaluation is begun. This evaluation, consisting of neurological consultation, EEG and imaging studies, may or may not reveal the cause of the seizure, but should be accomplished as promptly as possible. If it is imprudent or clinically risky to stop medication totally, half doses should be used until further information is obtained.

If neurological disease, head trauma, substance withdrawal or epilepsy is discovered, any decisions about restarting psychotropic medication must be made in concert with the medical/neurological treaters. If no other obvious cause for the seizure is found, it still does not prove that the psychotropic is the cause but suspicion is raised, particularly if the patient:

- has been recently started on the psychotropic
- has been on high doses
- has had the dose recently increased
- is on one of the medications listed in Table 20.14.

If continued psychotropic medication is clinically necessary, it is generally wise to change medications and, when possible, change to a medication with a low potential for seizure induction. If no alternative exists, or other alternatives are clinically ineffective, the clinician may have no choice but to restart the potential offending medication. If so, begin at low doses, increasing slowly. If possible, the clinician should aim for a lower final target maintenance dose, at least for several months, to observe for further seizure activity. If no further seizures occur within 90 days and the lower maintenance dose is clinically insufficient, the dose can gradually be raised to the previously effective level. In this clinical situation, written informed consent must be obtained from the patient, describing the acknowledged risk of seizure. In the chart, the clinician should document the lack of available alternatives and the clinical decision-making process.

Notes and references

1 Preskorn SH *et al.* (2002) Physician perceptions of drug–drug interactions and how to avoid them. *Journal of Psychiatric Practice* 8(2): 112–115.
2 DeVane CL and Nemeroff CB (2002) 2002 guide to psychotropic drug interactions. *Primary Psychiatry* 9(3): 28–57.
3 Strouse TB (2001) Interactions between psychotropics and other prescription medications: a focus on antidepressants. *Essential Psychopharmacology* 4(1): 1–22.
4 Ogasawara H *et al.* (1999) Simultaneous measurement of venlafaxine and its major metabolite. *Clinical Chemistry* 47: 1061–1067.

5   Martin TG (1996) Serotonin syndrome. *Annals of Emergency Medicine* 28: 520–526.

6   Mills K (1995) Serotonin syndrome. *American Family Physician* 52: 1475–1482.

7   Brown T *et al.* (1996) Pathophysiology and management of serotonin syndrome. *Annals of Pharmacotherapy* 30: 527–532.

8   Lappin RI and Auchincloss EL (1994) Treatment of the serotonin syndrome with cyproheptadine. *New England Journal of Medicine* 331: 1021–1022.

9   Shader RI and Greenblatt DJ (1972) Belladonna alkaloids and synthetic anticholinergics: uses and toxicity. In RI Shader (ed.), *Psychiatric Complications of Medical Drugs* (pp. 102–147), Raven Press.

10 Shader RI and Greenblatt DJ (1977) Clinical implications of benzodiazepine pharmacokinetics. *American Journal of Psychiatry* 134: 642–645.

11 Tune L (1980) Serum levels of anticholinergic drugs in treatment of acute extrapyramidal side effects. *Archives of General Psychiatry* 37: 293–297.

12 Hidalgo HA and Mowers RM (1990) Anticholinergic drug abuse. *Annals of Pharmacotherapy* 24: 40–41.

13 Adcock EW (1971) Cyclopentolate (Cyclogyl) toxicity in pediatric patients. *Pediatric Pharmacology and Therapeutics* 79: 127–129.

14 Ananth JV and Jain RC (1973) Benztropine psychosis. *Canadian Psychiatric Association Journal* 18: 409–414.

15 Granacher RP and Baldessarini RJ (1975) Physostigmine: its use in acute anticholinergic syndrome with antidepressant and antiparkinsonian drugs. *Archives of General Psychiatry* 32: 375–382.

16 Greenblatt DJ and Shader RI (1973) Anticholinergics. *New England Journal of Medicine* 288: 1215–1219.

17 Duvoisin RC and Katz R (1968) Reversal of central anticholinergics syndrome in man by physostigmine. *Journal of the American Medical Assocation* 206: 1963–1965.

18 Aggrawal A (2000) Lithium toxicity: a review. *Anil Aggrawal's Internet Journal of Forensic Medicine and Toxicology* 1(2).

19 The facts about lithium toxicity, available at: www.healthline.com/health/lithium-toxicity

20 Haddad LM and Winchester TF (1990) *Clinical Management of Poisoning and Drug Overdose*, 2nd edn., WB Saunders, p. 658.

21 Groleau G (1994) Lithium toxicity. *Emergency Medicine Clinics of North America* 12: 511.

22 Hansen HE and Amdisen A (1978) Lithium intoxication (report of 23 cases and review of 100 cases from the literature). *Quarterly Journal of Medicine* 47: 123.

23 El-Mallakh RS (1986) Acute lithium neurotoxicity. *Psychiatric Developments* 4: 311–328.

24 Krishel S and Jackimczyk K (1991) Cyclic antidepressants, lithium, and neuroleptic agents: pharmacology and toxicology. *Emergency Medical Clinics of North America* 19: 53.

25 Kech PE and McElroy SL (2002) Clinical pharmacodynamics and pharmacokinetics of antimanic and mood stabilizing medication. *Journal of Clinical Psychiatry* 63 (Suppl. 4).

26 Thomsen K and Schou M (1968) Renal lithium excretion in man. *American Journal of Physiology* 215: 823–827.

27 Glassman A and Bitter JT (2001) Antipsychotic drugs: prolonged QTc interval, torsades de pointes and sudden death. *American Journal of Psychiatry* 158: 1774–1782.

28 Gelenberg A (2001) Ziprasidone (Geodon). *Biological Therapies in Psychiatry* 24 (6): 21–22.

29 Woosley RL *et al.* (2021) QTdrugs list, available at: https://crediblemeds.org/ (accessed April 14, 2021), AZCERT, Inc. 1822 Innovation Park Dr., Oro Valley, AZ 85755.

30 Ray WA *et al.* (2009) Atypical antipsychotic drugs and the risk of sudden cardiac death. *New England Journal of Medicine* 360: 225–235.

31 Schneeweiss S (2007) Risk of death associated with the use of conventional versus atypical antipsychotic drugs among elderly patients. *Canadian Medical Association Journal* 176(5).

32   Wang PS *et al.* (2005) Risk of death in elderly users of conventional vs. atypical antipsychotic medications. *New England Journal of Medicine* 353: 2335–2341.

33   Maher AR *et al.* (2011) Efficacy and comparative effectiveness of atypical antipsychotic medications for off-label uses in adults: a systematic review and meta-analysis. *Journal of the American Medical Association* 306(12): 1359–1369.

34   Kales HC *et al.* (2012) Risk of mortality among individual antipsychotics in patients with dementia. *American Journal of Psychiatry* 169(1): 71–79.

35   Corbett A and Ballard C (2012) Antipsychotics and mortality in dementia. *American Journal of Psychiatry* 169: 7–9.

36   *The Maudsley Prescribing Guidelines* (2009), 10th edn., Martin Dunitz, p. 105.

37   Marsden CD and Jenner P (1980) The pathophysiology of extrapyramidal side-effects of neuroleptic drugs. *Psychological Medicine* 10: 55–72.

38   Ayd FJ (1961) A survey of drug-induced extrapyramidal reactions. *Journal of the American Medical Association* 175: 1054–1060.

39   Tarsy D (1983) Neuroleptic-induced extrapyramidal reactions: classification, description, and diagnosis. *Clinical Neuropharmacology* 6: 9–26.

40   Gelenberg AJ (1983) Treating extrapyramidal reactions. *Biological Therapies in Psychiatry* 6: 13–16.

41   Gelenberg AJ (1987) Treating extrapyramidal reactions: some current issues. *Journal of Clinical Psychiatry* 9 (Suppl.): 24–27.

42   Addonizio G and Alexopoulos GS (1988) Drug-induced dystonia in young and elderly patients. *American Journal of Psychiatry* 145: 869–871.

43   Swett C (1975) Drug-induced dystonia. *American Journal of Psychiatry* 132: 532–534.

44   Sheppard C and Merlis S (1967) Drug-induced extrapyramidal symptoms: their incidence and treatment. *American Journal of Psychiatry* 123: 886–889.

45   Man PL (1973) Long-term effects of haloperidol. *Diseases of the Nervous System* 34: 113–118.

46   Boyer WF *et al.* (1987) Anticholinergic prophylaxis of acute haloperidol induced acute dystonic reactions. *Journal of Clinical Psychopharmacology* 7: 164–166.

47   Miller CH *et al.* (1996) The prevalence and severity of acute extrapyramidal side effects in patients treated with clozapine, risperidone or conventional antipsychotics. In *New Research Program and Abstracts of the 149th Annual Meeting of the American Psychiatric Association* (Abstract NR542: pp. 217–218), APA.

48   Rosebush PI and Mazurek MF (1999) Neurologic side effects in neuroleptic-naïve patients treated with haloperidol or risperidone. *Neurology* 52: 782–785.

49   Kapur S *et al.* (1999) Clinical and theoretical implications of 5-HT2 and D2 receptor occupancy of clozapine, risperidone and olanzapine in schizophrenia. *American Journal of Psychiatry* 156: 286–293.

50   Donlon PT and Stenson RL (1976) Neuroleptic induced extrapyramidal symptoms. *Diseases of the Nervous System* 37: 629–635.

51   Chouinard G *et al.* (1987) Long-term effects of l-dopa and procyclidine on neuroleptic-induced extrapyramidal and schizophrenic symptoms. *Psychopharmacological Bulletin* 23: 221–226.

52   Friis T *et al.* (1983) Sodium valproate and biperiden in neuroleptic-induced akathisia, parkinsonism and hyperkinesias. *Acta Psychiatrica Scandinavica* 67: 178–187.

53   Fann WE and Lake CR (1976) Amantadine versus trihexyphenidyl in the treatment of neuroleptic-induced parkinsonism. *American Journal of Psychiatry* 133: 940–943.

54   Borison RL (1983) Amantadine in the management of extrapyramidal side effects. *Clinical Neuropharmacology* 6 (Suppl.): S57–S63.

55   Gagrat D *et al.* (1978) Intravenous diazepam in the treatment of neuroleptic-induced acute dystonia and akathisia. *American Journal of Psychiatry* 135: 1232–1233.

56   Caroff SN *et al.* (2000) Atypical antipsychotics and neuroleptic malignant syndrome. *Psychiatric Annals* 30: 314–321.

57   Velamoor VR *et al.* (1994) Progression of symptoms in neuroleptic malignant syndrome. *Journal of Nervous Mental Disease* 182: 168–173.

58   Caroff SN and Mann SC (1993) Neuroleptic malignant syndrome. *Medical Clinics of North America* 77: 185–202.

59   Caroff SN and Mann SC (1988) Neuroleptic malignant syndrome. *Psychopharmacological Bulletin* 24: 25–29.

60   What is NMSIS?, available at: www.mhaus.org/nmsis/about-us/what-is-nmsis/

61   Davis JM *et al.* (1991) Electroconvulsive therapy in the treatment of the neuroleptic malignant syndrome. *Convulsive Therapy* 7: 111–120.

62   Serfertova D (1997) Treatment of the neuroleptic malignant syndrome by electroconvulsive therapy. *Biological Psychiatry* 42: 1835.

63   Brasic JR (2018) Tardive dyskinesia, available at: https://emedicine.medscape.com/article/1151826-overview

64   Goetz DG (1997) Tardive dyskinesia. In RL Watts and WC Koller (eds.), *Movement Disorders: Neurologic Principles and Practice* (pp. 519–526), McGraw-Hill Professional.

65   Sherr JD (2002) The prevention and management of tardive dyskinesia in the elderly. *Psychiatric Annals* 32(4): 237–243.

66   Beasley CM *et al.* (1996) Olanzapine versus placebo: results of a double-blind, fixed dose olanzapine trial. *Psychopharmacology* 124: 159–167.

67   Ereshefsky L *et al.* (1991) Clozapine: an atypical antipsychotic agent. *Clinical Pharmacy* 8: 691–709.

68   Lieberman JA *et al.* (1989) Clozapine guidelines for clinical management. *Journal of Clinical Psychiatry* 50: 329–338.

69   Safferman AZ *et al.* (1991) Update on the clinical efficacy and side effects of clozapine. *Schizophrenia Bulletin* 17: 247–261.

70   Safferman AZ *et al.* (1992) Clozapine and akathisia [letter]. *Biological Psychiatry* 31: 749–754.

71   Cohen LJ (1994) Risperidone. *Pharmacotherapy* 14: 263–265.

72   Chouinard G *et al.* (1993) A Canadian multicenter placebo-controlled study of fixed doses of risperidone and haloperidol in the treatment of chronic schizophrenic patients. *Journal of Clinical Psychopharmacology* 13: 25–40.

73   Casey DE (1999) Tardive dyskinesia and atypical antipsychotic drugs. *Schizophrenia Research* 35: 561–566.

74   Driesens F (1998) Neuroleptic medication facilitates the natural occurrence of tardive dyskinesia: a critical review. *Acta Psychiatrica Belgica* 88: 195–205.

75   Alexander B and Lund B (1999) Tardive dyskinesia, Clinical Psychopharmacology Seminar, Virtual Hospital, University of Iowa; see also Movement disorders, available at: https://uihc.org/movement-disorders

76   Fernandez HH *et al.* (2017) Randomized controlled trial of deutetrabenazine for tardive dyskinesia: the ARM-TD study. *Neurology* 88(21): 2003–2010.

77   Anderson KE *et al.* (2017) Deutetrabenazine for treatment of involuntary movements in patients with tardive dyskinesia (AIM-TD): a double-blind, randomised, placebo-controlled, phase 3 trial. *Lancet Psychiatry* 4(8): 595–604.

78   Jus A *et al.* (1976) Epidemiology of tardive dyskinesia, part 2. *Diseases of the Nervous System* 37: 257–261.

79   Kane JM (1988) Tardive dyskinesia: prevalence, incidence and risk factors. *Journal of Clinical Psychopharmacology* 8: 52S–56S.

80   Graham PM *et al.* (1982) Combination monoamine oxidase inhibitor/TCA interaction. [letter]. *Lancet* 2: 440.

81   White K and Simpson G (1984) The combined use of MAOIs and tricyclics. *Journal of Clinical Psychiatry* 45: 67–69.

82   Grossman E *et al.* (1996) Should a moratorium be placed on sublingual nifedipine capsules given for hypertensive emergencies and pseudo emergencies? *Journal of the American Medical Association* 276: 1328–1331.

83   Cates M and Powers R (1998) Concomitant rash and blood dyscrasia in geriatric psychiatry patients treated with carbamazepine. *Annals of Pharmacotherapy* 32(9): 884–887.

84   *The Maudsley Prescribing Guidelines* (2009), 10th edn., Martin Dunitz, pp. 197–198.

85   Garcia-Pando AC *et al.* (2002) Hepatotoxicity associated with new antidepressants. *Journal of Clinical Psychiatry* 63(2): 135–137.

86   *The Maudsley Prescribing Guidelines* (2009) 10th edn., Martin Dunitz, pp. 120–124.

87   *British National Formulary* (2002) 43rd edn., British Medical Association, p. 189.

88   Pisani F *et al.* (2002) Effect of psychotropic drugs on seizure threshold. *Drug Safety* 25(2): 91–110.

89   Janicak TG *et al.* (1997) *Principles and Practice of Psychopharmacotherapy*, 2nd edn., Williams & Wilkins, p. 195.

90   Gross A *et al.* (2000) Psychotropic medication use in patients with epilepsy: effect on seizure frequency. *Journal of Neuropsychiatry and Clinical Neuroscience* 12(4): 458–464.

91   Toth P and Frankenburg FR (1994) Clozapine and seizures: a review. *Canadian Journal of Psychiatry* 39(4): 236–238. doi: 10.1177/070674379403900409

21 Medication allergies

• Identification of allergic responses	378
• Management of allergy symptoms	380
• Other issues of evaluation when allergy is suspected	380
• Stopping the offending medication	381
• What else to do	381
• Pills contain more than just the active ingredient	382
• Reference	382

Although allergic responses to psychotropic medications are fundamentally no different from allergic responses to any other medication, it is helpful to review the management principles of allergic reactions as they present to the prescriber of mental health prescriptions.

An allergic reaction to a medication can occur:

- with any medication
- at any time
- with any practitioner.

Such reactions can occur regardless of the purpose for prescribing, the dosage, the length of time the patient has been taking the medication or the practitioner's skill level. Therefore, the clinician always must be aware of the possibility of allergic reactions when medications are being prescribed.

While allergic reactions often occur within the first 30 days of usage, allergic responses can occur at a much later date, even after several years of treatment. Although allergic responses are more likely to occur when medication dosages are increased, they may also occur when doses have not changed. Unfortunately, allergic responses may occur when the medication is helping the patient considerably, although they also occur when there is little therapeutic response.

Identification of allergic responses

Patients will both underestimate and overestimate the occurrence of an allergy. While often believing that they know what an allergy is and how it might present, patients are not always correct and may overlook a true allergy unless it is identified for them. There are also many individuals who have a heightened sensitivity to allergies and assume that any adverse effect that occurs from a medication is an "allergy." A commonly mistaken example is often found with traditional antipsychotics. Patients who experience extrapyramidal symptoms (EPS) have often labeled themselves as being "allergic" to traditional antipsychotics, when in fact they are not allergic at all. They have experienced a significant and unpleasant side effect, but it is not an allergic reaction. Distinguishing a side effect from an allergy is significant in that side effects can be managed and may be temporary, permitting the patient to continue taking the medication. Most allergies, however, do not resolve with time, and, when severe, may present life-threatening symptoms. Therefore, when a patient is experiencing a true medication allergy, that patient should discontinue the medication and, in general, not be re-challenged.

Some patients do have true multiple drug and food allergies. For those patients who are, in fact, allergic to many different medications, a gradual institution of small doses of medications will lessen the likelihood of a dramatic allergic reaction that might ensue if a full dose is given initially. Other individuals have labeled themselves "allergy prone," and will often describe a long list of allergies in the initial evaluation interview. Even if it is the clinician's assessment that many of these "allergies" are really side effects, such patients are anxious about starting a medication. Generally, they are reassured if any new medication is started in very small doses. By doing so, the clinician recognizes the patient's sensitivities to medications. Typical medication allergy symptoms are listed in Table 21.1.

The core allergic symptom is a rash. It is often itchy and reddened and may or may not be raised. Drug allergies typically begin centrally, that is on the trunk, and spread to the extremities. The spread of the rash may occur over several hours or several days. Typically, the rash does not remain confined to one extremity or one area. Rashes that affect only a small area of the skin and do not spread are often from another cause. Similarly, a rash with a sharply defined circumscribed pattern may not be a true drug allergy (for example, a rash that occurs only in those areas exposed to sunlight may be a sun sensitivity, not an allergy). Rashes confined to an area solely covered by clothing may be the result of allergy to soap products or to the material in the clothing.

In addition to a rash, the patient may have urticaria or hives. Hives, large blotchy spots that itch, may have variable diameters and may be present with or without a finer rash.

Swelling and edema of various body parts often accompanies a rash and urticaria. Such swelling can occur around the eyes and face, and there may be dependent edema in the ankles.

Certain patients, sometimes fueled by practitioners who specialize in "allergic problems" or "environmental sensitivity," will believe that allergies are the cause for behavioral symptoms, psychiatric illness or mental reactions. While true allergies may not be totally ruled out, if the patient's symptoms do not include at least one of those

Table 21.1 Common allergy symptoms

- Rash – starts centrally and spreads
- Itchiness
- Reddened skin
- Urticaria (hives)
- Swelling/edema
- Respiratory distress, in more serious allergic reactions

Table 21.2 Drug allergy assessment and treatment

- Examine the rash directly.
- If a drug allergy is a likely cause, stop the offending medication as soon as possible.
- Give diphenhydramine (Benadryl) 25–100 mg daily by mouth. An alternative would be Loratadine (Claritin) 10 mg/day.
- Suggest a tepid bath or damp cloth soaks and, if necessary, a topical steroid cream for the rash.
- Do not start any replacement medication until the allergy symptoms are resolved, unless the mental health target symptoms being treated create an emergency.

---

identified in Table 21.1, the presence of a true medication allergy should be highly suspect. In general, within our current state of knowledge, mental health symptoms, syndromes and conditions are not primarily allergic in origin.

Management of allergy symptoms

The practitioner's response to possible allergy symptoms is summarized in Table 21.2.

Of primary importance is that the practitioner be able to observe directly the rash and/or urticaria. Based on the previous discussion, it may be relatively apparent, when seen, whether or not the rash is likely a drug allergy. The patient should be seen as soon as possible by the practitioner, particularly if he/she is telephoning with complaints suggestive of an allergic response. Small or very circumscribed rashes can often be ruled out as being unlikely to be due to drug allergies simply by inspection. On the other hand, significant and spreading rashes, which can occur from a drug allergy, can also be highly suspected solely through observation. When in the office, the patient should be asked to disrobe only sufficiently to allow the practitioner to see some of the affected areas. If the rash is present on the breast, groin or buttocks areas in either sex and these areas need to be observed, it is safest to have another staff member present when the observation is made.

Other issues of evaluation when allergy is suspected

At the time of the observation of the rash, the patient should be questioned about any changes in foods, other over-the-counter preparations, prescription medications or lifestyle changes within the several weeks prior to the emergence of the rash. Even when a drug allergy is likely identified, it may turn out that it is not the psychotropic medication prescribed that is the cause. Other substances to which the patient is exposed – fabrics, detergents, colognes, foods, new over-the-counter compounds or prescriptions written by other practitioners – may also be responsible for the allergy diagnosed.

The patient should also be specifically questioned about the presence of shortness of breath, wheezing or difficulty in breathing.

Box 21.1 Danger

Any breathing difficulties observed by the clinician or described by the patient constitute a potential emergency. *Such patients should be sent directly to the emergency room for assessment of breathing capacity, and need for oxygen and/or mechanical ventilation.*

While the rash and urticaria may be uncomfortable, the potentially lethal outcome in an allergic reaction is respiratory arrest. While respiratory problems from medication allergy are not routine, when present they are of immediate concern.

Stopping the offending medication

If it is the assessment of the practitioner that a drug allergy is present, the medication should be stopped immediately. Strong, uncomfortable rashes, large areas of urticaria and/or breathing problems mandate that any offending medication be stopped immediately, even from a relatively high dose, risking the possibility of rebound symptoms. If the symptoms are minimal, tolerable, no breathing problems are present and the medication is one that could precipitate a discontinuation syndrome (see Chapter 8), a rapid taper can be a somewhat more comfortable recommendation for the patient. In any case, the medication should be stopped quickly.

If allergy symptoms are questionable, assume it is a drug allergy until proven otherwise. From a medico-legal viewpoint, it is much safer for a practitioner to stop a medication on the assumption that an allergy is present, and discover later that it was not. The riskier course would be to continue a medication only to learn that a patient is truly allergic and have possible serious symptoms ensue.

Allergic reactions will subside within several days to a week. Even the most severe allergic reaction should be totally resolved within a 10-day period. Many patients require little or no treatment during this period, other than having the offending medication removed. For some patients, however, itchiness can be quite uncomfortable and can disrupt sleep. For these patients, the use of 25–100 mg diphenhydramine or another antihistamine daily will minimize the discomfort. *Tepid* baths or tepid, moist cloth soaks on areas of urticaria and rash will also diminish the itchiness. Hot baths or soaks will likely aggravate the rash. For particularly uncomfortable rashes, betamethasone 0.5 percent topical cream or a similar agent may be used.

What else to do

Documentation of the allergy, and of the practitioner's response to it, is crucial to good medical practice and may prevent any allegation of mismanagement. The clinician should *document, in writing: the symptoms described* by complaint and/or on examination; *when* the patient *made* the clinician *aware* of these symptoms; *when* the patient was *seen in person* and *by whom*; and *what recommendations* were made regarding treatment and/or further assessment.

Following an initial evaluation in which medication allergies are suspected or confirmed, the clinician should be in contact with the patient within several days to ask whether the symptoms are improving, and document the follow-up contact. If it is not convenient to have a face-to-face follow-up evaluation and the allergic reaction is mild, a telephone assessment is satisfactory as long as documentation is completed and improvement is noted.

If the clinician assesses that a drug allergy to his or her prescription has occurred, the patient should be clearly informed that this was a drug allergy and advised that this medication should not be taken again. The appropriate portion of the patient's chart should be labeled for future reference. Some facilities or practitioners will paste a brightly colored stick-on to the front of the chart noting any allergies. Another useful tool is to make a list of patient allergies on the patient's medication list. Thus, when going to document any new medication or prescription, it is easy for the clinician to glance at these medicines to which the patient is allergic and avoid them. Although resolution of the allergic symptoms with discontinuation does not prove the connection, it is usually assumed to be true.

In unusual circumstances (e.g., another more likely cause than the psychotropic is discovered for the symptoms, or the clinician feels the patient must be retried on this medication for lack of viable alternatives), a re-challenge with the suspected offending agent may be tried. If attempted, the drug should be reintroduced very gradually, with frequent clinical re-evaluation for the onset of rash, urticaria or respiratory difficulties. If the symptoms recur, the re-challenge is generally abandoned.

Pills contain more than just the active ingredient

Some patients are allergic to dyes, additives, food coloring, flavoring or preservatives used in the preparation of capsules or pills, but not to the psychoactive compound. A particularly common allergy is to tartrazine (FD&C yellow #5). A fairly recent study[1] showed that approximately 3.8 percent of patients exposed to tartrazine-containing compounds developed allergic reactions. These allergic reactions subside within 24–48 hours after stopping the tartrazine and none of these patients showed allergy to non-tartrazine containing brands. A history of aspirin sensitivity is a marker toward possible tartrazine sensitivity, as *tartrazine allergy occurs in 13.2 percent of those with aspirin sensitivity.*

Box 21.2 Danger

Aspirin sensitivity may predict tartrazine allergies. Medications containing tartrazine should be relegated to second-line treatment in such patients. If chosen, small doses should be used initially and frequent follow-up ensured.

The identification of tartrazine allergies is important, since the patient may not be truly allergic to the underlying psychotropic compound. Such a patient may be changed to a different preparation or a different brand of the same psychotropic that does not include tartrazine, and may well be able to tolerate the psychotropic drug. Another strategy is to investigate whether other pill strengths of the same brand are manufactured without the dye. For example, a patient who is sensitive to the 150 mg strength pill that contains tartrazine, could, perhaps, take three 50 mg pills which are a different color and do not contain the dye.

Reference

1   Bhatia MS (2000) Allergy to tartrazine in psychotropic drugs. *Journal of Clinical Psychiatry* 61: 7.

Part V
Competent clinical practice

22 Misuse of medication – taking too much and taking too little

• How medication misuse presents	387
• Accidental and careless overutilization	388
• Intentional overdose	389
• Serious overdose	390
• Minor overdose	391
• Using too little medication	392
• Fraud and abuse with psychotropic medications	392
• Practitioner protections against abuse of prescription medications	393
• The development of abuse	396
• If abuse is suspected	396
• The pharmacist as ally	397
• What to do when abuse occurs	397
• References	399

Despite our best efforts and conscientious practice, patients don't always take medications as prescribed. In order to properly assess and manage this problem, it is important to distinguish several key terms, and understand how they overlap or are distinct. While overutilization of medication is generally of more urgent concern to the clinician, under usage of medication can also occur and will be discussed later in the chapter.

Misuse of medication occurs in every clinical setting and in every practitioner's practice. No setting is immune. Particularly high-risk populations for medication misuse include:

* predominantly adolescent populations, especially if adolescents are housed together
* patients with personality disorders, particularly with sociopathic or borderline traits
* forensic settings, such as prison or the penitentiary
* people who abuse alcohol, recreational drugs or other substances.

It is a common misconception that if the patient takes too much medication it is abuse, and the clinician has been deceived. This is not always the case, and knowing the various categories of overuse will help the clinician to understand when, and when not, to be concerned. Table 22.1 will serve as an outline for important terms and a framework for this chapter.

Table 22.1 Misuse of medication

Overutilization of medication
1 Accidental over usage:
   • from carelessness or confusion
   • by persons who believe they are following directions
   • "chronic overdose"
2 Intentional over usage:
   • acute overdose
   • substance abuse
   • substance dependence (addiction)

Underutilization of medication
   • because of fear
   • as a symptom of the illness being treated
   • because the patient can't afford the medication

Separate clinical issues that may overlap with misuse
   • physiological (physical) dependence
   • intoxication

Misuse of medication is a general term describing the use of medication in an unauthorized or non-recommended manner. Misuse may be chronic or acute, accidental or intentional, and involve over usage or under usage. It may or may not include withdrawal or tolerance. It may be a part of "self-treatment" with a belief on the part of patients that they know what is "right" for them and what they "need," regardless of what the clinician prescribes. Patients' misuse of medications may occur in an effort to self-treat a psychiatric symptom or physical symptom. It may be a part of universal feelings about medications in general, be related to psychotropic medications only or be limited to one particular medication. Misuse may be rationalized by patients ("if one pill is good, then four pills must be better"), or come from a belief about their physiological tolerance to medication ("I always need more medication than everyone else"). The broadest subtypes of misuse involve *overutilization* (using more medication than the clinician prescribes) and *underutilization* (using less medication than the clinician prescribes).

Overutilization may be accidental and unrealized by patients. On the other hand, it may be a conscious decision on their part to take excessive amounts of a drug. This can lead to an excess of medication that may occur gradually over a period of time (*chronic overdose*), and sometimes leads to gradually increasing signs of medication intoxication. Overdose may also occur all at once in an intentional ingestion of a large amount of medications for various reasons (referred to, in this text, as an *acute overdose*).

Substance abuse is a maladaptive pattern of medication usage manifested by recurrent and significant adverse consequences related to the use of a substance or medication. There may be physical debilitation, a decrease in school/work performance, neglect of family duties, legal problems or other behavioral reactions accompanying substance abuse, but continued use of the medication occurs despite having persistent and recurrent social or interpersonal problems. *The term "substance abuse" does not automatically include physical tolerance, withdrawal or a pattern of compulsive use; instead it includes only the harmful consequences of repeated usage.*[1]

Substance dependence (commonly referred to as "addiction") not only shows a pattern of repeated self-administration of a drug, but also results in physical tolerance, compulsive drug-taking behavior and withdrawal when the medication is stopped. There may be a pattern of cognitive, behavioral and physiological reactions that result as the person continues to use increasing amounts of medication.[2]

Physical tolerance (the need for increased amounts of medication to achieve intoxication or the desired effect, or a diminished effect with continued use of the same amount of the substance) is common in substance dependence. Physical tolerance is, however, neither a necessary nor a sufficient condition to warrant the diagnosis of substance dependence (addiction). Similarly, *withdrawal*[3] (a maladaptive behavioral change with physiological and cognitive components, which occurs when blood or tissue concentrations of a substance diminish quickly in an individual who has maintained prolonged heavy use of the substance) also may or may not be present in a person with substance dependence. Persons with substance dependence (addiction) often use the substance in larger amounts over a long period of time. They spend a great deal of time obtaining the substance, using it or recovering from its effects. Often their daily activities revolve around obtaining, using or withdrawing from the use of the substance. They often have marked social, recreational and occupational changes because of substance use. They may express a desire to decrease or regulate the amount that they use, and often have many unsuccessful attempts to decrease or stop using it. Despite recognizing the pattern of usage in their overall life and the negative consequences thereof, they are unable or unwilling to discontinue use. *The crucial component of substance dependence is not over usage, but the inability to abstain from using despite having ample evidence that continued use is harmful.*

Physiological dependence is a physiological state that occurs when the individual has taken doses of medication for a long enough period of time that when the medication is stopped, symptoms of physiological withdrawal occur. It is not automatically a sign of drug abuse, substance abuse or inappropriate practice by the clinician or the patient. *Physiological dependence is a physical state based on usage of medication at a high enough dose for a long enough period of time.* It does not necessarily translate into substance abuse if it occurs from conscious rational decisions, made in partnership between the clinician and the patient, in order to treat certain psychiatric or medical problems. For example, a patient with chronic anxiety disorder treated over a long time with a benzodiazepine may become physically dependent on the medication (i.e., withdrawal will occur when the drug is stopped suddenly), but the patient is not necessarily abusing the medication.

Intoxication is a substance-specific syndrome that occurs shortly after ingestion of a substance, and may include symptoms of maladaptive behavioral and psychological changes, including impaired cognitive abilities, judgment, coordination, social or work functioning as well as perceptual changes and belligerence. The manifestations can vary greatly between individuals, and may depend on the substance ingested and the setting in which it occurs. Intoxication can occur acutely or chronically.

How medication misuse presents

Evidence of medication misuse may present to the clinician from a variety of sources:

- from the patient volunteering a report
- from direct questioning by the clinician
- from investigating side effects and how the patient is dealing with them

- from an urgent telephone call from the patient saying, "I took too much"
- from emergency room staff or other medical clinic personnel treating your patient
- via reports from a family member, caretaker or friend who is concerned about the patient's behavior
- after the clinician observes symptoms such as slurred speech, irregular gait or sedation
- from high serum blood levels of a medication on a laboratory report
- from a pharmacist's call requesting early renewal of a prescription by the patient
- after the fact, when the over usage is no longer occurring.

Whatever the reason, when a clinician becomes aware that the patient is taking too much medication, he or she must assess the cause, document the assessment and take necessary action.

Accidental and careless overutilization

Many confused, anxious, elderly or visually impaired patients may accidentally take too much medication – occasionally or chronically. Patients with poor memory may not realize that they have already taken a dose, or may be oblivious to how much medication they have taken. Some patients will confuse various medications they are taking, overutilizing one medication and underutilizing another. Patients with visual problems may confuse one pill or pill bottle for another. Some patients feel that medications can be taken "whenever I need it," and do not keep track of how often they are dosing themselves. Patients who use medications along with alcohol or street drugs can become further confused and, when intoxicated, misuse their medications unintentionally.

If it is determined that the patient is accidentally but carelessly taking too much medication, resulting in chronic overdose:

- The clinician should verbally reinforce the specific instructions as to how much medication should be taken and how often.
- Written instructions should be reissued and the patient educated about the risks of continued overutilization.
- The clinician may wish to use the help of family members – a spouse, parent, adult or child – to oversee the usage of medication. Elderly, confused patients, or minors who are overutilizing medication, may need supervision, with the responsibility of medication administration delegated to another person.
- The use of a "pill minder," in which pills can be filled into a partitioned container organized by days of the week and times, can often help forgetful patients to know whether or not they have taken their doses. These may also be useful for any patient who takes chronic medication, particularly with complicated regimens of medication. Such devices usually consist of a series of compartments which are manually filled and opened when needed. More recently developed electronic devices will sound a notification alarm and automatically open a compartment to dispense the correct quantity of the appropriate medication.
- Patients with visual problems should have an optometric exam, use a magnifying glass and/or use color-coded bottles for their medications.

Accidental overdose when patients believe they are following instructions

Despite written instructions, repetition and education, many patients still misunderstand instructions for dosing psychotropics. In some cases, patients may have left the clinician's office correctly understanding directions, but may be told by other family members or healthcare professionals that they should change their psychotropic dosage, and do so without contacting the prescriber. Occasionally, the patient is given the wrong pill from the pharmacy or the medication is mis-labeled. The patient follows the instructions, not knowing they are incorrect.

In these circumstances, the clinician should re-emphasize the correct instructions or reissue a correct, written schedule of dosing. If necessary, the patient or a family member should bring the pill bottle or read the label over the telephone. It may be necessary to call the pharmacy to verify that the correct medication, in the correct dosage, has been dispensed. If incorrect instructions are coming from the family or another healthcare provider, the clinician should contact that party to explain the rationale for the dosing schedule and ask that future dosing matters be left solely to the prescribing clinician, so as to eliminate confusion for the patient.

Intentional overdose

When the patient is not suicidal

When patients intentionally take a large dose of medication, their conscious (or unconscious) intent may not always be to harm themselves. Other reasons that patients may intentionally take a large amount of medication include:

1 to treat intolerable symptoms such as:
   * frequent, significant insomnia
   * excruciating anxiety
   * emotional pain
   * physical pain
   * hallucinations
2 to show anger or make a point ("I'll show you") which may be part of an argument, and often occurs impulsively
3 to attempt to make someone feel guilty ("You'll be sorry") – although most often this is a family member, a boyfriend/girlfriend or a spouse. Occasionally it may be the clinician!
4 to escape temporarily from what is perceived as an intolerable situation ("I just wanted to get away from it all and sleep")
5 for psychotic reasons – for example, patients may feel that by taking a large amount of medication they can escape delusional persecution, observation or taunting. They may also be responding to command hallucinations.

With suicidal intent

Suicide is a complex phenomenon with many facets, and the causes of suicide vary among cultures (e.g., use of firearms is most common in the United States, hanging is most common in Eastern Europe and drug overdose most common in Northern Europe and the United Kingdom). Attempted or completed suicide through self-poisoning by inges-tion of medications is a common methodology worldwide – more so by females, whereas hanging and asphyxia are more common in males. By definition, when prescribing psy-chotropic medications to a patient, the prescriber has enabled one of the risk factors for suicide (easy access to lethal toxins – prescription medications).[4] While it is beyond the scope of this book to explore all the causative, evaluative and risk factors involved in suicide, this section explores the practical issues facing the practitioner when a current medication patient presents having possibly intentionally overdosed on medication.

On occasion, the patient appears in person directly after taking an intentional over-dose. More commonly, the clinician receives an emergency telephone call after hours. The recommended evaluation procedure for the medicating clinician, whether on the telephone or in person, is to do a brief screening of the patient's condition, including any elements of physical danger, patient lucidity and ability to communicate. Questions that should be asked at this time are:

- How much of your psychotropic medication did you take?
- When did you take the medication?
- Did you take any other medicines with the psychotropic?
- Did you take any alcohol or other street drugs with the medication?
- Are you having trouble breathing?
- What, if any, symptoms do you have now?
- Are you feeling sleepy?
- Have you vomited, or do you feel like vomiting?
- Are you having trouble walking or performing other coordinated actions?
- Are you feeling dizzy, lightheaded or faint?
- Is anyone else present with you now?

If the patient is sufficiently alert and the clinician is not current with the patient's other possible medical conditions or medication regimens, the clinician should ask about the presence of any other medical problems and regularly taken non-psychotropic medications. Responses to the above questions in a lucid patient will dictate the clinician's immediate response. Any patient who cannot speak clearly and/or respond to initial questions presents a medical emergency. An urgent evaluation and/or trans-portation to an emergency room setting should be arranged for any patient who cannot respond clearly or sounds intoxicated.

Serious overdose

Because of potential serious medical sequelae, overdoses that include the following psy-chotropic medications should *always* have emergency medical clearance through face-to-face evaluation:

- MAO inhibitors
- tricyclic antidepressants
- lithium

Physical signs which, when present, should concern the clinician and necessitate a face-to-face evaluation, include:

- slurred speech
- fluctuating level of consciousness
- inability to remain awake
- mental confusion.

Other situations that mandate a medical evaluation include:

- a mixed medication overdose with more than one prescription medication, or pre-scription medication plus an over-the-counter compound
- medication overdose mixed with alcohol, recreational drugs or toxins
- any patient who cannot convince the clinician that the amount of medication ingested was small
- when the patient is vague, manipulative or gamey
- any overdose of more than three times the daily dose of medication
- any patient who is excessively worried and cannot be reassured. (For medico-legal reasons, it is generally safer to have such a patient evaluated than have the clinician assume the full burden of responsibility, even if the risk is small.)

If a patient or a family member calls about an overdose, and the clinician cannot get a clear and convincing response that the overdose is minor, the patient should be sent to the emergency room or medical clinic for medical clearance. It is always better to be safe than sorry. With any serious overdose, in addition to arranging for the patient to go for medical evaluation, the clinician should assure that safe transportation is available. This can be another driver, Uber, Lyft, taxicab or ambulance. If there is concern about the patient's ability to get to the hospital without further symptoms, it is best to call 911 for emergency ambulance transportation (999 in the UK).

Once the patient has been instructed to get to an emergency evaluation and trans-portation has been assured, the clinician should call the emergency room or clinic to provide historical data obtained from the patient or family, and any pertinent history from the patient's record. Once the patient has arrived and has been evaluated, the emergency staff should be asked to call the clinician with the results of their evaluation. It is important for the clinician to write down details of the contact(s) and actions taken. Such written records should include the *time* of the first contact and when notification of the overdose was received by the clinician, along with the results of his or her evaluation and recommendations made for treatment or evalu-ation, including emergency room referral, if made. Documentation of any follow-up care that is to be provided, based on the emergency room's evaluation, should also be recorded.

Minor overdose

A healthy patient

- without the presence of a medical disorder
- in the absence of alcohol or illicit drugs
- in the absence of other medications
- who is not alone
- who did not ingest a high-risk medication

can generally tolerate up to two to three times the usual daily dose of many medications without medical sequelae. Patients who meet the above criteria may have some increased side effects, but these are generally not life-threatening ones. SSRI antidepressants, other newer antidepressants, typical and atypical antipsychotics, as well as benzodiazepines in minor amounts may cause sleepiness, gastrointestinal upset or a confused feeling. As long as such patients are observed and are not alone, they generally do not need emergency care. If more than 6 hours have passed since the patient ingested the overdose and there are no side effects, it is unlikely that further effects will emerge.

Following such a minor overdose, if the clinician intends to continue the patient on the medicine prescribed, he or she should hold at least one dose, order the next scheduled dose at half the usual amount, and then resume regular dosing.

Using too little medication

While generally less urgently significant than taking too much medication, taking less medication than prescribed may lead to an inadequate therapeutic effect, and partial or sporadic response. Reasons why patients take less medication than the clinician prescribes include:

- fear of excessive response ("it will control me," "change me" or "make me feel something I don't want to feel")
- fear of side effects
- as a symptom of the illness being treated – patients with panic disorder or obsessive–compulsive disorder frequently catastrophize possible outcomes; they assume that medication response will be negative and seek to avoid problems by minimizing their medication dose
- the patient feels that "I'm medication sensitive" and always need less than the recommended dose
- the patient does not have enough money to pay for full therapeutic doses.

See Chapter 14 for a further discussion of underdosing in the geriatric patient.

Fraud and abuse with psychotropic medications

Any clinician who prescribes medications that have the potential for abuse is a potential target for patients who will fraudulently use and abuse medication. No practitioner is immune from this abuse potential. As has been described earlier, the vast majority of psychotropic medications are not abused or abusable. However, stimulants, sedative/ hypnotics, benzodiazepines and anticholinergics are medications that some patients may obtain under false pretenses or use in inappropriate amounts. Although many people equate the fraudulent obtaining of prescriptions with personal drug abuse, this view is not always correct – there are exceptions. While the vast majority of patients seeking medication illegally are, in fact, abusing medications themselves, other reasons include:

- obtaining medication for sale on the street
- using the medications to moderate the effect of other recreational or prescribed drugs (for example, using benzodiazepines to "come down" from abuse of stimulants, or using anticholinergics to increase the "high" of narcotics)
- obtaining medications for others who may be abusing.

Table 22.2 Methods of obtaining medication fraudulently

- Altering a written prescription, particularly the number of pills dispensed
- Falsely posing, by telephone, as a current patient in need of a refill to off-hours covering practitioners
- Theft of blank prescriptions
- Direct theft of medication
- Falsely presenting symptoms that could be treated with abusable medications
- Requesting excessive amounts of medication
- Trading medications with others

One might assume that the primary method of obtaining medication fraudulently is through altered, fake or illegally copied prescriptions. This certainly does occur, and given that 4.55 billion prescriptions were filled in the United States in 2020,[5] when even a small percentage of prescriptions are fraudulent, it constitutes a large number. There are, however, multiple other ways that medications including psychotropics are fraudulently obtained. The most common methods of prescription fraud and abuse are shown in Table 22.2.

By following a few simple techniques and practices, clinicians can minimize the majority of these causes of fraudulent use of prescription medications. Any prescriber, however, no matter how diligent, will occasionally find that he or she has been fraudulently utilized.

Practitioner protections against abuse of prescription medications

To avoid prescription alteration

When stocking office supplies, alter-proof prescription pads should be ordered. While these are slightly more expensive than plain paper prescriptions, these alter-proof prescriptions will blur or smudge if there is an attempt to erase or rewrite the name of the medication or the number of pills prescribed. Any alteration will usually be obvious to the pharmacist, who will often call the practitioner prior to dispensing. When writing the prescription, the clinician should always clearly write the number of pills in *words* rather than in *numbers*. It is very difficult to alter the wording "dispense one hundred" whereas it is relatively easy to add a zero to "10" to make "100." It is also best to give a patient a prescription without cross-outs or alterations in the writing. If a mistake is made in writing a prescription, write a new prescription. If there is a large blank space on the prescription under the handwriting, draw a diagonal line to fill the space. Although it is not advisable, if prescriptions for a controlled substance must be left for pick-up, leave them in a sealed envelope with the patient's initials (not the full name) on the outside.

To make photocopying prescriptions more difficult, some medical practitioners use prescription pads that contain security measures similar to those used on bank checks, and in some cases, these are mandated by law. Some states help control stolen prescriptions by requiring special "prescriptions in triplicate" for certain drug classes. Blank triplicates are only available from the regulating agency and are individually numbered. The practitioner retains a copy, the second and third copies are given to the patient to give to the pharmacist. The State of California has replaced triplicate forms with a newer format that is impossible to photocopy or fax: the background is printed with repetitions of the word *void* in a color that shows up as black on a photocopy.

When forgery is suspected, pharmacists will call the practitioner (see below) to verify the authenticity of the prescription.

Off-hours coverage issues

Most practitioners assume that the largest risk for medication abuse is altering prescriptions. While it does occur, an even more frequently practiced means of fraudulently obtaining medications occurs when somebody poses as an active patient of a clinician who is out of town or off-call. The drug-seeker will telephone the covering prescriber, requesting a renewal prescription for an abusable medication. Frequently stated reasons are that he or she has unexpectedly "run out," has had to cancel an appointment "just before" the clinician's absence or has "lost" a prescription. If the off-hours call is for an abusable medication, this often presents a dilemma for the covering clinician. If the patient requests a large amount of medication, it is usually an ominous sign. The more intelligent abuser will call for smaller amounts of medications from a number of different clinicians covering the practices of multiple off-call providers. There are medication-abusing individuals who regularly and repeatedly spend weekends and holidays phoning numerous mental health practitioners and fraudulently requesting "reasonable" amounts of controlled substance medications.

Remedying this situation requires the agreement of those practitioners who work together providing off-hours coverage. A ground rule for the group is that *any patient who calls off-hours for abusable medications must provide the covering prescriber with the telephone number of a pharmacy at which the regular prescriber has written a prescription that can be verified.* When the off-hours prescriber calls the pharmacy, it is an easy matter to verify if and when this patient has received previous prescriptions written by the clinician of record and when the most recent prescription was filled. If there is no record of this patient having received previous prescriptions, no medication is authorized. If the patient cannot give a pharmacy telephone number where previous prescriptions can be verified, the off-hours clinician simply refuses to prescribe any medication.

It is not uncommon for the abuser to offer a variety of excuses, such as: "I must have used a different pharmacy" or "the pharmacy I use is closed" or "I'm traveling and I need to have it filled here." In general, the off-hours clinician should ignore these excuses and simply refuse to provide medication until the primary clinician returns. On rare occasions, the covering clinician may be convinced to provide some amount of medication. If so, only enough pills should be provided to get the patient through until the regular clinician returns. Prescriptions for large amounts of abusable medications should not be written off-hours, regardless of the reasons presented. Drug-seekers can often protest strongly when refused medication, in an effort to badger the clinician. When routinely enforced, these procedures give the abuser the message that this prescriber is not vulnerable to prescription fraud. These procedures also have the benefit of reinforcing to the legitimate patient that waiting until the last minute to refill medications may be problematic.

Another common ploy of abusers is to request refills for several medications, one or more of which are non-abusable and one that may be abusable. If the clinician renews all the medications, the individual will then pick up only the abusable medication, feigning to the pharmacy that he or she lacks the money to pay for all the medications.

Therefore, the above-outlined guidelines should apply even if multiple medications are requested.

Since the vast number of psychotropic medications, particularly antidepressants, antipsychotics and mood stabilizers, are generally not abused or abusable, a clinician covering for an off-duty provider can generally prescribe refills of these medications comfortably with at least enough medication until the return of the regular prescriber. Likewise, the patient will need to provide a phone number of the "regular" pharmacy so that the on-call provider can confirm that the person is an active patient and that the prescription from the regular provider is ongoing. If the caller cannot provide this information, it is an ominous sign and likely represents fraud or abuse.

Theft of prescriptions

Simple preventative measures can easily address the issue of stolen blank prescriptions. Careful, locked storage of blank prescriptions is crucial. The clinician must take care not to leave prescription pads or blank prescriptions in easily accessible places. Common locations that are vulnerable to theft include:

- on a desk that may be available to the patient when the clinician leaves the room
- in an unlocked drawer
- in an unlocked car
- at home, in the practitioner's residence.

Despite reasonable precautions, it is still possible that prescriptions may be accidentally lost or stolen. Unfortunately, there is relatively little recourse if this occurs, and missing prescriptions may fall into the hands of an abuser. When fraudulently filled out and presented for filling, a pharmacist is often unlikely to recognize the problem.

The new patient who requests large amounts of abusable medicines

The clinician may be presented with a new patient requesting a large amount of an abusable medication. A typical scenario involves the patient who has recently relocated or is changing clinicians and now needs a "usual" dose of a benzodiazepine or stimulant. Some patients may ask specifically and exclusively for one particular abusable medication, refusing other non-abusable preparations. While some of these individuals are abusers, a certain number of them are legitimately seeking continuity of care. After a diagnostic evaluation, and if the request appears justified, the clinician may choose to prescribe a small amount of a controlled medication initially. It is incumbent upon the clinician at this first visit to obtain a release of information from the patient for the previously prescribing clinician. *The previous treater should be contacted before the next patient visit.* The previous prescriber can give relevant information – verifying the patient's legitimate medication profile and conscientious use of medications – or, on occasion, identifying the patient as an abuser. If the patient cannot provide the name of a previous clinician or verifiable treatment information, the clinician should be quite cautious in prescribing abusable medications, and may refuse to do so at all. Regardless of the new patient's request, as with any treatment plan, it is not reasonable to prescribe large amounts of abusable medication with many refills, or to provide a long-term prescription without regular follow-up appointments to assess the patient's response and continued need.

The development of abuse

Some patients who begin using habit-forming medication during appropriate prescription may gradually slip into abuse. When this begins to occur, behaviors will emerge that suggest to the clinician that this problematic situation is developing. Common tip-offs include:

1   *Frequent early requests for renewal* of medication. This practice may initially occur with refill requests a few days early, but can worsen to the stage where requests come weeks or months early. The patient will usually have a rationale for needing an early renewal, such as the pills having been destroyed, lost or damaged.
2   *Frequently missed appointments* with telephone contact (often after hours) requesting medication refills. Patients who are abusing medication may try to avoid face-to-face contact with their regular provider.
3   *Repeated requests for dose increases*, particularly beyond a safe dosage range.
4   *Requests for multiple abusable medications*, such as a tranquilizer plus a hypnotic, or a tranquilizer to counteract the effects of a stimulant.

If abuse is suspected

When the clinician begins to suspect abuse, direct and prompt action is necessary. The initial clinical response is not always to refuse to prescribe or refill prescriptions. *The first step is the identification of the problem and the setting of firm limits with the patient.* These may include clear timeframes at which renewals will be authorized, and parameters as to when a lost or missing prescription will be replaced. Some patients will accept these limits and guidelines without protest; others may become overtly angry, act insulted or threaten to change providers.

While some clinicians will refuse, under any circumstances, to rewrite lost prescriptions for abusable medications, it is not unreasonable to rewrite a lost prescription for an abusable medication on one occasion to an otherwise stable patient. Further requests for replacement prescriptions, however, should be refused. This policy should be given in written form, together with other office policies, usually at the initial patient contact.

If a patient requests and/or insists on increasing doses of abusable medications, the clinician needs to clearly outline the parameters of the treatment dosage. For example, a scenario can occur when an anxious patient repeatedly complains of feeling more anxious unless he or she takes a larger benzodiazepine dose. If the patient's dose reaches the maximum level at which the clinician is comfortable, other non-abusable medications with an anti-anxiety effect (an SSRI, gabapentin, valerian root or buspirone) can be added or substituted. The clinician should explore possible precipitants to the increased anxiety and offer counseling directly or through the psychotherapist working with the patient. If these remedies are ineffective, sometimes the clinician's best response is to indicate that the patient may, unfortunately, continue to be mildly anxious at times, and that further escalation of doses is not advised or permitted. Fortunately, the latter situation is not typical of the majority of anxiety disorder patients, who will use medications responsibly. It is generally the anxiety disorder patient with a history of substance abuse who misuses benzodiazepines.

The pharmacist as ally

The pharmacist can be of great assistance in both identifying and dealing with patients who abuse medications. It is not uncommon for a pharmacist to call the prescriber to verify the accuracy of a prescription for a large number of habit-forming pills. This is a reasonable precaution that the prescriber should welcome and reinforce. Likewise, the pharmacist may question any apparently altered or suspiciously written prescription. The pharmacist is also in the best position to recognize a patient using multiple prescribers for the same medication, or who is prescribed multiple habit-forming medications. The call from the pharmacist noting this concern may be the first indication to prescribers that they are prescribing psychotropic medications while other providers are prescribing further psychotropics, pain medication or other habit-forming medications. A pharmacist can also alert the clinician to requests for early refills or other suspicious behavior. The clinician can then contact the appropriate state regulatory agency for the list of prescriptions for habituating medicines that have been filled for this patient.

What to do when abuse occurs

When abuse occurs, the clinician should observe the following guidelines.

With the patient

- Educate the patient about the dangers of medication overuse and possible consequences.
- Set clear limits of dosage to be prescribed and frequency of any refills.
- Once possible abuse is identified, do not provide any further replacement prescriptions regardless of the reason. If a prescription is "lost," "stolen" or otherwise missing, the patient will have to go without medication until the next regularly scheduled renewal. It becomes the patient's responsibility to safeguard medications.
- If, despite education and clear limits, further excessive medication requests or abuse continues, stop prescribing that medication.
- If you have a release of information and intend to contact other providers about the abuse problem, remind the patient of this. If the patient "revokes" this release, use clinical judgment as to whether this revocation can be overridden. In general, mild to moderate drug over usage without emergency health or safety concerns does not justify overriding this revocation to release information. If there is an emergency or safety risk present with acute danger to the patient or other individuals, and you choose to override the lack of consent to release information, document the decisions and reasoning clearly. In the UK, the requirement for reporting suspected drug abuse is different from that in the United States (see the last section of this chapter).

- Decide if you are comfortable continuing to see the medication-abusing patient for any other services besides psychotropic prescription. If so, outline the parameters of this continued treatment.
- If you are not comfortable continuing any contact, send the patient a brief written letter documenting the abusive behavior and stating that, despite your efforts to educate the patient about the dangers, medication overuse has continued. State the dates and facts of over usage and/or renewals. Document the decision to terminate any treatment relationship and specify a date when this will occur.
- If, at the time of termination, the patient is at risk for serious withdrawal phenomena from the medication prescribed, offer to coordinate drug rehabilitation treatment or admission.

With the pharmacy

- You may receive and welcome information provided by the pharmacist about abuse of medications by a patient or information about prescriptions from other providers. While you certainly will want to cooperate with any questions about a specific, perhaps fraudulent prescription, the information you may divulge to the pharmacist without a release of information is limited (see below).
- A signed written release of information from the patient to speak with the pharmacist is unusual. The fact that you wrote a prescription for a patient does not constitute a release. When contacted by a pharmacist, the only information you may provide is your intent to have your specific prescription or future prescriptions filled for this patient or not. If the pharmacist asks about a questionable prescription, you can, and should, also verify if you wrote a particular prescription.
- Although you may be tempted to do so, you are not permitted to discuss your knowledge of drug abuse, improper usage of medications, diagnoses, clinical symptoms, behavioral or legal history with the pharmacist without a release of information.

With other prescribers

- Preferably, the patient's release of information will have been obtained at the beginning of treatment so that contact with other treaters/prescribers is authorized. If not, this release of information must be obtained from the patient in order to contact other medical or mental health providers. If the patient is willing to permit it, you may then contact other healthcare providers about medication overuse. If the patient is unwilling to consent, and no emergency situation exists, you may not violate confidentiality.
- If you are contacting other providers and have written consent, talk directly with any other prescribers of medication. Do not leave voicemail messages, or speak through intermediaries or other staff members.
- If joint decisions are made regarding further prescriptive action, discuss and document the plan and who will notify the patient of the plan.
- One particularly effective strategy is to have the patient call other providers in your presence, from your office, informing the other providers of the abuse problem with a request that these providers stop prescribing abusable medications.

Table 22.3 Reporting drug misuse in the UK

England
malcolm.roxburgh@nta-nhs.org.uk
Telephone: (020) 7972 1964

Scotland
Telephone: (0131) 275 6348

Northern Ireland
Dr. Ian McMaster
Ian.mcmaster@dhsspsni.gov.uk
Castle Buildings
Belfast BT4 3FQ
Telephone: (028) 9052 2421

Source: Adapted from *British National Formulary* (2020), 80th edn., BNF Publications.

With the authorities

In the United States:

- contacting the police or other law-enforcement authorities is only appropriate for clear criminal behavior such as theft of blank prescriptions, medication supplies or other personal items
- simple medication abuse is not justification for a police report.

In the UK:

- practitioners are expected to report cases of drug misuse on a standard form to their regional or national drug misuse center. All types of problem drug misuse, including opioid, benzodiazepine and CNS stimulant abuse, should be reported via the regional telephone numbers listed in Table 22.3

References

1 American Psychiatric Association (2013) *Diagnostic and Statistical Manual of Mental Disorders*, 5th edn., American Psychiatric Association, pp. 192–204.
2 Ibid.
3 Ibid.
4 Tondo L and Baldessarini RJ (2002) Suicide: an overview. In *Psychiatry Clinical Management*, Vol. 3, Medical Education Collaborative.
5 Total number of retail prescriptions filled annually in the U.S. 2013–2025, available at: www.statista.com/statistics/261303/total-number-of-retail-prescriptions-filled-annually-in-the-us/

23 "Difficult" medication patients and how to treat them

• Overriding principles of managing difficult patients	400
• The patient who abuses the telephone	403
• The overly anxious patient	404
• The patient preoccupied with side effects and negative reactions	405
• The minimal contact patient	407
• The non-adherent patient	408
• The patient who needs to be in charge	410
• The information overload patient	412
• The "naturalist"	413
• The borderline patient	414
• Consultation and disengagement	419
• The patient is not always the problem	420
• Notes and references	420

If the principles in this book are followed, the majority of patients for whom clinicians prescribe psychotropic medications will be easily managed and successfully treated. There are, however, some patients who present special problems for a clinician in the medication prescriptive process. Often, the difficulty in treatment is a reflection of the patient's personality. When negative personality traits are strong, these may color the entire interaction with the prescriber. Clinicians may, at times, find themselves frustrated and wishing to avoid treating such patients. While these traits are annoying, knowledgeable clinicians can work within the limits that they present. This chapter focuses on the most common "difficult patients" (see Table 23.1), and makes recommendations for clinical management.

Overriding principles of managing difficult patients

Some general principles that are useful in dealing with all "difficult" patients are listed in Table 23.2.

With time, each clinician develops his or her own personal style of dealing with patients. Special patients, however, may need a modification of the prescriber's style in order to achieve successful treatment. While it may take some amount of work and commitment on the part of the clinician, such minor modifications of interaction and approach will pay off with increased adherence and fewer points of friction.

Table 23.1 Some "difficult" medication patients

- The patient who abuses the telephone
- The overly anxious patient
- The patient preoccupied with side effects
- The minimal contact patient
- The non-adherent patient
- The patient who needs to be in charge
- The information overload patient
- The "naturalist"
- The borderline patient

Table 23.2 Principles of treating "difficult" medication patients

---

- Be prepared to modify your usual interactional style. To be successful with problem patients, you may need to take a slightly different approach.
- You do not have to change a patient's personality to work with him/her; you need only prescribe in a safe and effective manner. It is unlikely that your interventions will change underlying, fundamental personality traits.
- If there is friction with a patient, carefully choose the issues on which you must stand firm, and those on which you can be flexible.
- Distinguish issues of safety and necessity from issues of personal style – yours and the those of the patient.
- When possible, find a way to give the patient acknowledgement and a measure of respect for their "difficult" behavior (see below).
- When necessary, identify a patient's pattern of behavior gently, without criticism, and *after* acknowledging the "value" of their style.
- Keep your focus narrowed to the elements of the prescriptive process itself, and avoid the tendency to generalize critique and feedback.
- For particularly resistant patients, you do not need their agreement that your rules for treatment are correct. During prescriptive interactions, you need only gently but firmly insist on adherence with your guidelines and expectations.
- Consider enlarging "the team" treating the patient.
- Engage the patient in trying to fix the "problem."
- Limit the number of "difficult" patients you treat.

Some clinicians are reluctant to change their style, feeling that they are "conceding" to the patient's personality. This is not true. As long as safety and clinical necessity are not compromised, the ability to modify style is a sign of the experienced and wise clinician.

At times, friction or irritation between clinician and patient may rise to the point that almost all interactions appear to be negative. Here, clinicians should realistically acknowledge to themselves that a particular patient is frustrating them, making them angry and/or leaving them feeling unable to help them as they would like. It is important for clinicians to distinguish those areas of interaction that must be insisted upon from those matters where they can accede to a patient's wishes. *Clinicians should choose their battles carefully. It is important to separate issues of clinical safety and necessity from issues of interactional style.*

If some small issues of style or "the usual way of doing things" are not critical and can be changed, it is much easier to insist on those points of safety and good clinical care on which there is no compromise. Clinicians who refuse to budge on even small issues may get grudging adherence temporarily, but this usually results in a major power struggle, or in the patient looking for care elsewhere.

Be positive where possible

One particularly useful technique in dealing with problem medication patients is to understand and verbally recognize those parts of the patient's personality style that, even though exaggerated, may provide positive benefit for the patient. To help bring these issues to light, clinicians can ask themselves:

- What does this style accomplish for the patient?
- Are there elements of how this patient is relating to me that can be interpreted as elements of positive, rational or helpful behavior?

Once understood, it becomes possible for the clinician to approach the patient with verbal interactions that are interpreted positively by the patient as being both understanding and respectful. Many of these patients have had chronically abrasive, troublesome and unsuccessful relationships with healthcare providers, and a clinician's display of understanding can diminish conflict and start the process of alliance with the patient that may have been difficult to achieve in the past. For example:

- a suspicious patient can be labeled as "careful"
- a patient who swamps the clinician with data and articles is "someone who wishes to be informed"
- a patient who avoids appointments is "busy and trying to be efficient"
- a patient who overutilizes medication is someone who "wants to feel good – as most of us do."

The team approach to problem patients

Difficult patients, even when skillfully managed by a primary clinician, often need the talents of multiple types of care providers. Coordinated assistance from several individuals or clinics not only provides multifaceted support and help, but also dilutes the difficult, sometimes abrasive, effects of these patients over several providers. If they are not already part of the patient's care, the clinician should consider using other medical specialists, a mental health counselor, a psychopharmacology provider, a social worker, a visiting nurse, a dietitian or an occupational/vocational specialist. Conversely, but also true, these patients often do not do well seeing a different primary care provider with every visit (even though the providers themselves may see this as a benefit since each provider does not see the patient often). Trust needs to be built with one primary provider who coordinates care. If the patient has changing or multiple primary medical care providers, it is worthwhile to solidify and coordinate the primary medical care with one central provider who, when needed, will use others with specific expertise as noted above.

The "team" should always include the patient when deciding how to manage problem behaviors.

Box 23.1 Talking to patients

Particularly if progress is minimal and tensions are high, the clinician should not hesitate to engage the patient with interventions such as:

- *"What do you think is wrong?"*
- *"What do you think would help?"*
- *"Here is the problem that I observe [describe the behaviors]; help me figure out a way that makes this situation better for you and provides the help you need, but also works for me (and my staff)."*
- *"I am willing to adjust how I work with you [specify what you are doing or are willing to do]. In what ways can you change to make our working together go more smoothly?"*

Box 23.2 Primary care

If the problem patient is a person with multiple somatic complaints whose diagnosis remains elusive and/or does not improve with standard therapies, consider a mental health etiology. Many patients with large numbers of vague, changing somatic symptoms have an underlying mood or anxiety disorder. Begin inquiring into the patient's mood state with two useful screening questions:

1 During the past month, have you often been feeling down, depressed or hopeless?
2 During the past month, have you often been bothered by little interest or pleasure in doing things?

Consider referral to, or collaboration with, a mental health specialist. Such patients often will not take a mental health referral smoothly and will show resistance, anger or a feeling of being misunderstood. Use the techniques outlined in Chapter 6 for making a mental health referral.

The patient who abuses the telephone

Abuse of the telephone is covered in Chapter 28, and will be reviewed only briefly here. Of critical importance is understanding the reason that the patient is abusing the phone. The clinician's approach will vary depending on the cause for phone overutilization. Once a clear pattern of overuse is seen (this is often signaled by the clinician's frustration at receiving yet *another* phone call from this particular patient), the clinician should speak directly to the patient about the issue. Identify the pattern rather than waiting for patients to see "the error of their ways" – patients may not view their behavior in the way that the clinician does. Without direct action, the patient may continue to overutilize the clinician's time, increasing the clinician's frustration and perhaps leading to a future angry, explosive or inappropriate interaction. The following guidelines should be observed:

- If the patient is calling about an issue that is not an emergency, identify this fact and that the matter can wait until the next scheduled visit.
- Define what are appropriate issues for phone consultation, and what can be postponed until the next face-to-face consultation.
- If necessary, set specific regular times for calls, and the length of time that you can spend on the telephone.
- If repeated inappropriate telephone calls continue, label the call as inappropriate and minimize the length of the call.
- If the patient continues to call inappropriately, it is reasonable to interrupt at the beginning of the call, and insist that the patient bring the subject matter to the next session, without continuing the conversation.

Specific "Talking to patients" interactions for telephone abusing patients are detailed in Chapter 28.

The overly anxious patient

Patients who have an anxiety-prone personality can show marked concern about the use of medication as one aspect of their treatment. The very notion that a clinician is recommending medication may make them more anxious. They may have multiple questions about suggested prescriptions. These persons are also anxious about many other issues in their life – job, children, parenting, finances, risk of an accident, tragedy or death. They often catastrophize and assume the worst outcome of a situation, even if its likelihood is rare. In applying this way of thinking to the use of medication, they expect a problematic, uncomfortable or disastrous response to medications.

Several strategies are useful in dealing with overly anxious patients. Whenever possible, medication should be *started only when such patients are ready*. Anxious patients may need to ponder the clinician's recommendation before they are willing to begin taking medication. Faced with mild to moderate symptoms, it may be totally appropriate to allow a patient to digest and consider the suggestion for medication before the prescription is actually written or filled. In the long run, even if the clinician would prefer that the medication be started sooner, it is often preferable to wait for a patient to become ready (albeit still hesitantly), than to insist on beginning a medication with an overly anxious patient who is not ready to accept the recommendation. If the patient is fundamentally not prepared to begin medication and the clinician insists, the person will usually find a reason for never starting or quickly stopping the medication. Initially, when beginning medication, *more frequent appointments* with these patients may provide the opportunity to ask questions and receive reassurance. When a change in medication is contemplated, it is often useful to *identify the need for this change as far in advance as possible* to give the patient time to adjust. It may take a very anxious person several visits to be ready to change medication or even change doses.

Box 23.3 Talking to patients

As a way of recognizing a patient for his or her anxiety, it can be useful to say: *"I can see that you are a person who wants to be very, very sure about the safety and effectiveness of anything you would take. This is a useful way of thinking, and I share your wish to ensure that any medicines you use are taken safely without serious adverse effects. Let's work together to make sure this happens."*

Even when clinicians feel they have provided sufficient education and reassurance to anxious patients, those with an over anxious personality style often require repeated reassurances. Such a patient may arrive at the next visit asking virtually the same questions that the clinician has previously answered. The person will again ask for reassurance that the medication is necessary, safe and in the appropriate dose. While it can be tedious, particularly if repeated multiple times, this behavior is intrinsic to the patient's style. It cannot be ignored, or the patient will likely stop medication. Even if the clinician identifies this behavior pattern and describes it to the patient, the underlying personality style will seldom disappear.

For the exceptionally anxious patient who continues to call frequently between appointments for education, reassurance and questions about the medication, a useful strategy is to ask the patient to call on a regularly structured schedule. By using a brief scheduled contact, the clinician decreases the patient's anxiety, keeps the patient on medication and avoids frequent annoying off-hours calls for reassurance. For example, the clinician could tell the patient to call every Thursday between 1 p.m. and 2 p.m. with any accumulated questions they have, but to hold routine questions at other times. Gradually, as the patient becomes more comfortable, the interval between telephone check-ins can be increased or the telephone calls perhaps discontinued.

The patient preoccupied with side effects and negative reactions

Patients with this behavior pattern will often have many of the same traits as the overly anxious personality style described above. Many of the principles of medication management of these two types of person will also overlap. Patients solely preoccupied with negative side effects, however, are not, in general, overly anxious about other areas of their life. They may be particularly preoccupied with the effects of psychotropics on their mind or body. It should not be assumed that patients who ask many questions prior to taking medication will automatically become problem patients preoccupied with side effects. Some patients, once they have received answers to their initial questions and the necessary reassurances, will proceed comfortably with taking medication. Once medicated, they have few questions and do not develop the level of concern associated with the side-effect preoccupied patient. If, however, over several appointments it becomes clear that the patient has a long list of possible concerns about medication, and at each appointment presents the clinician with a long list of possible "side effects" that they attribute to this psychotropic, it may be necessary to take management steps.

First, it is important to listen carefully and *differentiate true or possible side effects from effects that are not likely to be related to the medication.* Early in the prescriptive process, this level of active listening reassures the patient that the clinician, too, will be diligent in looking for negative effects of the medication, and that the patient has an active partner in evaluating any discomfort experienced. It is seldom helpful to simply dismiss all the patient's concerns as "unrealistic" or "overreaction." The clinician should be clear and direct with such a patient as to which effects may, in fact, be side effects and which are probably unrelated.

It is not uncommon for these patients to bring a printed list of potential side effects that they have taken from a book or the Internet, or have heard from relatives or friends, without any sense of how likely it is that such effects will occur. When possible, in discussing the likelihood of possible side effects, actual percentages of incidence taken from source materials should be used (e.g., "This reaction does occur, but has been reported in 0.1 percent of people taking this drug. This means that for every 1000 patients, 999 will never have this problem.")

Box 23.4 Talking to patients

One way of approaching a patient like this would be to say: *"Of the list you bring, these are potential side effects ... [specify]. These are not likely side effects of this medication ... [specify]. We will have ample warning if and when they are going to occur. Together we will be watching for these problems and certainly will consider stopping the medication if there any signs or symptoms that are dangerous. I know you are a very careful person; so am I. I doubt very much that these rare possibilities are going to be problems for you. If it were me, knowing what I know about the medication, and having the symptoms that you have, I would take the medication. I would not let these concerns prevent me from trying a medication that could be very helpful."*

Early in treatment, more frequent appointments with such patients will allay fears and deal with their concerns. Gradually, as they become more comfortable with the effects of the medication, intervals between appointments can be increased. It is also useful to have patients chart the occurrence and frequency of any negative effects that they perceive. Have the patient include day, date, time and severity This provides them with a sense of being actively involved in their own medication management. Such a chart or list additionally gives the clinician a rapid way to see if a particular side effect occurs frequently, or has any pattern of occurrence.

Patients who have continually persistent and changing complaints about their medication can also be approached in a manner similar to the process of dealing with the hypochondriacal patient. In this model, the clinician has regularly spaced appointments with the patient while using simple benign interventions without major changes in the medication regimen. This permits the patient to continue the medication, maintain a relationship with the clinician and yet perceive that some "active" intervention is occurring. Small changes in timing or dosage, or the use of benign over-the-counter remedies, can be a temporizing measure. An occasional laboratory measurement to test for organ safety can also be reassuring to the patient. While these small changes or tests are performed, the central medication regime is neither discontinued, nor changed in a major way. The patient is allowed a longer time to identify the beneficial therapeutic effects of the psychotropic and to forge an increasingly strong alliance with the clinician.

When a patient has been identified in the clinician's mind as a "complainer," a "whiner" or a "worry wart" about negative medication effects, it may unfortunately be assumed that any new complaint about the medication is automatically a result of the patient's hypersensitive style. Even the most "side-effect preoccupied" patient may, at times, have genuine unwanted effects from the medications that are significant or troublesome. While it can be time-consuming, each claim of a new side effect must be evaluated on its own merit. At times, it may be necessary and very appropriate to change medications for these patients because of a problematic side effect.

The minimal contact patient

Patients with this style do not see the value of, or need for, follow-up medication appointments. Such patients will feel and, at times, verbalize: "You have seen me. I'm doing fine. I don't see why my prescription just can't be renewed without having to see you again." Although the underlying, driving force is their personality style, such patients will often cloak their resistance in the need to spend long hours at work, having multiple personal commitments, extensive travel or a changing schedule, any of which will not permit making and keeping appointments. Even when scheduled, such patients may cancel a follow-up appointment and "forget" to reschedule it. When their prescription is nearly exhausted, they will often call the pharmacy for a refill and avoid talking to the clinician directly. If the clinician is willing to continue to renew prescriptions by telephone, the patient is likely to continue this pattern of behavior indefinitely.

Dealing with the minimal contact patient involves recognition of this pattern and, at times, insistence on appropriate follow up. As outlined in the earlier chapters of this book, the clinician must see a patient face-to-face periodically for safe, effective prescribing practice. Once stabilized, the patient should be seen at a minimum of every 3 months for at least the first year. In times of area-wide or worldwide illness requiring quarantine, the practitioner may modify this schedule or use telemedicine contacts. While slightly less beneficial than in-person meetings, telemedicine appointments can in most situations provide the clinician with the observation that they need for safe practice. It is totally appropriate for clinicians to require that they become acquainted with patients for whom they are prescribing, and these visits accomplish this task in addition to managing the prescription. When the minimal contact pattern is first discovered (often when the pharmacy calls for a refill at the request of a patient who has not made or kept follow-up appointments), the prescription should be filled for a small number of pills and the pharmacy is requested to have the patient contact the clinician prior to further refills. If the patient continues to request telephone refills, the clinician should deny the requests and require a face-to-face visit. Clinicians should not allow an inappropriate interval between visits if they feel a face-to-face appointment is necessary for safe management.

For the patient who consistently delays or fails to keep face-to-face appointments, the pattern should be identified, and the parameters of safe care laid out. Many minimal contact patients will use off-hours coverage providers to avoid making or keeping appointments with the primary clinician. This pattern, if involving controlled substances, can also be part of patient medication abuse. When the medication prescribed is not a controlled substance, it is more likely that the patient does not like to make or keep regular appointments. See Chapter 22 on the misuse of medication for further information on dealing with this situation.

 Box 23.5 Talking to patients

"I know it may be inconvenient for you to come to the office for a visit. You have a very busy schedule and the last thing you need is another appointment. It is, however, essential for me to see you in person to prescribe safely and responsibly. I need to get to know you, assess your condition, order appropriate lab tests and monitor the safety of your prescription. Here is the frequency with which I can work with you..."

For appointment-resistant patients who are on long-term maintenance medication, it is possible to stretch out the intervals between their face-to-face visits to a frequency of every 4–6 months. Such longer intervals should only be permitted if:

- the clinician knows the patient, his or her clinical history, the diagnosis and any complicating medical conditions
- the patient is on a stable, uncomplicated regimen of medication
- the patient does not have a rapidly changing or brittle medical condition
- the patient does not have a rapidly changing or brittle psychological condition
- the patient is responsible in taking medications
- the patient does not abuse alcohol or drugs.

The non-adherent patient

There are multiple ways in which a patient can be non-adherent, and multiple reasons why this occurs. Some patients do not follow through with appointments or do not take their medications on schedule. Others do not follow through with requested serum blood levels, or run out of medications and fall into a symptomatic crisis. Several patient types described elsewhere in this book, such as the substance abusing patient, the minimal contact patient and the confused patient, include non-adherence as part of the clinical picture.

Patients who are not adherent but do not fall into the above-mentioned categories often present to the clinician not for themselves, but because others have insisted upon treatment. These patients may be frankly involuntary, or simply not personally motivated. Some non-adherent patients feel they have no reason to improve and are reluctant to follow a medication regimen. It is these resistant individuals who do not fall into other categories that are discussed in this section.

Principles that cover the management of non-adherent patients include the following:

1   *Distinguish less than ideal treatment from unsafe treatment.* Although some patients may participate only partially in a medication regime, it does not automatically mean that they have markedly compromised their safety or health.

2 *Symptoms or discomfort may not constitute an unsafe situation.* Patients who stop medication prematurely or take medication irregularly may develop symptoms of the underlying illness for which they are being treated, or they may develop a discontinuation syndrome. When symptoms emerge, patients may be a bother to their family, friends, neighbors or co-workers. While this may be inconvenient and problematic for others, it does not necessarily constitute an unsafe situation or one in which the clinician must intervene, beyond encouragement, elucidation of the reasons for the behavior and continued recommendations for more consistency.

Particularly when a patient is being treated at someone else's insistence, the clinician should make efforts to uncover reasons for taking a medication that would benefit the patient, regardless of the reasons why the family, the work supervisor, the courts or other agencies have brought the patient to treatment. It is worthwhile trying to discover aspects of the patient's life that could be benefited by medication, even if such benefit is not the prime motivation for other people, or the primary reason the patient is being seen. For example, a person may be court-ordered to treatment for psychosis, but be motivated to take medication because it allows him/her to keep a job that makes money for the car he or she wants to buy. A patient may come seeking medication for depression at the insistence of his spouse, but continue to take it because when not depressed, his sexual performance is better. A bipolar adolescent may not be motivated to take medication for her parents or teachers, but will do so because when medicated she does not "say weird things" that drive her friends away.

3 *Some treatment is often better than no treatment.* Some non-adherent patients fail to comply in ways that result in less than optimum treatment. While it is clear to many people around them that the ultimate outcome would likely be better if they were more adherent, patients still refuse to participate fully with medication recommendations, even despite clinician encouragement. Rather than withdraw from prescribing or becoming angry with such patients, the treater should decide if some measure of adherence is better than none at all – which it often is. This does not mean that the treater would support non-adherence or would not be diligent in attempts to improve patient adherence; it simply means that medication treatment need not be all or nothing.

4 *Some non-adherent patients will behave in ways that result in arrest, incarceration or other sanctions.* Even if such behaviors are a direct result of non-adherence with medication, it may ultimately be in such a patient's best interest to suffer the discomfort of incarceration or punishment in order to facilitate future adherence.

Parents dealing with adolescents and young adults who are disobedient, truant or are involved in frankly illegal activities are often reluctant to involve the police or jail. Even when these behaviors are the result of a mental illness that could be treated with medication, the patient does not comply with medication recommendations and prescription. The clinician must often counsel the family that the use of the appropriate authorities may not only be necessary, but also advisable, to reinforce negatively the problematic behavior, including non-adherence.

5 *Non-response does not necessarily equate to non-adherence.* Having prescribed many medications to a patient with minimal or no success, some clinicians assume that because the patient has not responded, he or she must not be following the clinician's advice. While a majority of patients will respond, at least partially, to

an aggressive psychopharmacological regimen targeted to an accurate diagnosis, some patients simply do not. Despite multiple medication trials, they are minimally better. This does not indicate that they are not complying with the prescriber's recommendations. Unfortunately, some mental health symptoms remain stubbornly non-responsive despite adequate and full patient adherence.

6   *Written documentation of the patient's non-adherence is important.* The practitioner should record that non-adherence is occurring and the evidence (unfilled prescriptions, pharmacy records, family reports, etc.) to support this conclusion. If this has been ongoing, the practitioner should document the efforts to encourage adherence including communication of potential risks/negative effects. Fortunately, it is rare that a person who commits a crime, has an accident or has some other negative outcome, attempts to blame the practitioner or claim that these events occurred in spite of his or her "adherence" to medication doses and frequency. The written record can be the most important factor supporting the practitioner's interactions with this patient.

The patient who needs to be in charge

Many executives, supervisors, leaders in business or persons having a strong need for control may come to the prescriptive interview with difficulty because it signifies giving control or power to another person. They maintain a lifestyle of control – of themselves and of others. They want, and need, to be in charge, and feel unsettled when someone else is making decisions about them, and for them. Once begun on medication, these patients will often return in a follow-up session having altered the timing, dose or start date of the medication. It will rapidly become clear to the clinician that such a patient needs to "run the show."

When such a pattern of control and subsequent unilateral decision-making becomes apparent to the clinician, several behavioral responses are useful.

First, the clinician should take his or her ego out of the prescriptive process. The clinician need not always make all the decisions about the prescription but can allow the patient to be in charge, at least partially, of some portion of the medication process. With such a patient, it is particularly important that a rigid, set medication regimen is avoided. If the clinician requires a set schedule of medication, and insists upon it with such an individual, a power struggle will be inevitable. Because these patients need to be in charge and make decisions, they cannot, and will not, relinquish control totally to another person. While clinicians cannot abdicate responsibility for medication decisions and schedule, they can allow the patient some choices while retaining the larger decision-making position.

Once areas of limited choice within which the patient can make decisions have been identified, the clinician can outline broad limits of safe prescription while allowing the patient a limited choice that will permit him or her to feel more in control. There may be a dosage range within which the clinician will allow flexibility. The patient may be in charge of how many "as needed" (or "PRN") doses they need to take, within certain limits. The clinician can also permit patient input about when a regular dose is changed.

Box 23.6 Talking to patients

Here is an approach to an "in-charge" patient when beginning a new medication. As can be seen in the following dialogue, the clinician makes references to the patient being in control and in charge: *"We are going to begin ... [name of medication]. Here are some general guidelines about when and how to take the medication, but I'd like you to be in charge of some elements of this. Let's start with 25 mg, and I'd like you to remain on that dose for several days. When you feel ready, and only when you feel ready, increase to 50 mg. Once you've adjusted to 50 mg you can, if you like, increase to 75 mg. My recommendation is that you do not go beyond 75 mg until our next visit. Obviously when you leave the office, you'll be the one taking the pills, but I think you'd be taking an added risk of side effects if you increase the medicine dose too fast."*

   To a patient who, during a follow-up session, has returned having taken several extra doses more than was prescribed: *"I know you're just trying to feel better as rapidly as you can, but I think you were actually fortunate that you didn't have any adverse effects of increasing the dose too fast. Had we talked, I might not have disagreed with your decision to increase your dose, but I think for future reference it would be best if we make this decision together."*

With sensitivity and tact, most of these individuals can be treated in a safe and effective manner. In the rare instance where such a person clearly and repeatedly takes medication in an unsafe manner or dose, the clinician may need to be more forceful, as shown below.

Box 23.7 Talking to patients

"We have discussed the parameters of using your medication and I had hoped we could see eye-to-eye about this. You have continued to make decisions about how and when you are taking your medication without our making these decisions together. What you are doing is not medically safe. We will need to agree on a plan of how you will use the medication in order for me to continue working with you. I would like to hear your thoughts about how you are making the decisions about medication, so we can negotiate a schedule that will not compromise your health." After this discussion and your proposal for a schedule, write down what you agree upon, give a copy to the patient and keep one in his/her chart. In the unusual circumstance when no agreement can be reached, or the patient makes an agreement but does not adhere to it, jeopardizing safety, the clinician will need to break off contact: *"I had hoped we could be a team in making decisions about your medication, but since you continue to violate our agreement, I think it best that you see another practitioner."*

The information overload patient

While many patients will, on occasion, bring articles about medication or mental health treatment to the clinician, there are some patients who take this to an extraordinary level. At virtually every appointment such patients arrive with a new article or set of data, asking "Is this appropriate for me?" or "Have you seen this?" Such patients are continually looking to refine their medication regimen or are hoping for an improved outcome. Their behavior can be independent of the adequacy of their medication response. Even when they are doing quite well, they seek "just a little bit more." These individuals may spend hours on the Internet, or in the library looking at journals or other sources for information about their illness and possible new treatments. For some patients, it appears to be their hobby or a vocation. Although most patients are genuinely trying to help themselves and to improve their treatment response, some are trying to show their intelligence or diligence, or match what they perceive as the practitioner's level of knowledge.

Requesting that patients cease bringing in articles or references is counterproductive and often misinterpreted. No matter how gently stated, the underlying message is that patients should not be involved in improving their level of care and this puts the clinician in a negative light. Therefore, the clinician should allow this behavior to continue without trying fundamentally to change such a patient's style. Although the prescriber should evaluate the pieces of information presented, there are keys to doing so in a time-efficient and useful way. The principles involved in dealing with this type of person include the following.

The clinician should ask the patient to always send or bring full copies of the articles or books to the office. If the patient brings only references, citations or website addresses for the clinician to follow up, he or she should ask the patient to make a hard copy and bring it at the next visit. Searching out such materials from the patient's suggestions can be quite time-consuming! Asking that the patient do the legwork also invites the patient to be selective in distinguishing material that is particularly relevant from "general information."

Sometimes an article is short and can be evaluated during a face-to-face session. At other times, it may be appropriate to peruse a lengthy article between appointments, which will allow the clinician to decide if more detailed reading is necessary. Usually this is not the case, and scanning of selected parts of the material is all that is needed to assess the material. It is not necessary to read in detail all the information that the patient has culled with hours of searching. The clinician can then correctly say at the next session that the material has been read, and make any appropriate comments regarding its applicability for this patient.

Many "information-seeking" patients find non-mainstream sources for their information. They may have connected to dubious Internet sites of biased, self-serving groups or organizations. The information may be primarily homeopathic in nature, or relate to "hormones," "vitamins," "natural" substances, herbal remedies or medications available only in other countries. Some of the information may come from print advertisements or Internet sites that are trying to sell products for profit. Some sources advertise "comprehensive remedies" that will treat almost any condition. The clinician can then point out the obvious fact that, if such a "miracle cure" were genuinely as effective as claimed, it would very quickly have become the common, mainstream standard of care.

At times, articles brought by a patient are genuinely useful and will inform even the knowledgeable clinician about a possible treatment that had not been considered. Despite any clinician's diligence to be updated and current with all medications, the number of sources of information on psychotropics available at this time is nearly overwhelming. Even the most well-read clinician can be challenged to stay current with all information available, and patient suggestions can be very helpful.

Box 23.8 Talking to patients

One way of recognizing and "crediting" the patient for this behavior would be to say: *"I appreciate your interest in getting better. Most patients are not willing to go to the lengths that you are to investigate new possibilities. I'll take a look at this article and see if there is anything that applies to my treatment of you."* Clinicians need not feel compelled to prescribe a remedy or medication that they are unfamiliar with or doubt will be effective. It is quite acceptable to decline to act on a patient's request for an obscure, unusual or potentially dangerous form of treatment just because it is requested (and possibly supported by "research" obtained by the patient). If the information is markedly complex, non-mainstream or inaccurate, the clinician could say: *"This is interesting, but I know of no research to support this treatment currently beyond this one website. You may be a little ahead of your time."*

The "naturalist"

This section is a brief summary of the concepts covered in more depth in Chapter 11 titled "'Natural' substances – do they help?"

For some persons, herbs, potions, hormones and plant products are deemed to be "natural," and therefore better and safer than synthetic medications, which are considered "chemical." Often these individuals will first try the use of health food stores, herbalists, practitioners of Eastern medicine, over-the-counter medications, "home remedies" and vitamins to treat their symptoms. They may not arrive at a more traditional medical office until they have unsuccessfully tried many other alternatives. Even when they do come to the clinician's office, they are reluctant to accept a recommendation for prescription medicines, which they perceive to be artificial and potentially dangerous.

Box 23.9 Talking to patients

In talking with a patient who has a strong preference for natural remedies, a clinician could use the following dialogue: *"You clearly want a treatment that is going to work in harmony with your body. I do, too. If there was a plant or herbal product that had sufficient research to support its use, I would suggest it. With your level of symptoms, however, I think that we should use a prescription medication which we know is pure, in a dose that is reproducible*

> *and for which we have solid research evidence to support its results. I know that this is probably not your first choice, but there are some things we need to remember:*
>
> - *a chemical is a chemical whether it's made by a plant or in a laboratory*
> - *many 'natural' products have markedly varying amounts of active ingredient in each pill, and it is difficult to standardize the dose you are receiving*
> - *many things that come out of the ground I would not put in my mouth (for example, many types of mushrooms)*
> - *just because something grows in the ground does not mean it is healthy."*

If such a person has very mild symptoms or insists on a "natural" remedy, a clinician may choose to try one of the remedies listed in the text below. While research evidence for their effectiveness is limited and, at times, contradictory, some patients who are fixated on natural remedies will insist on a trial of any possible "natural" compounds before being willing even to try a prescription. Practitioners may, if they choose, initially use one of these "natural" medications in a mildly symptomatic patient, if for no other reason than to obtain a stronger alliance with the patient and demonstrate the willingness to work effectively together.

If the patient symptoms are moderate or severe, however, there is some medico-legal risk in pursuing an unproven natural remedy when other proven prescription medications exist. Therefore, with a more severe symptom picture, a clinician should be skeptical of using unproven "natural" alternatives.

Box 23.10 Clinical tip

For mildly depressed patients who insist on a natural remedy, the use of St. John's Wort[1-3] may provide some benefit, although research is contradictory. Use of omega-3 fatty acids (fish oil)[4-6] has also been shown to be of some benefit in patients with affective disorders. Hoodia can be tried for medication-induced weight gain. For individuals with bipolar disorder who insist on a "natural" remedy, consider the use of lithium carbonate. In prescribing it, stress the fact that lithium is a natural element that is mined from the earth, and not a synthetic chemical. (In contrast to St. John's Wort, for which the research is contradictory, lithium has a long and strong track record in treating bipolar disorder and can be used with confidence, even in a patient with significant symptoms.) Valerian root has been used with some success to diminish anxiety and promote sleep.[7-9] There are no known successful herbal remedies for psychosis.

The borderline patient

The person with borderline personality disorder (often referred to as "a borderline") is one of the most challenging types of patient with which to interact and treat with medication. The majority of these individuals are young women, with a prevalence as high as

2 percent of the population.[10-11] The disorder is marked by frequent crises, self-harmful and markedly disruptive behavior ("acting out").[12] Such behavior is often repetitive, and these patients can rapidly become well known within a clinic, emergency department or group practice for difficult, problematic and, at times, seemingly outrageous behavior. Even when well-managed, they engender strong reactions and responses from clinicians. Poorly managed, they can cause clinicians to experience intense anger, frustration and self-doubt.

The reader may notice that these patients are covered somewhat more in depth than other "difficult" patients. Although not necessarily seen on a day-to-day basis, the intensity engendered by borderline patients, much of which emerges over medications and their prescription, merits a more thorough review. Clinicians currently treating one or more borderline patients will quickly recognize the issues presented here. When a clinician first becomes involved with such a patient (as is likely over time), the detailed information presented in this section will be welcome and deserving of review.

Medication prescription for borderline personality

Initially characterized in 1938 as a diagnosis that stood on the borderline between neurosis and psychosis, borderline personality disorder was later conceptualized to be a mild version of schizophrenia. This was reframed to the modern understanding of borderline personality disorder (BPD) by Kernberg in 1975.[13]

He characterized a person with BPD as a person who has problems maintaining consistent internal images and memories of people (poor "object relations") and displays primitive psychological defenses, including:

- splitting (a person is seen as all good or all bad)
- magical thinking
- projective identification (the projection of the person's own unpleasant characteristics on to others and trying to elicit in others feelings that the person him- or herself is experiencing).

The DSM-V now lists nine characteristics of persons with BPD, of which five must be present to make the diagnosis.[14] These diagnostic criteria comprise:

1 frantic efforts to avoid real or imagined abandonment
2 a pattern of unstable and intense interpersonal relationships characterized by alternation between extremes of idealization and devaluation
3 identity disturbance with a marked and persistently unstable sense of self
4 impulsivity in at least two areas, which can be self-damaging (such as spending, sexual behavior, substance abuse, reckless driving or binge eating)
5 recurrent suicidal behavior, gestures or threats, or self-mutilating behavior
6 affective instability due to marked mood reactivity lasting several hours, and rarely more than several days
7 chronic feelings of emptiness or boredom
8 inappropriate and intense, poorly controlled anger, including frequent displays of temper or recurrent physical fights
9 transient, stress-related paranoid ideation or dissociative symptoms.

Although the exact etiology of BPD is unclear, many patients diagnosed with this condition have strong histories of physical, sexual or mental abuse during their upbringing, and have experienced parental neglect and/or inconsistent parenting.[15–16] There is some evidence from brain-imaging studies that persons with BPD inconsistently activate areas of their frontal cortex, which would normally be expected to inhibit or suppress negative emotions.[17]

Because of their primitive defenses, if a borderline patient perceives that the clinician has been non-understanding, it is as if there has been no previous contact with the clinician. The patient cannot see the currently perceived problem in the context of a greater pattern of positive and therapeutic interaction, and the clinician is often defined by how he or she last acted with the borderline person. If the medicating clinician is not providing primary psychotherapy, there may be frequent attempts to split the primary psychotherapist and the medicating clinician. The patient may report behaviors or negative interactions with the psychotherapist, inviting the medicating clinician to intervene or join in the patient's outrage. Also, the medication clinician should not be surprised to hear that the psychotherapist has at times received information about the medication clinician that is negative, degrading or distorted.

Because of the idealizing/devaluing ("black-and-white") thinking of persons with BPD, the medicating clinician can be initially idealized as the "best," "most understanding" or "most knowledgeable" practitioner with whom the patient has ever dealt, often accompanied by denigration and devaluation of previous medication clinicians. This belief and interaction may persist for weeks, months or even years, only to change suddenly and unexpectedly. Change can occur when the patient perceives the clinician to have been absent when needed, to have prescribed a medication that was not successful, not to have "understood" the patient's needs satisfactorily or to have engaged in some other behavior that the patient perceives to represent lack of connection.

Because of strong affective fluctuations, particularly with anger and depression, the patient may repetitively request or demand a medication solution to his or her intense discomfort. Many borderline patients have a strong placebo response to medication. Therefore, there may be brief, overly positive responses to a medication intervention that are quickly lost. The patient may request further dosage increases in order to reclaim the initially perceived effect, at times requesting dosage levels beyond those normally given or safe. Persons with BPD have strong "oral" characteristics, and often will ingest medications, alcohol, drugs or other substances in hopes of remediating their intense affect. Using the philosophy that "if one pill is good, then three or four must be better," they may accidentally overdose in an attempt to self-medicate their emotional state.[18–19]

Because of their inability to self-soothe and manage crises, patients will often call the medicating clinician for help in calming themselves or for direct advice on how to manage interpersonal crises. These patients often feel "entitled," in that they can call the clinician whenever, and about whatever subject, they please. Some borderline patients can significantly overutilize the phone with the medicating clinician, if firm boundaries are not set.

Suicidal threats are common with borderline individuals, often in response to having perceived negative behavior on the part of someone important in their lives. At times, the source of their wrath or disappointment is the clinician and their suicidal threats can have a transparent, manipulative or angry message. Despite the seeming obviousness of these angry messages, it is not wise to ignore suicidal threats in borderline patients, since serious suicide attempts and death by overdose are common. Even when suicide attempts are repeated or are perceived to be manipulative, borderline patients will need to be evaluated in an emergency department and/or be psychiatrically hospitalized short term in the face of serious overdose or threat.

Behaviors of self-harm can include burning, cutting and scratching or self-mutilation, in addition to frank overdose. It is estimated that 75 percent of borderline patients have had at least one deliberate episode of self-harm, and that up to 9 percent of these patients successfully commit suicide.[20] Patients with BPD have significant problems maintaining clear boundaries with many people in their lives, and this may emerge in the medication prescription process. These patients can ask for exceptions to normal prescriptive practice, such as:

- requesting unusual, large doses of medication
- setting appointments outside the regular treatment setting or after hours
- personal friendship or support beyond that of the normal clinician–patient relationship.

Borderline patients often see themselves as special, and feel they deserve or need special treatment from the clinician. Their requests for special treatment can be repetitive and recurrent, but should, in general, be resisted. When granted unusual or special treatment, such patients often respond poorly, or ultimately take advantage of these special privileges. Any intimate or sexual contact is, of course, strictly prohibited, and even the appearance of impropriety or physical affection should be assiduously avoided. Borderline patients may change dramatically and suddenly. The idealized clinician who was "the best" may suddenly become "the worst," and accusations may be made about the clinician's behavior even when there is no solid reason.

Medication treatment principles with borderline patients

Borderline patients are particularly vexing, and can be problematic for even the most experienced medication clinician. The clinician should not hesitate to utilize consultation with other colleagues early in the course of treatment to discuss the management of a borderline patient. In general, because of the difficulty managing such patients, clinicians should avoid medicating large numbers of them simultaneously.

No medication should be provided in the absence of psychotherapy. If the medication clinician is not the primary psychotherapy clinician, it should be insisted that the patient be solidly involved in a psychotherapeutic relationship with another therapist prior to any medications being provided. In general, therapy for BPD is long term and difficult, with frequent crises. Individual therapy with a dialectical behavioral therapy or psychodynamic focus is crucial to long-term progress.

Medications may have some symptomatic benefit, although they are not the primary treatment. Medications used in BPD do not treat the underlying, core personality itself. Target symptoms should be identified, and specific medications chosen to modulate these target symptoms. In general, the four most common target symptoms identified are:

1   impulsive behavior
2   affective dysregulation, particularly depression
3   anger management
4   short-term psychotic symptoms.

SSRI antidepressants have been the backbone of treatment for many persons with BPD.[21] They have usefulness in decreasing impulsive behavior and have some modest antidepressant activity. Even large doses, however, seldom preclude the intense dysphoric depressions that these individuals experience. There is some evidence that mood stabilizers have some value for affective dysregulation and impulsiveness, but the evidence is not strong.[22–23] Naltrexone can be used for dissociative states.[24]

Psychotic symptoms most likely evident in borderlines include hallucinations, distortion of body image and ideas of reference. Transient psychotic symptoms are generally treated with low doses of antipsychotic medications. In general, atypical antipsychotics, such as olanzapine or risperidone, are safer than traditional antipsychotics, with fewer extrapyramidal side effects, lowered incidence of tardive dyskinesia and increased safety in overdose. Olanzapine[25] and risperidone[26] have also been shown to be useful with symptoms of aggression and depression in the patient with BPD. Doses should be small and the medication continued for relatively short periods of time – usually several days to several weeks. Most borderline patients do not require chronic antipsychotic medication unless there is clear re-emergence of symptoms quickly after the medication is withdrawn.

When first evaluating a patient with a borderline personality disorder, it is important to attempt to *establish a strong initial medication contract with the patient*. The clinician should emphasize the necessity of psychotherapy as being the central treatment issue, with medications being a supplemental aid. The prescriber will need to be specific about any guidelines for appointment frequency, directions for medication usage and "lost" prescriptions. It is essential to obtain a clear agreement from the patient as to safe and controlled use of medications. The risk from overdose should be described in detail.

Despite a strong initial contract, many borderlines will inappropriately use medications – overutilizing them chronically, episodically or erratically. In the context of a deep depression or intense anger, such patients may transiently take large amounts of medications to compensate for their lack of the internal, psychological ability to soothe themselves.

In general, medications that are dangerous in overdose, are habit-forming, or have narrow therapeutic indices should be avoided with borderline patients. These include tricyclic antidepressants, MAOIs, lithium carbonate and benzodiazepines. Beyond their habit-forming potential, benzodiazepines have the added property of disinhibition, which may exacerbate impulsiveness – one of the central features of BPD.

A calm, even-handed demeanor is essential in dealing with borderline patients, who can be affectively excitable, demanding, irritable and manipulative. It is important to maintain adherence to good prescribing principles and medication safety, despite repeated requests, insinuations, manipulation or threats. Calm but firm reiteration of how much medication will be prescribed, for what period of time and for what indications may be periodically necessary. When a clinician is in doubt (as is common with these patients), firmness, consistency and predictability are more useful than "giving in" to inappropriate requests, even when minor. The overvaluation and/or devaluation of the clinician should not be taken personally, or be allowed to alter good prescribing practice.

When primary psychotherapy is provided by another individual, it is important to maintain *frequent communication with the psychotherapist* to minimize splitting.

Regardless of any information provided by the patient about the behavior of the psychotherapist, no action should be taken until that therapist has been contacted and the reality of the situation discerned. If the medication clinician acts on a negative report, the issues may actually be the patient's misinterpretation and be partially (or totally) untrue. Other issues that should be discussed with the primary clinician include which person is going to be available for telephone contact and when, and which treatment issues will be handled by each clinician. Since borderline patients are particularly sensitive to absence, issues of coverage and availability during vacations should also be clearly outlined between clinicians, and then with the patient.

Since there is strong co-morbidity of borderline personality disorder with substance abuse, eating disorders and medication abuse, the medicating clinician should be alert to signs and symptoms of these problems.

Consultation and disengagement

All difficult patients can upset, anger, frustrate and disorganize clinical staff. When such patients' behavior is intense and repetitive, clinicians may lose perspective on their role, their interventions and their goals. At any time, but particularly if the above interventions are not working, a consultation may be utilized. This may be with a colleague in the same discipline, or with a mental health specialist. A telephone call specifically for advice, a brief meeting or a meal with the expressed purpose of discussing a problem case will often yield more results than a "curbstone consult" in the hall or the parking lot.

Despite clinicians' best efforts, consultation, skill and tact, some patients will not match well with some providers. There are situations when a clinician will feel unable to work productively with a patient who is unwilling or unable to participate in working together as a team. While not generally the first, second or third alternative, there *are* times when a practitioner must explore whether another clinician could work more effectively with a patient. When a clinician begins to question his or her ability to prescribe effectively and safely, despite efforts to modify the situation, he or she should raise the issue with the patient directly *as a possibility* before actually implementing a termination.

If the patient cannot or will not comply, the patient should be sent written notice of the clinician's intent to stop providing care/medication as of a specific date, with advice to find another caregiver.

Box 23.11 Talking to patients

"Miss Carpenter, I have begun to wonder whether I am the best clinician to treat you. We have had some differences of opinion about your care and we have attempted to come up with a plan to work together. From my view, this is not working. How are you feeling about working with me? Unless things change, I will need to withdraw from prescribing for you. This is what I need from you in order to continue working with you." Be specific and list the behaviors that need to occur, change or stop.

The patient is not always the problem

If a clinician finds that gradually (or suddenly) there are many "difficult" patients to be dealt with in one's practice, clinician-centered difficulties, not the patients, may be the primary problem. Overwork, a large caseload, an excessive number of gravely ill, complicated patients, lack of sleep, inadequate personal time, failure to take vacations, as well as personal and family stresses, can all lead to clinician burnout. Initially, one sign of this problem can be frequent irritation with patients, intolerance for small patient idiosyncrasies or finding multiple patient management issues burdensome. This can be accompanied by other warning signs, including:

- regularly being unable to stop thinking about "problem" patients
- allowing feelings about "difficult" patient interactions to intrude on family or social relationships
- inability to sleep well or relax when not at work
- an uncharacteristic emotional outburst at a patient
- excessive irritability with office staff or colleagues.

The presence of any of these signs should raise the warning flag that some alteration of workload, caseload mix or amount of non-work personal time is necessary. Although sometimes painful to accept, the difficulty at the office may be most clearly seen in the mirror.

Notes and references

1   Phillip M *et al.* (1999) Hypericum extract versus imipramine or placebo in patients with moderate depression: randomized multicentre study of treatment for eight weeks. *British Medical Journal* 319: 1534–1538.
2   Shelton RC *et al.* (2001) Effectiveness of St. John's Wort in major depression: a randomized controlled trial. *Journal of the American Medical Association* 285: 1978–1986.
3   Laakman G *et al.* (1998) St. John's Wort in mild to moderate depression: relevance of hyperforin for the clinical efficacy. *Pharmacopsychiatry* 31 (Suppl. 1): 54–59.
4   Hibbeln JR (1998) Fish consumption and major depression. *Lancet* 351: 1213.
5   Tanskanen A *et al.* (2001) Fish consumption and depressive symptoms in the general population in Finland. *Psychiatric Services* 52: 529–531.
6   Stoll AL *et al.* (1999) Omega-3 fatty acids in bipolar disorder: a preliminary double-blind, placebo-controlled trial. *Archives of General Psychiatry* 56: 407–412.
7   Wagner J *et al.* (1998) Beyond benzodiazepines: alternative pharmacologic agents for the treatment of insomnia. *Annals of Pharmacotherapy* 32: 680–691.
8   Heiligenstein E and Guenther G (1998) Over-the-counter psychotropics: a review of melatonin, St. John's Wort, valerian, and kava-kava. *Journal of American College Health* 32: 680–691.
9   Santos MS *et al.* (1994) Synaptosomal GABA release is influenced by valerian root extract involvement of the GABA carrier. *Archives of International Pharmacodynamics* 327: 220–231.
10   Clarkin JF *et al.* (1983) Proptotypic typology and the borderline personality disorder. *Journal of Abnormal Psychology* 92(3): 263–275.
11   Kernberg PF (1975) *Borderline Conditions and Pathological Narcissism*, Jason Aronson.
12   *Diagnostic and Statistical Manual* (2013) 5th edn., American Psychiatric Association Press.
13   Kernberg PF (1975) *Borderline Conditions and Pathological Narcissism*, Jason Aronson.
14   *Diagnostic and Statistical Manual* (2013) 5th edn., American Psychiatric Association Press.

15 Zanarini MC and Frankenburg F (1997) Pathways to the development of borderline personality disorder. *Journal of Personality Disorders* 11(1): 93–104.

16 Zanarini MC (2000) Childhood experiences associated with the development of borderline personality disorder. *Psychiatric Clinics of North America* 23(1): 89–101.

17 Davidson RJ *et al.* (2000) Dysfunction in the neural circuitry of emotion regulation: a possible prelude to violence. *Science* 289(5479): 591–594.

18 Soloff PH *et al.* (1994) Self-mutilation and suicidal behavior in borderline personality disorder. *Journal of Personality Disorders* 8(4): 257–267.

19 Gardner DL and Cowdry RW (1985) Suicidal and parasuicidal behavior in borderline personality disorder. *Psychiatric Clinics of North America* 8(2): 389–403.

20 Lineham MM *et al.* (1993) Naturalistic follow-up of a behavioral treatment for chronically parasuicidal borderline patients. *Archives of General Psychiatry* 50(12): 971–974. [Published *erratum* appears (1994) in *Archives of General Psychiatry* 51(5:) 422.]

21 American Psychiatric Association (2001) Practice guideline for the treatment of patients with borderline personality disorder. *American Journal of Psychiatry* 158: 1–52.

22 Olabi B and Hall J (2010) Borderline personality disorder: current drug treatments and future prospects. *Therapeutic Advances in Chronic Disease* 1(2): 59–66. doi: 10.1177/2040622310368455

23 Zanarini MC and Frankenburg FR (2001) Olanzapine treatment of female borderline personality disorder patients: a double-blind, placebo-controlled pilot study. *Journal of Clinical Psychiatry* 62: 849–854; Rocca P *et al.* (2002) Treatment of borderline personality disorder with risperidone. *Journal of Clinical Psychiatry* 63: 241–244.

24 Lubit RH (2018) Borderline personality disorder, available at: https://emedicine.medscape.com/article/913575-overview

25 Zanarini MC and Frankenburg FR (2001) Olanzapine treatment of female borderline personality disorder patients: a double-blind, placebo-controlled pilot study. *Journal of Clinical Psychiatry* 62: 849–854.

26 Rocca P *et al.* (2002) Treatment of borderline personality disorder with risperidone. *Journal of Clinical Psychiatry* 63: 241–244.

24 Prescription writing and record keeping

• The written prescription	422
• Stylistic elements and recommendations	422
• Record keeping	424
• Elements of a clinician's prescriptive note	424
• Systems for note taking	426
• Style items in a medication note	426
• Separate medication lists	427
• Ongoing laboratory monitoring	427
• Confidentiality and security of records	429
• Discussing clinical matters	430
• Record every encounter, not every fact	430
• Documenting unusual treatment	431

The written prescription

A patient comes to a prescriber for the prescriber's knowledge, judgment, evaluation and thinking. The end product of these endeavors is a professional assessment and usually a written prescription. The essential elements, without which a prescription cannot be valid, are listed in Table 24.1. Additional elements that may or may not be included in a prescription are in Table 24.2. A model prescription is shown in Figure 24.1.

Stylistic elements and recommendations

Attention to several other items will help make prescriptions consistent, and less open to misinterpretation. The clinician should, therefore, observe the following guidelines:

- Use legible handwriting. If handwriting is not easily readable, consider printing prescriptions. It is extraordinarily easy for a pharmacist to confuse "Lamictal" for "Lamisil," "Ludiomil" and "Lomotil" or "Fluoxetine" for "Fluvoxamine." If writing is not clear, mistakes will be made by the pharmacist or the patient. Many U.S. states are now legislating for electronic prescribing. Particularly for refills of a current medication, electronic prescribing makes things significantly easier for the practitioner. The appropriate patient's name is searched for in a database which will include the medications that the patient is taking. It is usually easy for the

Table 24.1 The essential elements of a prescription

- *Patient name.* Include the patient's full first name. Do not use initials or nicknames.
- *Date the prescription is written.* Although the vast majority of prescriptions are dated on the day the prescription is written, it is legal to write a prescription for a future date. While it should not be standard practice, this could occur, for example, with a patient who is taking a stimulant. Since stimulant medications can be only dispensed in the United States for a month at a time, a practitioner might, when prescribing for a long-term, stable patient at a 90-day medication management visit, write two future prescriptions dated for subsequent months so that the patient need not return to the office. In general, however, most prescriptions are dated on the day they are written.
- *The medication to be dispensed.* Use the generic or brand name, as appropriate.
- The *strength* (usually in number of mg or µg) and *dosage* form of the medication (pills, capsules, liquid, suppositories or another format).
- The *number of units to be dispensed* preceded by "Dispense" or "Disp #." Spell out the number of units in words rather than using numbers (e.g., "one hundred tablets" instead of "100 tablets").
- The number of *refills* allowed, if any, in words, not numbers.
- *Specific directions for use*, including how many units are to be taken, how often they are to be taken and by what route (oral, intravenous, rectal, etc.). If the medication is to be given as needed (PRN), specify how often the dose is to be taken and for what purpose. Preface the exact directions with "*sig*" (Latin for sign or mark – literally, how the prescriber wants the vial marked for patient usage).
- Some American states may legislate other items to be included in the written prescription. Contact the licensing board relative to your specialty for this information.

Table 24.2 Optional elements on a prescription

- Patient age.
- Patient address.
- Generic substitution allowed. Some prescriptions contain a check-off box to permit generic substitutions. If generic substitution is to be specifically *disallowed*, write "DAW," or "dispense as written," on the prescription.

Sample Prescription

Christoper M. Doran, MD

Name: Mary Jones   Date: 06/15/03
              Lithium carbonate
              300 mg
              Disp # Ninety
              Sig: Three capsules by mouth at bedtime

Label ☒   _____   (signature) MD

Refill None Times

Figure 24.1 Sample prescription.

practitioner to refill the medications if the amount and directions remain the same. It is incumbent on the practitioner, however, to make sure that the information stored in the database is correct. Often such data are entered on a smart phone and practitioners should be particularly aware of potentially mis-entering information from touching two simultaneous keys or touching the wrong key since erroneous information will be repeated in future refills.

- Use the metric system for the amounts of medication, wherever possible.
- Avoid abbreviations of medications (e.g., "Lith" for lithium, "MOM" for milk of magnesia).
- Avoid the use of abbreviations in giving directions (for example, spell out "four times a day" rather than writing "qid," which can be easily confused with "qd" – once a day).
- Always use a zero before strengths of less than 1 mg (for example, use 0.5 mg not .5 mg).
- Avoid using a terminal or trailing zero after a decimal (for example, use 0.1 mg, not 0.10 mg).

Record keeping

Written records of the prescriptive process are crucial to treatment documentation. Whether the interaction process occurs in an outpatient office, a clinic or a hospital, written records should be consistently made for every patient contact no matter how brief. Specifically, there should be written documentation of *every*:

- face-to-face appointment
- telephone contact
- e-mail contact
- text message (saving the original message and not deleting it will be sufficient)
- message left on an answering machine for the patient about a clinical matter
- original prescription or prescription refill.

Elements of a clinician's prescriptive note

The elements of an initial prescriptive evaluation are covered in Chapter 3, including the elements necessary to the written record, and will not be repeated here. The elements of a note documenting a follow-up session or any other contact that results in a revision of the medication regimen are included in Table 24.3.

A signature is necessary on institutional records, unless the note is solely in an outpatient clinician's private files.

Taking and preparing notes

There are many equally useful methods of recording patient clinical notes. What is crucial, however, is that the clinician:

- has a system of taking, filing and storing notes that is used consistently
- makes a notation of every clinical encounter at the time of the contact, or directly thereafter, and does not wait until a later date or time. If delayed, notes will inevitably be vague, inaccurate or not produced.

Table 24.3 Elements of a prescriptive note

- Date of the contact.
- Patient data, including target symptoms and significant changes in the clinical state. This should include changes in psychological condition, medical condition or medication use.
- Pertinent negatives if important questions are asked and responded to negatively (e.g., patient denies suicidal ideation).
- Side effects present or denied.
- Laboratory results, including any psychotropic blood levels.
- Clinician assessment of the current condition. Is the patient improving, unchanged or regressing? Is the medication effective in the overall treatment? If not sufficiently effective, what changes are needed?
- Plan and recommendations.
- Specify:
  - Any change in medication regimen. If the patient is to maintain the current regimen, specify this in writing.
  - Any warnings or recommendations.
  - Any prescriptions written.
  - Any laboratory tests needed or consultations requested.
- Date of the next evaluation for medications.

Within these broad parameters which clinicians can adapt to their personal style, notes can be documented in various ways:

- handwritten
- typed
- dictated and transcribed by others
- spoken into a computer and transcribed automatically through voice recognition software.

Some clinicians take written notes during their face-to-face meeting with the patient. Others prefer more eye contact, a greater sense of connection to the patient and to wait until the end of the visit to compose and document their clinical thoughts. Some practitioners feel that it is useful to dictate the patient's note in the patient's presence so that he or she knows exactly what is being documented about the visit. Others are more comfortable waiting until after the session to dictate or write, particularly if sensitive material is to be documented or precise wording is necessary. Although it is desirable that all dictation be reviewed for accuracy and completeness, not all practitioners routinely review their dictated notes until the next time the chart is opened. If a dictated note documents a sensitive issue, involves a negative patient outcome or is to be sent to others outside the treatment setting, each dictation should be promptly reviewed for accuracy.

Some clinicians may delay writing notes that document negative outcomes, particularly serious ones in which the records could ultimately be scrutinized. The rationale often is to wait for complete information to compose a note as accurately and thoroughly as possible. While this practice is not totally without merit, it is generally preferable to document notes on negative outcomes contemporaneously or soon after the event. It is important to document clinical decision-making at the time, with as much data as are then known. Information that is pending or missing can be noted, then an additional note written subsequently. If new or additional data affect the treatment plan, clinical thinking or assessment, the clinical reasoning should be explained simply. It is perfectly reasonable for the clinician to refine his or her thinking or change an assessment based on new data. *Under no circumstances should a previously written note be altered, rewritten, deleted or otherwise changed* in an effort to make it "look better" or make the decision-making appear more accurate. Altered records or notes, written after the fact, can raise medico-legal suspicion, particularly if there are negative outcomes.

Box 24.1 Clinical tip

No matter how experienced or confident a clinician may be, *he/she must not attempt multi-tasking; i.e., trying to write a document about one subject while discussing another*. This applies to writing prescriptions, medical record notes, laboratory test requests or any other written document while talking to patients, office staff or using the telephone. In particular, if the clinician feels rushed, it can be tempting to try to do two tasks at once. This practice will inevitably result in errors on the written document and/ or poor verbal communication. For example, even experienced clinicians cannot satisfactorily write prescriptions while discussing side effects, order a lab test while giving the patient medication directions or make a clinical record note while making a referral to a colleague on the telephone.

It can, however, be valuable to clinician and patient alike for the clinician to say out loud what he or she is writing. For example, it is reinforcing to speak what is written on a prescription as it is being done: *"Mrs. Harrison, I am writing this prescription for [name of medication]. I am giving you 60 pills with two refills. You are to take two of these by mouth every night at bedtime."* This practice may improve the accuracy of both the written *and* the verbal communications.

Systems for note taking

Several systematized methods of writing progress notes have been devised and widely promulgated. Although the acronyms vary, the elements are similar. Each system includes information gathered, the clinician's assessment or impression of the data, the recommendations and the plan. Some of the common acronyms are:

* SOAP (Subjective data, Objective data, Assessment and Plan)
* DAP (Data, Assessment and Plan)
* DAR (Data, Assessment and Recommendations).

A beginning clinician would do well to adopt and maintain one of the systematized formats to ensure that all necessary elements are included.

Style items in a medication note

Medication notes should be targeted and concise. Very long notes are often not read. As to content and wording, a useful guideline is that the clinician *should not include words or items in a note that he or she would not want read aloud to the patient or to a colleague.* Slang, derogatory or disparaging terms should be avoided, as should assessments that cannot be documented by observation and fact.

Regardless of the format used, written or typed clinical notes are best recorded on standard-sized paper (8½ × 11" in the United States, A4 in the UK), which is easily copied. Clinicians who prescribe medications will often have need to copy their records for other clinicians, for insurance companies or as documentation of the session. If the size of the paper is other than standard, it is often cumbersome to copy. *Spiral notebooks* or other bound volumes, which cannot easily be copied, should be avoided. Notes must always be written in ink pen, not in pencil.

Separate medication lists

In addition to whatever clinical notes of patient contact are maintained, it is useful for the prescriber to maintain a current, easily modifiable list of all medications prescribed so that the entire regimen for each patient is easily viewed at one time. Additionally, such a medication list permits the clinician rapidly to see when medications were started, when they were stopped and previous medications that were utilized.

In modern psychopharmacology, when patients are often prescribed multiple medications, it is not only convenient, but also safe practice to list all medications on one document. If clinicians document medication data solely in the body of a written paragraph, or in the "Plan" section of a progress note, it is difficult to follow which medications have been used, their start and stop dates, and when combinations of medications may have been tried. While maintaining a separate medication list in an outpatient chart requires additional writing on the part of the clinician, it results in superior organization and safety. An example of such a medication sheet, which shows dates, names, doses and includes a space for serum blood level results, is shown in Table 24.4. By circling dates when a medication is stopped, it is clear which medications have been tried, when and for how long they were used.

Ongoing laboratory monitoring

Although not all psychotropics require periodic laboratory tests, some medications require serum blood levels of the psychotropic (see Chapter 25), periodic assessment of liver function, blood count or other parameters, as has been described in other sections of this text. During follow-up appointments and throughout the length of prescription, the clinician will need to devise a system to know when repeat tests need to be ordered and to manage outcome reports of lab tests in the client's chart. There are various ways to do this, but if some methodology is not followed, clinicians will have difficulty remembering to order necessary tests at appropriate times and consistently organizing their laboratory records. This becomes particularly problematic when a patient is on multiple medications and is seen over a long period of time.

Clinicians practicing in inpatient or clinic settings may have a standard chart format with dividers, one of which is usually reserved for laboratory results. In an outpatient setting, where such a system is not required, clinicians should organize their office records so that *lab test results and reports of any physical examinations/consultations are kept separately in chronological order* in one section of the patient's chart. This provides

Table 24.4 Sample medication list

Medication log of (name of patient) _____

Date	Name of medication	Dose/freq.	Disp #	Refills	Comments/blood level/lab tests

Note: Circle stop dates. List medical conditions, other medications from other prescribers, allergies/ sensitivities.

Table 24.5 Sample laboratory test results form

Laboratory monitoring for (patient's name) _____

Date	Test	Significant positive or negative results	Information conveyed to patient (Yes/No/Date)	Changes in treatment plan or medication	Date of next test

a consistent place from which to review past medical results, view any trends, see when exams or tests were performed, and collate any physical exam and laboratory information when needed; for example, when preparing a report of the patient's care for a third party.

Although the clinician will want to mention appropriate physical exams and lab results in a progress note, in general it is not wise to insert these actual reports haphazardly or "as they arrive" into the patient's progress notes. While this may seem intuitive or an easy way to file, chronological filing within the progress notes can lead to confusion and an increasing likelihood that important results may be overlooked, especially when the patient's file becomes large.

Some clinicians will prefer to record serum blood levels and/or other lab test results on the patient's medication list as mentioned above. Others may prefer to devise separate

Table 24.6 Sample laboratory test results form (filled in)

Laboratory monitoring for (patient's name) _____

Date	Test	Significant positive or negative results	Information conveyed to patient	Changes in treatment plan or medication	Date of next test
9/4/03	Chemistry profile CBC TSH	Wnl Wnl 1.05	✓ (Sept 6) ✓ ✓	Start lithium	1–2 weeks
09/14/03	Lithium level (on 900 mg)	0.47 meq/l	✓ (9/16)	Increase dose to 1200 mg	2 weeks
10/01/03	Lithium level (on 1200 mg)	0.70 meq/l	✓ (Oct 2)	Maintain dose	6 weeks
11/15/03	Lithium	0.68 meq/l	✓ (Nov 16)	Maintain dose	3 months
02/18/04	Lithium TSH	0.52 meq/l 2.1	✓ (Feb 19)	Increase dose to 1500 mg	1–2 weeks
3/1/04	Lithium (on 1500 mg)	0.91 meq/l	✓ (3/3)	Maintain dose	3 months
6/7/04	Lithium	0.85 meq/l	✓ (6/8)	Maintain dose	6 months
12/02/04	Lithium Chemistry profile TSH CBC	0.86 meq/l Wnl 2.0 Wnl	✓ (12/3)	Maintain dose	6 months

Note: Wnl = Within normal limits.

forms specifically for monitoring laboratory values, with prompts for the clinician in ordering subsequent tests. An example of such a system is shown in Table 24.5. When using this format, the clinician will necessarily be succinct and likely use abbreviations to save documentation time. Only significant findings need be documented, as long as a copy of the full lab report is contained elsewhere in the chart.

The form shown in Table 24.5 could be filled out as in Table 24.6, which is an example of a patient initially started on lithium, who later had the dose increased to treat breakthrough symptoms.

Confidentiality and security of records

All medical records require attention to confidentiality and safe storage. Because of the special nature of mental health records, including those of medication prescription, even more attention is required in ensuring that written records and conversations about patient treatment are kept confidential.

Any written records that include documentation of mental health prescriptions should always be kept safe and locked away. Whether active or in storage, such records are typically kept in locked file cabinets, locked offices or locked storage rooms. A breach of confidentiality can occur when records are carried away or left in unusual places where they can be read by others. Some common locations where records are accidentally left and their confidentiality endangered include:

- left open on a desk when the clinician leaves the room
- in patient exam rooms
- in a hospital room
- in a patient waiting room
- in cars
- in a personal residence
- in public areas such as a staff cafeteria or meeting rooms

It is only clinicians themselves or certain select clinical/clerical staff who should have access to records, especially in clinic settings. It is important to ensure that records are not observed by non-authorized individuals, including custodial staff, repairmen, package delivery persons or other patients.

Discussing clinical matters

Oral communication is another way in which confidentiality of clinical and medication information can be easily and inadvertently violated. In general, verbal communication about patients should only be undertaken within an office or over the telephone in private. Common situations that can lead to violation of confidentiality include:

- discussing one patient's status while a second patient is in the office
- discussing a patient's case in a room with an open door
- talking with clinic staff outside an office, in a hallway or another public area of a clinic
- talking about patients in a clinic waiting area
- discussing clinical material in an elevator
- discussing patient information at a hospital nursing station
- discussing a patient's condition "on rounds"
- discussing patient histories at a meeting or conference
- discussing patient information over lunch or dinner
- discussing patient information on a cell phone when others are present.

Record every encounter, not every fact

As has been outlined throughout this chapter, it is important for the prescriber to make a clinical record of each face-to-face patient contact, laboratory test, medication prescription, electronic or telephone communication with patients. This does not mean, however, that every fact or historical revelation need be included in the prescriber's record. As healthcare professionals, we are regularly and routinely privy to details about the patient's past and present life. History of exposure to a sexually transmitted disease, cosmetic surgery, marital infidelity, domestic violence or termination of an unwanted pregnancy are just some of the emotionally charged elements that patients may reveal to us.

We are, of course, bound to keep accurate medical records for patient safety and medico-legal reasons. Nonetheless, it is important that the prescriber think about the relevance of recording all behavioral and historical elements in the overall care of the patient. In addition to the clinician's judgment, sometimes the patient him-/herself will request that the provider not document a particular item. Fearing embarrassment, a negative outcome from a health insurance company or the possibility that a family member or employer might ultimately have access to the record, a patient may request that certain items not be documented by the practitioner.

Before recording any particularly controversial or embarrassing historical fact, the prescriber should consider if such documentation is essential to this patient and this prescribing interaction. In some situations, it may be appropriate to take a collaborative approach and ask the patient if he/she has strong feelings about recording any particular piece of data. In other situations, the prescriber may use generalized or vague terminology which will jog the practitioner's memory when necessary, but is not specific and detailed. For example:

- domestic abuse may be recorded as "severe family difficulties"
- marital infidelity can be recorded as "relationship problems"
- a therapeutic abortion can be documented as "while pregnant, the patient received further treatment from a healthcare professional"
- a lawsuit about being terminated from employment can be recorded as "severe work stress leading to a job change."

Inevitably, there may be some conflict between the complete inclusion of data in mental health charting and the patient's need for privacy. Unless there is a clear reason to record emotionally charged issues for patient safety, it is generally better to err on the side of being less specific and/or omitting certain elements of documentation altogether.

Documenting unusual treatment

In attempting to obtain a full remission or achieve a response in a previously non-responsive patient, extraordinary measures are at times appropriate and necessary. When taking such measures, a prescriber must pay special attention to documentation of treatment which may be considered outside traditional normative care. This could include unusually large or unusually small doses of medication, combinations of medications which carry known safety risks, use of experimental medications or treatments which have little or no evidence base and medications for non-FDA approved uses. It is incumbent on the practitioner to document such practice clearly and completely should there be any adverse outcome and/or the practitioner's judgment is subsequently called into question.

When undertaking an unusual, non-normative treatment strategy, or prescribing an unusually high or low medication dosage or off-label use of a medication, it is important to document:

- the reasons for utilizing this treatment and/or not utilizing more typical modalities
- the measures that have already been tried and perhaps failed
- the expected outcome and length of the treatment
- a discussion of side effects and warnings about the treatment given to the patient

- written informed consent from the patient for the treatment
- written informed consent from the patient's family and/or guardian if there is any question of the patient's competency to give consent for his/her own treatment, or if the patient is under the age of 18.

In some clinical situations of potentially high risk or controversial methodology, it is best to obtain a written consultation from a colleague before initiating the treatment.

25 Blood levels of psychotropics

• When blood levels help	433
• Instructions to patients	435
• Frequency of blood levels	436
• Using clinical judgment	437
• When blood levels do not help	437
• Necessary documentation	438
• References	438

A prime example of the mixture of art and science in mental health medication is the use of serum blood levels of psychotropic medications. The introduction and successful use of serum blood levels[1] (sometimes referred to as Therapeutic Drug Monitoring, or TDM) has scientifically "legitimized" psychiatry to both clinicians and patients. It supports the notion that mental health prescriptions are scientific and in line with other specialties of medicine. Utilizing the results of blood levels, however, still requires the art of flexibility and judgment, rather than rote decision-making based on numbers.

When blood levels help

Serum blood levels may have several clinical applications:[1]

- to increase efficacy by using the optimum amount of medication
- to increase safety by decreasing side effects and minimizing the likelihood of toxicity
- to monitor adherence
- to protect against medico-legal actions.

Those types of medications where blood levels can be of significance include:

- medications that have a narrow therapeutic index (a small difference between a therapeutic level and a level resulting in toxicity/side effects), such as TCAs or lithium
- medications where there is a proven, useful therapeutic range that can be correlated to clinical response, such as nortriptyline or clozapine
- medications that have a wide variability in absorption, metabolism or excretion between individuals (e.g., TCAs).

Table 25.1 Psychotropic medications for which serum blood levels are helpful

- Lithium
- Carbamazepine
- Valproic acid
- Clozapine
- Nortriptyline
- Imipramine
- Desipramine
- Amitriptyline
- Clomipramine

Table 25.2 Therapeutic serum blood levels of commonly used psychotropic medications

Medication	Therapeutic range (meq)	Toxic levels (where established)
Lithium[1]	0.6–1.2 meq/l	> 1.5 meq/l
Carbamazepine[1]	4–12 mg/ml	> 12 mg/ml
Valproic acid[1]	50–100 mg/ml	
Clozapine[2]	> 350 µ/ml	
Nortriptyline[3]	50–150 mg/ml	
Imipramine[4-5] (parent compound plus metabolite)	200–250 mg/ml	> 450 mg/ml
Desipramine[4]	110–180 mg/ml	
Amitriptyline[4]	150–250 mg/ml	
Traditional and atypical antipsychotics*		

Sources:

1 Bezchlibnyk-Butler K and Jeffries JJ (1999) *Psychotropic Drugs*, 9th edn., Hogrefe & Huber, pp. 111–124.
2 Kronig MH *et al.* (1995) Plasma clozapine levels and clinical response for treatment refractory schizophrenic patients. *American Journal of Psychiatry* 152: 179–182.
3 Perry PJ *et al.* (1987) The relationship between antidepressant response and tricyclic antidepressant plasma concentrations. *Clinical Pharmacokinetics* 13: 381–392.
4 Hales RE (1999) *Textbook of Psychiatry*, 3rd edn., American Psychiatric Association Press, p. 294.
5 Kaplan HI and Sadock BJ (1995) *Comprehensive Textbook of Psychiatry*, 6th edn., Lippincott, Williams & Wilkins, p. 1164.

*Note: Trough serum blood levels utilized in the treatment of psychotic illnesses can be useful in helping to determine adherence or the presence of intolerable side effects. These levels are listed by Jönsson *et al.* (2019)[2] in the references at the end of the chapter.

Specifically, the medications in which serum blood levels have been useful are listed in Table 25.1.

The therapeutic range for each of these medications is listed in Table 25.2. These data are also included in Appendices 2, 4 and 5.

Small changes in blood level are generally not of clinical significance, and it usually serves no purpose to adjust medications to change blood levels by less than 5–10 percent.

Instructions to patients

Fortunately, regardless of what medication is being monitored through blood levels, instructions to the patient are virtually identical. Clinicians measure *trough blood levels*, typically timed 12 hours after the last medication dose. Since the timing is critical to obtaining levels that are accurate, for most patients this means drawing the blood level in the morning (12 hours after an evening dose). The timeframe is approximate, and a level drawn within 10–14 hours from the last dose is generally accurate. There is no intrinsic reason why a patient could not have a blood level drawn in the early evening (12 hours after a morning dose), but most outpatient laboratories are not open to draw the level.

Most psychotropics will generate a steady-state blood level within four half-lives. Therefore, in order accurately to measure the amount of medication at steady-state, it is necessary for the patient to be on a consistent dose of medication for at least 4 days prior to the blood level. Inconsistent dosing before a blood level can have a variable effect on the result. If the only dose missed was on day 1 or day 2, some reasonable estimate of the blood level may still be obtained. However, if the missed dose occurs on day 4, just before the blood level, the value obtained can be affected by as much as 25–50 percent.

Written instructions are helpful for most patients to ensure that they follow the methodology necessary to obtain accurate values. A typical instruction sheet for serum blood level testing is shown in Table 25.3.

Although it may vary by locale and laboratory used, lithium levels, valproic acid levels and serum carbamazepine levels are generally returned within 12–36 hours. "Stat" levels may be obtained quickly in situations of crisis or serious toxicity. Serum tricyclic antidepressant levels and clozapine levels take 48–96 hours to return to the clinician, since these tests are often not performed locally and need to be sent to a specialty lab.

On occasion, patients will call urgently from the lab saying that they are there to have their blood level drawn, but now realize that they took their morning dose an hour or two before. Such patients should be advised *not* to have the blood level drawn that day, to continue taking their regular dose and to return on another day. Drawing a level 1–2 hours after the last oral dose registers a meaningless number that cannot be reliably extrapolated to yield valuable information.

Table 25.3 Instructions for blood level testing

---

1 Draw your first level on [date] _____. Blood levels require 4 days on the same dose of medication in order to be accurate. If your dose of medicine has been changed recently, maintain a consistent dose for at least 4 days before testing. Do not miss any doses in the 4 days before the test.

2 Have the level drawn approximately *12 HOURS AFTER YOUR EVENING DOSE* (a range of 10–14 hours is allowed, but not shorter or longer).

3 If you usually take a dose of medicine in the morning, *WAIT UNTIL AFTER THE BLOOD IS DRAWN TO TAKE YOUR MORNING DOSE ON THE DAY OF THE TEST*. If you forget and take your morning dose that day, the test will not be accurate. *Have the blood level drawn another day*.

4 You may eat a normal breakfast on the day of a blood level test. It is *not* necessary to fast for this test. You may also take any other prescribed medication (that is not being measured in the blood level) on the morning of the test.

Frequency of blood levels

How often a blood level is drawn depends on a number of factors, including the particular medication monitored, the medical health or fragility of the patient and the patient's level of improvement (or lack thereof). *Lithium levels* are ordered both more frequently and more regularly over the long term than are levels of other psychotropics. The serum level of lithium can be significantly affected by various prescription and non-prescription medications (such as NSAIDs and diuretics), changes in salt and fluid balance, and gastrointestinal illness, particularly diarrhea.

Lithium levels are typically measured in the outpatient clinic within a week after starting lithium, within a week of any dosage increase and every 1–2 weeks thereafter until the blood level and/or the patient's clinical condition is stabilized. Once stabilized, lithium levels should be drawn every 3 months for the first year. Thereafter, levels can be drawn every 3–6 months. A serum creatinine, BUN, CBC and TSH should be monitored every 6–12 months for changes in kidney function, blood count and lowered thyroid function.

Serum *carbamazepine, valproic acid or clozapine* levels should be drawn 5–7 days after an initial target dose is reached, and every 1–4 weeks thereafter until an appropriate blood level is stabilized. If the patient is doing well clinically, blood levels may then be monitored every 3–4 months during the first year. Clinicians have variable ways of dealing with blood levels for patients remaining on these medications over the long term. Some clinicians choose to check blood levels at regular intervals even if the patient is doing well, whereas other clinicians will not draw routine blood levels unless there is some clinical indication to do so. Even if clinicians choose not to check routine blood values when a patient is doing well, it is appropriate to check a panel of liver function tests and a CBC to monitor for hepatic or hematological side effects at least once a year.

For *tricyclic antidepressants*, an initial level is generally drawn 5–7 days after an initial target dosage of medication has been reached. Follow-up blood levels may be drawn every 1–3 weeks thereafter, depending on patient response and the presence or absence of side effects. Once stabilized, tricyclic levels need not be drawn on a regular basis provided the patient remains clinically stable and symptoms are in remission.

Some of the exceptions to these general time guidelines for serum blood monitoring are listed in Table 25.4.

A *clinical relapse* or the emergence of *new or troublesome psychiatric symptoms* is a clear indication to check the blood level of any psychotropic medication currently prescribed to the patient. Blood levels may have changed, and a simple adjustment of dosage may be all that is necessary to re-establish remission.

The *addition or removal of a medication* that might affect the serum level of a psychotropic is also a good reason to check a blood level. Many of these occur because of P-450 interactions (see Chapter 20). Common psychotropic medications with such potential interactions include adding an SSRI to a TCA (which can raise the blood

Table 25.4 Reasons to obtain more frequent serum psychotropic levels

- Clinical relapse
- Addition/removal of an interacting medication
- Emergence of new side effects
- When the patient is hospitalized or institutionalized
- Suspected non-adherence

level of the TCA), or adding an SSRI to carbamazepine (which can raise the level of carbamazepine).

A third reason for rechecking a blood level is the *emergence of new side effects*. Subtle or significant changes in blood levels over time may result in side effects that were not present when the patient initiated the medication. A check of a blood level and comparison with baseline blood levels on which the patient had no side effects may alert the clinician to decrease the dosage and possibly eliminate the side effect.

Occasionally, it is necessary for a clinician to monitor *medication adherence*. A blood level will give valuable information as to whether the patient is taking the medication at all. From the numerical value and comparison to previous levels, it can usually be determined if the patient is following the full regimen.

It is prudent to check a serum blood level of a measurable psychotropic at the time of a *psychiatric or medical hospitalization*. Regardless of the reason for hospitalization, by definition there has been a major change in health status, and it is useful at these times to know the baseline level of the psychotropic. A psychiatric hospitalization indicates that a psychiatric crisis has occurred. Decisions about medications may need to be made, and blood levels can be helpful with this determination. A very low or zero blood level may also indicate that poor adherence can have contributed to the crisis. If the hospitalization is medical, there may be a significant medical illness or the possibility of surgery. In either case, knowing the current blood level of the psychotropic is helpful to the medical/surgical team.

Although not frequent currently, there can be changes in absorption or pharmacokinetics with certain *generic medications* compared to the branded version. When a patient changes from brand name to generic or vice versa and the patient's clinical state changes close to that time, a check of blood level is indicated (see Chapter 26).

Using clinical judgment

The presence of numerical blood levels should not override the clinician's judgment and clinical observation. It is a simple but unfortunate error to assume that all patients will do best when a blood level is within the published therapeutic range. Ultimately, *the most important parameters to monitor are the patient's functioning, emotional state and the presence of side effects*, if any. If the clinician finds that either a higher or lower blood level provides solid, consistent clinical control of symptoms, the clinician may choose to maintain the patient on this dose of medication. It is important, however, when using a dose that gives higher or lower than "normal" published levels, that the clinician documents the rationale for this exception. Notably, lithium, valproic acid and carbamazepine can provide adequate clinical response even if a patient's blood level is technically "low." There are numerous examples of patients who show satisfactory mood stabilization on sub-therapeutic blood levels, and in fact get significant side effects when their blood levels are brought into the published therapeutic range.

When blood levels do not help

There are many psychotropic medications for which blood levels are either unavailable or yield no significant clinical information. A list of such medications appears in Table 25.5.

For these drugs, clinically it would be helpful to have valid therapeutic dose ranges or some other biological measure of the amount of medication absorbed for a given oral

Table 25.5 Psychotropic medications for which <u>serum blood levels are of no value</u>

- All SSRI antidepressants
- Bupropion, nefazodone, mirtazepine, venlafaxine
- Benzodiazepines
- Buspirone
- Anticholinergic medications
- Cholinesterase inhibitors
- Any medication used for alcohol abuse

dose. While the technology for *qualitatively* measuring the presence of these medications in the blood stream exists – *yes*, it is present or *no* it is not – clinically helpful *quantitative* (numerical) results are not possible. Technological methodologies for accurate lab values are not always possible, or the results may not be reproducible. Even more commonly, medication levels may be measured but there is no significant correlation between the numerical medication levels and the clinical response. This is especially true for SSRI antidepressants, and traditional and atypical antipsychotics, where patient A may respond very well to significantly low blood levels and patient B may require exceptionally high blood levels. In typical practice, a clinician would have no reason to draw a blood level of the medicines listed in Table 25.5 except to assess adherence.

Necessary documentation

Blood levels are only useful when seen and assessed by the clinician. The clinician needs to indicate that the results of a blood level have been noted, which is usually done by initialing the report. It is useful to comment on the results of the blood level in the progress note for that day or the appointment note for that session. It is also crucial to document what action was taken based on the blood level received, particularly if the blood level was outside the therapeutic range:

- Was the clinician satisfied with the blood level?
- If not, are there to be any changes in dosage?
- When is the next blood level to be drawn?

Serum blood level results outside the therapeutic norm that are not noted and/or acted upon can present a medico-legal risk. In the event of an untoward response, the presence of a blood level that was not noted, not acted upon and not documented may prove to be the legal undoing of the clinician. Similarly, a timely blood level noted by the clinician may be a strong legal defense against a poor outcome of medication.

References

1 Janicak PG *et al.* (2010) *Principles and Practice of Psychopharmacotherapy*, 5th edn., Williams & Wilkins.
2 Jönsson AK *et al.* (2019) A compilation of serum concentrations of 12 antipsychotic drugs in a therapeutic drug monitoring setting. *Therapeutic Drug Monitoring* 41(3): 348–356. doi: 10.1097/FTD.0000000000000585

26 Generic medications

- Generic substitution problems   441
- Generic change without the clinician's knowledge   442
- Tips for generic use   442
- Serum blood levels and generic substitution   443
- Mandated generics   443
- References   444

Brand-name medications are protected by a patent issued to the pharmaceutical company that develops the medication to compensate the firm for the time, money and testing invested in bringing the medication to market. When the patent expires 20 years after being issued, other companies may manufacture the same medication. Formulations of the same product are marketed and sold under its generic (chemical) name, which usually leads to lower prices (see Table 26.1). Most mental health medications are available as generics except when first introduced, but over time the patents of branded products expire and generic preparations may then potentially be manufactured and sold.

The generic share of the prescription market in the United States increased from 18.6 percent in 1984, to 41.6 percent in 1996 and 89 percent in 2018.[1-2] Generic usage is increasing by as much as 7.7 percent per year worldwide. When the first generic medication is introduced following the patent expiration of a brand-name medication, typically its cost is reduced only slightly. The first generic product has a 6-month marketing exclusivity. Thus, significant cost reductions are often not seen until 6 months after the generic begins to be sold. The introduction of a second generic equivalent, on average, reduces the cost to approximately half the brand-name cost. If a large number of generic manufacturers are attracted to market and introduce competing generic medications, the average cost may fall to 20 percent of the branded cost, and sometimes lower.[3]

The fate of a medication when its patent expires depends on the extent of usage of the medication and what, if any, alternatives exist. When a medication is little used and/or there are better alternatives, generic formulations seldom emerge. The medication can still be prescribed through its branded name, and the price for this branded preparation usually remains relatively high. When a medication is commonly used and/or there are few superior alternatives, one or more generic preparations will emerge. The medication can then be prescribed as a less expensive generic. The generic may continue to be prescribed even though the higher priced brand-name preparation remains available.

Table 26.1 Generic medications

- Are chemically identical to the branded medication in regard to their active ingredients, dosage recommendations, safety, effectiveness, stability and quality
- May have different bioavailability than branded products
- May contain different dyes, fillers or coatings from branded products
- Are usually plain in color and packaging
- Are usually less expensive than branded medications, but not always

---

When generic preparations are available, pharmacoeconomics often drives pharmaceutical manufacturers to try one of several strategies to ensure continued prescription of a branded version. A different preparation that still contains the same active ingredient (e.g., a unique combination of more than one product or a new delivery system) may be marketed. In the United States, if the Food and Drug Administration (FDA) deems the medication to be sufficiently different, unique and effective, a new patent is issued. An example of this is valproic acid sodium, which became available as a useful generic medication, but gave some patients significant side effects. It was reformulated with a special coating to ensure more gradual absorption of the drug, thus having fewer side effects than the generic version. This newly formulated version of valproex sodium was marketed in the United States under the brand name Depakote with significant success.

Other companies have developed and marketed stereoisomers (mirror images) of the initial product. If such an isomer is valuable, more targeted, has fewer side effects than a mixture of isomers or has some other advantage, a new patent may be issued for the preparation. An example of this is S-citalopram (marketed in the United States as Lexapro), which is a product containing just one stereoisomer of citalopram rather than the mixture of stereoisomers of citalopram contained in Celexa. The manufacturer touts a lower side-effect profile although whether this can be borne out by research remains an open question.

Another manufacturing option is to repackage a medication under a new name for a new indication. Examples of this include fluoxetine (Prozac) remarketed as Serafem for premenstrual dysphoric disorder, and bupropion (Wellbutrin) remarketed as Zyban for smoking cessation.

Table 26.2 lists commonly used mental health medications that have a generic preparation.

In general, the FDA reports that generic drugs are safe and effective. Clinically, this is also the experience of most practitioners. When generics are substituted for branded products, the majority of patients who have previously clinically responded will continue to experience positive therapeutic benefit. The one and only reason to switch to a generic preparation is cost. Some patients have a strong preference for branded versus generic preparations. When this is so, there is little reason not to prescribe the branded preparation if the patient is willing to pay the cost difference. From the practitioner's point of view in treating mental illness, prescribing either branded or generic preparations is neither exemplary nor a problematic practice.

To allow or specify a generic product, write the chemical name of the medication on the prescription. Some prescriptions have a check-off box that can be marked to allow generic substitutions for a branded product.

Table 26.2 Commonly used mental health medications that have a generic preparation

These include:
- TCAs, all
- MAOIs, all
- Lithium carbonate
- Carbamazepine (Tegretol)
- Traditional antipsychotics, all
- Benzodiazepines, all
- Antihistamines, virtually all
- Beta blockers, virtually all
- Valproic acid (Depakote, Depakote ER)
- Benztropine (Cogentin)
- Sertraline (Zoloft)
- Paroxetine (Paxil)
- Citalopram (Celexa)
- Escitalopram (Lexapro)
- Bupropion (Wellbutrin)
- Fluoxetine (Prozac)
- Clozapine (Clozaril)
- Quetiapine (Seroquel)
- Risperidone (Risperdal)
- Ziprasidone (Geodon)
- Olanzapine (Zyprexa)
- Methylphenidate (Ritalin)
- Amphetamine, dextroamphetamine mixed salts (Adderall)
- Disulfiram (Antabuse)

Table 26.3 Potential generic problems

- Non-bioequivalence of generic medication may lead to differing blood levels for a specific patient and, therefore, a changed clinical state
- Patient sensitivity to inactive ingredients (e.g., dyes, fillers) in the generic preparation
- Manufacturing/processing problems with the generic (uncommon)

If the clinician does not wish to allow generic substitutions for a brand-name product, the prescription should include the phrase "Dispense as Written" or "DAW" to instruct the pharmacist that a generic drug may not be substituted.

Generic substitution problems

Although most people tolerate generic preparations well, and receive comparable therapeutic effect, when problems do occur with generic substitutions, it is generally because of the reasons listed in Table 26.3.

An issue of concern with a generic versus a branded product is bioequivalence. Two medications are considered bioequivalent if they have the same biological effect in the body at equivalent doses. This is usually determined by equal bioavailability – that is, equal doses of both preparations become equally available to the target tissue in the body. For oral medications, this means that they will be equivalently absorbed from the gut, carried through the bloodstream to the target tissue in similar concentrations and metabolized equally. Preparations that are absorbed more quickly or slowly, transported at significantly different rates, or broken down and excreted at different rates may not be bioequivalent. Differences in any of these steps could result in varying amounts of drug at the tissue site, markedly different peak concentrations of drug, differing clinical response, as well as different levels of side effects.

The definition of what constitutes bioequivalence according to the FDA is somewhat complex, but average differences in drug concentration for generic drugs that gain FDA approval are 3–4 percent in absorption and maximum drug concentration compared to their branded products.

Because each person has variables in his or her gastrointestinal capacity for drug absorption, protein binding in the blood and metabolic capacity, there may occur significant differences in bioavailability and bioequivalence even when the drugs have been officially deemed "bioequivalent." This can occur because the capsule/pill coating or filler is different for the branded and generic products, leading to changed absorption rates or peak drug concentrations. When the amount of drug differs at the site of action, "too little" or "too much" drug effect may occur, and/or new side effects may emerge.

Occasionally a patient has an allergy or adverse effect to an inactive component of the generic, such as a dye, filler or capsule coating.

In the past, on rare occasions, the manufacturing process of a generic drug may have been poorly controlled, resulting in marked variability in the amount of active medication in each pill or, even more rarely, contamination. The most notable example of contamination occurred in the early 1990s. The manufacturing process for tryptophan was contaminated and the resulting medication produced eosinophilia – myalgia in some patients. The current preparations of tryptophan are now totally safe.[4]

Generic change without the clinician's knowledge

Patients may be switched to a generic preparation when the primary clinician is unaware of the change. Such unexpected transitions can occur in the situations listed in Table 26.4.

If a patient begins to experience a change in clinical state, the practitioner should investigate, as one possible reason for the clinical change, whether a new generic drug preparation was given to the patient.

Tips for generic use

When a generic preparation is available and the clinician chooses to prescribe it, some practitioners prefer to start with the generic and titrate blood levels and/or clinical response with the generic medication alone. Other clinicians prefer to start with the

Table 26.4 Common situations when different generics may have been substituted

These could occur when there is:
- A move to a new geographic location
- Admission or discharge from hospital
- Entrance into, or exit from, a nursing care facility or hospice
- A change to a new pharmacy or insurance plan

branded preparation, stabilize the clinical condition and blood level, then switch to a generic at a later date. Either method is valid and clinically responsible.

When prescribing a generic medication, it is useful to suggest that patients continue to receive the same brand of generic preparation throughout the time they continue to take it to minimize any likelihood of differing capsules and fillers that could affect absorption. This may be accomplished by suggesting that they always use the same pharmacy to obtain their generic medication. Get patients to ask the pharmacist to supply the generic from the same manufacturer and report to the clinician if their pills "look different."

If and when a clinician switches a patient from a branded product to a generic, most patients will do well clinically with no significant difference in their clinical state. It is, however, wise to suggest that the patient report any changes in therapeutic effect, or new or increased side effects.

Serum blood levels and generic substitution

When serum blood levels of a medication are available and accurate (see Chapter 25), they can be used to investigate the cause of an altered clinical state or change in side effects when a generic switch is undertaken. The result of a generic serum blood level can be easily compared to a level drawn when taking a branded preparation. A blood level change of greater than 5–10 percent could signify that the amount of drug in the serum is different with the generic preparation, even if the oral dose is the same. While the clinician may not know whether this represents a change in absorption, metabolism or excretion, the oral dose can be relatively easily adjusted to re-establish the previously useful blood serum level. Differences of less than 5 percent in blood level are generally not clinically significant for mental health effects.

If no clinically valid serum blood level test exists and a clinical change occurs when a generic alternative is substituted, the clinician may try to guess whether a larger or smaller oral dose is necessary to re-establish clinical equilibrium. If this procedure is not successful and the patient remains symptomatic, an empirical trial of returning to the branded product may be helpful.

Mandated generics

Some institutions, insurance plans or managed care entities will mandate that the clinician prescribe generic preparations when available. This is usually a cost-saving measure that may, or may not, create a problem for an individual patient. In general, a patient's simple desire to receive a branded product is an insufficient reason for the clinician to insist that the patient receive the branded product. It is usually not useful, or successful, to insist on branded products for all patients and all medications as a general principle. There may, however, be occasions when a clinician will choose to address the use of generics and insist on a branded product for a particular patient. Usually, this is best done after trying the patient on a generic version and documenting a poorer response from the generic product. Clinicians should choose their battles carefully for those patients for whom they feel it is indicated, clinically, to insist on a brand-name product. Information should be documented and reasons outlined when calling the person authorizing such decisions. If there is a particular patient for whom the clinician wishes to have a branded product, a carefully reasoned proposal will usually receive approval.

References

1 Manisses Communications Group (2001) The generic-ization of drugs: will patients benefit? *Psychopharmacology Update* 12(8): 1, 4–5.
2 Mikulic M (2020) Branded vs. generic U.S. drug prescriptions dispensed 2005–2019, available at: https://www.statista.com/statistics/205042/proportion-of-brand-to-generic-prescriptions-dispensed/
3 Shop around before you fill your prescription, available at: www.webmd.com/health-insurance/lower-med-costs-20/shop-around-prescriptions
4 Philen RM (1993) Tryptophan contaminants associated with eosinophilia-myalgia syndrome: the Eosinophilia-Myalgia Studies of Oregon, New York and New Mexico. *American Journal of Epidemiology* 138(3): 154–159.

27 The digital prescriber

- The Internet and the digital revolution   445
- E-mail and the medication prescriber   446
- Texting   449
- A Communications Information Sheet for patients   449
- Electronic medical records (EMRs)   450
- Electronic prescribing and prescriptions   452
- Telepsychiatry – medication management via the computer   453
- Internet-based mental health treatment modalities   454
- Internet-based medication reference and educational information for
  practitioners   455
- Internet medication information for patients   457
- Websites maintained by practitioners for patient information   457
- Data collection, protocols and oversight   459
- Online patient access to medical records   460
- Computer and Internet security   460
- Social media and the prescriber – gold mine or mine field?   461
- The nasty underside of the Internet   463
- Notes and references   464

The Internet and the digital revolution

The age of electronic communication, the Internet and digital information is upon us. Perhaps at no time since the introduction of television has a technological advance more thoroughly and more rapidly integrated itself into our lives. The latest statistics[1] reveal that 5.7 billion individuals worldwide have Internet access, up from 3.4 billion in 2016. The U.S. Federal Communications Commission now states, "Until recently, not having broadband [Internet access] was an inconvenience. Now, broadband is essential to opportunity and citizenship."[2]

Since the first edition of this text, the acceptance of, and uses for, technology in the prescribing process have emerged like a tidal wave. Seen as an interesting adjunct at the beginning of the twenty-first century, interaction via the Internet in some capacity has become virtually essential for the competent, up-to-date prescriber. This chapter will identify the common functions that technology can play in a prescriber's practice and

Table 27.1 Technological functions used by mental health prescribers and their patients

- E-mail
- Texting
- Electronic medical records (EMRs)
- Electronic prescription
- Medication management over the computer (telehealth)
- Computerized mental health treatment modalities
- Internet-based medication database programs for practitioners
- Access to continuing medical education
- Websites maintained by practitioners for patient information
- Internet medication information for patients
- Online patient access to medical records

give details as to appropriate safety, confidentiality and protocol issues for the psychotropic prescriber.

Some clinicians have embraced technology and utilized it for years. Others must be dragged kicking and screaming into the Internet age and are doing so with great reluctance. There is no doubt, however, that younger prescribers trained in the last 10–15 years have grown up with technology as an essential part of day-to-day life. They not only embrace technology, but expect and demand it to be part of their work environment. Many, if not most, practitioners at this time own at least one electronic device with access to the Internet. These devices can be desktop, laptop or tablet computers, so-called "smart phones" and electronic readers, to name a few. The development of hardware to access the vast resources of the Internet is changing rapidly. No doubt there will be considerable evolution of these devices continuously.

More important than hardware, however, are the practical and ever-increasing functional uses for technology in a prescribing environment. Current technological functions used by mental health prescribers are listed in Table 27.1 and will be discussed in more detail throughout this chapter. As with all aspects of technology, new uses are emerging regularly and, in general, the overall usage of technology is increasing exponentially. Many of these functions remain optional and voluntary for both practitioners and patients. That being said, certain of these functions are so valuable and provide such improvement over non-digital methodologies that they are gradually being incentivized to practitioners by regulatory agencies. With time there is likely to be a penalty for not using technology in certain segments of the prescribing process, and ultimately it may well become mandatory.

E-mail and the medication prescriber

The concept of electronic mail, or e-mail, began in the 1960s and standardized protocols for sending e-mails were developed in the 1970s. At that time, however, both sender and recipient needed to be online for successful connection. It was only in the 1980s that e-mail began its inexorable rise to the central form of communication that it is today. The number of people in the developed world who do not have an active e-mail account and do not use it at least to some degree is rapidly diminishing. In addition to its uses for personal communication, it has become a mainstay of interaction between professionals in all walks of life. Many clinicians and prescribers have embraced e-mail as one way to communicate with patients quickly and efficiently. However, there are pitfalls.

The emerging desire of patients and clinicians to use e-mail has several sources. E-mail can be sent and received at any time, day or night. Some patients find that e-mail is a useful way to communicate from their workplace, since they are already at computer terminals for much of the workday. In confined areas where telephone conversations can be overheard, patients may be more comfortable utilizing e-mail. Patients traveling overseas may find e-mail the most convenient way to communicate with a clinician at a distance. Patients with disabilities may have modified computers that allow them ease of use.

Regardless of the clinician's degree of computer sophistication, some decisions about the use of e-mail will need to be made. Depending on how a practice is organized, some practitioners preferentially respond to phone messages and others to e-mail. This preference should be communicated to patients. If the clinician does not wish to use e-mail as a potential medium for communication with patients, the clinician's e-mail address should not be made available. Even so, resourceful patients may find the address through Internet search engines. If the clinician does not wish to communicate via e-mail, he or she must directly indicate this to the patient as part of the "new patient orientation" process and/or office signage.

Even if practitioner-to-patient e-mail is not utilized, prescribers often find it convenient to communicate with other practitioners via e-mail. Assuming the e-mail is secure and there is a signed release from the patient, consultative information, evaluations, medical records, prescriber concerns and laboratory reports can be easily attached to an e-mail and sent quickly to another practitioner involved in the patient's care.

In general, unsecured e-mail presents more risks than benefits for the prescribing clinician in keeping patient matters confidential. *A secure line and/or encryption of e-mails* should be used. Despite using all precautions, communication via e-mail may not be confidential. With increasing frequency, secure e-mail systems are being provided to medical clinicians and this confidentiality issue may gradually diminish, although it will never disappear (see below in the section on "Internet and computer security"). Currently, commercially available e-mail, like many other facets of the Internet, is not confidential, and others may possibly gain access to the content of messages sent to the clinician. This may be of little significance if e-mail is used primarily for scheduling or other non-clinical communication, but rises to an important level if clinical symptoms, medical history, diagnoses, medication names or laboratory results are being transmitted.

Prescribers who utilize e-mail regularly and receive frequent clinical information should ensure regular and automatic backup of their e-mail messages to prevent accidental erasure or loss of data due to computer failure or power outage. Although it may appear to be duplication and somewhat wasteful, in most cases e-mail messages sent to the prescriber from patients that contain clinical material should be printed in hard copy rather than stored solely electronically. While utilization of appropriate computer backup minimizes the likelihood of data loss, it does not solve the problem of convenient access to important clinical information contained in these e-mails, particularly when a patient's medical record is totally or in part maintained in paper form. When a clinician's transition to full electronic medical records is complete, this issue will likely be minimized. Until such time as this occurs in any given prescriber's practice, however, these hard copies should be treated as patient notes and stored in the patient's file. Any responses that the clinician provides through e-mail should also be printed out and kept in the patient's file with other written documentation.

If e-mail is utilized, the clinician will need to decide when, and how often, to read and respond to messages. If patients have come to expect that the clinician will utilize e-mail regularly and/or preferentially, they can also come to expect that the practitioner will check for new messages relatively frequently. At a minimum, clinicians utilizing e-mail regularly should check their inbox once or twice per day personally or through office staff. A check for messages should be done just prior to leaving the office at the end of the workday. The schedule on this should be communicated to the patient to avoid frustration from some patients who expect virtually immediate responses, because that is the way they have come to expect replies from other sources.

Other useful guidelines to practitioners for using e-mail are:

- Maintain a professional e-mail address separate from one's personal e-mail account and conscientiously use only the professional account for work-related communication.
- Limit e-mail responses to 140 words (the length of a Twitter message or several sentences). This prevents patients from asking complicated and involved questions requiring excessively detailed responses. If a communication from a patient requires a response which is longer than 140 words, it is generally best to respond with a telephone call.
- Inform patients that e-mails are not read by the practitioner repeatedly during the day and they should expect no more than one response daily. Some individuals who use technology and "Instant Messaging" frequently expect e-mail to be read and replies given much like a back-and-forth social conversation. Practitioners are virtually never in a position to provide this level of e-mail contact. As above, complicated issues requiring repeated responses or clarification are generally handled more efficiently by telephone.
- E-mail correspondence is notoriously subject to errors of omission, commission and misinterpretation of meaning. It is wise to carefully re-read any e-mail communication to a patient to ensure that it is clear and complete.
- Almost all e-mail programs have the ability to provide "out of office" or "vacation stop" features. When activated, they give a message to the sender that the clinician is not picking up messages. In the same way that a clinician should place an "out of office" message on the telephone, clinicians who are going to be away from the office should utilize this e-mail feature. By doing so, patients will not send e-mail messages, perhaps of an urgent nature, and be unaware that the clinician is not on duty. Some clinicians prefer to include the name and contact information for the covering practitioner in the "out of office" message in case of emergency.
- Certain clinicians, in an effort to avoid repetitive typing, may utilize memorized responses which can easily be inserted as a reply to a particularly common issue or question. While this is neither a positive nor a negative practice, the prescriber should be sure that the final message which is sent to a patient is accurate for that patient, since that message carries the same weight as a face-to-face or telephone response.
- Most e-mail programs have an "auto reply" feature which tells a patient that an e-mail has been received by the practitioner. This is useful for healthcare professionals who utilize e-mail so that the patient will know right away if their message has arrived safely.

Texting

Text messaging on mobile devices, particularly smart phones, has come into wide usage for many reasons. It is fast, easy and can be performed by one hand. The most common format of texting – short message service (SMS) – is, however, not sufficiently safe and secure for a healthcare environment. SMS text messages are sent and stored on servers in plain language text and can be intercepted during transit. It is also possible for SMS messages to be sent to the wrong number unbeknownst to the sender. Likewise, there is no notification from the recipient as to whether the message was read or even received. While texting has become almost universal among younger practitioners and has virtually substituted for phone calling, it is best reserved for personal communications to friends and family. Privileged health information (PHI) should never be given through a text message.

A Communications Information Sheet for patients

The advice that most practitioners routinely have given to patients – namely, "Call the office if you have any problems" – is no longer adequate in the twenty-first century. With the advent of the Internet and e-mail, both the patient and practitioner have a choice of methodologies by which to communicate. Each clinician and healthcare office will have different needs and electronic availability. It should not be assumed that the patient will automatically know how the practitioner wishes to be contacted given today's choices.

Once the practitioner has decided how he/she wishes to maintain communication with patients, it is important to put this information in writing for the patient in a "Communications Information Sheet" that can be given to the patient at the first visit. By doing so, the practitioner will save time, avoid future confusion and potentially even avoid a malpractice suit. We are almost certain to see future lawsuits based on the following two statements:

- "Doctor, I sent you an e-mail about that serious problem, but you didn't reply."
- "The nurse practitioner in this case did not inform my client that e-mail messages between them were not confidential."

A sample "Communications Information Sheet":

To my patients:

During your treatment with me, it is important that we are able to communicate effectively. This information sheet will describe how and when to best communicate with me and my staff.

The office telephone number is … The office is open between the hours of 8 a.m. and 4:30 p.m. Monday through Friday except holidays. We will make every effort to answer your call in person during those hours. However, if you do not make contact with one of the staff in person, the recorded message will tell you what to do in the event of an emergency. Please do not leave emergency messages at this number. You may, however, leave information about routine matters such as appointment requests, appointment changes and billing questions on the recording and your call will be returned later that day.

I also do utilize e-mail to communicate with patients about routine matters. The office e-mail address is ... Although I make every effort to securely and confidentially handle e-mail messages, please be aware that at present, information sent to me via e-mail is **NOT SECURE**. Please do not send or expect return messages that contain sensitive or privileged information such as diagnoses, medication names, laboratory test results or potentially embarrassing symptomatology. A good rule of thumb is that no e-mail message should contain information that you would not feel comfortable saying loudly in a busy waiting room. Please limit the length of any e-mails to several sentences (about the length of this paragraph). If your message or inquiry is longer than this, please contact the office by phone.

I or my staff will retrieve and respond to e-mail twice a day, usually at the beginning and end of the workday. E-mail is not retrieved on weekends, holidays or after hours and I am unable to respond to more than one e-mail message per day.

Dr. Johnson

Alternatively, the third paragraph could be worded:

I do utilize e-mail to communicate with patients. The office e-mail address is ... Although the e-mail server utilized by the office is deemed secure, all transmissions through the Internet have at least some security vulnerability. Please be aware of this when deciding what information to transmit by e-mail.

Or:

I regret that I do not utilize e-mail or text messages for clinical issues. Although I realize that some people are accustomed to using e-mail routinely, I cannot, for a variety of reasons, use this modality in a secure and efficient way in my practice. Please use the telephone to contact me or my staff regarding clinical issues.

As with telephone calls, some patients may prefer to ask for prescription renewal via e-mail rather than by face-to-face interactions and follow-up meetings. If such requests become a pattern, it is recommended that the clinician does not provide renewals via these requests, since e-mail is one additional step removed from the patient than the telephone. Without voice and other behavioral signs and signals, it is even more difficult to accurately assess the patient's current state. If repeated prescription refills are provided with only e-mail contact, it is generally considered substandard practice.

Some unscrupulous clinicians have offered to prescribe medications for patients over the Internet without any face-to-face evaluation whatever. Usually this is an attempt to establish a high-volume prescription-writing business with profit as a motive. This practice is unacceptable and represents poor clinical care. A prescription written for medication constitutes a therapeutic relationship, and all the legal liabilities which accompany this relationship are in force. The clinician who prescribes without any face-to-face patient contact takes on serious legal risk.

Electronic medical records (EMRs)

The call for computerization of medical records into an electronic form – EMR (sometimes referred to as an electronic health record or EHR) – has been heard for several decades. Expected advantages of a transition to the use of an EMR are listed in Table 27.2.

Although many of these likely improvements are espoused by practitioners and regulatory bodies alike, the transition to an EMR has been spotty and slower than expected until recently. In the beginning in the United States, only one mega-organization, the U.S. Department of Veterans Affairs, mandates the use of electronic records in all its hospitals and clinics. Additionally, electronic health records are utilized in integrated medical groups such as Kaiser Permanente, the Mayo Clinic, the Cleveland Clinic, University of Pittsburgh Medical Center and other large organizations which have been able to bear the costs of start-up. At the time of this publication, 85.9% of all medical practices are utilizing an electronic record.[3]

The reasons for a rather slow implementation of EMRs were many – some institutional and some individual. Large-scale roadblocks include lack of a standardized protocol, lack of collaboration between competing EMR provider groups and the cost of implementation. Through financial and other incentives and sanctions, primarily through Medicare and Medicaid, such roadblocks have been overcome and EMRs have now become virtually routine.

In the UK, there has been an ongoing project to upload all of the medical records from the National Health Service (NHS) into a centralized databank. Originally scheduled to be completed in 2006, 25 million records had been uploaded as of 2010. Fifty million were scheduled to be uploaded by 2014 and the project was completed in the latter half of the decade.

The European Commission aimed to enable all Europeans to have access to online medical records anywhere in Europe by 2020. With the newly enacted Directive 2011/24/EU on Patients' Rights in Cross-border Healthcare due for implementation by 2013, a centralized European health record system is now a reality.

Table 27.2 Expected advantages of linked, computerized electronic medical records

---

- Overall improvement in the quality of healthcare through improved care coordination
- Increasing storage capabilities for longer periods of time
- Speed of access at multiple sites simultaneously
- Continuous updating possible
- Ability to provide medical alerts and reminders
- Built-in intelligence capabilities which can recognize abnormal lab results or potential life-threatening drug interactions
- Linking of the clinician to protocols, care plans, critical paths, literature databases, pharmaceutical information and other sites of professional knowledge
- Customized views of information relevant to the needs of different specialties allowing users to design and utilize reporting formats tailored to their special needs
- Decreased charting time and charting errors, therefore increasing the productivity of healthcare workers
- Decreased medical errors due to illegible notes
- Providing more accurate billing information which will allow providers to submit their claims electronically and receive payment more rapidly
- Increased patient empowerment to take a more active role in their health and in the health of their families by receiving electronic copies of their medical records and sharing their health information securely over the Internet with their families

---

Source: Advantages and disadvantages of the Electronic Medical Record, available at: www.aameda.org/MemberServices/Exec/Articles/spg04/Gurley%20article.pdf

Although individual prescribers may make a shift to Electronic Medical Records on their own, more often than not, the decision to implement an EMR is fueled by institutional and group practice policy. For mental health prescribers who do wish to implement EMRs, two criteria become important in choosing a system:

- choosing an EMR system which is specifically designed for mental health professionals since many generalized EMR systems match poorly with mental health needs
- in the United States, choosing an EMR program which is certified for what the government has called "meaningful use," thereby qualifying for the Medicare/Medicaid incentives noted above.

There are now many systems that meet both of these criteria:[4]

Electronic prescribing and prescriptions

This section covers two different, but related, entities. The first and simplest involves the printing and generation of prescriptions by a computer. This does not require Internet access and can be performed from a standalone computer with a printer in a prescriber's office. Using appropriate software (see below), the prescriber can enter and store information about specific patients, which, on command, can generate paper prescriptions for signature. While not as advantageous as the second methodology below, creating prescriptions in this way does have advantages over handwritten prescriptions. For patients who regularly need a long list of medications, renewal prescriptions can be printed quickly, accurately and legibly.

In setting up such a program, the prescriber should ensure that all necessary information is routinely included in the software template for a prescription. The prescriber is usually guided through this process by the software. Required information includes the patient's first and last name, current address, date of birth and the prescriber's name should be printed at the bottom of the prescription. In general, the software has a database of currently available branded and generic medications, formulations and dosage strengths which allows the prescriber to select the appropriate choices for a particular patient. Assuming the same computer is routinely used, these data are remembered for further renewals of prescriptions written for any one patient. A current active medication list for each patient is also generated and summary data for any one specific medication or any one prescribing date can easily be obtained.

The second methodology, which is more appropriately called electronic prescribing or "e-prescribing," has become much more common in twenty-first-century prescribing. It requires access to the Internet and cannot be performed by a standalone computer. It includes the advantages mentioned above for computer-generated paper prescriptions, but adds considerably more benefit. Specifically, e-prescribing supports:

- electronically transmitted prescription information to community or mail-order pharmacies, decreasing the time in which the medication is received by the patient, thus potentially increasing adherence
- multiple safety checks including automated prompts that offer information on the drug being prescribed, potential inappropriate dose or route of administration, drug–drug interactions, allergy concerns, warnings or cautions

- information can be provided related to the availability of lower-cost, therapeutically appropriate alternatives (if any)
- information on formulary or tiered formulary medications, patient eligibility and authorization requirements are received electronically from the patient's drug plan
- availability of the patient's medical and medication history from all providers at the time of prescribing
- reduced time spent on phone calls, call-backs and faxing prescriptions to pharmacies
- greater prescriber mobility including prescribing from multiple office sites or from remote locations using mobile devices
- improved drug surveillance/recall ability

To facilitate the transition to e-prescribing, the U.S. government has provided an incentive plan if a "qualified" electronic prescribing system is utilized and specific criteria are fulfilled. Incentives and disincentives have been provided to the prescriber or practice. The details can be accessed at the Centers for Medicare and Medicaid Services (CMS) website at www.cms.gov/ERxIncentive/

For all the reasons outlined above, similar measures to encourage and implement electronic prescribing are being undertaken in the UK and across Europe. As of 2018, 18 European countries had electronic prescribing and three more pilot programs in process.[5]

Telepsychiatry – medication management via the computer

Perhaps the most revolutionary electronic function in mental health prescribing is the advantage and common acceptance of conducting all medical appointments in all specialties via the computer. The practitioner and the patient can see one another electronically and hear each other's voice. Via the computer, completion of every aspect of the medication management process is possible even though the prescriber and the patient are in different locations. There is virtually no aspect of the procedures described in the rest of this text that cannot be successfully undertaken via the Internet with currently available hardware and software. Whether it is an initial medication evaluation, follow-up sessions which may or may not include psychotherapy, consultations or the provision of prescriptions, there is an available methodology to accomplish each task. For the purposes of this section, we will refer to this process as "telepsychiatry" (the mental health equivalent of "telemedicine").

Prior to 2020, there were already practical uses of telepsychiatry such as the necessity to interact with patients who may be in a rural setting where practitioners are scarce, or where patients lack transportation to reach the prescriber in person. Telepsychiatry can also be useful in more efficiently treating patients with disabilities where transport to the prescriber's office is a significant hardship. This use of the Internet has also permitted specialty consultation on difficult medication problems where an "expert" can both interact with a patient and discuss the patient with a clinician in a remote location. For other practitioners, telepsychiatry has been used solely for the convenience and/or preference of the prescriber or patient. There is no doubt, however, that with the worldwide pandemic secondary to COVID-19, telemedicine in general and telepsychiatry in particular have mushroomed. The risks of contracting this highly contagious virus have led many practitioners and many patients to utilize telepsychiatry for its ability to maintain the health of all practitioners and patients. Many people now assume that telepsychiatry is firmly entrenched in our society and will continue to be used when the pandemic is under control.

With the proliferation of broadband, high-speed Internet connections, the distance between practitioner and patient makes little difference. The patient can be halfway around the block or halfway around the world. With computer access available in almost all countries, this methodology also opens the possibility for patients to have an "appointment" with their practitioner while on vacation, on work-related trips or when they are temporarily relocated to another country.

While some practitioners may initially feel a lack of personal contact using telepsychiatry, almost all providers have become comfortable with this methodology. The patient's body movements, gestures, voice inflections, eye contact and other cues on which the practitioner relies are both seen and heard via the computer. Nonetheless, practitioners may choose to avoid telepsychiatry with some patients. Unless there is absolutely no other way to have therapeutic contact, profoundly psychotic patients, who may become delusional about electronic equipment, and patients who are acutely intoxicated on drugs or alcohol should be seen face to face.

The hardware and software setup to accomplish telepsychiatry can be elaborate and expensive, or relatively simple and inexpensive. Institutions such as university departments of psychiatry, the U.S. Department of Veterans Affairs, large hospitals or mental health centers often set aside specific rooms and equipment for telemedicine. Such institutions will have access to specialists in information technology to set up the camera, Internet connection and software at both the "home" site as well as the "remote" site where patients come. With the software described below, however, an individual practitioner with an Internet-connected laptop or desktop computer and a camera can achieve virtually the same outcome at a modest cost.

The software necessary for this form of interaction is not specific to telepsychiatry and can be any of a number of programs which produce video telephone calls or "video chat" via the Internet. Most of these software programs can be downloaded free of charge and the video phone calls are also free of charge, apart from the data subscription costs. A partial list of commonly used services includes:

> Zoom (https://zoom.us)
> Skype (www.skype.com/intl/en-us/home)
> Google video chat (http://mail.google.com/videochat)
> Windows Live Messenger (https://windows_live_messenger.en.downloadastro.com/ and other sites)

Internet-based mental health treatment modalities

In addition to Internet-based prescribing and medication management, other mental health treatment has begun to be offered over the Internet and via computer-based programs. It is the most complex and controversial use of the computer in mental health where the computer essentially replaces the psychotherapist.[6] A variety of diagnostic and therapeutic techniques have been modified to be utilized via the computer. It is likely that many more will appear in the coming years. Proponents as well as critics have voiced strong opinions about the use of computer-based psychotherapy without a live therapist. It is clear that considerable research will be necessary to evaluate the ultimate usefulness of these techniques in general, and their advantages or disadvantages when compared with person-to-person interactions. A sampling of computer-based psychotherapeutic treatment which prescribers may recommend in addition to medication includes:

- cognitive behavioral therapy for obsessive–compulsive disorder (OCD)[7–8] and depression[9–10]
- virtual reality (simulated real environments through digital media) to treat post-traumatic stress disorder (PTSD) and phobias[11]
- computer games to provide therapy for adolescents[12]
- use of cell phones for peer support.[13]

Internet-based medication reference and educational information for practitioners

Use of a computer and access to the Internet provides a rich and almost unlimited source of professional information for the prescriber. Whether in a consultation room, in the professional's office, on a hospital ward, in the emergency department, at home or when traveling, the prescriber can easily access specific information about particular psychotropics including doses, side effects, medication interactions, indications and risk factors.

Although some medication database lists are free, the most comprehensive and clinically useful software programs, which include much more information than simply medication names and dosages, are fee-based. Some of the most popular and well-used database sites include:

> Pubmed (https://pubmed.ncbi.nlm.nih.gov/
> Epocrates (www.epocrates.com)
> The Cochrane Medical Library (www.cochranelibrary.com/search?cookiesEnabled)
> Medline Plus (https://medlineplus.gov/)

In addition to these medication-related databases, the prescriber now also has rapid and simple access to ongoing continuing professional education. With the use of a laptop, tablet, desktop computer or a mobile device, the prescriber can read, watch or listen to a variety of educational presentations focused on specific diagnoses, medications, therapies or other topics of interest to the mental health practitioner. In some cases, the practitioner can log-in to a live presentation by an authoritative expert using video and/or audio methodologies. In these real-time presentations there is often the opportunity for questioning the expert on concerns or areas of interest. Many times, these live presentations are saved so that the practitioner can obtain them in their entirety at a later date or a more convenient time. In addition, there are large numbers of print educational offerings available on the Internet, many of which are certified for credit as Continuing Medical Education. These offerings are presented by a variety of authoritative sources including:

- professional Mental Health Associations
- medical education agencies such as Medscape (www.medscape.com) and
- CMEWebMD (www.reliasmedia.com/CMEweb)
- Practicing Clinicians Exchange for Nurses (PCE) (www.practicingclinicians.com/) and Nursing CEU (www.nurseceu.com/)

- hospitals
- prestigious educational institutions, including universities, medical and nursing schools
- governmental and regulatory agencies.

Search engines to find upcoming educational conferences include:
  In the United States:

> www.medical.theconferencewebsite.com/index4.php
> www.doctorsreview.com/meetings/
> www.laboure.edu/blog/nursing-conferences
> www.allconferences.com/Health/Nursing/

In the UK:

> www.emedevents.com/uk-medical-conferences
> www.rsm.ac.uk/
> www.rcn.org.uk/newsevents/events
> www.nursing-events.co.uk/

Prescribers of psychotropic medications should consider themselves on a life-long learning curve. With the advent of new medications, new treatments and new uses for various medications, clinicians will need to educate themselves continually in order to remain expert.

To maintain this level of currency, the practitioner should read psychopharmacology journals in print or online. Although there are many useful texts, some particularly helpful journals with direct prescriptive applicability include:

- *Biological Therapies in Psychiatry* (Gelenberg Consulting & Publishing LLC, PO Box 42650, Tucson, AZ; https://ascpp.org/resources/psychiatry-resource/journal-of-clinical-psychiatry/Biological Therapies in Psychiatry)
- In the UK, *The Maudsley Prescribing Guidelines*[14] provides yearly updated medication recommendations by disease entity, and contains a wealth of additional information. American prescribers should strongly consider obtaining an electronic or print copy of this book since the vast majority of information included is applicable to American practice, and there are few comprehensive, annually updated psychotropic medication guides in the United States.
- *Clinical Handbook of Psychotropic Drugs*[15] is in book format but is updated quarterly to remain current with new information.
- The journal of the American Psychiatric Association (*American Journal of Psychiatry*) also provides good research information and review articles.
- *Journal of Psychopharmacology* (http://jop.sagepub.com/).
- *Journal of Clinical Psychopharmacology* (http://journals.lww.com/psychopharmacology/pages/default.aspx).
- *JAMA Psychiatry* (formerly *The Archives of General Psychiatry*) (https://jamanetwork.com/).
- *The British Journal of Psychiatry* (http://bjp.rcpsych.org/).

In general, mental health nurse practitioners who prescribe will find specific psycho-pharmacology journals or psychiatric journals more helpful and comprehensive than nursing journals for prescribing information.

In the first edition of this text, 18 years ago, two references were cited which purported to give all the essential websites useful for the mental health professional.[16–17] One was already over 500 pages long! At the rate the Internet is growing, such books could easily be the size of a small encyclopedia!

Rather than attempt to provide a list of all possible mental health/prescribing/ medication websites here, the reader should utilize any of the following general and mental health-related search engines to find articles, references, books and data on a specific psychopharmacological topic:

- National Institute of Mental Health (NIMH), www.nimh.nih.gov/index.shtml
- American Academy of Child and Adolescent Psychiatry (AACAP), www.aacap. org/
- Medscape Psychiatry News, www.medscape.com/psychiatry
- *American Journal of Psychiatry*, http://ajp.psychiatryonline.org
- SAMHSA, The Substance Abuse and Mental Health Services Administration, www.samhsa.gov/
- *Journal of the American Medical Association* (JAMA), http://jama.ama-assn.org
- University of Iowa Family Practice Health Library, www.uihealthcare.org/
- American Association of Family Practice, www.aafp.org/
- Mayo Clinic Health Information, www.mayoclinic.com/patient-care-and-health-information
- MedlinePlus, www.nlm.nih.gov/medlineplus/

Internet medication information for patients

Beyond the information provided to clinicians, the Internet is a rich source of information for patients, provided that patients are prompted to use the Internet wisely. Many patients, unfortunately, do not adequately differentiate accurate, factual sites from sites with a bias or slant that may make the information therein suspect. When it comes to medications, patients may unfortunately assume that anything "in print" and published on the Internet is valid, and applies to them. Therefore, guidelines are necessary to help patients use this treasure trove of information selectively and effectively.

Websites maintained by practitioners for patient information

Practitioner-designed Internet websites now serve multiple functions for prescribers and patients. In their simplest form, they have supplanted the telephone "Yellow Pages" for many consumers and professionals alike. Accessible with a few keystrokes, websites can be easily constructed to provide practice location, hours, specialties, fees, the practitioner's educational background and other information about him/her and the office. In addition, the prescriber may choose to upload educational information about particular diagnoses, medications or instructions (for example, the procedure for obtaining an accurate psychotropic blood level, or a list of competent authoritative websites that could be used by patients who are pregnant and considering psychotropic medication).

While a website design professional could be employed to construct a practitioner-specific or group-specific website, it is no longer necessary to do so. There are many easy-to-use, free, customizable website design software programs which can be downloaded from the Internet and utilized successfully by practitioners with even limited computer skills. In some cases, the website may be maintained free of charge for an indefinite period. In other cases, the practitioner must pay a monthly or yearly fee to keep the website up and running. In any case, it is relatively simple to change or update information as needed. A sampling of popular programs for website construction includes:

- Blogger from Google (www.blogger.com/home)
- Open Software Design (www.oswd.org/)
- Net Objects Fusion (http://netobjects.com/html/essentials.html)

Whether on a personal or professional website, many individuals have started "blogs" (an abbreviation for "web logs"). Blogs are easy to construct, can be written about any topic and can contain pictures or videos. Many individuals find it refreshing to express their experiences, beliefs and opinions in written form.

When the blog is started as part of a professional website, the practitioner must be aware what blog content is appropriate and professional, and what material is not. On the other hand, if a blog was opened for purely personal reasons and targeted toward friends and family, some material may have been recorded which the prescriber would prefer that patients or colleagues do not see. As with the cautions detailed later in this chapter on using social media, all practitioners should be aware that Internet search engines have considerable ability to find documents related to a particular practitioner's name. Once published on the Internet, a blog will generally be easy to discover by anyone doing a simple search.

A handout to patients left in the waiting room, such as the following, can be helpful.

Box 27.1 Talking to patients

"There are ever-increasing numbers of sites on the Internet that seek to give information about mental health problems, medications, possible side effects and general health/medical issues. In general, I am supportive of you having information about your treatment and any medications that you are taking. Some sites are quite helpful and informative, while others contain opinions without adequate factual backup, biased information disguised as "fact" and, occasionally, information that is simply inaccurate. Even solid, authoritative sites may present data or mention side effects that are highly unlikely, or will not apply.

Here are some tips on assessing the possible usefulness of Internet sites:

- Your "search engine" results do not guarantee quality.
- Just because information is "in print" on a website says nothing about its accuracy, or relevance to you, even if it appears authoritative, colorful and appealing to the eye.
- Even sites allegedly "sponsored" by official-sounding organizations may be biased.

- Who sponsors the site? Most reliable sites are sponsored by those with credible credentials, including medical and nursing associations, hospitals, medical centers and accredited schools of medicine and nursing.
- Is the information factual or opinion?
  - Does the site have a vested interest? Does it attempt to get you to buy a product or service? This is usually a sign of possible bias.
- How current is the information? When was it last updated? The date of the most recent revision should be clearly evident on the site, usually at the bottom. Sites that are the most accurate and medically valid are updated regularly, but even recent updates may not necessarily guarantee quality content.
- What is the privacy policy? How does the site treat any personal information given?
- If the site offers the services of a healthcare provider or group, what are their credentials? Can you verify them?
- Competent mental health treatment is not assured by a "professional looking" website.
- Pure and authentic medications are not sold at bargain basement prices. You get what you pay for.
- If a site offers to sell medications without a prescription or face-to-face evaluation, go elsewhere. The site is at best low quality, and at worst fraudulent and/or illegal.

PLEASE DO NOT MAKE ANY CHANGES IN YOUR TREATMENT REGIMEN OR THE MEDICINES THAT I PRESCRIBE FOR YOU BASED ON INTERNET INFORMATION WITHOUT DISCUSSING THE ISSUE WITH ME FIRST."

Data collection, protocols and oversight

One of the less direct but significant effects of EMRs and electronic prescriptions is the ability to track prescribing trends for specific medications and specific practitioners. A corollary trend is to utilize specific protocols for treatment and medication prescription (for example, in certain payer systems, the patient must have failed drugs X and Y before drug Z can be prescribed). The use of protocols has multiple supporting rationales including attempts to standardize treatment and ensure that effective treatment techniques are not overlooked. It is also true, however, that some protocols are primarily instituted for financial reasons to require generic or cheaper medications to be tried before more expensive ones are utilized.

Not all prescribers and clinicians feel positively about increased oversight and data collection in their practice. Some practitioners hold strongly to the concept that treatment and prescribing decisions are to be made solely between clinician and patient within the confines of the consultation room. "Big Brother" should not be looking over one's shoulder. The advent of electronic medical records has not initiated this oversight process; it merely has made data collection significantly more streamlined, rapid and real-time. Managed care entities, third-party payers and regulatory agencies have long had the ability to observe clinician prescribing patterns. This allows the truly negligent and/or fraudulent prescriber to be more easily identified from prescribing data. Such clinicians can be watched more closely or placed on performance improvement plans.

Regardless of one's personal viewpoint on the issue of prescriber oversight, it is highly likely that as electronic records and prescriptions become the rule rather than the exception, we can expect more rather than less oversight.

The ability to scan, sort and accumulate data from electronic prescribing will also produce useful, evidence-based information for all practitioners. As we are better able to measure patient improvement, medication choices will be tied to the extent of therapeutic outcome. Useful data can be gathered which will help elucidate future treatment decisions that will have a solid evidence basis.

Online patient access to medical records

In recent years, as access to one's medical records has come to be seen as a right rather than a privilege, there has been a progressive movement to allow patients easy access to their medical charts. The move to electronic medical records will permit a significant improvement in the ease with which patients (or patients' families, when permitted to do so) can view their records. Virtually all of the EMR systems mentioned earlier in this chapter allow a patient free online access to his/her medical records, prescriptions and appointment times.

In the UK, patients are currently required to ask their general practitioner (GP) for permission to view their records and provide a valid reason for doing so. Access to all medical records from the NHS is free and one's practitioner must allow access. Instructions can be found at: www.nhs.uk/using-the-nhs/about-the-nhs/how-to-access-your-health-records/

Computer and Internet security

The issue of data security in the age of computers and the Internet has been a major and ongoing concern for virtually all who use them. Despite a large and ever-growing industry solely dedicated to the security of computer data and equipment, transmitted information of all kinds can be accessed inappropriately and unlawfully. Hardly a month goes by that a major database of financial, commercial, credit card or other data is not "hacked into" by sophisticated computer thieves. Medical data are no different. No matter what sophisticated security measures are put in place, one should assume that computer data are not fully secure and private.

Some healthcare professionals deal with this issue by refusing to use computers for any professional healthcare purpose, feeling that this ensures the security of patient data. While this prevents computer "hacking," multiple ways still exist for the loss of paper and oral patient information. Despite the risks, most practitioners have moved or are moving to utilization of the computer in their professional practice. Although an individual prescriber or group practice cannot fully eliminate sophisticated computer intrusion into a medical database, there are simple and necessary security precautions that all practitioners should take. These include:

- Double-password protect any computers that contain patient data (i.e., two steps must be used to enter the site).

- When leaving a desk or work site even briefly, turn the computer off so that other individuals cannot view sensitive data. This also obviously applies when leaving the office at the end of the day.
- Be sure to carry any mobile devices that contain medical information on your person and guard them carefully.
- Do not access medical data when using "public" wireless connections such as in airports, meeting spaces, coffee shops, stores or commercial offices. When doing so, nearby individuals with mobile devices may have access to these data.
- As mentioned below, do not post privileged healthcare information (PHI) on public websites including social media unless specific consent has been given by the patient.

Social media and the prescriber – gold mine or mine field?

The technological advances discussed in this chapter are of significant assistance to the prescriber when used safely and professionally. Social media sites, while enjoying worldwide popularity, contain as many risks as advantages for the clinician. Although the term continues to evolve, "social media" currently refers to forms of electronic communication on the Internet through which users create online communities to share information, ideas, personal messages and other content such as pictures and videos. Such media are epitomized by the current giants of social connectedness – Facebook, LinkedIn, Instagram, Snapchat, Pinterest, Reddit and Twitter – but include many other groups such as YouTube, Myspace and Medscape Physician Connect. It is unreasonable to expect that healthcare professionals will exempt themselves from this worldwide social phenomenon. Clear thinking is necessary, however, to assure that this powerful force is used positively and with minimal risk to one's professional status.

First and foremost, a prescriber should decide if the use of social media is desirable at all. From a professional perspective, utilizing the other methodologies in this chapter provides many of the benefits of the digital age without entering social media groups. If the prescriber does decide to participate in social media, the clinician should be clear as to his/her purpose in using these sites. There are four common reasons to use social media, each of which bears elaboration:

- social – to connect an individual to friends, family or others who have common interests
- professional – to connect the practitioner to the general public
- professional – to establish peer-to-peer communication regarding professional matters
- professional – to establish and/or maintain clinician–patient communication.

In general, the use of social media primarily entails individuals wishing to use the Internet to *maintain social contact with people they know* or who are important to them. If a clinician wishes to do this, he/she should establish a personal account under his/her personal name which is separate from any professional account which may be established. For privacy purposes, some clinicians use a pseudonym or nickname. Even when doing so, it is important to remember that with the extensive capabilities of Internet search engines, it is quite easy for patients, colleagues and potential employers to find and access a clinician's personal accounts on social media sites. We have already entered an age in which pictures, writings, opinions and other items attributable to us – our so-called "digital footprint" – exist in cyberspace essentially indefinitely. Postings and pictures/videos which may have been thought to be cute, witty, endearing, sexy or sassy may come back to haunt practitioners at a later time. There is simply nothing positive that can be gained if other professional or patient contacts see insensitive comments, risqué photos or off-color jokes from a present or past time. Professionals, therefore, should be particularly careful about the text or pictures that are posted to any personal accounts within a social media site.

Some clinicians may wish to use social media to *broadcast information about their practice and gain visibility within the community*. Not unlike advertising in the telephone book "Yellow Pages," practitioners can describe specialty professional interests, familiarity with specific treatment modalities, therapeutic techniques and business practices. When doing this, the prescriber should set up a specific business/practice account on a social media modality separate from any personal accounts.

Individual practitioners or practice groups may choose to make videos regarding clinical procedures or patient teaching which can be more successfully shown in video format than in text. When appropriate, such videos may be posted to a video site such as YouTube for ease of accessibility. Several professional organizations routinely upload videos showing a variety of patient education topics.

Additionally, some professionals may seek to set up formal electronic "discussions" between patients and/or non-patients about specific disease entities, treatment modalities, medications or other topics. While this conceivably may provide a service to some patients, the clinician should be aware that any comments that he/she makes on such a "discussion board" or "Chat Room" can be construed as medical advice and subject to all the obligations entailed when advising patients. There are many existing discussion groups and "bulletin boards" maintained by professional and non-professional groups that already serve the same purpose. It is often better for prescribers to refer patients to those sites rather than attempt to duplicate them.

Practitioners can utilize the worldwide reach of social media sites *to communicate with other professionals* about matters of mutual clinical interest. Now with the click of a mouse, clinicians can make contact with practitioners throughout the globe in ways that were unthinkable in the past. It is generally more secure and more focused when undertaking this type of communication to utilize professionally focused social media sites such as LinkedIn, Sermo or Medscape Physician Connect.

Clinicians who choose to use social media for specific *clinician–patient communication* should be exceptionally cautious as it is easy to violate legal or ethical privacy considerations mandated by the Health Insurance Portability and Accountability Act (HIPAA) and state laws. The simple act of accepting a "friend request" likely would not constitute an adequate consent to the disclosure of patient information under HIPAA and other state privacy laws. Without patient consent, healthcare providers should not use social media to share health information that could be linked to an individual patient, such as names, pictures and physical descriptions. It is best in general that a medication practitioner does *not* seek such consent to utilize social media for this purpose. Individual e-mails between the clinician and patient are considerably more secure and appropriate for the exchange of clinical information than social media, although as mentioned above, they too are not totally secure. Healthcare organizations which maintain a presence on a social media network should ensure that they have policies covering what information can or cannot be shared by their employees on a social media site.

Any clinician who chooses to interact with patients on a social media site should also be able to clearly distinguish between "medical data" and protected/privileged health information (PHI). Information that patients collect about themselves is simply "medical data." However, once a patient *shares* that information with a clinician, it becomes PHI. The clinician is required to safeguard PHI information and can share it with others only after receiving permission from the patient.

The take-home message for prescribers is that the use of social media for direct communication with patients is littered with pitfalls and potential legal hazards. Given that there are other ways for clinicians and patients to communicate electronically, most practitioners should be hesitant to use social media outlets to communicate with patients.

The nasty underside of the Internet

As exciting and almost miraculous as the introduction of the computer and the Internet have been to the practice of prescribing mental health medications, the advent of the Internet has also spawned inappropriate, illegal and dangerous uses with which the practitioner needs to be familiar. Three old adages still remain true:

- There is no such thing as a free lunch.
- If it seems too good to be true, it probably is.
- You get what you pay for.

With the ease of constructing a glamorous, professional-looking website, substandard and even unlicensed practitioners can promote themselves to patients on the Internet. No matter what the text of a website reads, and how polished it may look, mere publication does not automatically confer accuracy or truth. The Internet is unregulated and virtually anyone can put up a website offering any mental health service including prescription. The recommendations cited above for patients when they are seeking authoritative *medication* sites on the Internet also apply when deciding to use an *online practitioner*. Patients should be encouraged to seek documentation of professional qualifications, membership in professional organizations, any reported instances of substandard care and, when possible, direct patient comments from others who have dealt with this practitioner. Many times, substandard practitioners will utilize audio chat or real-time text chat rather than video interaction. It is virtually impossible for a patient to determine by voice or typing alone whether this is a practitioner who is qualified and professional or a fraud sitting in a dimly lit basement in their pajamas. While there are useful treatment resources available on the Internet, patients should maintain a healthy dose of skepticism when utilizing online resources.

Of particular concern is the prescriber who offers to provide medication for an online patient without any face-to-face meeting. Often such providers require only cursory medical history from the patient and are willing to provide a prescription of any medication for a fee. *High-quality practitioners do not prescribe psychotropic medications for a patient without at least an initial in-person visit.*

A final caveat for patients using the Internet is the possibility of counterfeit medications being provided by an online pharmaceutical source. Recent estimates suggest that global sales of counterfeit medications are reaching more than $75 billion, doubling in the 5 years between 2005 and 2010.[18] While any medicine or class of medicines can be counterfeit, often there will be a sudden increase in medicines to treat a new or well-publicized illness (e.g., the recent spate of medications to treat COVID-19). Such medication bought from an unverified Internet site can lack the active ingredients claimed, have distinctly variable amounts of the active ingredient or, in some cases, contain dangerous materials or toxins. A UK study of 96 websites selling painkillers found that 76 percent of these sites were offering to provide medication without a prescription. Similarly, a U.S. study of 159 sites offering controlled substances showed that 85 percent of the sites did not require a prescription. In the UK, it has been reported that 33 percent of the physicians surveyed said they had "treated" or "likely treated" a patient for side effects of substandard medications purchased online.[19]

In addition to recommending that patients use mainstream, well-known and verifiable sources to obtain medication, they should be encouraged to disregard any e-mail solicitations to purchase medications. Competent, above-board suppliers of medication do not send out mass e-mails soliciting patients. These e-mails are virtually always from questionable pharmaceutical sources. Any Internet pharmacy offering medications without a prescription provided by a licensed provider is suspect. Medications offered at substantial price discounts are also worrisome. "If it seems to be too good to be true, it usually is."

For reasons of cost or availability, some patients choose to get prescriptions filled by pharmacies outside the United States or the UK. There are reputable pharmaceutical providers in other countries that may, because of national law, be able to sell certain brand-name medications cheaply or have access to certain medications that are not available within one's country of residence. As with any online medication supplier, references should be checked. Medications sold at "cut rate" prices are likely to be counterfeit.

Notes and references

1 *Report U.S. Media Trends by Demographic*, available at: www.nielsen.com/us/en/insights/article/2012/report-u-s-media-trends-by-demographic/
2 FCC (2010) National Broadband Plan, available at: www.broadband.gov/plan/1-introduction/
3 National Electronic Health Records Survey (2017) Percentage of office-based physicians using any electronic health record (EHR)/electronic medical record (EMR) system and physicians that have a certified EHR/EMR system, by U.S. state; see also: When patients fear EHR, available at: www.informationweek.com/healthcare/electronic-health-records/when-patients-fear-ehr/a/d-id/1297519
4 Where can I find a list of HER products that have been certified or certified EHRs?, available at: www.healthit.gov/faq/where-can-i-find-list-ehr-products-have-been-certified-or-certified-ehrs; Frentz DA and Carlat D (2011) Which electronic health record should you buy? A review of three products. *Carlat Report 9*, December 12.
5 The state of national electronic prescription systems in the EU with special consideration given to interoperability issues, available at: www.sciencedirect.com/science/article/abs/pii/S1386505620302367?via%3Dihub
6 Cavanagh K and Shapiro DA (2004) Computer treatment for common mental health problems. *Journal of Clinical Psychology* 60(3): 239–251.
7 Andersson E *et al.* (2011) Internet-based cognitive behavior therapy for obsessive compulsive disorder: a pilot study. *BMC Psychiatry* 11: 125.
8 Greist JH *et al.* (2002) Behavior therapy for obsessive-compulsive disorder guided by a computer or by a clinician compared with relaxation as a control. *Journal of Clinical Psychiatry* 63(2): 138–145.

9   Wright JH *et al.* (2005) Computer-assisted cognitive therapy for depression: maintaining efficacy while reducing therapist time. *American Journal of Psychiatry* 162: 1158–1164.

10 Foroushani PS *et al.* (2011) Meta-review of the effectiveness of computerized CBT in treating depression. *BMC Psychiatry* 11: Article 131.

11 Rizzo A *et al.* (2006) A virtual reality exposure therapy application for Iraq war military personnel with post-traumatic stress disorder: from training to toy to treatment. In M Roy (ed.), *NATO Advanced Research Workshop on Novel Approaches to the Diagnosis and Treatment of Posttraumatic Stress Disorder* (pp. 235–250), IOS Press.

12 Coyle D *et al.* (2005) Personal investigator: a therapeutic 3D game for adolescent psychotherapy. *Journal of Interactive Technology & Smart Education* 2(2): 73–88.

13 Goss S *et al.* (2010) Using cell/mobile phone SMS to enhance client crisis and peer support. In KA Anthony *et al.* (eds.), *The Use of Technology in Mental Health: Applications, Ethics and Practice* (pp. 56–67), Charles C. Thomas Pub. Ltd.

14 *The Maudsley Prescribing Guidelines* (2009) 10th edn., Informa Healthcare.

15 Prochyshyn RM, Bezchlibnyk-Butler KZ and Jeffries JJ (eds.) (2019) *Clinical Handbook of Psychotropic Drugs*, 23rd edn., Hogrefe.

16 Slavney PR (consulting ed.) (2000) *Psychiatry 2000: An Internet Resource Guide*, eMedguides.

17 Stamps RF and Barach PM (2001) *The Therapist's Internet Handbook*, Norton Publishing.

18 Growing threat from counterfeit medicines, available at: www.who.int/bulletin/volumes/88/4/10-020410/en/#:~:text=Worldwide%20sales%20of%20counterfeit%20medicines,States%20of%20America%20; see also Jackson G *et al.* (2012) Assessing the problem of counterfeit medications in the United Kingdom. *International Journal of Clinical Practice* 66(3): 241–250; Blackstone EA *et al.* (2014) The health and economic effects of counterfeit drugs. *American Health Drug Benefits* 7(4): 216–224.

19 Kirby M *et al.* (2012) The counterfeit conundrum. *International Journal of Clinical Practice* 66(3): 229–231.

28 The prescriber and the telephone – mainstay and millstone

• Being available by telephone	466
• Appropriate use of the telephone by clinicians	467
• Telephone appointments	467
• Inappropriate use of the telephone	468
• When a patient calls too much	471
• Clinicians' over usage of the phone	472

Even as the world moves to digitalization and the methods of advanced technology, the telephone remains the most frequently used method of communication between clinician and patient. Its clinical and administrative uses are almost taken for granted. Telephone contact with the provider or office staff often provides the first impression that a patient receives of the clinician and his/her office. Used wisely and appropriately during medication management, the telephone can speed up assessments of medication changes, provide the prescriber with rapid feedback and perhaps save the patient an unnecessary trip to the office. At the same time, when used inappropriately or overutilized, the telephone can be both the bane of the practitioner's existence and medico-legal quicksand. This chapter describes the intelligent use of the telephone, its potential pitfalls and how to manage patients who use it inappropriately.

The telephone can be used to efficiently manage many clinical needs, including questions about response, side effects, dosage and interaction with other medications. The patient may be asked to call the clinician on a particular day to give feedback on the effectiveness of a new medication or dosage change. Further clinical refinement of dosage can be accomplished in a brief telephone call, thus saving both clinician and patient significant time and energy. When a patient calls with a question about a drug interaction or side effect, the clinician can quickly intervene, saving the patient discomfort and perhaps avoiding premature discontinuation of medication.

Being available by telephone

Telephone service is a lifeline to the clinician from the patient. There is an old adage: "If patients know they can call, they won't; if they feel they cannot call, they will." In the practice of medication prescription, this is extraordinarily true. Patients feel reassured when they know they can reach the clinician. If patients know that urgent questions will be responded to quickly and consistently, they can often tolerate minor side effects and need not bother the clinician with trivial issues. When patients feel the prescriber is unavailable, does not return calls or cannot be reached, their anxiety increases and they often magnify minor complaints into "crises." By making themselves available to patients by telephone, clinicians can effectively manage time and gain a reputation as a practitioner with whom patients have a solid alliance.

Appropriate use of the telephone by clinicians

- The prescriber should always return all clinically related telephone calls from a patient personally or through office staff promptly, but always by the end of the business day.
- If unable to speak with the patient directly, the clinician should leave a message indicating when a return call was made, and the next step to establish communication. If the patient's message machine is confidential, brief replies to questions can be left. Clinical information must not be left on a message machine or voicemail unless it is known that confidentiality will be maintained.
- Having pre-arranged blocks of time available for telephone contact with patients is useful, but not always possible. If such times are publicized, the clinician must be sure to be available during those specified times.
- The patient can expect medication management 24 hours a day, 7 days a week. When the clinician is not personally available, competent coverage with other providers needs to be arranged.
- If an emergency exists and it cannot be evaluated satisfactorily over the telephone, an appointment should be made for a face-to-face evaluation and/or the patient sent to an emergency department.
- When clinical care issues are involved, all telephone contacts should be documented. Such documentation should include the date and time of the call, the reason the patient called and any response given including medication alterations, dosage changes or any other treatment recommendations.
- Medication for new patients must not initially be prescribed over the telephone without a face-to-face evaluation. In general, major medication regimen changes should also not be made over the telephone.

If office staff answer the telephone for the clinician, it is important to ensure that they:

- are trained in professional, courteous and prompt response
- are trained in triage to recognize urgent matters
- can quickly reach the clinician personally, when necessary
- maintain appropriate patient confidentiality
- keep a log of the time and content of all calls
- have been appropriately trained and credentialed if they are to provide clinical information/guidance to patients or authorize prescription refills. Purely clerical staff should not be allowed to provide clinical recommendations without documented approval/input from the clinician.

Telephone appointments

On occasion, it may be reasonable to have a "telephone appointment" with the patient. While this should not be routine, it can, at times, be both expedient and clinically appropriate. Conditions that might justify a telephone appointment include inclement weather, infirmity of the patient, patient travel difficulties, a suddenly emergent clinical matter or other need for patient contact when a face-to-face evaluation or a telemedicine appointment is not possible.

A telephone follow-up appointment can be conducted using a similar structure to a face-to-face appointment (see Chapter 6). Although the clinician is deprived of facial gestures, body movements or other signs that might help in assessing the patient, safe evaluation and treatment can be accomplished. Particularly for a patient who has a stable medication regimen, it is possible to cover the items of a usual follow-up appointment and provide a renewal prescription. Documentation of a telephone visit should be similar to that for the typical face-to-face evaluation, and should include all the elements normally contained in a written note for such a visit. The vast majority of patients will not abuse the offer of a telephone appointment, and will be grateful for the opportunity when the situation warrants.

A regular pattern of prescribing over the telephone, or repeated telephone appointments, does not generally constitute safe, medically sound practice. If the clinician is thinking about giving medical/medication advice or prescribing over the telephone, the following questions should be considered:

1   Is this an established patient?
2   Do you know this patient well enough to treat over the telephone?
3   When was the last face-to-face visit?
4   How does this telephone treatment fit into the overall treatment of this patient?
5   How often is phone treatment occurring?
6   If a prescription is authorized:
   •   Is it for a limited time?
   •   Is it for the least amount of medication?
   •   When will the next face-to-face visit occur?
7   Is the telephone appointment a pattern for *this patient*?
8   Is the telephone appointment a pattern for *me*?

If the patient has moved away and requests telephone follow up, further questions should be considered:

1   Can I provide safe, high-quality evaluation and treatment without personal interaction?
2   Can I evaluate the patient's changing status over time?
3   What measures are in place for emergency care in the new locale?
4   Would a clinician in the new locale better serve the patient's condition?

When a patient has made a decision to relocate permanently, it is almost invariably preferable to transfer prescriptive care to a local practitioner if medication needs will continue.

Inappropriate use of the telephone

There are temptations, both to the patient and clinician, to overutilize the phone. Each of these considerations will be addressed separately.

Patient's over usage

Patients may misuse the phone in various ways, including:

* inappropriate frequency
* for inappropriate reasons
* at inappropriate times.

Causes for patient overutilization of the telephone include:

* anxiety
* mania
* personality disorder, particularly borderline personality
* it is sometimes "easier" to reach the mental health prescriber than other primary care medical clinicians
* lack of funds to pay for appointments
* the patient feels it is inconvenient to come to the office
* the patient feels a follow-up appointment is not necessary
* the patient feels embarrassed to come to a mental health office.

Depending on the reason overutilization occurs, each situation requires an individualized response from the clinician.

Anxious patients may telephone the clinician to interpret possible side effects or solely for reassurance in taking their prescribed medication. Mentally scattered or extremely nervous patients who have little support in their lives may call the prescriber frequently with medication questions. They will reach for what they perceive as their "life preserver" – the clinician – when they feel overwhelmed and anxious. Despite this anxiety, it is not therapeutic for them to relentlessly seek reassurance through repeated telephone calls.

Manic patients can overutilize the telephone with many individuals including family, friends, neighbors, acquaintances or even strangers. A prescriber may be caught in a manic pattern of verbosity and hyperlogia. At times, manic patients can call frequently, unaware that their repeated calls are inappropriate.

Some patients with personality disorders, particularly those with *borderline personality disorder*, feel "entitled" and special. They feel they can expect immediate access to the prescriber at whatever time and about whatever issue comes to their minds. Repeated or inappropriate access to the prescriber is just one part of what they perceive as their special rights (see Chapter 23 for a more in-depth discussion of borderline patients).

Some patients' use of the phone is inappropriate not because of frequency, but because of the nature of the call. These patients may call a medication prescriber about *issues that can and should be dealt with elsewhere*. When the patient has a regular psychotherapist, psychotherapy issues, marital issues, parenting issues or other issues relative to the patient's life should be referred to the psychotherapist. The medication prescriber is not the most direct (or most appropriate) resource. If, however, the prescriber is seen as an interested, available and knowledgeable resource, the patient may choose to bypass the regular therapist and call the prescriber. Gently redirecting the patient to the regular therapist is the appropriate intervention.

Patients may call the prescriber for medically unrelated issues. Patients may wish to use the mental health prescriber as a general practitioner, calling about headaches, blood pressure, rashes, pain, coughs, antibiotics or other medical issues. If the prescriber has a minimal telephone barrier, patients may perceive that he or she is easier to reach than a busy primary care provider. Some patients may call the mental health prescriber rather than attempting to deal with what they perceive as a difficult maze of resistance to reach a family practitioner or specialist in a large office. It is not uncommon for a patient to request a renewal for a non-mental health prescription just because "I can never reach Dr. X" or because "my nurse practitioner is out of town." Rather than attempting to reach the appropriate clinician's backup or coverage person, such patients will call the mental health prescriber.

Anxious or desperate individuals who are not current patients may telephone requesting medications for anxiety, sleep, depression or other mental health symptoms without an in-person evaluation. Although a practitioner may empathize with the patient's plight, *prescription without face-to-face evaluation is inappropriate and dangerous*. These requests should be denied, and such patients referred to an emergency department or a more available colleague.

There are occasions when a previous patient, well known to the clinician but who has not been seen in months or years, calls in a crisis. For a responsible patient, it may be reasonable to re-institute a temporary, small amount of medication until the patient can be seen in person. At the time of this telephone contact, the clinician should ask about intervening medical issues that may have changed before automatically restarting a previously utilized medication:

- Have there been any medical changes?
- Are there new or ongoing medications or allergies?
- Is there ongoing suicidal ideation or substance abuse?
- Face-to-face follow up should be arranged as soon as possible.

In other situations, patients who have neglected to arrange a follow-up visit will telephone requesting prescription renewals. This is usually done when a patient's medications are nearly depleted. Initially when this happens, the clinician may appropriately ensure continuity of medication by providing a short-term prescription to cover the patient until the face-to-face evaluation is performed. Although this may be reasonable for an occasional lapse, if the situation becomes repetitive, the clinician will need to define the rules of safe prescription. When the patient continually fails to make or keep appointments, and repeatedly asks for telephone renewals, the clinician should give a clear message that further renewals will not be provided over the telephone without face-to-face evaluation. This should be documented in the patient's record (see further elaboration in Chapter 22).

Some patients may also abuse the telephone by deliberately calling the clinician after regular business hours. They call off-hours, reaching coverage personnel, in hopes of gaining further medication renewals without the need for face-to-face evaluation from the primary clinician. This behavior must be addressed by a coordinated effort between the primary clinician and coverage clinicians. Standard practice for weekend or holiday coverage personnel should be to provide only enough medication to last the patient until the primary clinician becomes available. On the next regular workday, the primary clinician can then appropriately assess the situation for further prescription.

When a patient calls too much

Some general principles are helpful for managing inappropriate telephone usage in a medication practice.

First, the clinician should ensure that there is an established pattern of inappropriate telephone usage before setting rules. One unnecessary call does not automatically mean that a patient is being inappropriate. Particularly early in treatment, a patient may not know what is, and what is not, an appropriate call. Education about the use of the telephone will lay the groundwork for a workable agreement between patient and clinician.

If inappropriate phone calls become a pattern, the clinician must deal promptly and directly with the patient about this behavior.

Box 28.1 Talking to patients

"We need to talk about your telephone calls to me and your treatment plan."

The discussion should be specific regarding the issues of frequency of calls, nature of calls, timing of calls or any other telephone issue that is problematic. The clinician should be firm, but not display anger. A specific outline of therapeutic use of the telephone should be detailed, including specifics about *when* the clinician can be called, *how often* and *about what issues*. It is important that the clinician also adheres to the newly established parameters. If for some reason the clinician deviates from the outlined plan for a telephone-abusing patient, this instance must be identified as a deviation and the clinician must explain why it is being done. It is quite reasonable, at times, to tell the patient to bring certain issues to the next face-to-face appointment, and that these issues do not require an extra-session telephone call.

Clinicians should not cut off all telephone contact with an active patient, even though with some particularly troublesome patients they may wish to do so. While medications are being prescribed, the patient must continue to have emergency access to the clinician. It may be necessary, however, for the prescriber to define what constitutes an "emergency." Once outlined, the plan should be documented in the written notes and a copy given to the patient.

Box 28.2 Talking to patients

If telephone calls continue to be abused after initial parameters are set and reinforced, the clinician can state: *"We have talked about your use of the telephone, and you have continued to use it in ways that I do not feel are helpful. This is the last time I will discuss the matter. If you do not use the phone appropriately, in the ways I have outlined in our plan, you are putting your relationship with me in jeopardy and we may need to stop your treatment."* Then, reiterate the parameters.

When repeated last-minute telephone requests for medication renewal have been identified as problematic, further telephone requests for medication renewal should be refused, even if the patient may run short of medication or experience some rebound side effects from having a medication-free interval.

When the clinician identifies a particular telephone call as inappropriate from a patient who has done it before, the clinician should interrupt the dialogue and identify it as a non-urgent one. Identification of the call as an inappropriate one is the only necessary response; such an interruption is quite professional and necessary. Usually, this intervention will alter the behavior of even intractable patients. However, if a patient continues to use the telephone inappropriately and ignores guidelines, the therapist may need to terminate the relationship. The patient should be given written notice that his/her treatment, therapy and/or medication relationship with the clinician has ended, along with a date after which the clinician will provide no further prescriptions. It is appropriate to provide several weeks of medication to allow the patient time to find another prescriber. The patient will have the responsibility of finding a new prescriber.

Clinicians' over usage of the phone

When a *clinician* finds that he or she is scheduling frequent telephone appointments without face-to-face evaluations, it is a warning sign that the clinician may be overutilizing the telephone. The busy clinician may see telephone therapy as a way of fitting large numbers of patients into a small space of time. While useful as a temporary measure, it should not become standard practice. Clinician overutilization of the telephone is often accompanied by offering an excessive number of medication refills over an extended period without re-evaluation.

29 The pharmacist, the pharmaceutical industry and the clinician

- Interacting with the pharmacist   473
- Preauthorization – a fact of American practice   474
- The pharmaceutical industry   474
- Indigent care medication programs   476
- Media advertising and mental health medications   476
- Reference   477

Interacting with the pharmacist

When utilized appropriately, the pharmacist can be a significant resource in the practice of psychopharmacology. An experienced pharmacist can often answer queries about drug interactions, dosage forms or strengths, and identify possible medication substitutions. Today's pharmacies are busy places, but most pharmacists are eager to be of help to practitioners.

When pharmacists telephone the clinician, it is often because they have some concerns about a prescription. It may be as simple as being unable to read the clinician's handwriting and needing clarification, or an important element of the prescription may have been inadvertently omitted. Which drug is required? How many pills were prescribed? What is the dosing schedule?

The pharmacist may also have clinical concerns about what has been written; a dose may be higher than usual or the number of pills to be dispensed may be of concern. At times the pharmacist may see an aberration, crossed-out writing or some other indication that raises suspicion, and calls to document the authenticity of the prescription. Some of these issues may be largely resolved in the near future as we move toward the era of computer-generated electronic prescriptions sent directly from the clinician's office to the pharmacy across the street or across the country.

Many pharmacies at this time have computer-generated programs that produce complete patient medication profiles, with drug interaction and safety information about the medication prescribed. This information can be given to the patient as a print-out, and contains warnings, precautions, possible side effects and interactions with other medications. Such programs also contain a list of patient drug allergies and a chronological medication prescription history from all prescribers. Some programs automatically highlight possible drug interactions. When the program identifies a possible interaction, the pharmacist's call can provide useful information to the prescriber, who may be unaware that the patient is using a medication from another prescriber. It is important to know, for example, that a patient who is starting lithium is already taking large doses of a prescription non-steroidal, anti-inflammatory medicine that could, in some instances, raise the patient's lithium level by 50–100 percent. An episode of toxicity can then be avoided by starting the lithium at lower-than-normal doses.

Pharmacists' calls based on computer programs and the notifications they generate do not, however, create a mandate for the clinician, or automatically require a change of prescription. Such programs may highlight very rare interactions that, while possible, are quite unlikely for a particular patient. Sometimes only one case of an interaction may have been suspected, but never proven. At other times, the potential interaction highlighted is common, but the clinician, in concert with the patient, has decided to accept any possible interactional risk for reasons of clinical necessity. If there is good justification for the medication regimen prescribed, and the clinician is aware of the possible interactions with other medications, he or she may reassure the pharmacist about proceeding with filling the prescription. When proceeding with a combination of medications that may carry some additional risk, the clinician should document the clinical rationale for this decision.

Preauthorization – a fact of American practice

In the United States, where many patients receive medication coverage as an insurance benefit, the pharmacist will call if the medication prescribed is not on the approved list covered by the patient's insurance. The pharmacy will require "preauthorization" of a medication from the insurance plan before the insurance company will pay for the medication. Sometimes the pharmacist will ask if the clinician wishes to prescribe another medication that is covered by the insurance, almost as if the medications were interchangeable. The medications on the approved list will vary from insurance plan to insurance plan, and may change over time. Such approval has much to do with corporate decisions based on cost, and does not necessarily reflect the clinical value, safety or utility of medications covered. If the clinician has good reasons for prescribing the original medication, he or she may not want to change medications just because it is not on the patient's formulary. If this is the case, it is necessary for the clinician to call the insurance company to receive "pre-approval." If other medications on the approved list have been previously prescribed and have failed, or if there is a good clinical reason for using a specific medication without substitution, it will usually be approved if the clinician takes the time to justify the clinical necessity.

The pharmaceutical industry

The presence of the pharmaceutical industry is a highly visible factor in clinical practice. A delicate balance exists between the practitioner and pharmaceutical manufacturers with regard to the prescription of medications. Pharmaceutical firms are large, multinational companies with enormous budgets. These manufacturers must have the alliance of practitioners to prescribe their products, since there is no direct way to distribute their medications except through licensed, trained professionals. In turn, practitioners depend on the pharmaceutical industry to develop new medications and test them for safety. Industry-sponsored research has become a large segment of the medication data on which clinical decisions are made.

Since the field of mental health has been "discovered," increasing expenditures of pharmaceutical dollars are devoted to research into mental health medications. Mental illnesses that improve with the use of medication may require medication recurrently or, at times, on a life-long basis. With this incentive, it can be expected that, over the next 10–20 years, research into psychotropics will continue to be one of the dominant forces in pharmacological research. Unfortunately, individual practitioners are likely to have little influence on the focus of research, how it is funded or the ultimate cost of medications to the patients.

Pharmaceutical representatives

The relationship between clinicians and the pharmaceutical industry is primarily structured through interaction with pharmaceutical representatives. These representatives will be eager to meet with practitioners as often as possible. Pharmaceutical representatives are, first and foremost, employees of the pharmaceutical company and promoters of their products. Additionally, however, they are educators in the use of their products and facilitators of clinical practice. The services they offer are listed in Table 29.1.

The practitioner's interface – opportunities and risks

The practitioner's level of connection with one or more pharmaceutical companies is an issue that has stimulated much controversy and many differences in practice. Some clinicians or institutions will refuse to have any contact with pharmaceutical representatives, feeling that it is unnecessary, or may bias their prescriptive decisions. Others will see representatives on a regular basis, obtaining samples and attending sponsored educational conferences. Clinicians will need to decide what level of comfort they have with pharmaceutical industry interaction. Some guidelines about interaction with pharmaceutical companies are provided in the American Medical Association policy (see Appendix 7). Although issued years ago, it still provides useful guidance.

In 2008, the Pharmaceutical Research and Manufacturers of America (PhRMA), a voluntary trade association of pharmaceutical companies, adopted a revised "Code of Interactions with Healthcare Professionals." Although it does not represent all companies, the group's adoption of a set of standardized principles has minimized excessive and inappropriate inducements to prescribing professionals. The code was revised and strengthened from its original version issued in 2002. The text of the revised Code and a list of the signatories is contained in Appendix 7. It may also be viewed along

Table 29.1 Services provided by pharmaceutical representatives

---

- Printed literature about their products and about mental illnesses in general
- Access to educational material, diagnostic and treatment aids, including a wide variety of paper, audio and video products for the clinician, the patient and families
- Access to professional educational opportunities taught by experts in the field and sponsored by the pharmaceutical company
- Availability of research studies on questions about the use of their products in various clinical illnesses
- Free medication samples for professional distribution
- Access to indigent care programs to provide low- or no-cost medications to needy patients

---

with clarifying questions and answers on the Internet at www.phrma.org/en/Codes-and-guidelines/Code-on-Interactions-with-Health-Care-Professionals

Regardless of what level of contact is maintained, some potential pitfalls for the clinician should be highlighted:

- It may be easy to be drawn into ethically questionable practices with pharmaceutical companies. Even well-intended clinical decisions can be affected by meetings, inducements or dinners. Involvement in non-educational entertainment inducements is of particular concern. Attending a theater, sporting event or trip sponsored by a pharmaceutical company with no educational agenda is now prohibited by the Code. At the same time, avoidance of industry-sponsored educational programs may unnecessarily limit the clinician's exposure to useful clinical information. When attending such a program, it is important during the presentation to identify a speaker who is truly objective and is presenting unbiased material. Some presenters may be employed by the pharmaceutical company, or be speaking primarily to promote a particular product. These talks must be labeled as "Promotional" talks. Other CME (Continuing Medical Education) talks should not, in theory, have a promotional aspect or bias.
- The availability of product samples can be a convenient and money-saving way for patients to begin an initial trial of a new medication. Making decisions about which product to prescribe solely on the convenience of having samples available, however, is not sound clinical practice.

Indigent care medication programs

Many pharmaceutical companies provide indigent care programs for low-income patients. These can be quite helpful for a patient who benefits significantly from a particular medication, but cannot afford it. Although there is paperwork involved for the clinician, the patient can be maintained on medication at no cost, at least on a time-limited basis. Although each company's procedure may vary slightly, once the clinician fills out the appropriate request, a medication supply is shipped to the prescriber who then distributes it to the patient.

A list of indigent care medication programs by manufacturer, with contact addresses and telephone numbers, can be seen on the Internet at www.pparx.org/

Media advertising and mental health medications

Direct marketing of pharmaceuticals began in 1981. Since the relaxation of regulations on such advertising in 1997, however, television, radio and print media (especially in the United States, but worldwide as well) have begun to accept an ever-increasing stream of direct-to-consumer medication advertisements. While initially limited to allergy products, gastrointestinal remedies and cholesterol-lowering medications, the practice has now spread to a wide variety of drugs, including many mental health medications. Companies have also now changed a previous long-standing policy that refrained from advertising scheduled, potentially habit-forming medicines, by running print and television advertisements about the use of stimulants for ADHD or hypnotics for sleep. It is rare to watch a television program now without at least one pharmaceutical advertisement.

Professionals have varying responses to such advertisements, and there are both benefits and drawbacks for mental health. When such advertising applies to mental health medication, the positives are that it can legitimize mental health problems and de-stigmatize seeking help for emotional problems. Some patients who would not otherwise do so will seek treatment solely because they have seen symptoms mentioned on television that correspond to what they have been feeling. Given that we, as professionals, continue to treat only a fraction of those people who suffer with most mental health conditions, advertising has some value for societal mental health management.

Negatives to this advertising include trivializing prescriptions and the prescription process itself. Patients often arrive in the office with their mind set on receiving a medication that they have seen advertised. Patients who expect a prescription for medicine A seen on TV may be less favorably disposed to medicine B, even if the prescriber thinks it is more appropriate. Valuable prescriber time can be consumed discussing with a patient why medicine A is less appropriate or even harmful for them. Additionally, the cost of such media advertising (which some suggest is greater than the companies' research and development budget)[1] ultimately contributes to the high overall cost of pharmaceuticals for patients.

Reference

1   Gagnon M-A and Lexchin J (2008) The cost of pushing pills: a new estimate of pharmaceutical promotion expenditures in the United States. *PLoS Medicine* 5(1): e1.

30 Preparing an office for mental health prescribing

• Mandatory issues	478
• Optional measures	481
• Personal presentation	482
• Periodic re-evaluation of image	483
• References	483

A clinician may open an office for prescribing mental health medication within an organization, clinic or hospital, in a government-sponsored setting or as an independent practitioner. Depending on the clinician's discipline and training, it may be as an independent practitioner with independent prescribing authority or as a collaborative practitioner requiring consultation or collaboration with another professional.

Depending on the setting, basic necessities and paperwork may be set up and provided by an institution. When opening an independent practice, however, clinicians will need to arrange for each item themselves. This chapter will provide a checklist of important issues to be addressed by the provider of mental health prescriptions.

Mandatory issues

Clinicians must:

1 *Consult state or national law* regarding the limits of their practice and prescriptive authority. Contact the State Board which regulates your professional discipline and fulfill all requirements required by the state(s) in which you will be practicing.
2 *If not covered by their license itself, maintain a copy of their prescriptive authority agreement* and any legal limitations on their prescriptive authority at the office site.
3 If practicing within a group, devise and sign a contract with any other group members and specify any contractual arrangements. This agreement should be in writing, and a copy maintained at the practice.
4 *Obtain malpractice insurance for prescription*. This should include limits of a minimum of $1 million per occurrence and $3 million per event. Ensure that premises liability insurance is included, for any accidental occurrences that happen in the office (such as the patient who trips, falls and suffers an injury). *Under no circumstances should the clinician begin writing prescriptions until malpractice insurance coverage has been obtained in writing*.

5   In the United States, *obtain a Controlled Substance Registration Certificate* from the Drug Enforcement Administration of the Department of Justice for prescription of scheduled medications. Although it is possible to prescribe without such registration, a practitioner without this certificate will not be able to write for benzodiazepines, sedative/hypnotics or stimulants, resulting in a limited practice. In the United States, an application may be obtained by calling the DEA's Diversion Control Division at 1-800-882-9539 or via the Internet: www.deadiversion.usdoj.gov/index.html

In the UK, doctors and dentists can prescribe all controlled medicines to treat illness or injury. However, doctors must hold a license from the Home Office to prescribe controlled medicines to treat addiction. Specially trained nurses can prescribe some controlled medicines for specific conditions, such as pain relief in palliative care. Midwives may use a limited range of controlled medicines, for example, to relieve pain during childbirth. Other healthcare professionals, including nurses and pharmacists, may prescribe controlled medicines as part of an agreed care plan for a specific patient.

Issues of prescribing scheduled medications are handled at the Home Office, Direct Communications, Unit 2, Marsham Street, London, SW1P 4DF, telephone 020 7035 4848 or via the Internet: www.gov.uk/guidance/controlled-drugs-personal-licences#apply-for-a-licence

6   If required by their licensure, *choose a consultant*. Although it may vary by state law, a consultant for a nurse practitioner can be any physician or in some cases an experienced advanced practice nurse. When possible, a psychiatrist with psychopharmacological expertise is a desirable choice as consultant. Depending on location and availability, a family practitioner, internist, pediatrician or other medical specialist may also serve as a consultant. Such physicians, in general, do not have advanced psychopharmacology expertise. While they are within the limits of the law, such consultants may not be able to provide in-depth consultation about psychotropics. The clinician should keep a copy of the consultative agreement on the office premises.

7   *Lease or sublease office space.* It is not advisable to work out of a personal residence. Although in times past this was popular for certain mental health practitioners, mixing personal life with professional life is not, in general, competent safe practice. Of considerable importance is an office that maintains *adequate soundproofing.* Patients generally feel much more comfortable if they know their verbalizations cannot be heard in the waiting room or in another office. To maintain adequate confidentiality, special soundproofing may be needed in ceilings and walls. Use of a radio, fan or "white noise" machine in the waiting room also reduces sound from the office to the waiting room.

8   *Establish coverage with other licensed practitioners, for 24-hours a day, 7-days a week coverage,* as medication prescription requires availability by a qualified practitioner around the clock for emergencies. Practitioners may be of the same discipline or other disciplines with prescriptive authority. This is considerably different from standard psychotherapy practice, in which some practitioners may not require (or provide) such emergency availability. A patient who experiences a medication emergency and cannot reach a qualified practitioner may have grounds for medico-legal action.

9   *Establish a telephone service,* including a means of off-hours and weekend notification such as an answering service, pager, answering machine, cell phone or other

method. The prescription of medications does require the availability of rapid access to the clinician or to covering personnel off-hours. The system should be tested periodically to make sure it operates consistently and smoothly.

10 Establish *Internet access* via computer, smart phone, tablet or another device.

11 *If not covered by their license, arrange to have laboratory tests ordered* through their consultant or another provider/clinic if their licensure does not allow for independent ordering of laboratory tests directly at a laboratory.

12 *Obtain pads of prescriptions.* Personalized prescriptions written on alter-proof paper are preferred. Many medical supply houses in the United States provide these at reasonable prices and can be found via the Internet. Some clinicians prefer to have their address, BNDD number (required to prescribe potentially habit-forming medications), state license number or other information on the prescriptions, while others do not. Non-personalized prescriptions with no identifying information are legal, but are perhaps more open to fraud. Some states require specialized prescription blanks (such as triplicate prescriptions) for prescriptions in their state.

13 *Obtain reference books* such as the *Physician's Desk Reference (PDR),*[1] *The Maudsley Prescribing Guidelines,*[2] *The USP D1,*[3] *Drug Facts and Comparisons*[4] and this text! Obtain the latest version of the *Diagnostic and Statistical Manual (DSM),*[5] with a list of mental health diagnoses and their code numbers (American Psychiatric Association, 1400 K Street, NW, Washington, DC 20005).

14 *Devise paperwork* for medication prescription (see below under Optional Measures), which should include:
  • A consent to treatment form.
  • A consent to share clinical information with a consultant, colleague and/or family member.
  • A consent to leave clinical information on an answering device at a designated number.
  • A patient registration form (this may be devised by the clinician or pre-printed). Clinicians vary in how much information they wish to be completed by the patient on a registration form. Some prefer very simple forms with name, date, address, phone (and perhaps e-mail address) and name of emergency contact. Others prefer spaces for payer information, medical insurance identification and consent to treat statement. Still other clinicians wish to have the patient fill out a medical/psychiatric history including chief complaint, past medical and psychiatric history, current and past medications, known allergies and name of psychotherapist, if any. Use of more comprehensive forms when reviewed and initiated by the prescriber may allow a clinician to maximize the time spent at an initial evaluation session. Whatever form is used, it should be retained in the patient's chart.
  • A sheet describing fees, including missed appointment charges.
  • Written instructions for commonly prescribed medications, which should include side effects, interactions and warnings (these may be pre-printed from a manufacturer or self-composed).
  • Laboratory test request forms – obtain a list of codes for commonly used tests from the laboratory.
  • Patient instruction sheets for having laboratory tests drawn.

- Checklists of various symptoms for commonly diagnosed conditions (such as depression, bipolar disorder, obsessive–compulsive disorder, panic disorder, etc.) to serve as an outline for initial evaluations by the clinician.
- Medication record forms to document medications prescribed (these may be pre-printed or self-devised; see Chapter 5 for examples).
- Initial evaluation and progress note forms, unless the plan is to use plain notepaper.
- Appointment cards with the address and telephone number of the office.
- Letterhead stationery for reports and other correspondence.
- A fax cover sheet.

15 *Devise a system for organizing and storing medical records* that maintains privacy, safety and confidentiality of records, and consider how the capacity can be expanded as further patients are seen.

16 Obtain folders, charts, file cabinets, paper, notebooks, a clock, calendar and appointment book.

17 For safe storage of medication samples, *obtain locked cabinets* or identify a locked storage room.

Some clinicians utilize an electronic device for a number of functions including clock, calendar, appointment book and Internet access. Certain devices allow for speech recognition and, therefore, can serve to create office notes and letters when attached to a printer. As discussed in Chapter 24, if such a device is used, make sure that at least one backup system is in place and utilized regularly. All such devices are subject to malfunction, virus contamination and loss. Without a backup, days, weeks, months and even years of vital and irreplaceable information can be lost.

Optional measures

Optional measures that may be helpful and recommended, but are not essential, include the following:

1 *Interview and hire clerical help* to perform reception work, telephone answering, typing, billing, accounting and/or insurance preparation.

2 *Obtain a blood pressure cuff* for convenient monitoring of blood pressure or a standard cuff and stethoscope.

3 *Obtain pharmaceutical samples* from drug company representatives, if these will be used. Local representatives' names and telephone numbers can generally be obtained through a pharmaceutical company's central phone number. These are listed by company at the front of the *Physician's Desk Reference*.

4 *Obtain a fax machine* to receive faxed lab work, medical records, consents for treatment and other data from practitioners and insurance companies.

5 *Obtain a computer* with Internet access and printer for word processing and online information gathering.

6 *Obtain a printer* for making hard copies of electronic information as well as printing faxes.

7 *Begin subscriptions to psychopharmacology journals* or journals relative to your specialty. If it is preferred, subscribe to an Internet-based program to access up-to-date psychopharmacological information (see Chapter 27).

8 Obtain a scale for measurement of the patient's weight.
9 Some clinicians may opt for obtaining additional forms and checklists. There are several texts from which such forms can be viewed and copied. These include:

- Zuckerman EL (2008) *The Paper Office: Forms, Guidelines, and Resources to Make your Practice Work Ethically, Legally, and Profitably: The Clinician's Toolbox*, 4th edn., Guilford Press.
- Wiger DE (2010) *The Clinical Documentation Sourcebook: The Complete Paperwork Resource for your Mental Health Practice*, 4th edn., Wiley.
- Wyatt RJ and Chew RH (2005) *Wyatt's Practical Psychiatric Practice: Forms and Protocols for Clinical Use*, 3rd edn., American Psychiatric Publishing, Inc.

10 Consider the use of a financial advisor, accountant and/or a lawyer to become familiar with issues of practice structure and legal issues referable to opening a practice. Especially for the practitioner who is coming directly out of training, attendance at a medical practice seminar and/or taking a tutorial on billing, billing computer software and financial record keeping can be useful. Performing an Internet search on "billing seminars for healthcare," "healthcare practice management," "medical billing tutorial" or a similar subject will reveal opportunities available in one's local area.
11 If you are planning to medicate children, set up a play area and obtain toys, age-appropriate dolls and other suitable materials.
12 Talk with other clinicians about their experience of prescriptive practice, office set-up and management.

Before beginning the prescription process, the clinician should have a clear understanding as to the limits of his or her own ability. Together with the consultant, the clinician should identify and document which patients, if any, will be restricted by a collaborative agreement. For example, without consultation and oversight, the inexperienced practitioner might be limited from prescribing to:

- the seriously active suicidal patient
- the acutely psychotic patient
- the patient with acting out borderline personality
- the patient in acute alcohol withdrawal
- the complicated medical patient with multiple physical illnesses and multiple non-psychiatric medications.

Personal presentation

Clothing and grooming are part of the personal image that a prescriber presents to a patient. First impressions count, and can color the way in which patients view the clinician's treatment. Consider carefully the style of dress and level of formality of office clothing. With the advent of "casual Fridays" and a trend toward less formal clothes in many offices, this has seeped into mental health offices. While remaining true to your sense of style, consider how you would regard a clinician seen for the first time dressed as you intend. Shorts, tank tops, muscle shirts, t-shirts, ripped/torn clothing or badly worn shoes do not have a place in a prescriber's office. Similarly, short skirts, baggy low pants, excessively tight, low-cut or revealing outfits give an erroneous and inappropriate message to the patient. What may be considered upscale and fashionable at a club or party may be quite inappropriate in an office. While not required, shirt and tie for men or skirt and blouse for women never go out of style and convey an air of professionalism and competence which goes a long way to instilling confidence in the patient. Whenever there is a choice between too formal and too casual, there is little downside to formality. If you find yourself asking "Could this be too casual, too short, too revealing, too tight or too stained?" assume that it is and wear something else.

Grooming also plays a part in the overall presentation. Combed hair, neatly trimmed facial hair, appropriate makeup if desired, brushed teeth without bad breath, clean hands and neatly trimmed nails complete the appearance of a clinician with whom the patient will feel comfortable.

The one possible exception to the above suggestions about personal appearance can be for the clinician who solely sees children. In this circumstance, some clinicians prefer a more casual outfit which may be less imposing to a child. Also, clothes that are flexible enough to permit getting on the floor and participating in play therapy may be more functional.

Periodic re-evaluation of image

As with any business or organization, a healthcare provider's building, office and physical presentation to a patient reflects positively or negatively on the quality of care to be delivered. This is particularly true for the psychotropic medication prescriber. For all the reasons listed in the first two chapters of this book, mental health medications and the persons who prescribe them are not automatically or universally accepted without doubt, apprehension and skepticism. A professional, organized office and care delivery system in an up-to-date building can start the prescriptive process off on the right foot. The appropriate atmosphere gives a sense that quality, safe, professional decisions are made in this practitioner's setting. When the office and environs are disorganized, cluttered or non-professional, it may predispose the patient to wonder if the quality of care is likewise.

Even when the parameters detailed in this chapter are followed, time passes and circumstances change. Buildings age, offices can become shabby and furnishings outdated. Professional forms can become obsolete or inaccurate. Service provision by office staff may not meet the standards originally set. *It is extraordinarily valuable periodically to view the office, the staff and the service provided through the eyes of a potential patient.* What building will they see? Whom will they encounter? What is the level of interaction with the clinician or any staff by telephone or in person? Do all these elements meet the desired professional image? Are education materials (print, videotape, audio tape, CD-ROM, computer program) current and accurate? Are available medication samples within printed expiration dates?

References

1 *Physician's Desk Reference*, Medical Economics Inc., published annually.
2 *The Maudsley Prescribing Guidelines*, Informa Healthcare, published annually.
3 *U.S. Pharmacopeia*, USP–NF, published annually.
4 *Drug Facts and Comparisons*, Walters and Kluwer, published annually.
5 *Diagnostic and Statistical Manual*, American Psychiatric Association, published periodically.

31 The way forward

• Practice guidelines	484
• Genetics – the next big frontier	485
• Lifestyle prescribing	486
• Summary	487
• References	487

Practice guidelines

As the science of psychopharmacology and mental health treatment has become more evidence-based and scientific, numerous practice guidelines have been developed for the treatment of various illnesses. These practice guidelines include decision trees for the use of medications, or combinations of medications and non-pharmacologic therapies in the treatment of specific illnesses. Some guidelines are rapidly becoming standards against which competent practice is measured.

These practice guidelines can provide a number of advantages. They are useful to novice prescribers or practitioners who prescribe infrequently in providing a framework for thorough and consistent treatment of mental illnesses. More experienced practitioners may find such practice guidelines periodically helpful to review their own competence and practice patterns. In treatment-resistant patients, a review of practice guidelines may unearth a treatment possibility that the clinician had not considered. As the clinician gains more experience, he or she may not need to use the guideline as a regular tool, but may do so only intermittently or in particularly difficult cases.

The American Psychiatric Association, various state agencies and numerous managed care organizations have devised many such guidelines after multidisciplinary input. Copies of practice and medication guidelines for many mental health conditions may be obtained via the Internet at:

- American Psychiatric Association (APA) Practice Guidelines, at: http://psychiatryonline.org/guidelines.aspx
- Expert Consensus Guidelines, at: www.psychguides.com/
- The International Psychopharmacology Algorithm Project, at: www.ipap.org/
- Psychopharmacology Algorithm Project at the Harvard Medical School, at: http://psychopharm.mobi/

Genetics – the next big frontier

There is little doubt among clinicians, researchers, teachers and theoreticians that the next big breakthrough in mental health assessment and treatment will likely be fueled, at least in part, by genetic sequencing. While exciting to anticipate, clinically useful information derived from an assay of a person's genome and gene-based *"personalized medicine"* is clearly in its infancy for mental health.

Knowing the makeup of all or specific sections of a person's genome could be helpful to a prescribing clinician in four ways:

- genetic assay to determine a person's ability to metabolize a particular medicine
- pharmacogenomics or genetic testing which would predict a patient's likelihood of responsiveness to a particular drug
- psychogenomics or genetic testing which would identify the genetic underpinnings of human behavior and mental illness – this might lead to a categorization of illnesses or subtypes of illnesses based on a genomic pattern
- gene therapy or treatment of illness by genetic repair or substitution.

At present, we can easily obtain a sample from which aspects of a person's genetic profile can be ascertained via a buccal swab or other tissue source. Only the first of the above four measurements, however, is currently available and *this test has not yet been shown to be clinically useful for most patients*. The cytochrome P-450 enzyme system is the predominant method of metabolizing psychotropic drugs in the body (see Chapter 20 for a full discussion). Theoretically, knowledge about how well or poorly an individual will metabolize a particular compound would provide helpful data on initial dosing, predicting side effects and helping a prescriber treat a non-responding patient. To date, research in this area has focused on patients taking antipsychotics and SSRI antidepressants. By using the test, extensive metabolizers, poor metabolizers, intermediate metabolizers and ultra-rapid metabolizers have been identified. Unfortunately, commercially available tests of this trait, such as the AmpliChip CYP450 Test by Roche Molecular Diagnostics[1] have failed to prove their ability to affect clinical decision-making or to improve clinical outcomes for most patients.[2–5] Many potential patients (even knowledgable ones) expect that practitioners can use this test to provide specific recommendations for medications to be used. Such patients need to be educated about what this testing can and cannot reveal.

Not to be deterred by the modest current discoveries, let us speculate how genetics might practically assist the mental health prescriber in the future. Much research is now being performed to connect an individual's genome with their responsiveness to particular psychotropic drugs, so-called *pharmacogenomics*. Analogous to antibiotic sensitivity testing, the hope is to perform genetic screening on an individual prior to the initiation of treatment and use this information to predict the likelihood that they will respond to a given medication. When and if this becomes a reality in mental health, it is unlikely that such testing would reveal black/white, yes/no responsiveness and sensitivity. It is more probable that the results of such tests for psychiatric conditions would suggest, for example, that a patient has an "80 percent chance of responding to medication A" and a "30 percent chance of responding to medication B." While not perfect, this would nonetheless be an important step forward for patients and clinicians in minimizing the "trial and error" approach so common in psychotropic prescription today.

Such information would also be a major boon to pharmaceutical companies. Drug manufacturers could offer clinicians testing data which would be an enhanced predictor for the successful use of their products. These companies, therefore, have invested considerable financial resources in this regard. If successful, one would expect that this would be a use of genetic testing with considerable relevance to clinical practice.

With our current level of understanding, knowledgeable experts in the field concur that mental health diagnoses are not likely the result of single-gene abnormalities. Even in the simplest genetic profile associated with a mental health diagnosis, multiple genetic abnormalities are involved. The entire causative process of a particular condition may be significantly more complex and not be based on genetic factors alone. Gene expression and protein production based on genetic structure may be substantially influenced by environmental factors and/or experiential factors. Therefore, the last two areas relating to the genome and mental health, *psychogenomics* and *gene therapy*, are much less likely to occur any time soon. Although, if and when they do become a reality, such discoveries will revolutionize the practice of clinical mental health treatment. Assume, for example, that large numbers of patient genetic maps are collected both from mentally ill patients and from people free from mental illness. If a consistent set of genetic abnormalities could be correlated with clinical symptom patterns, such research could lead to more scientifically based definitions of psychiatric illnesses (for example, depression or schizophrenia). It is further possible that genetically definable subtypes of these illnesses could be delineated. With reliable identification of illness subtypes through genetic mapping, targeted medication therapies for particular subtypes could be devised.

Even further in the future is the possible identification of abnormal DNA sections which predictably produce specified mental health conditions regardless of other factors. If this emerges as a reality (and it is not at all clear that it is going to), such identification has the potential to lead to gene alteration, repair or substitution which could treat symptoms when they occur via the CRISPR process. CRISPRs are specialized stretches of DNA. The protein Cas9 (or "CRISPR-associated") is an enzyme that acts like a pair of molecular scissors, capable of cutting strands of DNA. Therefore, the CRISPR process involves identifying a spur of DNA which is responsible for a problematic outcome, snipping it out using Cas9 and replacing it with a "normal" piece of DNA, resulting in repair of the abnormal outcome. Even more desirable, such "gene therapy" early in life might prevent the ultimate manifestation of a disease before it occurs.

Lifestyle prescribing

One of the most interesting conundrums that the prescriber of mental health medications (and indeed all healthcare prescribers) now faces is the gradual but inexorable move to lifestyle prescribing – writing prescriptions not to treat diagnosable illness, but to enhance a patient's life. Most workers in healthcare entered it to relieve suffering and treat disease. By and large that is what we continue to do. Gradually, however, we are moving into the arena of prescribing medications for other purposes. When a patient has a diagnosable condition with painful mental and/or physical symptoms, we prescribe medication to alleviate them. But how then are we to respond when a patient *wants* to feel better or have his or her life improved by medication, but has *no diagnosable illness*?

Lest we say to ourselves this is a question for "down the road" and not in our current practice, we must think clearly about what we already do. As healthcare prescribers, we already write prescriptions to regrow hair, improve penile erections, improve sleep, lose weight and help a patient with attention and mental focus. While at times we may believe that all our prescriptions for these problems can be justified by making a diagnosis, we often continue to prescribe even when the primary diagnosis has been treated. If a depressed patient has no further symptoms other than a continuing sleep disorder, do we not continue to prescribe sleeping medications because without them, the patient remains fatigued? It may ease our minds if we feel that a patient's erectile dysfunction is caused by psychotropics which we are prescribing or by a vascular or neurological disease. More often than we may care to realize, the patient wants continued prescriptions for sildenafil simply to improve his sex life. Many students complain of attention deficit disorder with symptoms of poor concentration, lack of focus and disorganization. Are we absolutely sure when writing a stimulant prescription that the patient does not simply wish for a stimulant prescription to stay up longer, have more energy and get better grades? Plastic surgeons already perform body enhancing surgery on a daily basis for no other reason than that the patient wishes to have his/her body look different or "better." Is it reasonable for us to prescribe orlistat, recommend hoodia or even a "stomach stapling" for a patient who is 150 pounds overweight especially if we feel that some of our own medications have contributed to the obesity? What about the patient who is 40 pounds overweight? Or 20 pounds overweight? What then?

Do we react differently if the patient in an honest and straightforward manner says to us "I want to have a better sex life but I am not sick," or "I want to be mentally sharper and be able to get by with little sleep, but I don't have Attention Deficit Hyperactivity Disorder?" Society today is bombarded with advertisements to buy products to provide "five-hour energy" or enhance memory. Some people take laxatives because they're constipated, others simply because they want "a clean colon." Such over-the-counter products are sold to the general population as a way to enhance lifestyle. Will direct patient requests for prescription medications to perform similar functions be far behind? It is not that we are approaching a line in the sand between prescribing for disease and prescribing for lifestyle. We have already crossed it.

As prescribers and practitioners, we need to think about the issues raised by the above questions before we are confronted by patients with these requests; they are already sitting in our waiting rooms. The age of lifestyle prescribing is not coming, it is here. It is part of the way forward, whether we like it or not.

Summary

If you have followed and applied the principles in this book you will be a competent and knowledgeable practitioner of psychopharmacology. Your wisdom and expertise will help countless patients to ease the burden of mental health problems and provide increased satisfaction in their lives. Whether you have this book at the beginning of your career or mid-career to sharpen your skills, if you, make an effort to incorporate these principles as part of your standard practice habits, you will soon be seen as a knowledgeable and compassionate practitioner by both patients and fellow clinicians.

References

1   de Leon J *et al.* (2006) The AmpliChip CYP450 genotyping test: integrating a new clinical tool. *Molecular Diagnosis and Therapy* 10(3): 135–151. doi: 10.1007/BF03256453

2   Mrazek DA (2010) Psychiatric pharmacogenomic testing in clinical practice. *Dialogues in Clinical Neuroscience* 12: 69.

3   Porcelli S *et al.* (2011) Genetic polymorphisms of cytochrome P450 enzymes and antidepressant metabolism. *Expert Opinion on Drug Metabolism and Toxicology* 7(9): 1101–1115.

4   Zandi PP *et al.* (2010) The promise and reality of pharmacogenetics in psychiatry. *Psychiatry Clinics of North America* 33: 181.

5   Fleeman N *et al.* (2011) Cytochrome P450 testing for prescribing antipsychotics in adults with schizophrenia: systematic review and meta-analyses. *Pharmacogenomics Journal* 11: 1–14.

Appendix 1: Mental status testing

The de facto standard for a brief mental status exam, often used by primary care professionals and mental health clinicians alike, when a rapid, repeatable assessment of mental status is necessary, is the Mini Mental Status Exam (MMSE) as shown below. It takes less than 10 minutes to administer.

Instructions for administration of Mini Mental Status Exam

Orientation

1 Ask for the date. Then ask specifically for any parts omitted, e.g., "Can you also tell me what season it is?" 1 point for each correct answer.
2 Ask in turn "Can you tell me the name of this hospital?" (town, country, etc.). 1 point for each correct answer.

Registration

Ask the patient if you may test his memory. Then say the names of three unrelated objects, clearly and slowly (about 1 second for each). After you have spoken all three, ask him to repeat them. This first repetition determines the score (0–3), but keep saying them until he can repeat all three correctly, up to six trials. If he does not eventually learn all three, recall cannot be meaningfully tested.

Attention and calculation

Ask the patient to begin with 100 and count backward by 7, stop after five subtractions (93, 86, 79, 72, 65). Score the total number of correct answers. If the patient cannot or will not perform this task, ask him to spell the word "world" backward. The score is the number of letters in correct order, e.g., dlrow = 5, dlorw = 3.

Recall

Ask the patient if he can recall the three words you previously asked him to remember. Score 0–3.

Language

Naming. Show the patient a wristwatch and ask him what it is. Repeat for pencil. Score 0–2.

Repetition. Ask the patient to repeat the sentence "No ifs, ands or buts" after you. Allow only one trial. Score 0 or 1.

Three-stage command. Give the patient a piece of plain blank paper and give the following instructions: score 1 point for each part correctly executed.

- *Reading*: On a blank piece of paper, print the sentence "Close your eyes" in letters large enough for the patient to see clearly. Ask him to read it and do what it says. Score 1 point only if he actually closes his eyes.
- *Writing*: Give the patient a blank piece of paper and ask him to write a sentence.
- Do not dictate a sentence; it is to be written spontaneously. It must contain a subject and verb and be sensible. Correct grammar and punctuation are not necessary.
- *Copying*: On a clean piece of paper, draw intersecting pentagons, each side about 1", and ask him to copy it exactly as it is. All ten angles must be present and two must intersect to score 1 point. Tremor and rotation are ignored.

Estimate the patient's level of sensorium along a continuum, from alert on the left to coma on the right.

More detailed evaluation

When a more detailed evaluation of a patient's mental status is necessary, it is often useful to document a more thorough examination, which is outlined here. It contains some elements used in the MMSE with elaboration and the addition of other measurements. The basics of this mental status exam can be completed in approximately 10 minutes once the technique is mastered. Optional elements listed at the end may be added for further detail. Principles of performing this mental status exam are as follows:

- A significant portion of the exam involves educated observation of the patient's appearance, behavior, speech and mood, and can be done during the course of history taking or in the course of performing the specific mental status tests below.
- Each of the questions should be asked in a routinized way that the clinician states consistently each time the questions are asked. Examples of how to word these questions are listed with each item below.
- When recording the responses to the mental status examination, make brief notes, which may be elaborated upon at a later time for purposes of the patient's chart. A report generated by this mental status exam should "paint a picture" of the clinician's observations and experience of this patient, such that a reader of the evaluation can visualize, as clearly as possible, how the patient presented and interacted. Examples of such reports are included below.

Table A.1 Mini Mental Status Exam

EXAM A: MINI MENTAL STATUS EXAM (MMSE)		
Maximum score	*Score*	*Orientation*
5	( )	What is the (year) (season) (date) (day) (month)?
5	( )	Where are we: (state) (country) (town) (hospital) (floor)?
		Registration
3	( )	Name 3 objects: 1 second to say each. Then ask the patient all 3 after you have said them. Give 1 point for each correct answer. Then repeat them until he learns all 3. Count trials and record trials.
		Attention and calculation
5	( )	Serial 7s. 1 point for each correct answer. Stop after 5 answers. Alternatively, spell "world" backward.
		Recall
3	( )	Ask for the 3 objects repeated above. Give 1 point for each correct answer.
		Language
9	( )	Name a pencil and watch (2 points). Repeat the following: "No ifs, ands or buts" (1 point). Follow a 3-stage command: "Take a paper in your right hand, fold it in half, and put it on the floor" (3 points). Read and obey the following: close your eyes (1 point); write a sentence (1 point); copy design (1 point).

——— Total score

Assess level of consciousness along a continuum: ☐ ☐ ☐ ☐

                                                  Alert   Drowsy   Stupor   Coma

Source: Folstein MF *et al.* (1975) Mini-Mental State: a practical method for grading the state of patients for the clinician. *Journal of Psychiatric Research* 12: 189–198.

Appearance and behavior

Look for:

- dress, grooming
- gait, motor activity
- relatedness to the interviewer
- eye contact, expression
- somnolence, fluctuating attention
- hyperventilation, nervous gestures

- autonomic reactions (sweating, flushing)
- personality traits (effort level/apathy, response to difficulties, attempts to please or resist).

Speech

Look for:

- pace (slowed or rapid, pressured)
- volume
- grammar (for education)
- dysarthria (slurring)
- amount of verbalization
- organization
  - circumstantial
  - tangential
  - overinclusiveness
- neologisms (new, nonsensical words)
- clanging (rhyming associations)
- blocking (abrupt stoppage of thought or speech).

Affect

Look for:

- appropriate reactions to speech content
- flattened, monotone
- exaggerated reactions
- labile (changing affect)
- circumstantial – starts an answer but does not complete it and moves to minimally connected issues, but eventually returns to the appropriate answer.
- tangential – starts an answer but does not complete it and moves to minimally connected issues, but never returns to an appropriate answer.

Although a question is answered, patient includes excessive, unnecessary detail and irrelevancies.

Mood

Look for:

- sadness
- elation, grandiosity
- anxiety
- anger, rage
- fear
- suspiciousness.

Verbal introduction to memory tests

- "Now I'm going to ask you some questions that will help me evaluate your memory and concentration. Some will be easy and others may be difficult; I want you to do your best."
- Give the patient a motive to try hard on the testing (e.g., "This will help me to determine if you can handle your money matters or manage your own medications, etc…").

Concentration and memory
Three objects:

- "Now I'm going to give you three things to remember, and I'll ask you to repeat them in a few minutes." (use three unrelated objects, with at least two elements in each object – e.g., a blue fountain pen, a pair of used roller skates and the address 37 South Broadway)
- "Can you repeat them for me now, just to make sure you have them?" (immediate recall)
- 5 minutes later – "What were those three things I asked you to remember?" (recall).

In the interim, you can go on to other questions assessing orientation, memory and calculations. Don't forget to ask for recall of the three objects before you complete the exam.

Orientation

- "What is the date today?" (date, month, year)
- "What is the day of the week?"
- If necessary, "What is the season?"
- "Where are we right now?"
- "What is your full name and birth date?"

Concentration and memory
Serial 1s, 3s and/or 7s (choose one test or all):

- "Now I am going to have you do some counting. Start at 100 (50 or 30) and count backwards by 7s (3s or 1s). I want you to subtract 7 from 100 and keep subtracting 7 (3 or 1) from the total." (If the patient looks for reassurance after one or more answers, "I won't tell you if you are right or wrong, just keep going.")
- Note the responses, time, consistency, response to errors, perseveration.
- Presidents (United States):
  - "Who is the president of the United States right now?"
  - "Name the presidents before him in order, as far as you can go." (Biden, Trump, Obama, George W. Bush, Clinton, George Bush, Reagan, Carter, Ford, Nixon, Johnson, Kennedy)
- Prime Ministers (UK):
  - "Who is the prime minister now?"
  - "Name the prime ministers in order as far as you can go." (Johnson, May, Cameron, Brown, Blair, Major, Thatcher, Callaghan, Wilson, Heath, Wilson)

Calculations

- "Let's say you were going to the store and wanted to buy ... (e.g., a can of beans) and it costs ... (e.g., 57 cents). If you gave the clerk a dollar, how much change would you get?" (43 cents)
- "If you wanted to buy (four) cans of (e.g., soup) and they cost (e.g., 28 cents) each, how much would you have to pay?" ($1.12)

Other helpful tests

- "Spell the word 'world' backwards."
- "Repeat the phrase, 'no ifs, ands or buts'."
- "Trail test" of numbers and letters. Write a random array of numbers from 1 to 10 and letters from A to H at various places on a sheet of paper. Ask the patient to connect the numbers in order from 1 to 10 with a pencil. Then connect the letters in order from A to H in order with another pencil line.
- Fill in a clock face. Ask the person to draw the way a clock face looks. Ask them to draw the hands of the clock so it shows the time 10 minutes after 7 o'clock.
- Name common objects in the room (pen, pad, computer, picture).
- Follow a two- or three-step command (e.g., place your left hand on your right ear, then cross your legs).
- Write a sentence (e.g., I expect I will be feeling much better within a few weeks).

Often it is best to start with serial 1s in the hope of giving the patient confidence with a simpler task, then progress to serial 3s and 7s. If the patient has significant difficulties and/or multiple errors with the simpler task, there is no benefit to trying the more difficult tasks.

Psychosis

Look for:
- darting glances
- apparent response to internal stimuli
- illusions
- delusional thought content.

Ask:
- Do you see or hear things that other people don't see or hear?
- Do you hear voices when no one is around?
- Do you get "big ideas" that you, or other people, think are "too much" or not accomplishable? (grandiosity)
- Do you ever feel people are watching or following you?
- Do you ever feel people are always talking behind your back planning you harm? (paranoia)

Other information

Assess presence or absence of:

- suicidal ideation
- homicidal ideation (as outlined in Chapter 3).

Optional elements

Judgment:

- "What would you do if you were in a movie theater and suddenly smelled smoke?" (Walk to the exit; alert the manager)
- "What would you do if you were walking along the street and came upon a letter on the ground with an address and stamp on it?" (Put it in a mailbox)

Abstraction:

1   "How are the following pairs of objects alike?"
    - an apple and an orange (fruits)
    - a bathtub and the Atlantic Ocean (they both hold water)
    - a table and a chair (pieces of furniture)
    - a fly and a tree (living things).
2   "Listen to these sayings, and tell me what is the most general meaning they have to most people" (proverbs – ability to abstract)
    - Don't count your chickens before they hatch. (Don't expect something to come true before it actually happens.)
    - Even monkeys fall out of trees. (Even experts can make mistakes or fail.)
    - People who live in glass houses shouldn't throw stones. (If you have faults, you shouldn't criticize others.)

Intellectual functioning (United States)

- "How far is it from New York to Los Angeles?" (about 3000 miles)
- "Name the five largest cities in the United States." (New York, Los Angeles, Chicago, Houston, Philadelphia)
- "Who is the governor (mayor) of …?" (the state or city you are in)
- Intellectual functioning (UK)"How far is it from London to Birmingham?" (about 150 km)
- "What are the five largest cities in Britain?" (London, Manchester, Birmingham-Wolverhampton, Leeds-Bradford, Glasgow)

Examples of possible Mini Mental Status Exam reports

A person with minimal impairment and "normal" mental status

A person need not answer all questions perfectly to be considered as having a "normal" mental status. An isolated erroneous calculation or other minor incorrect answer is not uncommon in the absence of other signs and symptoms. Being faced with being "tested" by the clinician will create sufficient anxiety for some people not to perform perfectly. Multiple problems should, however, raise the clinician's suspicion of some mental deficits.

A depressed man

Mr. Jones is a 64-year-old Caucasian male who was evaluated for pharmacotherapy on November 8, 2013. He looks older than his stated age, walks slowly with labored steps coming into the office and appears to be in a modest amount of physical pain. He has a worried, apprehensive look on his face, and sits slumping in his chair. He can maintain eye contact with the interviewer, but often looks down at the floor or at his lap. He is alert and oriented to person, place and time; however, he shows psychomotor slowing in his speech and body movements. He wrings his hands at times and grips the arms of the chair tightly. His affect is moderately constricted and his mood is moderately depressed. He is tearful several times during the interview when talking about the death of his wife. At these times, it takes him several minutes to compose himself to go on with the rest of the interview. He says that he has had thoughts of killing himself by shooting, but does not own a firearm. He denies any homicidal ideation. He is able to recall three of three objects immediately after being given them, and two of three objects at 5 minutes. He does serial 7s with three errors out of 15 subtractions done in a 2-minute span. He knows the current president of the United States and is able to name three presidents in order before Biden. He is able to make change correctly from $1 and is able to spell the word *world* backwards without error, although he struggles to remember each letter. He denies any auditory or visual hallucinations, or paranoid ideation.

A psychotic young man

Mr. Abernathy is a 21-year-old man of Jamaican extraction who was seen for a medication examination on Thursday, June 10, 2012. He was dressed in tattered pants, worn shoes and a dirty t-shirt. His hair was tousled, and he had several days' growth of beard. His eyes were widened. He was markedly agitated, and had difficulty sitting in the chair to complete the evaluation. He showed frequent agitated movements and darting glances around the room, looking suspiciously off into corners. He talked primarily in a monotone, except when he glanced around the room, when he appeared anxious and agitated. He maintained a perplexed facial expression and displayed thought blocking. When asked about this, he initially denied it was of any significance. When asked a second time, he said that "I thought I saw something that scared me," but would not elaborate. He was oriented to person and place, but thought it was July instead of June. On specific questioning, he admitted to hearing voices, which he thought were those of his father, telling him that he was "no good" and a "failure." He appeared to be responding to internal stimuli, although he denied this. He stated that he had tried to kill himself 2 weeks ago by "eating himself to death," but said he had no plans to try to kill himself at this time. He denied any homicidal thoughts or behavior. He believed that several people in his apartment building had been watching him closely "to see if I was working for the government, but I'm not." Further, formal mental status testing was attempted, but the patient became increasingly agitated. He expressed concern that perhaps the interviewer was also trying to find out if he was "working for the government," and he refused to answer any further questions.

The Mini-Cog assessment instrument for dementia

The Mini-Cog assessment instrument combines an uncued three-item recall test with a clock-drawing test (CDT). The Mini-Cog can be administered in about 3 minutes, requires no special equipment and is relatively uninfluenced by level of education or language variations.

Administration

The test is administered as follows:

1 Instruct the patient to listen carefully to and remember three unrelated words and then immediately repeat the words.
2 Instruct the patient to draw the face of a clock, either on a blank sheet of paper, or on a sheet with the clock circle already drawn on the page. After the patient puts the numbers on the clock face, ask him or her to draw the hands of the clock to read a specific time, such as 11:20. These instructions can be repeated, but no additional instructions should be given. Give the patient as much time as needed to complete the task. The CDT serves as the recall distractor.
3 Ask the patient to repeat the three previously presented words.

Scoring

Give 1 point for each recalled word after the CDT distractor. Score 1–3.

A score of 0 indicates positive screen for dementia.
A score of 1 or 2 with an abnormal CDT indicates positive screen for dementia.
A score of 1 or 2 with a normal CDT indicates negative screen for dementia.
A score of 3 indicates negative screen for dementia.

The CDT is considered normal if all numbers are present in the correct sequence and position, and the hands readably display the requested time.

It should be mentioned that the Mini Mental Status Exam, the Mini-Cog or those items in a full mental status exam will not consistently identify subtle, minor memory/mental status changes in a well-compensated individual. A person who is not having significant behavioral abnormalities and who functions adequately in a work/school environment, but complains of poor memory or decreased concentration, may give "normal" responses to the tests mentioned here. When present, subtle memory, concentration and retention problems may only be revealed through a formal battery of neuropsychological tests administered by a psychologist trained in neuropsychological evaluation.

Appendices 2–5

Appendices 2–5 present the same data organized in different ways for easy reference.

Appendix 2 lists commonly prescribed psychotropics by medication function with subgroups of chemical class listed alphabetically by generic name.

Appendix 3 lists common psychotropic medicines alphabetically by generic name.

Appendix 4 lists common psychotropics available in the United States listed alphabetically by brand name.

Appendix 5 lists common psychotropics available in the UK listed alphabetically by brand name.

Each list includes starting doses and standard therapeutic dosage ranges.

Abbreviations

STD	Standard release preparation
-SR	Sustained release preparation
-XR	Extended release preparation
NA	Not available
Ng/ml	nanograms per milliliter
µg/ml	micrograms per milliliter
meq/l	milliequivalents per liter
QD	once a day
BID	twice daily
TID	three times daily
QID	four times daily

Collated from

1 *British National Formulary* (2011), Vol. 62, Pharmaceutical Press.
2 Schatzberg AF *et al.* (2010) *Manual of Clinical Psychopharmacology*, 7th edn., American Psychiatric Publishing, Inc.
3 *The Maudsley Prescribing Guidelines* (2009), Informa Healthcare.
4 Pharmaceutical company product package inserts.
5 Albers LJ *et al.* (2010) *Handbook of Psychiatric Drugs*, 2011 edn., Clinical Strategies Publishing.

Appendix 2: Common psychotropic medications by class

These drug categories list those compounds commonly used in mental health treatment or in amelioration of mental health medication side effects. They are not exhaustive of every medication in each category.

Chemical (generic) name	USA brand name(s)	UK brand name(s)	Starting dose (mg) Standard	Standard therapeutic dose (mg)	Useful blood levels
Antidepressants *Non-SSRI new generation*					
Bupropion	Wellbutrin, Wellbutrin-SR, Zyban		100 QD (STD)	200–450 (STD)	No
Bupropion Hbr	Aplenzin		174	348	No
Desvenlafaxine	Pristiq		50	50–400	No
Duloxetine	Cymbalta	Cymbalta	30–40	40–120	No
Mirtazepine	Remeron	Zispin	15	15–45	No
Nefazodone	Serzone	Dutonin	100 QD-100 BID	200–600	No
Reboxetine	NA	Edronax	4 BID	8–12	No
Venlafaxine	Effexor-XR, Effexor	Efexor-XR, Efexor	37.5 BID (STD) 37.5–75 (-XR)	75–375 (STD) 75–225 (-XR)	No
Vilazodone	Viibryd	Viibryd	10–20	40	No
Zyban			150 mg QD (-SR)	150–400 (-SR)	
SSRIs					
Citalopram	Celexa	Cipramil	20	20–60	No
Escitalopram	Lexapro	NA	10	10–20	No
Fluoxamine	previously Luvox, generic	Faverin, generic	50	50–300	No
Fluoxetine	Prozac, Serafem, generic	Prozac, generic	20	20–80	No
Paroxetine	Paxil, Paxil CR	Seroxat	20	10–60	No
Sertraline	Zoloft	Lustral	50	50–200	No
Vilazodone	Viibryd	Viibryd	10–20	40	No
Tricyclic					
Amitriptyline	Elavil, generic	Lentizol, Triptafen, generic	25–50	50–300	120–250 ng/ml
Amitriptyline + chlordiazepoxide	Limbitrol	NA	1 tab TID	1 tab-2 tabs TID	No

Amitriptyline + perphenazine	Etrafon, Etrafon Forte	NA	2–25 tab TID	2–25 tab BID-QID	No
Amoxapine	(previously Asendin), generic	Asendis	50 BID	50–600	No
Clomipramine	(previously Anafranil), generic	Anafranil, Anafranil SR, generic	25–100	25–250	100–250 ng/ml
Desipramine	Norpramin, generic	Pertofrane	25 TID	100–300	115–180 ng/ml
Dothiepin/Dosulpein	NA	Prothiaden, generic	75	150–225	No
Doxepin	Sinequan, generic	Sinequan	25 TID	75–300	200–250 ng/ml Blood level of parent compound plus metabolite
Imipramine	Tofranil, generic	Tofranil, generic	25 TID	75–300	200–250 ng/ml Blood level of parent compound plus metabolite
Lofepramine	NA	Gamanil, generic	70	40–210	No
Nortriptyline	(previously Pamelor), Aventyl, generic	Allegron, Motipress, Motival	50–100	75–150	50–150 ng/ml
Protriptyline	Vivactil	Concordin, generic	15	15–60	70–250 ng/ml
Trimipramine	Surmontil	Surmontil	75	50–300	No
Heterocyclics					
Maprotiline	(previously Ludiomil), generic	Ludiomil	25 TID	75–225	No
Mianserin	NA	generic	30–40	30–90	No
Selegiline	Ersam	generic	6	6–12	No
Trazodone	(previously Desyrel)	Molipaxin, generic	50–100	150–600	No
MAO inhibitors					
Doxepin	Silenor	generic	3–6	3–6	No
Isocarboxazid	NA		10	20–60	No
Meclobemide	NA	Manerix	100–300	300–600	No
Phenelzine	Nardil	Nardil	15	15–90	No
Selegiline	Ersam		6	6–12	No
Tranylcypromine	Parnate	Parnate	10	30–60	No
Mood-stabilizing medication					
Carbamazepine	Tegretol, generic	Tegretol, Teril, Timonil, generic	100–400	400–1600	4–12 1-g/ml

(continued)

Chemical (generic) name	USA brand name(s)	UK brand name(s)	Starting dose (mg)/ Standard	Standard therapeutic dose (mg)	Useful blood levels
Lamotrigine	Lamictal	Lamictal	25	100–400	No
Lithium carbonate	Eskalith, Eskalith CR, Lithobid, generic	Liskonum, Camcolit	300–600	600–1800	0.6–1.2 meq/l
Oxcarbazepine	Trileptal	Trileptal	300 BID	600–2400	No
Topiramate	Topamax	Topamax	25	200–400	No
Valproic acid	Depakote, Depakote-ER, Depakene, generic	Epilim, Convulex, Depakote, generic	250 TID	750–4200	50–100 1-g/ml
Verapamil	Verelan, Calan, Isoptin, generic	Cordilox, Securon, Univer, Verapress, Vertab, generic	40 TI	80–120 TID	No

Anti-anxiety/hypnotics
Benzodiazepines

Chemical (generic) name	USA brand name(s)	UK brand name(s)	Starting dose (mg)/ Standard	Standard therapeutic dose (mg)	Useful blood levels
Alprazolam	Xanax, generic	Xanax, generic	0.25 TID	0.25–10	No
Chlorazepate	Tranxene	Tranxene	7.5	7.5–60	No
Chlordiazepoxide	Librium, generic	Tropium, Librium, generic	10 TID	15–100	No
Clobazam	NA	Clobazam	20	20–60	No
Clonazepam	Klonopin, generic	Rivotril	1	1.5–20	No
Diazepam	Valium, generic	Valium, Rimapam, Tensium	2–4	4–40	No
Doxepin	Silenor		3–6	3–6	No
Estazolam	Prosom		0.5	0.5–2	No
Flunitrazepam	NA	Rohypnol	0.5–1	0.5–2	No
Flurazepam	Flurazepam (previously Dalmane)	Flurazepam	15	15–30	No
Loprazolam	NA	(previously Dormonoct)	1	1.5–2	No
Lorazepam	Ativan, generic	Ativan, generic	1–2	1–10	No
Lormetazepam	NA	generic	0.5	0.5–1.5	No
Nitrazepam	NA	Somnite, Mogadon generic	5	5–10	No
Oxazepam	(previously Serax) generic	generic	10	30–120	No

Sodium Oxybate	Xyrem	Xyrem	2.25 twice at night	4.5–9	No
Temazepam	Restoril	generic	15	7.5–30	No
Triazolam	Halcion	N/A	0.125	0.125–0.5	No
Non-benzodiazepine anti-anxiety medication					
Buspirone	Buspar, generic	Buspar, generic	5–10 TID	30–60	No
Sedative hypnotics					
Chloral Hydrate	generic	Chloral Elixir, Welldorm	500	500–2000	No
Clomethiazole	NA	Heminevrin	1 capsule	1–2 capsules	No
Zaleplon	Sonata	Sonata	5	5–20	No
Zolpidem	Ambien	Stilnoct	5	5–10	No
Zopiclone	N/A	Zimovane	3.75	3.75–7.5	No
Antipsychotics					
Traditional					
Benperidol	NA	Anquil, generic	0.25–1.5	0.25–1.5	No
Chlorpromazine	Thorazine, generic	Largactil, generic	25 TID	30–800	No
Flupentixol	NA	Depixol	3–9 BID	6–18	No
Fluphenazine	generic (previously Prolixin)	Moditen, Modecate	2.5–10	1–40	No
Haloperidol	Haldol, generic	Haldol, Dozic, Serenace, generic	1–3 BID	1–100	No
Levopromazine	NA	ozinan	25–50	100–200	No
Loxapine	Loxitane	Loxapac	10–25 BID	20–250	No
Mesoridazine	Serentil	NA	50 TID	100–400	No
Molindone	Moban	NA	50 TID	15–225	No
Oxypertine	NA	generic	80–120	80–300	No
Pericyazine	NA	Neulactil	25 TID	75–300	No
Perphenazine	Trilafon, Etrafon, generic	Fentazin	4 TID	12–64	No
Pimozide	Orap	Orap	2	2–20	No
Promazine	NA	generic	25–30 QID	400–800	No

(continued)

Chemical (generic) name	USA brand name(s)	UK brand name(s)	Starting dose (mg) Standard	Standard therapeutic dose (mg)	Useful blood levels
Sulpiride	NA	Dolmatil, Clopixol, Sulpital, Sulpor, generic	200–400	400–2400	No
Thioridazine	generic (previously Mellaril)	Mellaril, generic	50–300	20–600	No
Thiothixene	Navane	NA	2 TID	6–60	No
Trifluoperazine	Stelazine, generic	Stelazine, generic	5 BID	2–40	No
Zuclopenthixol	NA	Clopixol	20–30	20–150	No
Atypical					
Amisulpride	NA	Solian	50–100	50–1200	No
Aripiprazole	Abilify	NA	10–15	10–30	No
Clozapine	Clozaril, generic	Clozaril	12.5 BID	12.5–900	>350 mg/ml
Dexmethylphenidate	Focalin, Focalin-XR	Focalim	5–10	30–40	
Dextroamphetamine	Dextrostat		1–4	5–60	No
Guanfacine	Intuniv	Intuniv	1	1–4	
Iloperidone	Fanapt	Fanapt, Zomaril	1 BID	6–12 BID	No
Lisdexamfetamine	Vyvanse		30	30–70	No
Lurasidone	Latuda	Latuda	40 with food	40–160	No
Methylphenidate			10	10–30	
Olanzapine	Zyprexa aytrana	Zyprexa	2.5–10	2.5–20	No
Paliperidone	Invega	Invega	6	3–12	
Quetiapine	Seroquel	Seroquel	25	50–750	No
Risperidone	Risperdal	Risperdal	0.5	0.5–16	No
Ziprasidone	Geodon	NA	20–40	40–160	No
Zotepine	NA	Zoleptil	25 TID	50–300	No
Miscellaneous					
Anticholinergics					
Benztropine	Cogentin, generic	Cogentin (generic as benztropin or Benzatropin)	0.5–1	1–8	No
Biperidon	Akineton	Akineton	1 BID	2–8	No

(*continued*)

Procyclidine	NA	Arpicolin, Kemadrin, generic	2.5 TID	7.5–20	No
Trihexyphenidyl	Artane, generic	Broflex, generic	1	2–15	No
Antihistamines					
Cyproheptadine	Periactin, generic	Periactin	4 TID	4–32	No
Diphenhydramine	Benadryl, generic	generic	25 BID	50–400	No
Hydroxyzine	Atarax, Vistaril, generic	Atarax, Cerax	25	50–100	No
Beta blockers					
Atenolol	Tenormin generic	Tenormin	50	50–100	No
Pindolol	generic	Viskin, Viskaldix	5 BID	15–45	No
Amphetamine					
Anti-obesity agents					
Appetite suppressants					
Orlistat	Xenical	Xenical	120 TID	120 TID	No
Phentermine	Ionamin, Apidex	NA	37.5	18.75–37.5	No
Sibutramine	Meridia	Reductil	10	5–15	No
Stimulants					
Dexmethylphenidate	Focalin, Focalin-XR	Focalin	5–10	30–40	
Dextroamphetamine	Dextrostat		1–4	5–60	
Guanfacine	Intuniv	Intuniv	1	1–4	No
Lisdexamfetamine	Vyvanse		30	30–70	No
Methylphenidate	Minipress	Minipress	1	1–4	No
Other medications mentioned in this book					
Diphenoxylate and Atropine	generic	Lomotil	1 tab QID	2 tabs Q 6 hours	No
Docusate	Colace, Peri-Colace, generic	Dioctyl, Docusol	50	50–200	No
Ispaghula husk	NA	Fybogel, Isogel, Ispagel, Konsyl, Regulan	1 packet BID	1 packet QD–TID	No
Levothyroxine	Levoxyl, Levothroid, Synthroid, Unithroid	Levothyroxine, Liothyronine, Terroxin	12.5–50 1-g	12.5–500 1-g	No
Loperamide	Immodium	Immodium, generic	4	6–16	No

Chemical (generic) name	USA brand name(s)	UK brand name(s)	Starting dose (mg) Standard	Standard therapeutic dose (mg)	Useful blood levels
L-Tryptophan	NA	Optimax	1 TID	6	No
Meprobamate	Miltown, Equagesic, generic	Equagesic, generic	400 TID	1200–1600	No
Neurontin	Gabapentin	Neurontin	300	1500–3600	No
Prazosin	Minipress	Minipress	1	1–4	No
Psyllium husk	Metmucil, generic		1 tsp in water	1 tsp in water	No
Senna	Senekot	Manevac, Senekot, generic	15	15–30	No
Sildenafil	Viagra		50	25–100	No

Appendix 3: Common psychotropic medications listed alphabetically by generic name

These drug categories list those compounds commonly used in mental health treatment or in amelioration of mental health medication side effects. They are not exhaustive of every medication in each category.

Chemical (generic) name	USA brand name(s)	UK brand name(s)	Class of medication
Acamprosate	NA	Campral EC	Medication for alcohol abuse
Alprazolam	Xanax, generic	Xanax, generic	Benzodiazepines
Amisulpride	NA	Solian	Atypical Antipsychotic
Amitriptyline	Elavil, generic	Lentizol, Triptafen, generic	Tricyclic Antidepressant
Amitriptyline + chlordiazepoxide	Limbitrol	NA	Tricyclic Antidepressant
Amitriptyline + perphenazine	Etrafon, Etrafon Forte	NA	Tricyclic Antidepressant
Amoxapine	(previously Asendin), generic	Asendis	Tricyclic Antidepressant
Atenolol	Tenormin	Tenormin	Beta Blocker
Benperidol	NA	Anquil, generic	Traditional Antipsychotic
Benztropine	Cogentin, generic	Cogentin (generic as benztropine or benztropine)	Anticholinergic
Biperidon	Akineton	Akineton	Anticholinergic
Bupropion	Wellbutrin, Wellbutrin-SR, Zyban	Zyban	Non-SSRI New Generation
Buprion Hbr	Aplenzin		Antidepressant
Buspirone	Buspar, generic	Buspar, generic	Non-Benzodiazepine Anti-anxiety
Carbamazepine	Tegretol, generic	Tegretol, Teril, Timonil, generic	Mood Stabilizer
Chloral Hydrate	generic	Chloral Elixir, Welldorm	Sedative Hypnotic
Chlorazepate	Tranxene	Tranxene	Benzodiazepines
Chlordiazepoxide	Librium, generic	Tropium, Librium, generic	Benzodiazepines
Chlorpromazine	Thorazine, generic	Largactil, generic	Traditional Antipsychotic
Citalopram	Celexa	Cipramil	SSRI Antidepressant
Clobazam	NA	Clobazam	Benzodiazepines
Clomethiazole	NA	Heminevrin	Sedative Hypnotic
Clomipramine	(previously Anafranil), generic	Anafranil, Anafranil SR, generic	Tricyclic Antidepressant
Clonazepam	Klonopin, generic	Rivotril	Benzodiazepines
Clozapine	Clozaril, generic	Clozaril	Atypical Antipsychotic
Cyproheptadine	Periactin, generic	Periactin	Antihistamine
Desipramine	Norpramin, generic	Pertofrane	Tricyclic Antidepressant
esvenlafaxine	Pristiq		Antidepressant
Detroamphetamine and amphetamine examphetamine	Adderall, Concordia	NA	Stimulant
Dexmethylphenidate	Dexedrine	Dexedrine	Stimulant
Dextroamphetamine	Focalin, Focalin-XR	Focalin	Stimulant
	Dextrostat	NA	Stimulant

Diazepam	Valium, generic	Valium, Rimapam, Tensium	Benzodiazepines
extroamphetamine	extrostat		Stimulant
Diphenhydramine	Benadryl, generic		Antihistamine
Diphenoxylate and atropine	generic	generic	Other medications
Disulfiram	Antabuse, generic	Lomotil	Medication for alcohol abuse
Docusate	Colace, Peri-Colace, generic	Antabuse	Other medications
onepezil	Aricept	Dioctyl, Docusol	Cholinestrase Inhibitor
othiepin/Dosulpein	NA	Aricept	Tricyclic Antidepressant
Doxepin	Sinequan, generic	Prothiaden, generic	Tricyclic Antidepressant
Doxepin	Silenor	Sinequan	Hypnotic
Duloxetine	Cymbalta	Cymbalta	Antidepressant
Escitalopram	Lexapro	NA	SSRI Antidepressant
Estazolam	Prosom	NA	Benzodiazepines
Flunitrazepam	NA	Rohypnol	Benzodiazepines
Fluoxamine	previously Luvox, generic	Faverin, generic	SSRI Antidepressant
Fluoxetine	Prozac, Serafem, generic	rozac, generic	SSRI Antidepressant
Flupentixol	DA	Depixol	Traditional Antipsychotic
Fluphenazine	generic (previously Prolixin)	Moditen, Modecate	Traditional Antipsychotic
Flurazepam	Flurazepam (previously Dalmane)	Flurazepam	Benzodiazepines
Gabapentin	Neurontin	Neurontin	Other medications
Galantamine	Reminyl	Reminyl	Cholinestrase Inhibitor
Guanfacine	Intuniv	Intuniv	ADHD treatment
Haloperidol	Haldol, generic	Haldol, Dozic, Serenace, generic	Traditional Antipsychotic
Hydroxyzine	Atarax, Vistaril, generic	Atarax, Cerax	Antihistamine
Iloperidone	Fanapt	Fanapt, Zomaril	Antipsychotic
Imipramine	Tofranil, generic	Tofranil, generic	Tricyclic Antidepressant
Isocarboxazid	NA	generic	MAOI
Ispaghula husk	NA	Fybogel, Isogel, Ispagel, Konsyl, Regulan	Other medications
Lamotrigine	Lamictal	Lamictal	Mood Stabilizer
Levopromazine	NA	Nozinan	Traditional Antipsychotic
Levothyroxine	Levoxyl, Levothroid, Synthroid, Unithroid	Levothyroxine, Liothyronine, Terroxin	Other medications
Lisdexamfetamine	Vyvanse		Stimulant

(continued)

Chemical (generic) name	USA brand name(s)	UK brand name(s)	Class of medication
Lithium carbonate	Eskalith, Eskalith CR, Lithobid, generic	Liskonum, Camcolit	Mood Stabilizer
Lofepramine	NA	Gamanil, generic	Tricyclic Antidepressant
Loperamide	Immodium	Immodium, generic	Other medications
Loprazolam	NA	(previously Dormonoct)	Benzodiazepines
Lorazepam	Ativan, generic	Ativan, generic	Benzodiazepines
Lormetazepam	NA	generic	Benzodiazepines
Loxapine	Loxitane	Loxapac	Traditional Antipsychotic
L–Tryptophan	NA	Optimax	Other medications
Lurasidone	Latuda	Latuda	Antipsychotic
Maprotiline	(previously Ludiomil)	Ludiomil	Heterocyclic generic Antidepressant
Meclobemide	NA	Manerix	MAOI medications
Meprobamate	Miltown, Equagesic, generic	Equagesic, generic	Other
Mesoridazine	Serentil	NA	Traditional Antipsychotic
Methamphetamine	Desoxyn	NA	Stimulant
Methylphenidate	Daytrana, Ritalin, Ritalin SR, Concerta, Concerta extended release, Metadate, Metadate ER, Methylin, Methylin ER, generic	Ritalin, Equasym	Stimulant
Mianserin	NA	generic	Heterocyclic
Mirtazapine	Remeron	Zispin	Non-SSRI New Generation Antidepressant
Modafanil	Provigil	Provigil	Stimulant
Molindone	Moban	NA	Traditional Antipsychotic
Naltrexone	Depade	Nalorex	Medication for alcohol abuse
Nefazodone	Serzone	Dutonin	Non-SSRI New Generation Antidepressant
Modafanil	Provigil	Provigil	Stimulant
Molindone	Moban	NA	Traditional
Naltrexone	Depade	Nalorex	Medication for alcohol abuse
Nefazodone	Serzone	Dutonin	Non-SSRI New Generation
Nitrazepam	NA	Somnite, Mogadon	Benzodiazepines
Nortriptyline	(previously Pamelor), Aventyl, generic	Allegron, Motipress, Motival	Tricyclic Antidepressant

Olanzapine	Zyprexa	Zyprexa	Atypical Antipsychotic
Orlistat	Xenical	Xenical	Anti-obesity agent
Oxazepam	(previously Serax), generic	generic	Benzodiazepines
Oxcarbazepine	Trileptal	Trileptal	Mood Stabilizer
Oxypertine	NA	generic	Traditional Antipsychotic
Paliperidone	Invega	Invega	Antipsychotic
Paroxetine	Paxil, Paxil CR	Seroxat	SSRI Antidepressant
Pemoline	Cylert	NA	Stimulant
Pericyazine	NA	Neulactil	Traditional Antipsychotic
Perphenazine	Trilafon, Etrafon, generic	Fentazin	Traditional Antipsychotic
Phenelzine	Nardil	Nardil	MAOI
Phentermine	Ionamin, Apidex	NA	Appetite Suppressant
Pimozide	Orap	Orap	Traditional Antipsychotic
Pindolol	generic	Viskin, Viskaldix	Beta Blocker
Prazosin	Minipress	Minipress	Other medications
Procyclidine	NA	Arpicolin, Kemadrin, generic	Anticholinergic
Promazine	NA	generic	Traditional Antipsychotic
Propanolol	Inderal	Inderal, generic, Inderetic, Inderex	Beta Blocker
Protriptyline	Vivactil	Concordin, generic	Tricyclic Antidepressant
Psyllium husk	Metmucil, generic		Other medications
Quetiapine	Seroquel	Seroquel	Atypical Antipsychotic
Reboxetine	NA	Edronax	Non-SSRI New Generation
Risperidone	Risperdal	Risperdal	Atypical Antipsychotic
Rivastigmine	Exelon	Exelon	Cholinestrase Inhibitor
Selegiline	Emsam		Antidepressant
Senna	Senekot	Manevac, Senekot, generic	Other medications
Sertraline	Zoloft	Lustral	SSRI Antidepressant
Sibutramine	Meridia	Reductil	Appetite Suppressant
Sildenafil	Viagra	Viagra	Other medications
Sodium Oxybate	Xyrem	Xyrem	Hypnotic
Sulpiride	NA	Dolmatil, Clopixol, Sulpital, Sulpor, generic	Traditional Antipsychotic
Tacrine	Cognex	NA	Cholinestrase Inhibitor
Temazepam	Restoril	generic	Benzodiazepines
Thioridazine	generic (previously Mellaril)	Mellaril, generic	Traditional Antipsychotic

(*continued*)

Chemical (generic) name	USA brand name(s)	UK brand name(s)	Class of medication
Thiothixene	Navane	NA	Traditional Antipsychotic
Topiramate	Topamax	Topamax	Mood Stabilizer
Tranylcypromine	Parnate (previously Desyrel)	Parnate Molipaxin, generic	MAOI
Trazodone	Oleptro		Heterocyclic Antidespressant
Triazolam	Halcion	NA	Benzodiazepines
Trifluoperazine	Stelazine, generic	Stelazine, generic	Traditional Antipsychotic
Trihexyphenidyl	Artane, generic	Broflex, generic	Anticholinergic
Trimipramine	Surmontil	Surmontil	Tricyclic Antidepressant
Valproic Acid	Depakote, Depakote ER, Depakene, generic	Epilim, Convulex, Depakote, generic	Mood Stabilizer
Venlafaxine	Effexor-XR, Effexor	Efexor-XR, Efexor	Non-SSRI New Generation Antidepressant
Verapamil	Verelan, Calan, Isoptin, generic	Cordilox, Securon, Univer, Verapress, Vertab, generic	Mood Stabilizer
Vilazodone	Viibryd	Viibryd	SSRI Antidepressant
Zaleplon	Sonata	Sonata	Sedative Hypnotic
Ziprasidone	Geodon	NA	Atypical Antipsychotic
Zolpidem	Ambien	Stilnoct	Sedative Hypnotic
Zopiclone	NA	Zimovane	Sedative Hypnotic
Zotepine	NA	Zoleptil	Atypical Antipsychotic
Zuclopenthixol	NA	Clopixol	Traditional Antipsychotic

Appendix 4: Common psychotropic medications available in the United States, listed alphabetically by brand name

These drug categories list those compounds commonly used in mental health treatment or in amelioration of mental health medication side effects. They are not exhaustive of every medication in each category.

USA brand name(s)	Chemical (generic) name	Starting dose (mg) except as specified	Standard therapeutic dose (mg)	Useful blood levels
Abilify	Aripiprazole	10–15	10–30	No
Adderall	Dextroamphetamine and amphetamine	2.5–5 BID	5–60	No
Akineton	Biperidon	1 BID	2–8	No
Ambien	Zolpidem	5	5–10	No
Anafranil	Clomipramine	25–100	25–250	100–250 ng/ml
Antabuse	Disulfiram	250	125–500	No
Apidex	Phentermine	37.5	18.75–37.5	No
Aplenzin	Bupropion Hbr	174	348	No
Aricept	Donepezil	5	5–10	No
Artane	Trihexyphenidyl	1	2–15	No
Asendin	Amoxapine	50 BID	50–600	No
Atarax	Hydroxyzine	25	50–100	No
Ativan	Lorazepam	1–2	1–10	No
Aventyl	Nortriptyline	50–100	75–150	50–150 ng/ml
Benadryl	Diphenhydramine	25 BID	50–400	No
Buspar	Buspirone	5–10 TID	30–60	No
Calan	Verapamil	40 TID	80–120 TID	No
Celexa	Citalopram	20	20–60	No
Clozaril	Clozapine	12.5 BID	12.5–900	>350 mg/ml
Cogentin	Benztropine	0.5–1	1–8	No
Cognex	Tacrine	10 QID	40–160	No
Colace	Docusate	50	50–200	No
Concerta	Methylphenidate	5–10 BID	10–60	No
Concerta extended release	Methylphenidate	5–10 BID	10–60	No
Concordia	Dextroamphetamine and amphetamine	2.5–5 BID	5–60	No
Cylert	Pemoline	37.5	37.5–112.5	No
Cymbalta	Duloxetine	30–40	40–120	No
Daytrana	Methylphenidate	10	4–12	No
Depade	Naltrexone	25	50	No
Depakene	Valproic acid	250 TID	750–4200	50–100 1-g/ml
Depakote	Valproic acid	250 TID	750–4200	50–100 1-g/ml
Depakote ER	Valproic acid	250 TID	750–4200	50–100 1-g/ml

(*continued*)

Desoxyn	Methamphetamine	5 BID	5–25	No
Desyrel	Trazodone	50–100	150–600	No
Dexedrine	Dexamphetamine	10	10–60	No
Dextrostat	extroamphetamine	10	10–60	No
		10–5	22037	
Effexor-XR	Venlafaxine	37.5 BID (STD)	75–375 (STD)	No
		37.5–75 (-XR)	75–225 (-XR)	
Elavil	Amitriptyline	25–50	50–300	120–250 ng/ml
Emsam	Selegiline	6	6–12	No
Equagesic	Meprobamate	400 TID	1200–1600	No
Eskalith	Lithium carbonate	300–600	600–1800	0.6–1.2 meq/l
Eskalith CR	Lithium carbonate	300–600	600–1800	0.6–1.2 meq/l
Etrafon	Amitriptyline + perphenazine	2–25 tab TID	2–25 tab BID-QID	No
Etrafon	Perphenazine	4 TID	12–64	No
Etrafon Forte	Amitriptyline + perphenazine	2–25 tab TID	2–25 tab BID-QID	No
Exelon	Rivastigmine	1.5 BID	6–12	No
Fanapt	Iloperidone	1 BID	6–12 BID	No
Focalin, Focalin-XR	Dexmethylphenidate	5–10	30–40	No
Flurazepam	Flurazepam	15	15–30	No
Geodon	Ziprasidone	20–40	40–160	No
Halcion	Triazolam	0.125	0.125–0.5	No
Haldol	Haloperidol	1–3 BID	1–100	No
Immodium	Loperamide	4	6–16	No
Inderal	Propanolol	10–20 BID-TID	20–320	No
Intuniv	Guanfacine	1	1–4	No
Invega	Paliperidone	6	3–12	No
Ionamin	Phentermine	37.5	18.75–37.5	No
Isoptin	Verapamil	40 TID	80–120 TID	No
Klonopin	Clonazepam	1	1.5–20	No
Lamictal	Lamotrigine	25	100–400	No
Latuda	Lurasidone	40 with food	40–160	No
Levothroid	Levothyroxine	12.5–50 1-g	12.5–500 1-g	No
Levoxyl	Levothyroxine	12.5–50 1-g	12.5–500 1-g	No
Lexapro	Escitalopram	10	10–20	No
Librium	Chlordiazepoxide	10 TID	15–100	No

USA brand name(s)	Chemical (generic) name	Starting dose (mg) except as specified	Standard therapeutic dose (mg)	Useful blood levels
Limbitrol	Amitriptyline + chlordiazepoxide	1 tab TID	1 tab–2 tabs TID	No
Lithobid	Lithium carbonate	300–600	600–1800	0.6–1.2 meq/l
Loxitane	Loxapine	10–25 BID	20–250	No
Ludiomil	Maprotiline	25 TID	75–225	No
Luvox	Fluvoxamine	50	50–300	No
Mellaril	Thioridazine	50–300	20–600	No
Meridia	Sibutramine	10	-15	No
Metadate	Methylphenidate	5–10 BID	10–60	No
Metadate ER	Methylphenidate	5–10 BID	10–60	No
Methylin	Methylphenidate	5–10 BID	10–60	No
Methylin ER	Methylphenidate	5–10 BID	10–60	No
Metmucil	Psyllium husk	1 tsp in water	1 tsp in water	No
Miltown	Meprobamate	400 TID	1200–1600	No
Minipress	Prazosin	1	1–15 hs	No
Moban	Molindone	50 TID	15–225	No
Nardil	Phenelzine	15	15–90	No
Navane	Thiothixene	2 TID	6–60	No
Neurontin	Gabapentin	300	1800–3600	No
Norpramin	Desipramine	25 TID	100–300	115–180 ng/ml
Oleptro	Trazodone	150	150–375	No
Orap	Pimozide	2	2–20	No
Pamelor	Nortriptyline	50–100	75–150	50–150 ng/ml
Parnate	Tranylcypromine	10	30–60	No
Paxil	Paroxetine	20	10–60	No
Paxil CR	Paroxetine	20	10–60	No
Periactin	Cyproheptadine	4 TID	4–32	No
Peri-Colace	Docusate	50	50–200	No
Pristiq	Desvenlafaxine	50	50–400	No
Prolixin	Fluphenazine	2.5–10	1–40	No
Prosom	Estazolam	0.5	0.5–2	No
Provigil	Modafanil	100–200	200–400	No
Prozac	Fluoxetine	20	20–80	No
Remeron	Mirtazepine	15	15–45	No

Brand	Generic	Dose	Range	Blood level
Reminyl	Galantamine	4 BID	16–32	No
Restoril	Temazepam	15	7.5–30	No
Risperdal	Risperidone	0.5	0.5–16	No
Ritalin	Methylphenidate	5–10 BID	10–60	No
Ritalin SR	Methylphenidate	5–10 BID	10–60	No
Saphris	Asenapine	5–10 BID	5–10	No
Senekot	Senna	15	15–30	No
Serafem	Fluoxetine	20	20–80	No
Serax	Oxazepam	10	30–120	No
Serentil	Mesoridazine	50 TID	100–400	No
Seroquel	Quetiapine	25	50–750	No
Serzone	Nefazodone	100 QD–100	200–600	No
Silenor	Doxepin	3–6	3–6	No
Sinequan	Doxepin	25 TID	75–300	200–250 ng/ml Blood level of parent compound plus metabolite
Sonata	Zaleplon	5 BID	5–20	No
Stelazine	Trifluoperazine	5 BID	2–40	No
Surmontil	Trimipramine	75	50–300	No
Synthroid	Levothyroxine	12.5–50 1-g	12.5–500 1-g	4–12 1-g/ml
Tegretol	Carbamazepine	100–400	400–1600	No
Tenormin	Atenolol	50	50–100	No
Thorazine	Chlorpromazine	25 TID	30–800	No
Tofranil	Imipramine	25 TID	75–300	200–250 ng/ml Blood level of parent compound plus metabolite
Topamax	Topiramate	25	200–400	No
Tranxene	Chlorazepate	7.5	7.5–60	No
Trilafon	Perphenazine	4 TID	12–64	No
Trileptal	Oxcarbazepine	300 BID	600–2400	No
Unithroid	Levothyroxine	12.5–50 1-g	12.5–500 1-g	No
Valium	Diazepam	2–6	4–40	No
Verelan	Verapamil	40 TID	80–120 TID	No
Viagra	Sildenafil	50	25–100	No
Viibryd	Vilazodone	10–20	40	No

(continued)

USA brand name(s)	Chemical (generic) name	Starting dose (mg) except as specified	Standard therapeutic dose (mg)	Useful blood levels
Vistaril	Hydroxyzine	25	50–100	No
Vivactil	Protriptyline (synthetic)	15	15–60	70–250 ng/ml
Vyvanse	Lisdexamfetamine	30	30–70	No
Wellbutrin	Bupropion	100 QD (STD)	200–450 (STD)	No
		150 mg QD (-SR)	150–400 (-SR)	
Wellbutrin-SR	Bupropion	100 QD (STD)	200–450 (STD)	No
		150 mg QD (-SR)	150–400 (-SR)	
Wellbutrin-XR	Bupropion	300 qd		No
Xanax	Alprazolam	0.25 TID	0.25–10	No
Xenical	Orlistat	120 TID	120 TID	No
Xyrem	Sodium Oxybate	2.25 twice at night	4.5–9	No
Zoloft	Sertraline	50	50–200	No
Zyban	Bupropion	100 QD (STD)	200–450 (STD)	No
		150 mg QD (-SR)	150–400 (-SR)	
Zyprexa	Olanzapine	2.5–10	2.5–20	No

Appendix 5: Common psychotropic medications available in the UK, listed alphabetically by brand name

These drug categories list those compounds commonly used in mental health treatment or in amelioration of mental health medication side effects. They are not exhaustive of every medication in each category.

UK brand name(s)	Chemical (generic) name	Starting dose (mg) except as specified	Standard therapeutic dose (mg)	Useful blood levels
Akineton	Biperidon	1 BID	2–8	No
Allegron	Nortriptyline	50–100	75–150	50–150 ng/ml
Anafranil	Clomipramine	25–100	25–250	100–250 ng/ml
Anafranil SR	Clomipramine	25–100	25–250	100–250 ng/ml
Anquil	Benperidol	0.25–1.5	0.25–1.5	No
Antabuse	Disulfiram	250	125–500	No
Aricept	Donepezil	5	5–10	No
Arpicolin	Procyclidine	2.5 TID	7.5–20	No
Asendis	Amoxapine	50 BID	50–600	No
Atarax	Hydroxyzine	25	50–100	No
Ativan	Lorazepam	1–2	1–10	No
Broflex	Trihexyphenidyl	1	2–15	No
Buspar	Buspirone	5–10 TID	30–60	No
Camcolit	Lithium carbonate	300–600	600–1800	0.6–1.2 meq/l
Campral EC	Acamprosate	666 BID	2000	No
Cerax	Hydroxyzine	25	50–100	No
Chloral Elixir	Chloral hydrate	500	500–2000	No
Cipramil	Citalopram	20	20–60	No
Clobazam	Clobazam	20	20–60	No
Clopixol	Sulpiride	200–400	400–2400	No
Clopixol	Zuclopenthixol	20–30	20–150	No
Clozaril	Clozapine	12.5 BID	12.5–900	>350 mg/ml
Cogentin	Benztropine	0.5–1	1–8	No
Concordin	Protriptyline	15	15–60	70–250 ng/ml
Convulex	Valproic acid	250 TID	750–4200	50–100 1-g/ml
Cordilox	Verapamil	40 TID	80–120 TID	No
Cymbalta	Duloxetine	30–40	40–120	No
Depakote	Valproic acid	250 TID	750–4200	50–100 1-g/ml
Depixol	Flupentixol	3–9 BID	6–18	No
Dexedrine	Dexamphetamine	10	10–60	No
Dioctyl	Docusate	50	50–200	No
Docusol	Docusate	50	50–200	No
Dolmatil	Sulpiride	200–400	400–2400	No

Dozic	Haloperidol	1–3 BID	1–100	No
Dutonin	Nefazodone	100 QD–100 BID	200–600	No
Edronax	Reboxetine	4 BID	8–12	No
Efexor	Venlafaxine	37.5 BID (STD) / 37.5–75 (-XR)	75–375 (STD) / 75–225 (-XR)	No
Efexor-XR	Venlafaxine	37.5 BID (STD) / 37.5–75 (-XR)	75–375 (STD) / 75–225 (-XR)	No
Epilim	Valproic acid	250	50–4200	50–100 1-g/ml
Equagesic	Meprobamate	400 TID	1200–1600	No
Equasym	Methylphenidate	5–10 BID	10–60	No
Exelon	Rivastigmine	1.5 BID	6–12	No
Fanapt, Zomaril	Iloperidone	1 BID	6–12 BID	No
Faverin	Fluoxamine	50	50–300	No
Fentazin	Perphenazine	4 TID	12–64	No
Flurazepam	Flurazepam	15	15–30	No
Focalin	Dexmethylphenidate	5–10	30–40	No
Fybogel	Ispaghula husk	1 packet BID	1 packet QD-TID	No
Gamanil	Lofepramine	70	40–210	No
Haldol	Haloperidol	1–3 BID	1–100	No
Heminevrin	Clomethiazole	1 capsule	1–2 capsules	No
Immodium	Loperamide	4	6–16	No
Inderal	Propanolol	10–20 BID-TID	20–320	No
Inderetic	Propanolol	10–20 BID-TID	20–320	No
Inderex	Propanolol	10–20 BID-TID	20–320	No
Intuniv	Guanfacine	1	1–4	No
Invega	Paliperidone	6	3–12	No
Isogel	Ispaghula husk	1 packet BID	1 packet QD-TID	No
Ispagel	Ispaghula husk	1 packet BID	1 packet QD-TID	No
Kemadrin	Procyclidine	2.5 TID	7.5–20	No
Konsyl	Ispaghula husk	1 packet BID	1 packet QD-TID	No
Lamictal	Lamotrigine	25	100–400	No
Largactil	Chlorpromazine	25 TID	30–800	No
Latuda	Lurasidone	40 with food	40–160	No
Lentizol	Amitriptyline	25–50	50–300	120–250 ng/ml
Levothyroxine	Levothyroxine	12.5–50 1-g	12.5–500 1-g	No

(continued)

UK brand name(s)	Chemical (generic) name	Starting dose (mg) except as specified	Standard therapeutic dose (mg)	Useful blood levels
Librium	Chlordiazepoxide	10 TID	15–100	No
Liothyronine	Levothyroxine	12.5–50 1-g	12.5–500 1-g	No
Liskonum	Lithium carbonate	300–600	600–1800	0.6–1.2 meq/l
Lomotil	Diphenoxylate and atropine	1 tab QID	2 tabs Q 6 hours	No
Loxapac	Loxapine	10–25 BID	20–250	No
Ludiomil	Maprotiline	25 TID	75–225	No
Lustral	Sertraline	50	50–200	No
Manerix	Meclobemide	100–300	300–600	No
Manevac	Senna	15	15–30	No
Mellaril	Thioridazine	50–300	20–600	No
Minipress	Prazosin	1	1–15 hs	No
Modecate	Fluphenazine	2.5–10	1–40	No
Moditen	Fluphenazine	2.5–10	1–40	No
Mogadon	Nitrazepam	5	5–10	No
Molipaxin	Trazodone	50–100	150–600	No
Motipress	Nortriptyline	50–100	75–150	50–150 ng/ml
Motival	Nortriptyline	50–100	75–150	50–150 ng/ml
Nalorex	Naltrexone	25	50	No
Nardil	Phenelzine	15	15–90	No
Neulactil	Pericyazine	25 TID	75–300	No
Neurontin	Gabapentin	300	1800–3600	No
Nozinan	Levopromazine	25–50	100–200	No
Optimax	L-Tryptophan	1 TID	6	No
Orap	Pimozide	2	2–20	No
Parnate	Tranylcypromine	10	30–60	No
Periactin	Cyproheptadine	4 TID	4–32	No
Pertofrane	Desipramine	25 TID	100–300	115–180 ng/ml
Prothiaden	Dothiepin/dosulpein	75	150–225	No
Provigil	Modafanil	100–200	200–400	No
Prozac	Fluoxetine	20	20–80	No
Reductil	Sibutramine	10	5–15	No
Regulan	Ispaghula husk	1 packet BID	1 packet QD-TID	No
Reminyl	Galantamine	4 BID	16–32	No

Rimapam	Diazepam	2 TID	4–40	No
Risperdal	Risperidone	0.5	0.5–16	No
Ritalin	Methylphenidate	5–10 BID	10–60	No
Rivotril	Clonazepam	1	1.5–20	No
Rohypnol	Flunitrazepam	0.5–1	0.5–2	No
Saphris, Sycrest	Asenapine	5–10 BID	5–10	No
Securon	Verapamil	40 TID	80–120 TID	No
Senekot	Senna	15	15–30	No
Serenace	Haloperidol	1–3 BID	1–100	No
Seroquel	Quetiapine	25	50–750	No
Seroxat	Paroxetine	20	10–60	No
Sinequan	Doxepin	25 TID	75–300	200–250 ng/ml Blood level of parent compound plus metabolite
Solian	Amisulpride	50–100	50–1200	No
Somnite	Nitrazepam	5	5–10	No
Sonata	Zaleplon	5	5–20	No
Stelazine	Trifluoperazine	5 BID	2–40	No
Stilnoct	Zolpidem	5	5–10	No
Sulpital	Sulpiride	200–400	400–2400	No
Sulpor	Sulpiride	200–400	400–2400	No
Surmontil	Trimipramine	75	50–300	No
Tegretol	Carbamazepine	100–400	400–1600	4–12 1-g/ml
Tenormin	Atenolol	50	50–100	No
Tensium	Diazepam	2 TID	4–40	No
Teril	Carbamazepine	100–400	400–1600	4–12 1-g/ml
Terroxin	Levothyroxine	12.5–50 1-g	12.5–500 1-g	No
Timonil	Carbamazepine	100–400	400–1600	4–12 1-g/ml
Tofranil	Imipramine	25 TID	75–300	200–250 ng/ml Blood level of parent compound plus metabolite
Topamax	Topiramate	25	200–400	No
Tranxene	Chlorazepate	7.5	7.5–60	No
Trileptal	Oxcarbazepine	300 BID	600–2400	No
Triptafen	Amitriptyline	25–50	50–300	120–250 ng/ml

(*continued*)

UK brand name(s)	Chemical (generic) name	Starting dose (mg) except as specified	Standard therapeutic dose (mg)	Useful blood levels
Tropium	Chlordiazepoxide	10 TID	15–100	No
Univer	Verapamil	40 TID	80–120 TID	No
Valium	Diazepam	2 TID	4–40	No
Verapress	Verapamil	40 TID	80–120 TID	No
Vertab	Verapamil	40 TID	80–120 TID	No
Viibryd	Vilazodone	10–20	40	No
Viskaldix	Pindolol	5 BID	15–45	No
Viskin	Pindolol	5 BID	15–45	No
Welldorm	Chloral Hydrate	500	500–2000	No
Xanax	Alprazolam	0.25 TID	0.25–10	No
Xenical	Orlistat	120 TID	120 TID	No
Xyrem	Sodium Oxybate	2.25 twice at night	4.5–9	No
Zimovane	Zopiclone	3.75	3.75–7.5	No
Zispin	Mirtazepine	15	15–45	No
Zoleptil	Zotepine	25 TID	50–300	No
Zyban	Bupropion	100 QD (STD) 150 mg QD (-SR)	200–450 (STD) 150–400 (-SR)	No
Zyprexa	Olanzapine	2.5–10	2.5–20	No

Appendix 6: The National Institute of Mental Health Abnormal Involuntary Movement Scale (AIMS)

Examination procedure

Either before or after completing the examination procedure, observe the patient unobtrusively, at rest (e.g., in waiting room). The chair to be used in this examination should be a hard firm one without arms.

1. Ask patient to remove shoes and socks.
2. Ask patient if there is anything in his mouth (e.g., gum, candy), and if there is, to remove it.
3. Ask patient about the current condition of his teeth. Ask patient if he wears dentures. Do teeth or dentures bother the patient now?
4. Ask patient whether he notices any movements in mouth, face, hands or feet. If yes, ask him/her to describe these and to what extent they currently bother patient or interfere with his/her activities.
5. Have patient sit in a chair with hands on knees, legs slightly apart and feet flat on floor. (Look at entire body for movements while in this position.)
6. Ask patient to sit with hands hanging unsupported – if male, between legs, if female and wearing a dress, hanging over knees. (Observe hands and other body areas.)
7. Ask patient to open mouth. (Observe tongue at rest in mouth.) Do this twice.
8. Ask patient to protrude tongue. (Observe abnormalities of tongue movement.) Do this twice.
9. Ask patient to tap thumb with each finger, as rapidly as possible for 10–15 seconds; separately with right hand, then with left hand. (Observe facial and leg movements.)
10. Flex and extend patient's left and right arms (one at a time). (Note any rigidity.)
11. Ask patient to stand up. (Observe in profile. Observe all body areas again, hips included.)
12. Ask patient to extend both arms outstretched in front with palms down. (Observe trunk, legs and mouth.)
13. Have patient walk a few paces, turn and walk back to chair. (Observe hands and gait.) Do this twice.

Rating sheet

Patient name	Rater name	
Patient #	Data group: AIMS	Evaluation date

Instructions:
Complete the above examination
  procedure before making ratings.
  For movement ratings, circle the
  highest severity observed.

Code:
0: None
1: Minimal, may be extreme normal
2: Mild
3: Moderate
4: Severe

Facial and oral movements	1	Muscles of facial expression • e.g., movements of forehead, eyebrows, periorbital area, cheeks • Include frowning, blinking, smiling and grimacing	0 1 2 3 4
	2	Lips and perioral area e.g., puckering, pouting, smacking	0 1 2 3 4
	3	Jaw e.g., biting, clenching, chewing, mouth opening, lateral movement	0 1 2 3 4
	4	Tongue Rate only increase in movements both in and out of mouth, NOT the inability to sustain movement	0 1 2 3 4
Extremity movements	5	Upper (*arms, wrists, hands, fingers*) • Include choreic movements (i.e., rapid, objectively purposeless, irregular, spontaneous), athetoid movements (i.e., slow, irregular, complex, serpentine) • Do NOT include tremor (i.e., repetitive, regular, rhythmic)	0 1 2 3 4
	6	Lower (*legs, knees, ankles, toes*) e.g., lateral knee movement, foot tapping, heel dropping, foot squirming, inversion and eversion of the foot	0 1 2 3 4
Trunk movements	7	Neck, shoulders, hips e.g., rocking, twisting, squirming, pelvic gyrations	0 1 2 3 4
	8	Severity of abnormal movements	0 1 2 3 4
Global judgments	9	Incapacitation due to abnormal movements	0 1 2 3 4
	10	Patient's awareness of abnormal movements Rate only patient's report	0 1 2 3 4
Dental status	11	Current problems with teeth and/or dentures	0: No 1: Yes
	12	Does patient usually wear dentures?	0: No 1: Yes

Appendix 7: Pharmaceutical Research and Manufacturers of America (PhRMA) Code on Interactions with Healthcare Professionals (2008)

Preamble

The Pharmaceutical Research and Manufacturers of America (PhRMA) represents research-based pharmaceutical and biotechnology companies. Our members develop and market new medicines to enable patients to live longer and healthier lives.

Ethical relationships with healthcare professionals are critical to our mission of helping patients by developing and marketing new medicines. An important part of achieving this mission is ensuring that healthcare professionals have the latest, most accurate information available regarding prescription medicines, which play an ever-increasing role in patient healthcare. This document focuses on our interactions with healthcare professionals that relate to the marketing of our products.

Appropriate marketing of medicines ensures that patients have access to the products they need and that the products are used correctly for maximum patient benefit. Our relationships with healthcare professionals are critical to achieving these goals because they enable us to:

* inform healthcare professionals about the benefits and risks of our products to help advance appropriate patient use,
* provide scientific and educational information,
* support medical research and education, and
* obtain feedback and advice about our products through consultation with medical experts.

In interacting with the medical community, we are committed to following the highest ethical standards as well as all legal requirements. We are also concerned that our interactions with healthcare professionals not be perceived as inappropriate by patients or the public at large. This Code is to reinforce our intention that our interactions with healthcare professionals are professional exchanges designed to benefit patients and to enhance the practice of medicine. The Code is based on the principle that a healthcare professional's care of patients should be based, and should be perceived as being based, solely on each patient's medical needs and the healthcare professional's medical knowledge and experience.

Therefore, PhRMA adopts this updated and enhanced voluntary Code on relationships with U.S. healthcare professionals. This Code reflects and builds upon the standards and principles set forth in its predecessor, the PhRMA Code on Interactions with Healthcare Professionals that took effect on July 1, 2002. Like the 2002 edition, this Code addresses interactions with respect to marketed products and related pre-launch activities. PhRMA member companies' relationships with clinical investigators and other individuals and entities as they relate to the clinical research process are addressed in the PhRMA Principles on Conduct of Clinical Trials and Communication of Clinical Trial Results.

This updated Code will take effect in January 2009.

1 Basis of Interactions

Our relationships with healthcare professionals are regulated by multiple entities and are intended to benefit patients and to enhance the practice of medicine. Interactions should be focused on informing healthcare professionals about products, providing scientific and educational information, and supporting medical education.

Promotional materials provided to healthcare professionals by or on behalf of a company should: (a) be accurate and not misleading; (b) make claims about a product only when properly substantiated; (c) reflect the balance between risks and benefits; and (d) be consistent with all other Food and Drug Administration (FDA) requirements governing such communications.

2 Informational Presentations by Pharmaceutical Company Representatives and Accompanying Meals

Informational presentations and discussions by industry representatives and others speaking on behalf of a company provide healthcare providers with valuable scientific and clinical information about medicines that may lead to improved patient care.

In order to provide important scientific information and to respect healthcare professionals' abilities to manage their schedules and provide patient care, company representatives may take the opportunity to present information during healthcare professionals' working day, including mealtimes. In connection with such presentations or discussions, it is appropriate for occasional meals to be offered as a business courtesy to the healthcare professionals as well as members of their staff attending presentations, so long as the presentations provide scientific or educational value and the meals (a) are modest as judged by local standards; (b) are not part of an entertainment or recreational event; and (c) are provided in a manner conducive to informational communication.

Any such meals offered in connection with informational presentations made by field sales representatives or their immediate managers should also be limited to in-office or in-hospital settings. Inclusion of a healthcare professional's spouse or other guest in a meal accompanying an informational presentation made by or on behalf of a company is not appropriate. Offering "take-out" meals or meals to be eaten without a company representative being present (such as "dine & dash" programs) is not appropriate.

3 Prohibition on Entertainment and Recreation

Company interactions with healthcare professionals are professional in nature and are intended to facilitate the exchange of medical or scientific information that will benefit patient care. To ensure the appropriate focus on education and informational exchange and to avoid the appearance of impropriety, companies should not provide any entertainment or recreational items, such as tickets to the theater or sporting events, sporting equipment, or leisure or vacation trips, to any healthcare professional who is not a salaried employee of the company. Such entertainment or recreational benefits should not be offered, regardless of (1) the value of the items; (2) whether the company engages the healthcare professional as a speaker or consultant; or (3) whether the entertainment or recreation is secondary to an educational purpose.

Modest, occasional meals are permitted as long as they are offered in the appropriate circumstances and venues as described in relevant sections of this Code.

4 Pharmaceutical Company Support for Continuing Medical Education

Continuing medical education (CME), also known as independent medical education (IME), helps physicians and other medical professionals to obtain information and insights that can contribute to the improvement of patient care, and therefore, financial support from companies is appropriate. Such financial support for CME is intended to support education on a full range of treatment options and not to promote a particular medicine. Accordingly, a company should separate its CME grant-making functions from its sales and marketing departments. In addition, a company should develop objective criteria for making CME grant decisions to ensure that the program funded by the company is a bona fide educational program and that the financial support is not an inducement to prescribe or recommend a particular medicine or course of treatment.

Since the giving of any subsidy directly to a healthcare professional by a company may be viewed as an inappropriate cash gift, any financial support should be given to the CME provider, which, in turn, can use the money to reduce the overall CME registration fee for all participants. The company should respect the independent judgment of the CME provider and should follow standards for commercial support established by the Accreditation Council for Continuing Medical Education (ACCME) or other entity that may accredit the CME. When companies underwrite CME, responsibility for and control over the selection of content, faculty, educational methods, materials, and venue belongs to the organizers of the conferences or meetings in accordance with their guidelines. The company should not provide any advice or guidance to the CME provider, even if asked by the provider, regarding the content or faculty for a particular CME program funded by the company.

Financial support should not be offered for the costs of travel, lodging, or other personal expenses of non-faculty healthcare professionals attending CME, either directly to the individuals participating in the event or indirectly to the event's sponsor (except as set out in Section 9 below). Similarly, funding should not be offered to compensate for the time spent by healthcare professionals participating in the CME event.

A company should not provide meals directly at CME events, except that a CME provider at its own discretion may apply the financial support provided by a company for a CME event to provide meals for all participants.

5 Pharmaceutical Company Support for Third-Party Educational or Professional Meetings

Third-party scientific and educational conferences or professional meetings can contribute to the improvement of patient care, and, therefore, financial support from companies is appropriate. A conference or meeting is any activity, held at an appropriate location, where (a) the gathering is primarily dedicated, in both time and effort, to promoting objective scientific and educational activities and discourse (one or more educational presentation(s) should be the highlight of the gathering), and (b) the main incentive for bringing attendees together is to further their knowledge on the topic(s) being presented.

Since the giving of any subsidy directly to a healthcare professional by a company may be viewed as an inappropriate cash gift, any financial support should be given to the conference's sponsor, which, in turn, can use the money to reduce the overall conference registration fee for all attendees. When companies underwrite medical conferences or meetings other than their own, responsibility for and control over the selection of content, faculty, educational methods, materials, and venue belongs to the organizers of the conferences or meetings in accordance with their guidelines. Financial support should not be offered for the costs of travel, lodging, or other personal expenses of non-faculty healthcare professionals attending third-party scientific or educational conferences or professional meetings, either directly to the individuals attending the conference or indirectly to the conference's sponsor (except as set out in Section 9 below). Similarly, funding should not be offered to compensate for the time spent by healthcare professionals attending the conference or meeting.

6 Consultants

Consulting arrangements with healthcare professionals allow companies to obtain information or advice from medical experts on such topics as the marketplace, products, therapeutic areas and the needs of patients. Companies use this advice to inform their efforts to ensure that the medicines they produce and market are meeting the needs of patients. Decisions regarding the selection or retention of healthcare professionals as consultants should be made based on defined criteria such as general medical expertise and reputation, or knowledge and experience regarding a particular therapeutic area. Companies should continue to ensure that consultant arrangements are neither inducements nor rewards for prescribing or recommending a particular medicine or course of treatment.

It is appropriate for consultants who provide advisory services to be offered reasonable compensation for those services and reimbursement for reasonable travel, lodging, and meal expenses incurred as part of providing those services. Any compensation or reimbursement made in conjunction with a consulting arrangement should be reasonable and based on fair market value. Token consulting or advisory arrangements should not be used to justify compensating healthcare professionals for their time or their travel, lodging, and other out-of-pocket expenses. The following factors support the existence of a bona fide consulting arrangement (not all factors may be relevant to any particular arrangement):

- a written contract specifies the nature of the consulting services to be provided and the basis for payment of those services;
- a legitimate need for the consulting services has been clearly identified in advance of requesting the services and entering into arrangements with the prospective consultants;
- the criteria for selecting consultants are directly related to the identified purpose and the persons responsible for selecting the consultants have the expertise necessary to evaluate whether the particular healthcare professionals meet those criteria;

- the number of healthcare professionals retained is not greater than the number reasonably necessary to achieve the identified purpose;
- the retaining company maintains records concerning and makes appropriate use of the services provided by consultants;
- the venue and circumstances of any meeting with consultants are conducive to the consulting services and activities related to the services are the primary focus of the meeting; specifically, resorts are not appropriate venues.

While modest meals or receptions may be appropriate during company sponsored meetings with healthcare professional commercial consultants, companies should not provide recreational or entertainment events in conjunction with these meetings.

It is not appropriate to pay honoraria or travel or lodging expenses to non-faculty and non-consultant healthcare professional attendees at company-sponsored meetings, including attendees who participate in interactive sessions.

7 Speaker Programs and Speaker Training Meetings

Healthcare professionals participate in company-sponsored speaker programs in order to help educate and inform other healthcare professionals about the benefits, risks, and appropriate uses of company medicines. Any healthcare professional engaged by a company to participate in such external promotional programs on behalf of the company will be deemed a speaker for purposes of this Code, and the requirements of Section 7 apply to company interactions with that healthcare professional in his or her capacity as a speaker. Company decisions regarding the selection or retention of healthcare professionals as speakers should be made based on defined criteria such as general medical expertise and reputation, knowledge and experience regarding a particular therapeutic area, and communications skills. Companies should continue to ensure that speaking arrangements are neither inducements nor rewards for prescribing a particular medicine or course of treatment.

Speaker training is an essential activity because the FDA holds companies accountable for the presentations of their speakers. It is appropriate for healthcare professionals who participate in programs intended to train speakers for company-sponsored speaker programs to be offered reasonable compensation for their time, considering the value of the type of services provided, and to be offered reimbursement for reasonable travel, lodging, and meal expenses. Such compensation and reimbursement should only be offered when (1) the participants receive extensive training on the company's drug products or other specific topic to be presented and on compliance with FDA regulatory requirements for communications; (2) this training will result in the participants providing a valuable service to the company; and (3) the participants meet the general criteria for bona fide consulting arrangements (as discussed in Section 6 above). Speaker training sessions should be held in venues that are appropriate and conducive to informational communication and training about medical information; specifically, resorts are not appropriate venues.

Any compensation or reimbursement made to a healthcare professional in conjunction with a speaking arrangement should be reasonable and based on fair market value. Each company should, individually and independently, cap the total amount of annual compensation it will pay to an individual healthcare professional in connection with all speaking arrangements. Each company also should develop policies addressing the appropriate use of speakers, including utilization of speakers after training and the appropriate number of engagements for any particular speaker over time.

Speaker programs may include modest meals offered to attendees and should occur in a venue and manner conducive to informational communication. While speaker programs offer important educational opportunities to healthcare professionals, they are distinct from CME programs, and companies and speakers should be clear about this distinction. For example, speakers and their materials should clearly identify the company that is sponsoring the presentation, the fact that the speaker is presenting on behalf of the company, and that the speaker is presenting information that is consistent with FDA guidelines. Beyond providing all speakers with appropriate training, companies should periodically monitor speaker programs for compliance with FDA regulatory requirements for communications on behalf of the company about its medicines.

8 Healthcare Professionals who Are Members of Committees that Set Formularies or Develop Clinical Practice Guidelines

Healthcare professionals who are members of committees that set formularies of covered medicines or develop clinical practice guidelines that may influence the prescribing of medicines often have significant experience in their fields. That experience can be of great benefit to companies and ultimately to patients if these individuals choose to serve as speakers or commercial consultants for companies. To avoid even the appearance of impropriety, companies should require any healthcare professional who is a member of a committee that sets formularies or develops clinical guidelines and also serves as a speaker or commercial consultant for the company to disclose to the committee the existence and nature of his or her relationship with the company. This disclosure requirement should extend for at least two years beyond the termination of any speaker or consultant arrangement.

Upon disclosure, healthcare professionals who serve as speakers or consultants for companies should be required to follow the procedures set forth by the committee of which they are a member, which may include recusing themselves from decisions relating to the medicine for which they have provided speaking or consulting services.

9 Scholarships and Educational Funds

Financial assistance for scholarships or other educational funds to permit medical students, residents, fellows, and other healthcare professionals in training to attend carefully selected educational conferences may be offered so long as the selection of individuals who will receive the funds is made by the academic or training institution. "Carefully selected educational conferences" are generally defined as the major educational, scientific, or policymaking meetings of national, regional, or specialty medical associations.

10 Prohibition of Non-Educational and Practice-Related Items

Providing items for healthcare professionals' use that do not advance disease or treatment education – even if they are practice-related items of minimal value (such as pens, note pads, mugs and similar "reminder" items with company or product logos) – may foster misperceptions that company interactions with healthcare professionals are not based on informing them about medical and scientific issues. Such non-educational items should not be offered to healthcare professionals or members of their staff, even if they are accompanied by patient or physician educational materials.

Items intended for the personal benefit of healthcare professionals (such as floral arrangements, artwork, music CDs, or tickets to a sporting event) likewise should not be offered.

Payments in cash or cash equivalents (such as gift certificates) should not be offered to healthcare professionals either directly or indirectly, except as compensation for bona fide services (as described in Sections 6 and 7). Cash or equivalent payments of any kind create a potential appearance of impropriety or conflict of interest.

It is appropriate to provide product samples for patient use in accordance with the Prescription Drug Marketing Act.

11 Educational Items

It is appropriate for companies, where permitted by law, to offer items designed primarily for the education of patients or healthcare professionals if the items are not of substantial value ($100 or less) and do not have value to healthcare professionals outside of his or her professional responsibilities. For example, an anatomical model for use in an examination room is intended for the education of the patients and is therefore appropriate, whereas a DVD or CD player may have independent value to a healthcare professional outside of his or her professional responsibilities, even if it could also be used to provide education to patients, and therefore is not appropriate.

Items designed primarily for the education of patients or healthcare professionals should not be offered on more than an occasional basis, even if each individual item is appropriate.

12 Prescriber Data

Companies use non-patient identified prescriber data to facilitate the efficient flow of information to healthcare professionals. Such prescriber data, which does not identify individual patients, may serve many purposes, including enabling companies to: (a) impart important safety and risk information to prescribers of a particular drug; (b) conduct research; (c) comply with FDA mandated risk management plans that require drug companies to identify and interact with physicians who prescribe certain drugs; (d) track adverse events of marketed prescriptions drugs; and (e) focus marketing activities on those healthcare professionals who would most likely benefit from information about a particular drug.

Companies that choose to use non-patient identified prescriber data to facilitate communications with healthcare professionals should use this data responsibly. For example, companies should (a) respect the confidential nature of prescriber data; (b) develop policies regarding the use of the data; (c) educate employees and agents about those policies; (d) maintain an internal contact person to handle inquiries regarding the use of the data; and (e) identify appropriate disciplinary actions for misuse of this data. In addition, companies should respect and abide by the wishes of any healthcare professional who asks that his or her prescriber data not be made available to company sales representatives. Companies may demonstrate this respect by following the rules of voluntary programs that facilitate prescribers' ability to make this choice.

13 Independence and Decision Making

No grants, scholarships, subsidies, support, consulting contracts, or educational or practice related items should be provided or offered to a healthcare professional in exchange for prescribing products or for a commitment to continue prescribing products. Nothing should be offered or provided in a manner or on conditions that would interfere with the independence of a healthcare professional's prescribing practices.

14 Training and Conduct of Company Representatives

Pharmaceutical company representatives play an important role in delivering accurate, up-to-date information to healthcare professionals about the approved indications, benefits, and risks of pharmaceutical therapies. These representatives often serve as the primary point of contact between the companies who research, develop, manufacture, and market life-saving and life-enhancing medicines and the healthcare professionals who prescribe them. As such, the company representatives must act with the highest degree of professionalism and integrity.

Companies should ensure that all representatives who are employed by, or acting on behalf of, the companies and who visit healthcare professionals receive training about the applicable laws, regulations, and industry codes of practice, including this Code, that govern the representatives' interactions with healthcare professionals. In addition, companies should train their representatives to ensure that they have sufficient knowledge of general science and product-specific information to provide accurate, up-to-date information, consistent with FDA requirements.

Companies should provide updated or additional training in all of these areas as needed for their representatives who visit healthcare professionals. Companies should also assess their representatives periodically to ensure that they comply with relevant company policies and standards of conduct. Companies should take appropriate action when representatives fail to comply.

15 Adherence to Code

All companies that interact with healthcare professionals about pharmaceuticals should adopt procedures to assure adherence to this Code. Companies that publicly announce their commitment to abide by the Code and who complete an annual certification that they have policies and procedures in place to foster compliance with the Code will be identified by PhRMA on a public web site. The certification must be signed by the company's Chief Executive Officer and Chief Compliance Officer. The web site will identify the companies who commit to abide by the Code; provide contact information for their Chief Compliance Officers; and, at the appropriate time, publish the status of each company's annual certification.

Any comments received by PhRMA relating to a company's observance of the Code or conduct that is addressed by the Code will be referred by PhRMA to the relevant company's Chief Compliance Officer.

In addition, companies are encouraged to seek external verification periodically, meaning at least once every three years, that the company has policies and procedures in place to foster compliance with the Code. PhRMA will prepare general guidance for such external verification and will identify on its web site if a company has sought and obtained verification of its compliance policies and procedures from an external source.

The following is a list of all signatory companies that have announced as of March 23, 2012 that they intend to abide by the Code:

Abbott
Allergan, Inc.
Amgen Inc.
Amylin Pharmaceuticals, Inc.
Astellas US LLC
AstraZeneca LP
Bayer HealthCare Pharmaceuticals
Biogen Idec
Boehringer Ingelheim Pharmaceuticals, Inc.
Bristol-Myers Squibb Company
Celgene Corporation
Cell Therapeutics, Inc.
Cephalon, Inc.
Corcept Therapeutics
Covidien
Cubist Pharmaceuticals, Inc.
Cumberland Pharmaceuticals Inc.
CV Therapeutics, Inc.
Daiichi Sankyo, Inc.
Eisai Inc.
EMD Serono
Endo Pharmaceuticals, Inc.
Enzon Pharmaceuticals, Inc.
Ferring Pharmaceuticals, Inc.
Forest Laboratories, Inc.
Genentech, Inc.
Genzyme Corporation
GlaxoSmithKline
Ikaria, Inc.
Inspire Pharmaceuticals, Inc.
Johnson & Johnson (Pharmaceutical Companies)
LEO Pharma Inc.
Eli Lilly and Company
Lundbeck Inc.
Merck & Co., Inc.
Millennium Pharmaceuticals, Inc.
Novartis Pharmaceuticals Corporation
Noven Pharmaceuticals, Inc.
Novogyne Pharmaceuticals
Novo Nordisk Inc.
Optimer Pharmaceuticals, Inc.
Otsuka America Pharmaceuticals
Pfizer Inc

Purdue Pharma L.P.
Regeneron Pharmaceuticals, Inc.
Sanofi-Aventis U.S.
Shionogi Inc.
Shire Pharmaceuticals, Inc.
Sigma-Tau Pharmaceuticals, Inc.
Solstice Neurosciences, Inc.
Sucampo
Sunovion Pharmaceuticals Inc.
Takeda Pharmaceuticals North America, Inc.
Talecris Biotherapeutics
Theravance, Inc.
UCB, Inc.
Victory Pharma, Inc.
Zogenix, Inc.

Index

A, B, C, D, X classification of medication in pregnancy and lactation *183*
abnormal movement scale *see* AIMS scale
abuse of medication: what to do when medication abuse is suspected 395; what to do when medication abuse occurs 394; *see also* misuse of medication
abuse of stimulants *146*
abusing patient 398
access to medical records online 460
addiction: defined 386
adequate trial of medication 86
ADHD *see* Attention Deficit Hyperactivity Disorder
adherence: methods to increase 91
adolescents *see* children and adolescents
advertising of medication 476
agranulocytosis *see* bleeding and blood dyscrasias
AIMS scale for abnormal movements 35, 95, Appendix 6
akathisia as a side effect 14, 301–302
alcohol abuse: 234–240; laboratory tests in 240; signs of 239–240; treatment with medications 225
alcohol and psychotropic medication 240–249; routine warnings 216
alcohol detoxification: sample protocol for 249–250
alcohol use with psychotropics 234, 238
allergy: from medication 378–382; signs and symptoms of 378–380; treatment of 380
alopecia as a side effect *see* hair loss
alternative/home remedies for ADHD *282*
Alzheimer's dementia *see* Alzheimer's disease
Alzheimer's disease: causes of 266; medications for 267–268; treatment of 241
anti-anxiety medication: breastfeeding and 196
anticholinergic intoxication: causes of 344–345; prevention of 344; signs and symptoms of 345; situations of risk for 345; treatment of 346

anticonvulsants: use in the confused patient 363
antipsychotic medication: confused patient and 364
anxiety: as a side effect 299; checklist for 42; evaluation 41
anxious patient: and confusion 270; managing 26–27, 264, 404–405
appointments by telephone *see* telephone; appointments by
aspirin sensitivity: related to tartrazine sensitivity 382
asthenia *see* weakness
atropine psychosis *see* anticholinergic intoxication
Attention Deficit Hyperactivity Disorder 272–286; causes of 274–275; in adults 277; in children 276; medications for 279–280; non-medication treatments for 281–283
atypical: meaning of 136

benzodiazepine withdrawal 143–144
benzodiazepines, history of 140
benzodiazepines, uses of 141, 145; side effects of 141
bias, diagnostic 42
bias, medication 42–43
bipolar disorder: checklist for evaluation 42
bleeding and blood dyscrasias as a side effect 368–370
blood levels do not help 437
blood levels of medication 433–438; instructions for 435
blood sugar: elevation of as a side effect 325
borderline patient 414–418; principles of medication treatment 415–416
breast feeding: psychotropics and 196–202; antianxiety medications and 200; antidepressants and 199; antipsychotic medication and 200; mood stabilizers and 199

by 467; availability by 466; inappropriate use of 468–470; when patient calls too much 471

CAGE assessment tool 241
changeover sheet for changing medication 85, 86, 87
changing medication due to side effects 295
cholinesterase inhibitors 267–268
choosing a starting dose of medication 56
choosing medication 38–61; when the patient has previously been on medication 61; for kidney-impaired patient 63; for liver impaired patient 62
cognitive disorders *see* delirium; dementia; confused patient
cognitively impaired patient *see* confused patient
communications Information Sheet for patients 449
complex discontinuation 126
compliance *see* adherence
computer and Internet security 460
concurrence for a change of medication 137
confidentiality of records: possible breaches of 429–430
conflicting advice from others 138
confused patient 257–270; causes of 259–272; principles of treating 258
confusion, psychiatric diseases that may present as 270; *see also* delirium; dementia; confused patient
constipation as a side effect 304–305
consultation: in managing difficult patients 419; psychiatric in primary care 134
crisis in a stable patient; getting on TRAACCC 130–134

data collection, protocols and oversight 459
delirium: causes of 259–261; medical work-up of 261; symptoms of 237
dementia: Alzheimer's type *see* Alzheimer's disease; causes of 261; management of 262–264; medication for 263–264
depression means personal weakness 17
depression: checklist for evaluation 41; pregnant patient and 190–191; use of metaphor in 51
diarrhea as a side effect 305–306
difficult medication patients 400–420; positive approaches to 402; practitioner generated issues 420; principles of management 400–402; stopping treatment with 419–420; team approach to 418–419
digital prescriber 445–464

discontinuation syndromes 122–123, antipsychotic medication and 117–118; benzodiazepines and 119; management of 122; new episode of illness or not 124; SSRI's and 117–118; stimulants and 118; TCA's and 117–118; versus relapse 122–123
dry mouth as a side effect 319
dual diagnosis patient 242–245

e-mail and the medication prescriber 446–448
education as treatment 72
electronic medical records (EMR) 450–451
electronic prescribing and prescriptions 452
EPS *see* extrapyramidal symptoms
expiration dates of medication 96–97
extrapyramidal symptoms 356–358; causes of 356

falls as a side effect 324
five points of education about psychotropics 67
follow-up appointments 75–101; feedback from others in 89; goals of 78; inpatient 77; length of 76; preparing for 77; quantification of response in 79–82; side effect assessment in 87–88
fraud in obtaining medication 392; practitioner protection against 393

gastrointestinal problems as side effects *see* constipation; diarrhea; nausea
generic medication 439–444; blood levels with 443; changes without clinician's knowledge 442; common generic psychotropics Appendices 3, 4, 5, 498–524; tips for using 442
genetics and psychotropic medication 485
geriatric patients *see* older adults
gifts to practitioners: AMA guidelines for 529–530

hair loss as a side effect 319–320
headaches as a side effect 318
hepatotoxicity *see* liver toxicity
historical information from others 33
history taking 28–33
hyperprolactinemia as a side effect *see* prolactin elevation
hypomania as a side effect 302
hyponatremia as a side effect 326–327
hypotension as a side effect 304

inappropriate requests from patients: 134
indigent care medication programs 476
informational websites maintained by practitioners 457; mental health sites for the patient 457

informed consent for medication 70
initial evaluation for medication 23–44;
    assessment and formulation in 36–37;
    information from others in 33; medical
    work up in 34; mental status exam in 31;
    optional elements 32; required elements 30;
    time for 38
inpatient medication follow-up 77; *see also*
    follow-up appointments: inpatient
insufficient sleep syndrome 220
Internet and prescribers 445; risks and 460,
    473; security and 460; treatment protocols
    and 484
Internet and the digital revolution 445
Internet-based medication reference and
    educational information for treatment,
    based mental health treatment modalities
    454
Internet medication information for patients
    457
intoxicated and withdrawing patient,
    evaluating 242
involuntary medication 71

kidney-impaired patient: choosing medication
    for 69

lactation and psychotropics 196–200
levers for trying medication 49
lifestyle prescribing 486
lightheadedness as a side effect *see*
    hypotension
lipid elevation as a side effect 325
lithium toxicity: causes of 346–348
liver impaired patient: choosing medication
    for 62
liver toxicity as a side effect 368, 370, 371
loading doses 57; monotherapy 54; number of
    pills to prescribe 64; target of 56
long-term medication: who should receive 47,
    128
low blood pressure *see* hypotension
low sodium as a side effect *see* hyponatremia

MAOI reactions *see* monoamine oxidase
    inhibitor-reactions
MAOI's *see* monoamine oxidase inhibitors
me too concept of medication development
    145
media advertising and mental health
    medications 476
medical workup for medication 34; with
    children and adolescents 174
medication allergy *see* allergy: from
    medication
medication bias see bias medication
medication combinations, helpful 64–65

medication lists 427
medication: adequate trial of 86; blood
    levels of *see* blood levels of medication;
    borderline patient and 414–418
mental health medication statistics 6
mental health referral *see* referral to a mental
    health specialist
mental illnesses: practice guidelines for
    see practice guidelines for mental health
    treatment
mental status exam/testing: initial work up 31;
    full description 489–497
metaphor use in treatment of 51
mild cognitive impairment 268
missed doses of medication 97
misuse of medication 385–399; accidental
    overdose 388; fraud and abuse 392;
    intentional overdose 389–391; minor
    overdose 391
monoamine oxidase inhibitors 365–368
monotherapy 54
movement disorders as side effects 365–363
myths of mental health medication 9–19

narcolepsy 145, 220
nasty underside of the Internet 463
natural substances helpful 154–158; harmful
    159
naturalist patient 413
nausea as a side effect 304
necessary documentation in clinical note 424
necessity of follow-up 73–75
nervousness as a side effect *see* anxiety
neuroleptic malignant syndrome (NMS)
    359–360
new episode or relapse? 124
newer medication better? 135–136
NMS *see* neuroleptic malignant syndrome
non-adherence 210; older adults and 210
note taking: systems of 426; style elements of
    426
number of pills to prescribe 64

office for mental health prescribing: setting up
    478–483
older adults: medication interactions in
    212–213; principles of medication 211
online patient access to medical records
    460
other adjunctive therapies 107–108
other interventions for the prescriber with a
    substance abusing patient 249
over activation as a side effect 299–303
overdose of medication 385–399

P-450 interactions: conveyor belt analogy for
    334–335; use of a chart for 338–339

panic attacks 52; use of metaphor in 52
parenteral medications 99
parental power struggles with children about
    medication 173
parkinsonism as a side effect *see*
    extrapyramidal reactions
periodic limb movements (PLM) 220
periodic reassessment 137
personal presentation of practitioner 482
PHARMA code for healthcare professionals
    527
pharmaceutical representatives: clinicians and
    474–475
pharmacist: clinician interaction with 473;
    confidentiality issues and 473
physical tolerance to medication 46, 486–487
physiological dependence on medication 387
pill size 99
placebo: use of 72
polypharmacy, benefits of 64–65, inadvertent
    65–66
polysubstance abuse 241
positive comments: benefit of 83–85
power struggles over medication in children
    173
practice guidelines for mental health
    prescribing 484
preauthorization of medication 474
pregnancy: anxiety and 195; carbamazepine
    and 190; lithium and 191; psychotropics
    and 189; severely symptomatic patient and
    191; valproate and 192; when the patient is
    trying to get pregnant 187–188
prescribing psychotropics for older patients
    209–215
prescription writing *see* written prescription
prolactin elevation as a side effect 322
pseudo parkinsonism *see* extrapyramidal
    symptoms
psychotherapy: medication and 103–106;
    choosing in the first session 58–63
psychotropic medication, who prescribes? 105
psychotropic medication: alphabetically by
    brand name (UK) 519; alphabetically by
    brand name (USA) 520; alphabetically by
    generic name (USA and UK) 507
psychotropic medications and dual diagnosis
    patients 242–244
psychotropic medications by class 500
psychotropic medications by generic name
    507
psychotropic medications in the UK by brand
    name 519
psychotropic medications in the US by brand
    name 513
psychotropics in the treatment of alcohol
    withdrawal 249

psychotropics used in the treatment of
    substance use disorders 245–248

QTc interval issues 349–353

rash as a side effect *see* skin reactions
reasons patients take medication 50; children's
    reasons 173
reassessment of the patient: need for 137
record keeping 424–432; systems of 426
referring to a mental health professional 133
resistances to medication 46–47
restless leg syndrome (RLS) 220
routine warnings for recreational drugs 238
routine warnings regarding alcohol use and
    psychotropics in the non- substance abusing
    patients 238

sedation as a side effect 298; cause 299;
    pharmacotherapy of 305; psychotropics
    and 300
seizures as side effects 368; if a patient has a
    seizure on a psychotropic 368–369
selecting medication in the previously treated
    patient 61
serotonin syndrome 340–342; causes of 341
serum blood levels *see* blood levels of
    medication
sexual interference as a side effect 306–310
shopping bag presentation 152
side effects: assessment of severity 293–295;
    beginning clinician and 296; changing
    medication due to 293–294; clinical
    response and 296; discussing with patients
    291; medication combinations and 320–328;
    most frequent with skin reactions as side
    effects 321–322
sleep disorders, principles of treating 224
sleep latency: phase shifted 220; stages of
    220–221
sleep problems: definitions of 220; evaluation
    of 221–223; medications to treat 223–225;
    sleep apnea 220; in special populations 229;
    sleep efficiency 220, treatment of 224–228
smoking, tobacco and nicotine 233–255
social media and the prescriber 461
specific medicines and medication groups in
    breastfeeding 196–200
specific psychotropic medication
    considerations in the elderly 215–216
starting medication 53–73; art of choosing 58;
    choosing a starting dose 56
stimulant medication and its appropriate uses
    145
stimulant medication other uses of 279
stimulants 144–150, in ADHD 279; abuse of
    284; discontinuation syndrome with 118

stopping medication 113–126; side effects and 124; tapering in 116; unplanned 124–125; worsening during 116–117
stopping medication need to do more quickly 123
substance abuse defined 386
substance dependence defined 386–387
suicide and homicide assessment 32
suicide attempt *see* overdose, intentional
swallowing medication: difficulty with 176–177
symptomatic crisis *see* TRACCCC
synergy of medications 65

tapering medication need for 116
tardive dyskinesia (TD); causes of 361–363
target symptoms 33
tartrazine allergy 382
telephone use 466–472; abuse by clinician 472; abuse by patient 471; appointments
telepsychiatry, medication management via the computer 453
texting 449
therapeutic drug monitoring (TDM) *see* blood levels of medication

torsades de pointes see QTc interval issues
toxic delirium *see* anticholinergic intoxication
TRAACCC, getting on 130–133
traveling with medication 100
tremor as a side effect 290; medications that can cause 299–301
two simple, powerful questions 79

under usage of medication 392; in older adults 210
unplanned stoppage of medication *see* stopping medication: unplanned
unusual treatment: documentation of 431

weakness (asthenia) as a side effect 318
websites maintained by practitioners 457–458
weight gain as a side effect 300–308; approaches to treating 304; classes of medication that
what can medication do? 105
when pregnancy occurs 188
work–life balance 109
written prescription: required elements 423; optional elements 423–424

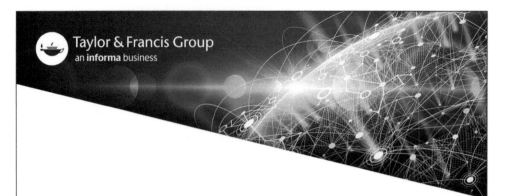
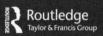
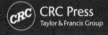

T - #0157 - 111024 - C143 - 246/174/27 - PB - 9780367466916 - Matt Lamination